Equipment for Respiratory Care

Teresa A. Volsko, MHHS, RRT, FAARC
Director, Respiratory Care, Transport, and the Communication Center
Akron Children's Hospital
Akron, Ohio

Robert L. Chatburn, MHHS, RRT-NPS, FAARC
Research Manager, Respiratory Institute, Cleveland Clinic
Professor, Department of Medicine
Lerner College of Medicine of Case Western Reserve University
Cleveland, Ohio

Mohamad F. El-Khatib, MD, PhD, MBA, RRT
Professor, Department of Anesthesiology
American University of Beirut School of Medicine
Director of Respiratory Therapy Department
American University of Beirut Medical Center
Beirut, Lebanon

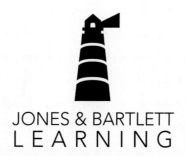

JONES & BARTLETT
LEARNING

World Headquarters
Jones & Bartlett Learning
5 Wall Street
Burlington, MA 01803
978-443-5000
info@jblearning.com
www.jblearning.com

Jones & Bartlett Learning books and products are available through most bookstores and online booksellers. To contact Jones & Bartlett Learning directly, call 800-832-0034, fax 978-443-8000, or visit our website, www.jblearning.com.

Substantial discounts on bulk quantities of Jones & Bartlett Learning publications are available to corporations, professional associations, and other qualified organizations. For details and specific discount information, contact the special sales department at Jones & Bartlett Learning via the above contact information or send an email to specialsales@jblearning.com.

0194-2

Production Credits

VP, Executive Publisher: David Cella
VP, Publisher: Vernon Anthony
Publisher: Cathy L. Esperti
Executive Editor: Rhonda Dearborn
Associate Editor: Kayla Dos Santos
Associate Editor: Sean Fabery
Production Manager: Carolyn Rogers Pershouse
Marketing Manager: Grace Richards

Art Development Editor: Joanna Lundeen
VP, Manufacturing and Inventory Control: Therese Connell
Composition: Cenveo Publisher Services
Cover and Interior Design: Michael O'Donnell
Manager of Photo Research, Rights & Permissions: Amy Rathburn
Rights and Photo Research Coordinator: Mary Flatley
Cover Image: © VikaSuh/ShutterStock, Inc.
Printing and Binding: RR Donnelley
Cover Printing: RR Donnelley

Library of Congress Cataloging-in-Publication Data

Equipment for respiratory care / edited by Teresa A. Volsko, Robert L. Chatburn, Dr. Mohamad F. El-Khatib.
    p. ; cm.
  Includes bibliographical references and index.
  ISBN 978-1-4496-5283-8 — ISBN 1-4496-5283-2
  I. Volsko, Teresa A., editor. II. Chatburn, Robert L., editor. III. El-Khatib, Mohamad F., editor.
  [DNLM: 1. Respiratory Therapy--instrumentation. 2. Respiratory Tract Diseases--therapy. WF 26]
  RC735.I5
  615.8ʹ3620284—dc23
                                2014020803

6048

Printed in the United States of America
18 17 16 15   10 9 8 7 6 5 4 3

Dedication

I dedicate this book to the respiratory students whose quest for knowledge inspired me to find new and innovative ways to maximize their educational experience, and to my family whose love and support allowed me to pursue my dreams!

Teresa A. Volsko

I dedicate this book to instructors around the world who strive for the best ways to describe and teach new technology. It is only through your tireless efforts that progress continues to be made and care continues to improve.

Robert L. Chatburn

To Mayssa, Farouk, Dina, and Manar—thanks for your love and support. You are the joy of my life.

To my mother Souad and to the soul of my father.

Mohamad F. El-Khatib

Brief Contents

Contents

Foreword

Throughout my career I have found that airway management is the major role of the respiratory therapist, whether this involves opening and maintaining a closed airway or sustaining breathing through mechanical ventilation. With this role comes an expectation of being the expert on all the equipment that is needed to maintain an airway and provide ventilation. This expertise is what sets respiratory therapists apart from other hospital personnel. Biomedical engineers know how equipment works by their mechanical design, and anesthesia personnel know how to ventilate patients in the controlled environment of the operating room, but troubleshooting skills and knowledge of airway and ventilation equipment separate the respiratory care professional from these other professionals.

Troubleshooting is an important skill for any respiratory therapy student to learn and for all practicing respiratory therapists to maintain. Troubleshooting involves locating and correcting technical problems related to the machinery used in patient care. Under most circumstances this requires logical reasoning, as opposed to problem posing and problem solving. Troubleshooting is always essential in clinical practice because members of the medical team in the ICU rely on respiratory therapists' technical expertise to advise, explain, and troubleshoot equipment used for airway management and mechanical ventilation. Respiratory therapists work in teams, but there are times when they must work without assistance. It is in such circumstances that troubleshooting respiratory care equipment is most crucial. The topic of troubleshooting in respiratory therapy is taught at a level that cannot be found in the core curriculum of medical schools or nursing schools. Thus, it is a unique skill of respiratory therapists that is not shared by other allied health clinicians, nurses, or physicians.

This new text covers most equipment topics addressed in respiratory therapy education. Respiratory therapy equipment courses are usually among the first courses in most respiratory therapy programs of study. Teresa A. Volsko, Robert L. Chatburn, and Mohamad F. El-Khatib bring their expertise and insights to the operation and indications for use of equipment used in respiratory care practice. The text provides information that builds on the respiratory therapist's knowledge of the physiology of the respiratory system as well as the electronic functionality of the equipment used, while experience is gained in the laboratory setting and on the job. I hope that students and practitioners alike will use this information and ask themselves, "How well do I use my troubleshooting skills when I work without assistance in my practice (for instance, when I make a home visit to a patient receiving mechanical ventilation)?" Our future patients are depending on us to be able to answer this question!

Lynda T. Goodfellow, EdD, RRT, AE-C, FAARC
Professor and Associate Dean
Byrdine F. Lewis School of Nursing and
Health Professions
Georgia State University
Atlanta, GA

Preface

Technological advances have made a significant impact on our profession. The equipment used to treat disorders of the respiratory tract no longer are simple machines. Many of the devices respiratory therapists use are governed by sophisticated operating systems.

In this inaugural edition the authors recognize that it is not just about the technology; it's about sharing knowledge and the key elements of information that will enable respiratory care professionals to distinguish between equipment malfunction and patient intolerance in order to effectively communicate recommendations for therapy or changes to the plan of care. The authors embraced this work as a mechanism to build a learning community and create a culture of professionalism.

> Therefore, it is essential for the respiratory care practitioner to have a thorough understanding of the theory and operation of equipment in order to effectively and safely match the therapeutic modality to patient need.

The approach or layout of each chapter is standardized, much like the format for a scientific research paper. Just as scientific papers commence with a thorough review of the literature, each chapter provides the reader with a purpose for the particular topic. The data from a variety of sources are summarized to provide equipment specifications, routine use, and limitations in a logical and uniform fashion. Rather than outlines of manufacturer specifications, the authors provide fundamental theoretical constructs for the categories of equipment described in each chapter.

> Therefore, our vision for this textbook was to change the paradigm of how respiratory care equipment books are written. Rather than presenting information in an encyclopedic reference form, each chapter in this text describes the structural and operational characteristics of respiratory care equipment in a practical, clinically relevant manner.

Finally, there is an in-depth discussion that ties in the clinical significance of the equipment presented. Similar to the discussion section of a scientific manuscript, this portion of the chapter establishes the practical relevance of the equipment discussed. The equipment selection and troubleshooting guides provide practical solutions to complex problems. These sections are presented in an easy to follow manner and provide the theoretical constructs, practical application, and algorithms to provide respiratory care students and professionals with the tools to distinguish equipment malfunction from patient intolerance. Understanding this difference is an essential critical thinking skill and instrumental when communicating with the interdisciplinary team. These skills are necessary in order to clearly articulate the need to initiate therapy or rationale for recommending modifications to the patient plan of care.

Chapter-by-Chapter Overview

The text is written in a clear and concise manner. Illustrations, tables, and figures are provided to enhance the learning experience.

Chapter 1, Introduction to Medical Gases, introduces the learner to the essential role medical gases play along the continuum of care. Essential elements in the selection, distribution, storage and safe handling of medical gases are presented. This chapter also highlights the safety standards required by credentialing bodies, such as the Joint Commission and the National Fire Protection Agency, that impact our clinical practice.

Chapter 2, Administering Medical Gases, provides clinically relevant information on the delivery systems and devices used to administer medical gas therapy. This chapter explores the ongoing debate regarding the best methods to safely deliver medical gases. Practical information, rooted in the evidence available in the literature, is presented to facilitate a systematic thinking approach to device selection.

Chapter 3, Hyperbaric Oxygen Therapy, explores the fascinating and rapidly expanding field of hyperbaric oxygen therapy. Because application of this therapeutic modality requires knowledge of the physics of gases, gas laws as well as different oxygen delivery systems will be presented. This chapter will also discuss the physiological principles of hyperbaric oxygen, as well as its indications, contraindications, complications, and hazards. A discussion of the different chambers, equipment, and monitoring used to evaluate oxygenation and ventilation as well as the use of concurrent mechanical ventilation is presented.

Chapter 4, Humidity and Aerosol Therapy, presents the principles of humidity and aerosol therapy. This chapter describes the various devices that are currently used in the clinical practice of providing humidity and aerosol therapies in spontaneously breathing and in mechanically ventilated patients. Information is provided to enable the learner to gain a firm understanding of the rationale, physiological basis, indications, and contraindications for humidity and aerosol therapies. Additionally, this chapter provides information in a manner that will facilitate comprehension of the technical considerations germane to the multitude of devices available for clinical use.

Chapter 5, Airway Management and Emergency Resuscitation Equipment, provides a clinical approach to the devices used to secure and maintain a patent airway. Because any device has the potential to help as well as cause harm, this chapter is designed to familiarize the learner with the indications, proper use, and limitations of airway management equipment. A practical approach to evaluating the plethora of equipment used in the routine and emergency care of the airway is also provided.

Chapter 6, Blood Gas and Critical Care Analyte Analysis, focuses on the equipment used for blood gas and analyte analysis. The types of equipment available in core labs and point-of-care testing are highlighted. The importance of and process for maintaining the integrity of a sample and assuring accuracy of results are detailed. Regulatory requirements from agencies such as the College of American Pathology (CAP) and the Joint Commission as well as federal requirements such as the Clinical Laboratory Improvement Amendments of 1988 (CLIA) are detailed.

Chapter 7, Patient Monitors, provides relevant information on noninvasive equipment used to measure and monitor clinical parameters important to the diagnosis and retreatment of cardiorespiratory system disorders. The appendices provide a unique way to compare performance characteristics and evaluate the utility or limitations of noninvasive monitors used for monitoring oxygen saturation and expired carbon dioxide concentrations, as well as mechanisms for identifying and quantifying hemoglobin disorders. This chapter will also provide a comprehensive review of equipment available for the evaluation and monitoring of lung mechanics.

Chapter 8, Measuring and Monitoring Pulmonary Function, describes types of devices used to evaluate and monitor pulmonary health. Stationary instruments used in a laboratory, as well as portable devices and those used at the bedside and in ambulatory and home care settings, will be characterized by their measurement methods. A comparison of methods to select devices that are useful in detecting airflow limitations, gas transfer impairment, volume limitations, and respiratory muscle weakness will be provided. This chapter will also highlight performance standards and regulatory requirements for training personnel and performing quality control procedures.

Chapter 9, Mechanical Ventilation, presents a unique and systematic approach to a complicated subject. The fundamental theory for understanding ventilator terminology is presented in a way that leads to a practical taxonomy for modes of ventilation. This approach facilitates the understanding of ventilator operation that transcends a mere proliferation of the trade names of the modes, minimizing confusion and the propensity for user error. Through the use of this taxonomy, the learner is able to classify, compare, and contrast the functional differences of the nearly 300 modes currently available on mechanical ventilators.

Chapter 10, Sleep Apnea Devices, provides clinically relevant information on the devices available for the treatment of sleep-disordered breathing. The principles of operation, safety, and technical considerations used for patient selection are provided. Key aspects of cleaning and maintenance as they relate to the safe and effective operation of these devices in the long-term care and home care environment are detailed.

Chapter 11, Cardiovascular Monitoring, focuses on the equipment used to monitor and assess the function of the cardiovascular system. The variety of devices used for cardiovascular monitoring, from the electrocardiogram (ECG) to those that measure intravascular pressures and cardiac output, are discussed. The clinical relevance of hemodynamic monitoring for mechanically ventilated patients is highlighted. In addition to the theory of operation, this chapter also familiarizes the learner with techniques used to troubleshoot technological problems.

Chapter 12, Hyperinflation Therapy, describes the devices used to perform lung expansion maneuvers, or equipment that subjects the lungs to volumes greater than normal in order to reinflate areas of collapse and improve gas exchange. Incentive spirometers, intermittent positive-pressure breathing devices, and positive airway pressure devices including positive expiratory pressure devices used to accomplish hyperinflation therapy goals are detailed.

Chapter 13, Airway Clearance, focuses on the mechanical devices used to clear airway secretions. Mechanical devices that assist with the cephalad mobilization of secretions in airways as well as those that assist with expectoration are discussed. Although some of the devices that are described in this chapter are also found in Chapter 12, the dual function of these devices and their operational characteristics that enable them to generate volumes greater than normal and expiratory flow rates that can move airway secretions cephalad are explored.

Chapter 14, Medicated Aerosol Delivery Devices, details the operational characteristics of a variety of devices used to deliver medication to the lung. An understanding of their function and limitations will enable respiratory therapists to appropriately select the device or devices that can make a positive clinical impact.

Chapter 15, Manual and Automatic Resuscitators, differentiates automatic resuscitators from mechanical ventilators and provides clinically relevant information on the different types of resuscitators available for manual ventilation. Key aspects for device use and selection are provided.

The authors of this textbook are distinguished educators, practicing clinicians, researchers, and internationally recognized experts in both pediatric and adult respiratory care. These authors have a passion for educating respiratory therapists, from the novice to the advanced practitioner, in order to optimize care, improve outcomes, and advance the practice of our profession. Their contributions will serve respiratory care students as well as credentialed practicing clinicians.

Instructor and Student Resources

For the Instructor

As a benefit of using this textbook and to save you valuable time in the preparation and instruction of this course, you will receive access to

- Slides in PowerPoint format
- Image bank
- Test bank
- Prepopulated midterm and final exams
- Chapter quizzes
- Sample syllabus
- Web links to computer-aided instructional materials to enhance the learning experience and ensure that the content is current and relevant to clinical practice, as well as online resources for students and faculty, which include:
  - AARC expert panel and evidence-based clinical practice guidelines
  - Comprehensive resources for medicated aerosol delivery
  - Practice guidelines from professional organizations

For the Students

- Laboratory exercises were designed to complement didactic instruction by providing reinforcement and providing opportunities to realistically simulate clinical scenarios and interdisciplinary team rounds.
- Case studies present scenarios and assessment items so students can apply their knowledge to real-life situations.

About the Authors

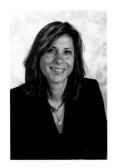

Teresa A. Volsko, MHHS, RRT, FAARC, is adjunct graduate faculty for Rush University and a fellow of the American Association for Respiratory Care. Currently, Terry is the Director of Respiratory Care, Transport, and the Communication Center for Akron Children's Hospital. Prior to joining the Akron Children's Hospital, Terry was an associate professor of health professions in the Bitonte College of Health and Human Services at Youngstown State University. She served as the program director for the Respiratory Care and Polysomnography programs for several years. Terry is the author of over 85 abstract and manuscript publications in peer-reviewed medical journals and several book chapters. She has served the profession in many capacities and is currently a member of the Board of Trustees for the National Board for Respiratory Care, the American Association for Respiratory Care Evidence-Based Clinical Guidelines Committee, and the Editorial Board of *Respiratory Care Journal*.

Terry was born and raised in the Youngstown, Ohio, area. She received her associate degree in respiratory therapy technology, and her Bachelor of Science and Master of Health and Human Services from Youngstown State University. She is currently completing her graduate work in the Master of Business Administration program at Youngstown State University. Terry's passion for the respiratory care profession and dedication to mentoring respiratory care students and professionals spans more than 3 decades.

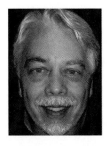

Robert L. Chatburn, MHHS, RRT-NPS, FAARC, is a professor at the Department of Medicine at Lerner College of Medicine of Case Western Reserve University and fellow of the American Association for Respiratory Care. Rob is currently the clinical research manager, Section of Respiratory Therapy, at the Cleveland Clinic. Previously he was the technical director of respiratory care at University Hospitals for 20 years. He is the author of 9 textbooks and over 300 publications in peer-reviewed medical journals. He is a member of the Editorial Board of *Respiratory Care Journal* and is recognized internationally for his contributions to mechanical ventilation research.

Rob, a native of Niles, Ohio, spent his career in the Cleveland, Ohio, area. He received an AS degree from Cuyahoga Community College and BS and MHHS degrees from Youngstown State University. He started his career at Rainbow Babies and Children's Hospital in 1977. In 1979 he was promoted to research coordinator. In 1986 he took the position of technical director of pediatric respiratory care and in 1995 annexed the adult division as well. In 1997 he became assistant professor of pediatrics at Case Western Reserve University and was promoted to associate professor in 1998. In 2006 Rob became clinical research manager, Section of Respiratory Therapy, at the Cleveland Clinic. Rob is a fellow of the American Association for Respiratory Care in 1998 and recipient of the Forrest M. Bird Lifetime Scientific Achievement Award.

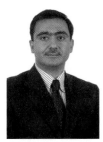

Mohamad F. El-Khatib, MD, PhD, MBA, RRT, is a professor of anesthesiology and director of respiratory therapy department at the American University of Beirut Medical Center. Dr. El-Khatib has published more than 115 peer-reviewed articles and abstracts in the fields of anesthesiology, critical care medicine, and respiratory care. Dr. El-Khatib's main area of interest is optimization of mechanical ventilation including newer and nonconventional modes of ventilatory support and strategies for liberation from mechanical ventilation. Dr. El-Khatib has lectured at many international and regional meetings. He is currently the managing editor of the *Middle East Journal of Anesthesiology*, and he is a reviewer for the journals of *Critical Care Medicine, Respiratory Care, Critical Care, American Journal of Respiratory and Critical Care Medicine, Lung*, and *Saudi Journal of Anesthesia*.

Contributors

Ehab Daoud, MD, FACP, FCCP
Assistant Professor of Medicine
University of New England
Biddeford, ME
Assistant Professor of Medicine and Surgery
Brown Alpert School of Medicine
Brown University
Providence, RI

Kathleen Deakins, MSHA, RRT, NPS, FAARC
Manager
Pediatric Respiratory Care
Rainbow Babies and Children's Hospital
Cleveland, OH

Maria Delost, PhD
Professor and Director, Clinical Laboratory Programs
Department of Health Professions
Youngstown State University
Youngstown, OH

William French, MA, RRT
Professor and Clinical Director,
Respiratory Therapy Program
Lakeland Community College
Kirtland, OH

David Grooms, MSHS, RRT
Respiratory Clinical Program Manager
Sentara Norfolk General, Leigh, and Bayside Hospitals
Suffolk, VA

Dean R. Hess, PhD, RRT
Assistant Director, Respiratory Care
Massachusetts General Hospital
Associate Professor, Anesthesia
Harvard Medical School
Boston, MA

Keith Hirst, MS, RRT-ACCS, NPS
Neonatal Respiratory Manager
Brigham and Women's Hospital
Boston, MA

Aanchal Kapoor, MD, FACP, FCCP
Associate Program Director for Critical Care Fellowship
    Program
Respiratory Institute
Cleveland Clinic
Cleveland, OH

Joseph Lewarski, BS, RRT, FAARC
Principal
RC Medical, Inc.
Wickliffe, OH

Eduardo Mireles-Cabodevila, MD
Assistant Professor, Department of Medicine
Lerner College of Medicine of Case Western Reserve
    University
Program Director, Critical Care Medicine Fellowship
Respiratory Institute
Cleveland Clinic
Cleveland, OH

Mohammad F. Siddiqui, MD, MPH
Houston Pulmonary Medicine Associates
Houston, TX

Steven Zhou, BA
Penn State College of Medicine
Hershey, PA

Reviewers

Wesley M. Granger, PhD, RRT, FAARC
Associate Professor
University of Alabama at Birmingham
Birmingham, AL

Rebecca A. Higdon, MS, RRT
Director of Clinical Education
Elizabethtown Community and Technical College
Elizabethtown, KY

Debra Kasel, EdD, RRT-ACCS, AE-C
Associate Professor, Respiratory Care
Northern Kentucky University
Highland Heights, KY

Thomas Lamphere, BS, RRT-ACCS, RPFT, FAARC
Instructor
Gwynedd Mercy University
Sellersville, PA

Michael Murphy, BA, RRT, EMT-P
Clinical Instructor
University of Hartford
Hartford, CT

Leslie Yancy-Meadows, MS, RRT
Senior Instructor/Clinical Coordinator
Shawnee State University
Portsmouth, OH

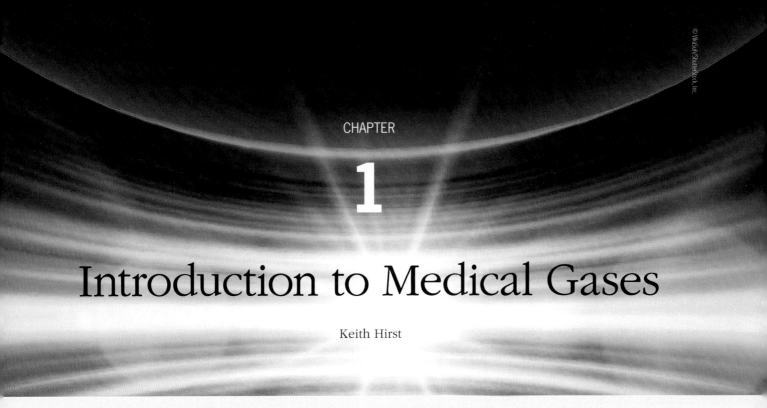

CHAPTER

1

Introduction to Medical Gases

Keith Hirst

OBJECTIVES

1. Define a medical gas.
2. Describe the types of gases used in respiratory care.
3. Explain how medical gases are delivered to the patient.
4. Describe how liquid oxygen is formed.
5. Describe how liquid oxygen is delivered to the patient.
6. Differentiate between liquid and compressed gas.
7. Describe the piping system used in acute care facilities.
8. Discuss the use of station outlets and the types of connectors used.
9. Explain the various methods of testing the hospital gas distribution system.
10. Identify problems with a hospital piping system.
11. Discuss how medical gases are stored and transported.
12. Identify the various cylinder sizes and colors and how they relate to the particular medical gas contents.
13. Discuss how oxygen concentrators work.

KEY TERMS

American National Standards Institute (ANSI)
American Standard Safety System (ASSS)
Diameter Index Safety System (DISS)
Diaphragm compressor
Direct-acting valves
Fractional distillation
Fusible plugs
Indirect-acting valves

Pin Index Safety System (PISS)
Piston compressor
Pressure relief valves
Quick connect adaptors
Rotary compressor
Rupture disks
Spring-loaded devices
Terminal units
Wood's metal
Zone valves

Introduction

Respiratory therapists have a wide range of medical gases at their disposal. Gases designated for therapeutic or diagnostic purposes must undergo rigorous testing and meet standards before use. The U.S. Pharmacopeia

(USP) provides the purification specifications manufacturers must abide by in order to distribute their products for human use. Therapeutic gases include oxygen, air, nitric oxide, and mixtures of helium and oxygen and oxygen and carbon dioxide. Gases may also be used to perform diagnostic tests or to calibrate the machines used to perform diagnostic testing. Helium, nitrogen, and carbon monoxide are commonly used for this purpose.

Medical-grade gases play an important role across the continuum of care. It is essential for the respiratory therapist to be knowledgeable not only of the types of gas used, but also how they are composed, manufactured, transported, and stored until needed. This chapter presents the principles of medical gas manufacturing, storage, transport, and use in a variety of healthcare settings.

Medical Gases

Oxygen (O_2)

Oxygen (O_2) is an elemental gas that is colorless, odorless, and tasteless at normal pressures and temperatures. It also supports life because oxygen makes up roughly 20.9% of the Earth's atmosphere by volume. It has a molecular weight of 31.9988 and a density of 1.326 kg/m^3 at standard temperature and pressure, dry (STPD).[1] When O_2 is in a liquid form, it has a pale bluish tint and is slightly heavier than water. A common misconception is that O_2 is flammable; it is not. It will, however, support combustion. Oxygen will accelerate combustion, causing the materials to burn at a higher temperature and more vigorously in its presence.[2] Substances that are combustible, such as oil, petroleum, and grease, will ignite more easily in an oxygen-enriched environment. Therefore, in the presence of oxygen, a small spark created by impact or caused by friction can ignite these highly combustible products very easily.[1] There is particular concern about fire risk in the operating room due in part to the extensive use of lasers, especially during head and neck surgery.[3,4]

Oxygen has a unique molecular bonding. When oxygen is added to certain elements and/or compounds, oxidation, or the breakdown of that substance, will occur. The rate of oxidation will vary depending on the substance, the temperature, and the amount of oxygen available.

Uses in Respiratory Care

Oxygen is used for diagnostic and therapeutic purposes. Diagnostically, it is used as a source gas to calibrate respiratory care monitoring equipment such as gas analyzers. It can also be used as a mixture for device calibration; for example, oxygen mixtures are used in the calibration of gas cylinders for transcutaneous oxygen monitors.

Due to its life-sustaining properties, O_2 is used in concentrations greater than ambient air to treat and/or prevent the manifestations or symptoms of hypoxia.[5] In the acute care setting, oxygen may be used when hypoxemia is suspected, such as during resuscitative efforts in response to trauma[6] or during cardiac arrest.[7] Oxygen also may be used in the acute care setting to prevent or treat the manifestations or symptoms associated with tissue hypoxemia.[8] It may also be used to provide long-term therapy to individuals with chronic illness.[9] Oxygen may also be administered to prevent or treat hypoxemia during surgical procedures[10] or when recovering from anesthesia.[11] It is used in a variety of patient populations from premature infants to adults. In some cases, supplemental oxygen may be needed for long-term use to treat hypoxemia associated with chronic lung conditions such as chronic obstructive pulmonary disease (COPD) or cystic fibrosis.[12]

Oxygen therapy is not without risk. There are detrimental effects from the delivery of high concentrations of oxygen and/or the presence of hyperoxemia for prolonged periods of time. In premature infants, the inability to regulate blood flow due to the vasodilation effects of oxygen and fluctuations in PaO_2 can alter cerebral blood flow and contribute to the development of intraventricular hemorrhages (IVH), as well as alter retinal blood flow and contribute to retinopathy of prematurity (ROP).[13,14] In adults, prolonged use at high concentrations ($F_IO_2 > 0.50$) may lead to oxygen toxicity, absorption atelectasis, and depression of ciliary and/or leukocyte function.[15–17]

Manufacturing

Oxygen is produced naturally by chlorophyll-containing plants through a process known as photosynthesis. Sunlight facilitates the production of glucose and oxygen when carbon dioxide and water combine within the chlorophyll-containing plants. Once transformed by this biological process, oxygen is released into the atmosphere.

Oxygen can be also be produced commercially by **fractional distillation** of liquefied air. This process for bulk production relies on a method known as the Joule-Kelvin principle, which states that when gases under pressure are released into a vacuum, the gas molecules will tend to lose their kinetic energy. The reduction of kinetic energy within the vacuum causes the temperature, as well as the cohesive forces between molecules, to decrease. This process is divided into three stages: (1) purification, (2) liquefaction, and (3) distillation.

During the purification stage, air is subjected to a series of compression and cooling cycles. At the beginning of this process air is compressed to 1,500 pounds per square inch (psi). Subjecting air to this increase in pressure also causes an increase in temperature. The conditioned gas is then passed through a water-cooled heat exchanger, which dissipates excess heat. The air is then compressed a second time at a higher pressure, 2,000 psi, after which the gas is passed through an after-cooler and delivered to a countercurrent heat exchanger at room temperature. Once this process is complete, the air is then cooled to −50°F (−45.6°C). This is the final cooling process in the purification phase. Waste nitrogen is used during this cooling process to freeze the water vapor and make it easier to remove.

Liquefaction is the next phase in the process. The gas passes through a series of heat exchangers and is cooled to extreme temperatures. This process eliminates any remaining water vapor. The initial pass through the first heat exchanger cools the air to −40°F (−40°C). The next pass through a third heat exchanger subjects the gas to a pressure of 200 psi and cools it to −265°F (−165°C). Liquefaction then takes place when the air is released into a separator and expanded to 90 psi. This release of pressure causes a further drop in temperature[1] and partial liquefaction of oxygen.

Distillation is the final stage of the process. In the separator, gas and liquid are pumped through separate streams into the distillation column. The liquid portion enters the top and passes through a series of cylindrical shells that contain metal trays. Vapor from the separator passes through the liquid as it travels across and through the metal trays. The liquid becomes richer in oxygen because this process enables nitrogen to be boiled off. As a result, the vapor that rises becomes very rich in nitrogen. Liquid oxygen forms at the bottom of the column; however, this oxygen is not free from impurities. The liquid oxygen may still contain krypton and argon. To remove any remaining impurities the oxygen is reboiled at a precise temperature and pressure. As the boiling points of these remaining gases are reached, they evaporate. The oxygen that is left through this process is 99.9% pure oxygen.[1]

Carbon Dioxide (CO_2)

Carbon dioxide (CO_2) is a chemical compound composed of two oxygen atoms covalently bonded to a single carbon atom. Its molecular weight is 44.01 and it has a density of 1.833 kg/m^3 at STPD.[1] Carbon is 27.3% and oxygen 72.7% of the total molecular weight of this compound. Carbon dioxide is a trace gas, comprising 0.039% of the atmosphere. It is colorless and, at low concentrations, is also odorless. At higher concentrations this gas has a sharp, acidic odor and can cause a sour taste in the mouth and irritation or stinging to the upper respiratory tract. Studies have demonstrated that inhalation of high concentrations of CO_2 (7.5%) was associated with increased heart rate and blood pressure as well as increased subjective scores of panic, anxiety, and fear[18,19] or even asphyxiation. This gas is heavier and more dense than both air and oxygen and is nonflammable and cannot support life. Because of these properties, CO_2 in its liquid form is sometimes used in fire suppression units in areas where water may damage sensitive equipment.[20] Solid CO_2 or dry ice can be used to ship medical and nonmedical items that would perish at normal temperatures.

Uses in Respiratory Care

Carbon dioxide has a limited role as a therapeutic gas. In lieu of adding mechanical dead space to a ventilator circuit, CO_2 has been titrated in small amounts to correct respiratory alkalosis for patients requiring full ventilator support. Typically, CO_2 is added to oxygen in concentrations of 5% or 10% CO_2, yielding 95% or 90% O_2, respectively, to form "carbogen." Inhaled carbogen (5% CO_2, 95% O_2) has been used to promote vasodilation and increase cerebral perfusion in patients with occlusive carotid artery disease.[21] When it is used therapeutically, the duration of therapy is relatively short, 10 minutes or less, and close patient monitoring is warranted. Pediatric cardiac patients have been given carbon dioxide postoperatively to manipulate pulmonary vascular resistance and thus reapportion pulmonary and peripheral blood flow.[22]

Carbon dioxide is most useful as a diagnostic or calibration gas in the clinical laboratory setting. It is also used for calibration of blood gas analyzers and transcutaneous partial pressure of carbon dioxide electrodes and capnographs. Carbon dioxide is added to membrane oxygenators for devices that bypass the heart and lungs, such as extracorporeal membrane oxygenation (ECMO) and cardiopulmonary bypass (CPB) machines. It has also been used as a shuttle gas for intraaortic balloon pumps (IABPs); however, most IABPs are now using helium.[23]

Manufacturing

Unrefined carbon dioxide is obtained either from geological reserves or as a by-product from the combustion of coal, coke, natural gas, and oil. It can also be obtained as a by-product from the fermentation of sugar during the production of alcohol.

Atmospheric CO_2 is refined for medical use. The refinement process removes impurities such as pollutants, water, and gas mixtures such as carbon monoxide, hydrogen sulfide, and nitric acid. The purity of medical-grade CO_2 must be at least 99.5%.

Helium (He)

Helium (He) may be the lightest gas used in respiratory care. Its molecular weight is 4 with a density at STPD of 0.165 kg/m^3.[1] It is a rare gas found in the earth's atmosphere at a concentration of 5 parts per million (ppm). Helium is colorless, odorless, and tasteless. This nonflammable gas does not react with biological membranes. It has excellent thermal conductivity and a high rate of permeability, and it is only slightly soluble in the bloodstream. It cannot support life because it is both chemically and physiologically inert.

Uses in Respiratory Care

Helium has a very low density—0.18 g/L compared to 1.29 g/L for air and 1.43 g/L for oxygen (STPD). Because of this low density, helium is used extensively to promote less turbulent gas flow and improve the distribution of gas in conditions where the airways are narrowed. Helium cannot support life and can be used for inhalation only as part of a gas mixture with oxygen. The helium–oxygen blend is often called "heliox." The literature reports the use of heliox decreases the work of breathing in conditions associated with increased airway resistance[24–26] by reducing the inspiratory pressure of the patient and hence reducing the work of breathing. Because helium is so light, it diffuses approximately four times faster than a mixture of nitrogen and oxygen, enhancing the effect on carbon dioxide elimination.[27]

Heliox is commercially available in He:O_2 concentrations of 80:20, 70:30, and 60:40. Typically, it is distributed in high pressure medical gas cylinders in the H, G, or E size. Because the gas density of heliox mixtures is less than that of air or oxygen, clinicians should be aware of the effect heliox may have on the functions of medical devices. Air and oxygen flowmeters, for example, are affected by gas density and will not correctly measure heliox flow. In this instance, a formula can be used to calculate the predicted heliox flow.

The predicted heliox flow is calculated by multiplying the diffusible factor for helium by the flow of gas set on the standard flowmeter. The conversion factor is 1.4 for a 60:40 mixture, 1.6 for 70:30, and 1.8 for an 80:20 blend.

If a 70:30 mixture were used for a patient and the flow set on a standard air/oxygen flowmeter were set to 10 L/min, the predicted flow of heliox can be calculated as:

Predicted flow of heliox = Conversion factor × Flow set on the flowmeter

Predicted flow of heliox = 1.6 × 10 L/min

Predicted flow of heliox = 16 L/min

Care should be taken when using heliox to power standard jet or vibrating mesh during medicated aerosol therapy. Heliox can negatively affect nebulizer function if the predicted flow does not match the manufacturer's recommended flow. Depending on the total predicted flow, a smaller particle size, altered nebulizer output, and/or longer nebulization time can result.[28–30]

The density, viscosity, and thermal conductivity of heliox may interfere with ventilator function. It is essential for the clinician to know whether a ventilator is calibrated to deliver helium–oxygen mixtures prior to use. The literature reports alterations in delivered and measured exhaled tidal volumes can occur when heliox is delivered through a ventilator that is not calibrated for use with gases other than air and oxygen.[31–33] To minimize the risks associated with ventilator malfunction, it is imperative for clinicians to consult the ventilator's operation manual and verify safe use of heliox.

Helium is an inert gas and will not interfere with human metabolism. This physical property facilitates the use of this medical gas with other medical devices and therapeutic interventions. Helium is used during surgical procedures to help expand patients' abdominal contents and make it easier for the surgeons to operate.[34] Helium is also used as a shuttle gas in intra-aortic balloon pumps to inflate the balloon. When used for this purpose, there is no risk of emboli or patient harm if the balloon were to rupture.[13]

Helium is also used diagnostically. It is used during pulmonary function testing to measure lung volumes and determine diffusion capacity.

Manufacturing

A small quantity of helium is naturally present in the atmosphere and can be obtained by fractionation. Most helium used is extracted from natural gas wells. It is obtained cryogenically and refined through a process of liquefaction and purification.

Compressed Air

Air is a mixture of several gases; the most prominent are nitrogen and oxygen, along with many other trace gases that support the atmosphere of Earth. The oxygen in air is needed to sustain most life forms because it is vital to the metabolic process in our bodies. Medical-grade air is colorless, odorless, and tasteless. It is also considered nonflammable, but like oxygen it can support combustion. It can have a blue tint if cooled and may have a milky appearance if it contains high levels of carbon dioxide. It has a molecular weight of 28.975 with a density of 1.29 g/L at STDP.

Uses in Respiratory Care

Medical grade air is most commonly blended with oxygen to provide a precise fractional inspired oxygen concentration (F_IO_2) or as a source gas to power small-volume nebulizers. Respiratory care equipment requiring a 50 psi gas source for operation, such as pneumatic percussors, may be more economically powered by compressed air. It can be supplied in several ways, including through piped systems, in high pressure compressed gas cylinders, or from portable compressors. Respiratory care equipment, such as mechanical ventilators, may have a built-in compressor to provide a self-contained medical-grade air source for blended gas. Small portable compressors are often used to power small-volume nebulizers for patients in their home or in facilities (clinics, nursing homes) that do not have a piped-in air source.

Manufacturing

Air is a gas that is in abundant supply and available in several different grades of purity. The grading system, developed by the Compressed Gas Association (CGA), ranges from A to N. Grade J is dry and free from oil and particulate and considered medical grade.

Compressed medical air for high pressure cylinders and/or bulk distribution through piping systems is manufactured in large quantities by the Claude or Linde process. Both methods compress and reexpand the air to cool it, which results in liquefaction. The Linde method requires much higher pressures (greater than 200 atm) to produce liquefaction. The pressure needed to produce liquefaction with the Claude method is only 30 atm.

When air is produced through portable compressors, filters and Teflon piston rings are used to ensure it is free from oil and particulates.

Nitrogen (N)

Nitrogen (N) is the most abundant gas, making up almost 78% of the earth's atmosphere by volume. It is an inert gas that is also colorless, odorless, and tasteless. It is nonflammable, non-life-supporting, and will not support combustion. It is less dense than air or oxygen, with a molecular weight of 28.01 and density of 1.25 g/L (STPD).

Uses in Respiratory Care

Nitrogen is used medically to provide gas mixtures of inspired oxygen at concentrations less than ambient (i.e., < 21%). The literature reports the use of subambient oxygen delivery to infants with unrepaired hypoplastic left heart syndrome (HLHS) or other single-ventricle lesions. The survival of these infants depends on success in maintaining patency of the ductus arteriosus, assuring adequate mixing of blood in the atria, and establishing and maintaining a balance between systemic and pulmonary blood flow at or near unity.[35] Oxygen concentrations less than 21% can be achieved by blending nitrogen with ambient concentrations of oxygen for infants requiring ventilator support;[36] for those not requiring ventilator assistance, devices, such as a hood or high flow nasal cannula, can be used. Titrating the subambient gas concentration may be a tedious and time-consuming task, but it is essential for the respiratory therapist to take the time necessary to determine the precise F_IO_2 necessary to alter the physiologic modifiers of pulmonary vascular resistance and maintain balanced circulation. Chatburn and colleagues have shown the Mini-OX III and the Teledyne TED-190 provide accurate and reliable F_IO_2 readings between 0 and 0.21 and are acceptable for delivering subambient oxygen concentrations.[37]

Nitrogen has also been used as a calibration gas for several types of gas analyzers. Typically it is used to provide a zero reference point. It can generally be found in pulmonary function laboratories as a diagnostic gas.

Manufacturing

Nitrogen is produced during the liquefaction of atmospheric air. Large quantities of this gas are separated from impurities by fractionation.

Nitric Oxide (NO)

Nitric oxide (NO) is a colorless, nonflammable, and toxic gas at room temperature. It is present as a trace gas in air; however, additional nitric oxide is produced as a byproduct of combustion and is thus considered an environmental pollutant. It is also a toxin produced by cigarette smoke. NO is typically odorless, but may carry a faint metallic smell. It is a very strong oxidizer and therefore supports combustion. Its molecular weight is 30.006 and at STDP has a density of 1.245 g/L.[1] At high levels it can contribute to the formation of methemoglobin and to tissue hypoxia. In the atmosphere, ozone readily changes nitric oxide to nitrogen dioxide (NO_2).

Uses in Respiratory Care

Nitric oxide is an important mediator of vasomotor control. Inhalation of NO at low doses (5–20 ppm) can be used to facilitate smooth muscle relaxation and pulmonary vasculature dilation. As a result, oxygenation improves through better ventilation/perfusion matching. At higher doses (< 80 ppm) it is a potent pulmonary vasodilator. Inhaled nitric oxide can effectively reduce pulmonary hypertension by lowering pulmonary artery resistance. Currently there is only one Food and Drug Administration (FDA) approved use for NO—for treatment of infants with hypoxic respiratory failure.[38] Term infants with persistent pulmonary hypertension, either as a primary cause or secondary to other disease processes, respond to inhaled nitric oxide with improvement in oxygenation indices and a decreased need for extracorporeal membrane oxygenation. In a study of 24 patients with congenital diaphragmatic hernia requiring surgical intervention and postoperative mechanical ventilatory support, inhaled NO contributed to a reduction of pulmonary hypertension, amelioration of respiratory symptoms, and recovery of pulmonary vascular function.[39]

The literature also reports positive patient outcomes with the use of NO with sickle cell disease[40] and for prevention of chronic lung disease in premature infants[41] and patients with acute respiratory distress syndrome (ARDS).[42,43]

Manufacturing

Nitric oxide is manufactured by the oxidation of ammonia at 932°F (500°C) in the presence of a platinum catalyst. It can also be produced when acid solutions of nitrates are reduced by metals.[1] Although rare and not a high yield for the amount of energy needed, at high temperatures (5,792°F/3,200°C) a direct combination of nitrogen and oxygen under energy-rich conditions can obtain 5% volume of nitric oxide. Nitric oxide is stored in aluminum cylinders with a final gas purity of 99.0%. To enhance safety, the cylinders have CGA 626 valve outlets.

Nitrous Oxide (N_2O)

Nitrous oxide is a colorless, odorless, and tasteless nontoxic gas that cannot support life. It is nonflammable but will support combustion. There are several grades for this gas. Grade A is acceptable for medical use. It has a molecular weight of 44.0128 and at STDP has a density of 1.947 kg/m³.[2]

Uses in Respiratory Care

Nitrous oxide is a central nervous system (CNS) depressant. Typically, it is used for general anesthesia during surgical procedures. Its use without at least 20% oxygen may cause asphyxia and patient demise.

Manufacturing

Nitrous oxide is obtained by the thermal decomposition of ammonium nitrate. It can also be recovered as a by-product from the steam from adipic acid manufacturing.[1]

Medical Gas Distribution Systems

Medical gases are used in the care of patients with respiratory disorders along the continuum of care. Therefore, it is essential for respiratory therapists to understand how medical gases are distributed to patient care areas. A bulk gas delivery system is any type of equipment assembly and interconnecting piping that has the capacity to store more than 20,000 cubic feet of medical grade gas for delivery to patient care areas.[2] Monitoring and alarm systems are built into the central supply and can take the form of (1) a high pressure gas cylinder supply or (2) a bulk supply system. The central oxygen supply system should be designed with features allowing backup and/or redundancy in the event of system failure.

Typically, little thought is given to this process by clinicians. Interest is generally peaked if a problem with the piping or bulk storage system occurs or new construction is planned. Malfunction of the gas distribution system within a hospital can contribute to serious patient safety events. The consequences of an oxygen failure extend to all patient care areas, from intensive to general care. Immediate identification of the areas affected and evaluation of the extent of the problem can minimize adverse patient outcomes. Man-made or natural disasters place a strain on resources available in our current healthcare system. The ability to provide adequate oxygen therapy could be disrupted if a disaster affected the institution's bulk supply. Should the manufacturing or delivery process be interrupted as well, the ability to provide medical gases would be further compromised because the consumption would outstrip the available supply. Delivering oxygen to patients requiring manual resuscitation, basic oxygen therapy, or positive-pressure ventilation during these scenarios would be very difficult.[44]

During new construction, attention should be focused beyond the nursing units. The need for piped medical gas extends to areas where special therapeutic and diagnostic procedures are performed. The need for a 50-psi gas source (for mechanical ventilators or high flow oxygen delivery systems) should be anticipated. Respiratory therapists are instrumental in the planning phase and will have valuable input regarding the number and location of compressed gas outlets. Therapist involvement in the initial planning and testing phase of new construction projects can minimize construction delays and the additional expense of unexpected and unbudgeted renovations. Operationally, poor planning can contribute to delays in care or safety events. For example, if piped-in gas was not available in interventional radiology, additional resources and planning would be needed to safely transport a mechanically ventilated patient to and from a procedure and care for them during the procedure. If the amount of compressed gas needed for the patient was not properly calculated, a mechanical failure of the ventilator due to an insufficient supply of source gas could cause the patient harm. Planning for and attending to patient needs may also require additional staff resources, all of which could have been avoided by adequate planning during the construction phase.

Usually, gases for bulk distribution to acute care institutions, such as hospitals or long-term acute care (LTAC) facilities, are stored in their liquid form in large reservoirs outside of the facility. High pressure cylinders banked together with a manifold system are too expensive and cumbersome for large acute care organizations and are more commonly seen in the long-term care venue. However, the potential for mass casualty and pandemic events has caused a resurgence in interest in and availability of a number of new systems.

In a survey of 35 hospitals in the greater Cleveland and Columbus, Ohio, metropolitan areas, Stoller and colleagues investigated the types of primary and reserve oxygen sources, and the presence and configuration of a backup system. Bulk liquid oxygen systems (with primary and reserve liquid reservoirs) were predominantly used as a main central supply source, with some providing manifold cylinders as backup.[45] Mishaps regarding the main supply line from the bulk oxygen reservoir were reported by 16% (5/32) of responding institutions.[45] The authors also reported that main and reserve tanks were contiguous and fed through a single line to the hospital facility, suggesting ongoing risk for interruption of the oxygen supply. Regardless of the type of central supply system a healthcare organization has, it is essential to formulate a contingency plan to lessen the risk of an interrupted supply of medical gas due to man-made or natural causes.

Bulk Gas Delivery Systems

Oxygen

The National Fire Protection Association (NFPA) defines a bulk oxygen system as one that has more than 20,000 ft³ of oxygen stored at atmospheric temperature and pressure.[3] This also includes all unconnected reserves on site. Most acute care institutions use bulk liquid systems to deliver oxygen to 50-psi outlets in patient-care areas. Generally, these systems are affordable, take up less physical space within the institution, and are robust and very reliable. Liquid oxygen is less expensive when shipped in bulk and stored in large insulated, double-walled, stainless steel containers, outside of but in close proximity to the healthcare facility (**Figure 1-1**). The construction of the containers is designed to keep the liquid oxygen in a liquid form. The storage container must maintain the contents at a temperature below −181.4°F (−118.6°C) in order to keep oxygen in a liquid state. Otherwise, a rise in temperature will cause oxygen to change from a liquid to a gaseous state. The bulk oxygen system takes up less physical space within the hospital or LTAC facility, when compared to systems that bank a series of large high pressure tanks.

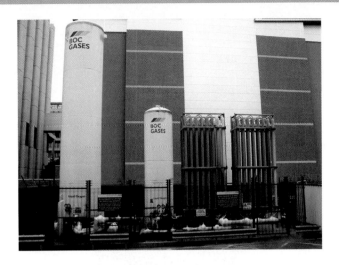

FIGURE 1-1 Liquid oxygen vessel used for bulk storage for an acute care facility. This illustration shows the bulk oxygen vessel at a distance from the facility surrounded by a protective fence, lighting and signage.

Courtesy of Captain-n00dle/Wikimedia Commons

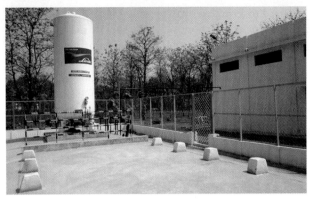

FIGURE 1-2 The NFPA Health Care Handbook provides guidelines for minimum distances for locating structures around bulk oxygen supply.

Courtesy of Bhakua/Flickr, https://creativecommons.org/licenses/by/2.0

The contents of the medical gas within the storage containers are closely monitored by electronic systems. Monitoring is the responsibility of either the medical gas vendor or the hospital maintenance department. Occasionally healthcare facilities have policies and procedures requiring that the vendor and the organization's maintenance department have joint monitoring responsibilities.

Large liquid-gas transport trailers are used to refill the external containers. Refilling typically occurs during the late evening or at night, to avoid congestion in the area surrounding the facility. The vendor delivery staff are trained and certified in the filling technique.

As the medical facility needs oxygen, the liquid oxygen passes through a vaporizer that also acts as a heat exchanger. The vaporizer absorbs the heat from the surrounding environment, raising its temperature to room temperature. This also raises the temperature of the gas and causes it to turn from a liquid to a gaseous state. As the oxygen turns from a liquid to a gas, the pressure increases within the container. Oxygen then passes through a reducing valve, which drops the pressure to a working pressure of approximately 50 psi.

Regulatory bodies govern the design and construction of bulk liquid oxygen systems. The NFPA regulates where the system can be located in relationship to buildings and other surrounding structures (**Figure 1-2**). (The NFPA Recommendations and Regulations for Bulk Oxygen Systems can be found in **Appendix 1-B**.) The American Society of Mechanical Engineers (ASME) controls how the system is designed and the construction of the storage containers. Lastly, the Bureau of Explosives regulates the pressure relief valves used within the system. The manner in which a healthcare facility complies with the standards established by these regulatory bodies is also important. The Joint Commission requires hospitals to comply with these standards and assesses compliance during regularly scheduled credentialing visits.

Air

Bulk delivery systems for air may also be part of the healthcare organization's gas distribution system. Two methods are commonly applied to this setting. As with oxygen, a large bank of high pressure cylinders can be used to provide medical-grade air for bulk distribution. However, similar to systems used for oxygen, this method is costly, time consuming, and impractical for large organizations such as hospitals. Therefore, most medical institutions will use industrial compressors to produce the air. Although high pressure tanks contain air that is drier and cleaner, air produced by industrial compressors meets the standards for medical grade and the system is much less expensive and cumbersome.

Medical industrial air compressors also are regulated by the NFPA. Typically, medical institutions are required to have at least two compressors on site. These compressors are motor-driven and run either in tandem or independent of each other. Regardless of how the compressors are set up, standards require that each compressor must be able to meet the complete needs of the institution during peak demand. This will minimize interruption of compressed air availability at the bedside in the event a compressor fails or requires service.

Each compressor must have its own pressure relief valve, check valves between the two compressors, as well as header and isolation valves to prevent pressure from one compressor form entering the other compressor. The compressors draw in air from the surrounding environment, filter and compress it, and reduce the working pressure to approximately 50 psi. The compressed air is then fed through an after-cooler and exposed to a sudden drop in temperature. As the air is cooled, any water vapor will rain out. This is an important process because ambient air contains moisture, and as air is compressed and pressure increases there is an increased risk of the air maintaining or holding onto that water vapor. Typically, as the air travels from the compressor through the piping system to the outlet at the bedside, the gas will cool. This will allow moisture to collect in the air piping, especially if the outlet has not been used. If the water vapor transferred through the piping reaches the compressed gas outlet, it can enter the respiratory care equipment and damage internal components.

Moisture collected as air is passed through the cooler is discarded. The dry air is stored in a reservoir tank until needed. This reservoir tank, also known as a receiver, must be equipped with a pressure gauge, relief valve, and automatic drain (for any condensate). A dryer is also located between the pressure regulator and receiver to further reduce moisture.

Although the systems in place remove most of the moisture and particulate matter, they are not entirely foolproof. Medical equipment requiring compressed air, such as ventilators, have filters to trap the particulate matter and prevent moisture from entering the device (**Figure 1-3**).

To prevent cross-contamination and the risk of a healthcare-acquired infection,[46] compressed medical air outlets should be used only for patient care equipment. The outlets should not be used to power engineering, maintenance, and other equipment that is nonmedical in nature.

Piping Distribution Systems

Bulk gases need to be distributed over zones that are located throughout the medical facility. The NFPA regulates the construction, installation, and testing of these systems. Gases are transported using seamless type K or L copper or brass pipes. These pipes are required to be labeled every 20 feet with the type of gas and direction of gas flow. A hospital may have bulk delivery systems for specialty gases, such as nitrous oxide, as well. Labeling allows for the gas within that piping to be easily identified and minimizes cross-connection within the facility's piping system. The diameter of piping used to deliver oxygen is 0.5 inch OD (outside diameter) and other gases are 0.375 inch OD.

The distribution of gases includes a series of pipe systems that include the pipes, pressure relief valves, zone valves, alarms, and station outlets or terminal units. Pipes are broken down into three categories and are described as follows:

- *Main line:* Pipes that connect the operating supply to risers, branch lines, or both

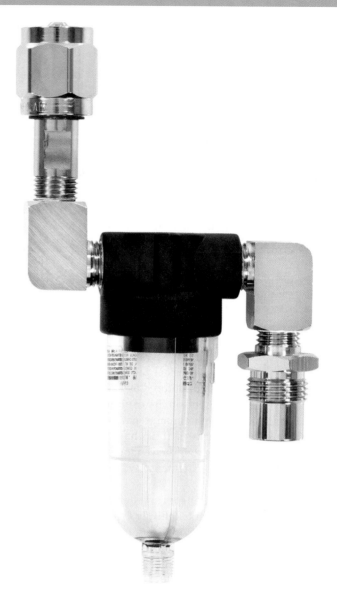

FIGURE 1-3 A water trap with a drain and filter are often used in line with the high pressure gas hose leading to moisture-sensitive equipment, such as mechanical ventilators and anesthesia machines.

Reproduced with permission from CareFusion.

- *Risers:* Pipes that are installed vertically that connect the main line with branch lines on each floor of the building
- *Branch (lateral) lines:* Pipes that travel from the risers to individual rooms or groups of rooms on the same floor of the building

Pressure Relief Valves

Pressure relief valves are a safety feature incorporated into the system. The valves allow for excess gas to vent from the system, should a buildup of pressure occur, preventing line damage. These valves are usually set at a pressure 50% greater than the normal line pressure. Pressure relief valves are located above each air compressor, downstream of the main line pressure regulator, as well as upstream of any zone valve.

Zone Valves

Zone valves are also known as shut-off valves, isolation valves, or section valves. They are located in the branch and riser lines and allow for a room, section of rooms, or entire floor to be isolated. Typically, zone vales are located in easily accessible areas where healthcare practitioners can access them in the event of an emergency, or should maintenance or repair of the central gas supply become necessary. Specifically, zone valves can be found near the operating supply gas, where the main line enters the building, at each riser supplied from the main line, adjacent to the riser connection, and in each branch line that serves non-life-support patient rooms as well as outside each critical care area. If a zone valve is activated, the affected zone is isolated from the central supply gas source, allowing the remaining areas of the facility to be unaffected.

Respiratory care practitioners should know the location of the zone valves in their facility, or at the very least in the unit in which the therapist is assigned. In many institutions, the respiratory therapist is responsible for activating a zone valve (shutting off the supply of gas to an area) in the event of an emergency such as a fire. Typically, zone valves are located near a central workstation like a nursing station. These valves are labeled and installed in boxes with a removable window (**Figure 1-4**). Typically, only a quarter turn

(from the 3 o'clock position to the 6 o'clock position) is necessary to activate a zone valve.

Pressure Gauges

Pressure gauges are an important feature of a gas distribution system because they allow healthcare workers/engineers to visualize the pressure of the gas in each line. Pressure gauges are installed in the main line adjacent to the actuating switch and in each area alarm panel. These gauges need to be labeled correctly, color coded, and readable from a standing position.

Alarms

All gas distribution systems require alarms to notify hospital personal of a system malfunction. Alarms need to monitor the operating supply, reserve supply, and pressure in the main line and local supply lines. Typically, there is a master alarm system that consists of two panels. Each of these panels incorporate audible and visual alarms to signify system problems. The alarms also have to be noncancelable if the operating pressure varies more than 20% from normal.[2] The alarms usually automatically reset after the issue has been resolved.

The following are common conditions activating an alarm on the master panel:

- Changing over from the primary to the secondary bank occurs as or just before the reserve supply goes into operation.
- Reserve supply is reduced to one average day's supply.
- Pressure in reserve supply is too low to allow proper function.
- Pressure in the main line increases or decreases from normal operating pressures.
- Level of liquid in the bulk liquid oxygen supply reaches a predetermined level.
- Dew point in the compressed air system exceeds a threshold.

There are also area alarm systems, which are common in critical care areas of the hospital such as the emergency department, intensive care units (ICUs), operating rooms (ORs), and postanesthesia care units (PACUs). Area alarms must also have an audible and visual noncancelable alarm if the operating pressure fluctuates from 20% of normal operating pressure. Usually these alarms are installed in the line specific to the unit they are servicing and are downstream of the zone valve.

Hospital personnel responsible for alarm surveillance should be skilled in troubleshooting the bulk gas delivery system, piping zone valves, and station outlets. It is also essential to have response plans in place to ensure that any medical equipment in the affected area(s) continues to work properly. When alarms have been activated, appropriate personnel should be notified, usually engineering and respiratory care.

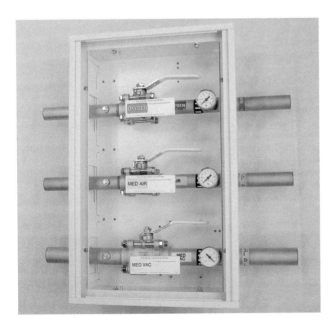

FIGURE 1-4 Oxygen, air, and vacuum zone valves.
Courtesy of Tri-Tech Medical Inc.

Station Outlets

Once the gas has traveled to the bedside, it goes to a station outlet or **terminal unit (Figure 1-5)**. This is the point at which medical equipment (i.e., high pressure lines from ventilators, flowmeters, etc.) connects to and disconnects from the central gas supply system. The station outlets are made up of several components, specifically a base block, faceplate, primary and secondary valves, and the connection point. The base block is the portion of the station outlet that connects to the piping system. It is similar in function to an electrical outlet at the end of an electrical wiring system. The faceplates cover the base block and are permanently labeled and color coded based on the gas being supplied to that end. The primary and secondary valves are safety valves that open and allow gas to flow into the device when a male end of the respiratory care equipment is placed in the female end of the faceplate. The valves also automatically shut off the flow of gas when the male and female ends disconnect, minimizing waste.

In order to prevent connection to the wrong gas source, each station outlet will accept only a gas-specific connector. Two types of systems are used: diameter index systems and quick connect adapters.

Diameter Index Safety System

A **Diameter Index Safety System (DISS)** is a threaded connection specific to the particular gas that is needed. The DISS was developed by the CGA for medical gases at 200 psi or less. A DISS connection consists of a body, nipple, and nut assembly. The body contains two specifically sized shoulders. The small bore (BB) mates with the small shoulder (MM), and the large bore (CC) mates with the large shoulder (NN). Each gas (air, oxygen, helium, and other gases) has its own corresponding size. This makes it very difficult to accidently switch gas lines for a mechanical ventilator. One drawback is that they are not quick to connect to because they have to be twisted on like a nut on a bolt. However, once seated they have a low risk for leaks (**Figure 1-6**).

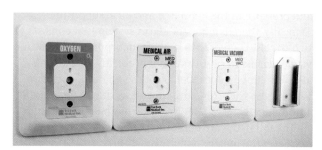

A

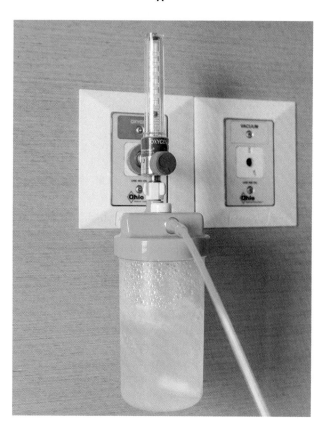

B

FIGURE 1-5 A. A typical quick connect station. B. An oxygen flowmeter attached to a quick connect station.

Photo A Courtesy of Tri-Tech Medical Inc. Photo B © Panom Pensawang/Shutterstock, Inc.

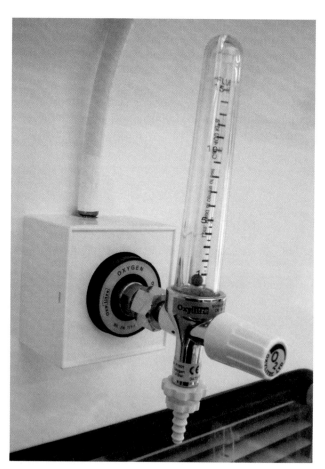

FIGURE 1-6 Oxygen and air DISS connections to an oxygen flowmeter.

Courtesy of Owain.davies/Wikipedia, http://creativecommons.org/licenses/by/3.0/deed.en

Quick Connect Adapters

Quick connect adapters allow the user to plug in and quickly access the gas source. There are two basic types, the National Compressed Gas (NCG) and the Ohio Diamond or Ohio Quick connecters. Both of these are nonthreaded and gas-specific male and female connections. They both work on the same principle: a plunger (female) is held by a spring. This spring prevents the gas from leaving the line. The probe (male) pushes the plunger back and gas is allowed to flow out. When the probe comes out, the spring pushes the plunger back into place. The advantage of this system is that the quick connectors are easier to connect than a DISS (similar to plug and play on a computer); however, they are more prone to leaks (**Figure 1-7**).

Testing and Verifying Medical Gas Distribution Systems

Once the gas pipes have been installed or serviced, testing must be conducted. It is important to verify the system is free from leaks and that no cross-connections have occurred. A visual inspection of the system is done

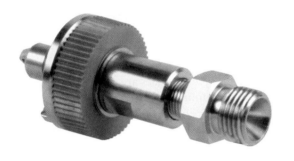

A

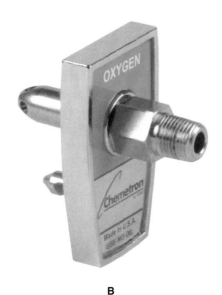

B

FIGURE 1-7 Examples of quick connect oxygen adaptors. A. Ohio Diamond. B. Chemtron.

Photos courtesy of Allied Healthcare Products, Inc..

to ensure the pipes are free from dirt, oil, grease, or other oxidized materials. It is also important to ensure the lines are not visibly damaged (dented, punctured, bent) or cross-connected with another type of specialty gas (e.g., the oxygen line is cross-connected with a nitrous oxide line).

Pressure Testing

Gas pipelines need to meet specific parameters and be leak free. A leak in a gas line could pose a fire hazard and cost money. To ensure that the gas pipeline is leak free, the system is pressurized using either dry air or nitrogen up to 150 pounds per square inch, gauge (psig). Each joint and connection is tested with a leak detection solution. Once a leak is detected and fixed, the system is tested again. When the system is determined to be free from leaks, and all alarm panels are installed and operational, the system is pressurized for 24 hours at 20% above normal operating pressure (typically around 60 psi). If any further leaks are found during this process, the leaks are repaired and the process repeated until the system remains leak free for 24 hours.

To ensure that cross-connections do not occur, each station outlet is tested to ensure that the outlet is delivering the gas the label specifies. For example, to test an air outlet, connect an air flowmeter to the outlet station. Direct a flow of gas into a bag containing an oxygen analyzer. The analyzer should read 21%. If it reads > 21%, cross-connection with an oxygen line may have occurred and needs to be corrected. Generally, each outlet station for each specialty gas is tested, one at a time. If all gas lines were tested at once, it would be difficult to know where the cross-connection occurred. Any suspicion of cross-connection should be explored and immediately corrected.

Component Testing

Testing should occur on all levels and include alarms and system function tests. The primary and secondary supply systems, as well as the switch from primary to reserve supply, need to be tested to ensure there is minimal interruption in gas flow service if a malfunction should occur or a supply system needs to be shut off for maintenance. The alarms associated with each of these systems also need to be checked for proper function. Verification that pressure relief valves vent off excess gas if the gas pressure rises above 50% of normal line pressure and reset when it drops back to normal levels is also important. The liquid oxygen low-level alarm should also be tested and confirmed. The compressed air system alarms need to be tested as well as the function of the safety valve and automatic drain.

Each zone valve should be shut off and terminal units tested to ensure the zone valve controls the units it is designed to. The valves should also be tested for tightness. This can be done by closing the zone valve and monitoring the downstream pressure for 30 minutes. If the pressure rises, then the valve is not shut or tight because gas is still flowing through and causing the pressure to rise.

Terminal units must also be tested for gas composition to confirm that all labeling is correct and no cross-connection has occurred. The station outlets also need to be checked annually for gas leakage, visual damage, and ease of insertion as well as locking and unlocking of the connector.

Periodic Testing

Testing of all components of the central bulk system should occur annually, and the results of the testing process documented. This documentation should include details of any problems encountered during testing, corrective actions taken, and verification that the problems have been resolved. The compressed air system intakes should be inspected quarterly for contamination. The function of the automatic drain and water from the receiver needs to be assessed daily.

Problems Associated with Medical Gas Distribution Systems

Although regulations and safeguards are built into bulk gas distribution systems, unexpected problems can still occur. Low or inadequate pressure can cause equipment malfunction, especially when 50 psi working pressure is required (i.e., for ventilators, anesthesia machines, air–oxygen blenders). Causes of low/inadequate pressure in the gas lines include the following:

- Inadvertent interruption of gas during construction
- Fire
- Motor vehicle accidents (usually involving the operating supply, causing a delay in the refill)
- Environmental forces (hurricane, tornado, earthquake, etc.)
- Damage or depletion of the operating supply
- Human error (inadvertent closure of zone valve and improper adjustment of main line regulator)
- Equipment failure (zone valve leaks, reserve supply failure, regulator malfunction, failure of switchover systems)
- Obstruction of the pipeline (by debris left behind during construction/installation)
- Quick connect failure (improper fit, breakage, obstruction of the connector, disconnection of the station outlet)

High pressures within the central gas system have the potential to cause serious safety events as well. However, if the pressure relief valves are properly installed and functioning then minimal harm to the equipment and/or the patient will result. Any system alarm, high or low, must be investigated. An alarm

may occur intermittently over a sustained period of time due to miscalibration or malfunctioning. Lack of communication between maintenance and clinical departments as well as a lack of understanding by hospital personnel and unfamiliarity with emergency measures contribute to delayed resolution of problems.

Gas Contamination

During construction and installation it is not uncommon for particulate matter such as oil, metal filings, solder flux, and other matter that contains hydrocarbons to enter the system. This can cause extreme damage to sensitive medical equipment and can pose a serious hazard if they are somehow inhaled by the patients. As discussed earlier, it is necessary that proper care is taken when cleaning and purging pipe lines.

Oil used to lubricate and maintain the compressors can easily contaminate air lines. Contamination can also occur from improperly installed air intake filters and/or if filters were cleaned but not fully dried.[4]

The moisture within the air system also can support bacterial growth that can be dispersed to patients.

Storage of Medical Gases
Cylinders Used for Gas Storage

Medical gases come in two forms, liquefied and non-liquefied. Nonliquefied gases are stored in cylinders made of steel, aluminum, or chrome molybdenum. Cylinders must be able to hold in excess of 2,000 psig of gas. Whereas liquefied gases come in specifically designed bulk liquid storage units, gas cylinders come in various colors depending on the gas they are holding and also have labels to indicate the type of gas. There are a host of agencies that govern and regulate the manufacturing, storage, transportation, and use of medical gas cylinders. (The NFPA and Compressed Gas Association [CGA] Recommendations for Compressed-Gas Cylinders can be found in **Appendix 1-A**.)

Construction

Medical gas cylinders are usually constructed of seamless, high-quality steel, aluminum, or chrome molybdenum. Steel and chrome molybdenum are more durable. Aluminum is lighter in weight and more often used in home care as well as for air or ground transport. Because aluminum cylinders are not affected by magnetic fields, they are also used in magnetic resonance imaging (MRI) suites.

The cylinders are formed by forcing a hardened steel press through a softer mass of cylinder material called a billet, shaping it into a tube-like structure. Once the tube is formed the bottom and top are heated, shaped, and closed. The top is threaded so that a valve stem can be fitted into the tank. The stem valve is what allows the cylinder to be filled with gas and the gas to be

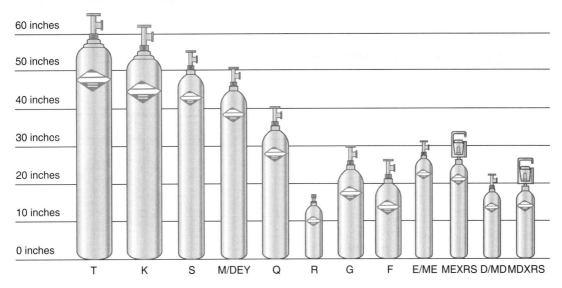

FIGURE 1-8 Sizes of high pressure cylinders approved for medical gas therapy.

released. The bottom is molded flat so they will stand up on their own.

Sizes

Medical gas cylinders come in various sizes depending on their intended use. To identify their size and capacity they are letter coded. The ML6 is the smallest and the T the largest (**Figure 1-8**). The most frequently used cylinders are the E and H sizes. E cylinders are commonly used for intrafacility transports or for home care. They are often seen attached to crash carts or in carriers secured to wheelchairs or gurneys (**Figure 1-9**). Medical gas cylinders are designed to hold 10% more than their actual filling capacity to allow room for the gas to safely expand with changes in ambient temperature.

Identification

Gas cylinders have several markings on them that healthcare providers should be familiar with. All tanks are color coded based on the gas contents (**Table 1-1**). These color codes are designated by the U.S. National Formulary. If the cylinder contains a mixture of two or more gases, then the proportion of each gas is colored on the cylinder; for example, a tank containing a mixture of 80% helium and 20% oxygen would have 80% of the tank colored brown and 20% colored green. The color system is only a visual guide. It is important for healthcare providers to check the label affixed to the cylinder to verify contents.

Printed labels are required by the CGA and **American National Standards Institute (ANSI)** (**Figure 1-10**) and include the name, gas/gas mixture, symbol, and volume of the cylinder in liters at a standard temperature (70°F or 21.1°C). The label should also indicate any hazards of the gas (i.e., flammable, oxidizer) as well as a statement

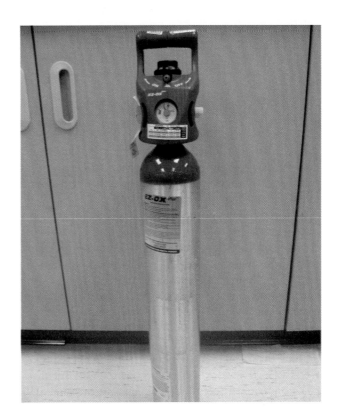

FIGURE 1-9 E-cylinder with a built-in pressure gauge and flowmeter and a handle. This design facilitates handling of the cylinder and minimizes the manipulation the respiratory therapist needs to do (i.e., attaching the regulator and seal ring) to administer oxygen therapy.

describing the dangers associated with exposure and avoiding injury. The name and address of the manufacturer or distributor should also be included.

Gas cylinders are typically engraved with information specific to the manufacturing and latest testing of the cylinder including the manufacturing point, material used in construction, service pressure of the

TABLE 1-1
Color Codes for Medical Gases

Gas	Chemical Symbol	Purity*	Color Code
Air		99.0%	Yellow or black and white[††]
Carbon dioxide	CO_2	99.0%	Gray
Carbon dioxide/ oxygen	CO_2/O_2	99.0%	Gray shoulder and green body[†]
Helium	He		Brown
Helium/oxygen	He/O_2	99.0%	Brown shoulder and green body[†]
Nitric oxide	NO	99.0%	Silver cylinder/teal and black
Nitrogen	N	99.0%	Black
Nitrous oxide	N_2O	97.0%	Light blue
Oxygen	O_2	99.0%	Green or white[††]

*National Formula Standards

[†]Always check labels to determine the percentage of each gas.

[††]International Color Code

cylinder, date of the original hydrostatic test, date the cylinder was reexamined and tested, and the manufacturer's name, owner's identification number, and size of the cylinder (**Figure 1-10**).

Compressed gas cylinders must undergo hydrostatic testing every 5 to 10 years. Hydrostatic testing is used to measure the thickness and durability of the tank. During testing the cylinder is placed into a water container. Both the cylinder and container are filled with water, and the water level in the cylinder is recorded when atmospheric pressure is met. The water pressure in the cylinder is increased to 3,000 psig while the water level in the container is measured and recorded. The volume of water displaced is equal to the expansion of the tank. If the water level rises, this means that the wall thickness has been reduced due to either damage or corrosion. If the tank fails this test it can no longer be used.

Filling a gas cylinder can be a dangerous situation and must follow strict guidelines. These guidelines are set and controlled by the Department of Transportation (DOT), the Food and Drug Administration (FDA), and the U.S. Pharmacopeia/National Formulary (USP/NF). Companies that fill gas cylinders must register with the FDA and are inspected on a biannual basis. Only properly trained personnel should fill a gas cylinder. Cylinders have to be clean and safe. Gases have to meet strict standards for purity according to the USP/NF. Each cylinder must have an intact label that is current and readable. All cylinders have to meet FDA and DOT specifications.

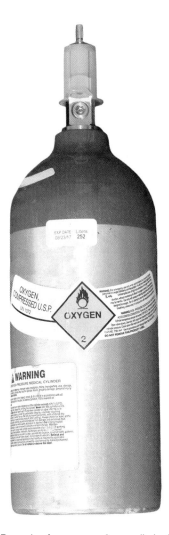

FIGURE 1-10 Example of compressed gas cylinder labeling. This photo denotes the typical markings on cylinders containing medical gases.

© L Barnwell/Shutterstock, Inc.

Four steps need to be followed for a cylinder to be filled. The first step is the cylinder prefill inspection. This makes sure that all residual gas is removed and that a visual inspection has occurred to make sure there are no signs of damage such as rust, dents, corrosion, or damage to paint. The visual inspection also verifies that the last hydrostatic test date meets DOT criteria and the cylinder is properly labeled. A hammer or "dead ring" test is performed at each refilling. To perform this test, a hammer is struck lightly on the side of the empty tank and one then listens to the tone it creates. If the cylinder is good, then the tone will be a clean ringing tone lasting approximately 3 seconds. If the tone is dull, flat, or fades quickly then the cylinder should be tested for damage.[2]

Step two is filling the cylinder with gas. This has to be done by a trained and certified person with certified equipment. The cylinder is attached to a manifold that is designed for filling, and then the tank is first purged and then filled with the appropriate gas from the supply

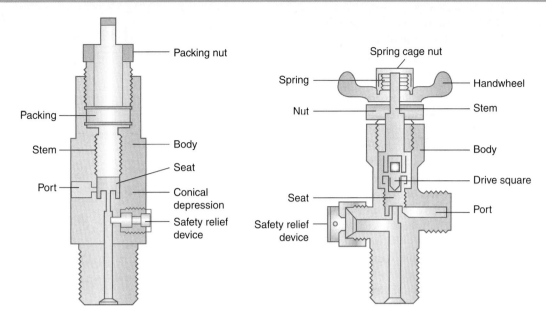

FIGURE 1-11 Cylinder valves.

source. There are special connections that are specific to the type of gas put in the tank. This makes it difficult to have a tank containing helium and oxygen to be filled with carbon dioxide. Gas is introduced so that the filling rate is not greater than 200 psig/min. Once filled to STP conditions, the valves are closed and the cylinders are removed.

After removal, the valves are checked for leaks and that the contents meet the purity standards set by the USP/NF. Then the tank, gas batch, and all the steps previously described must be carefully documented and recorded. The company must also have documentation on the daily gas calibration and that all connections and manifolds have been tested and inspected.

Cylinder Valves

To ensure that the gas does not accidentally leak or escape from the cylinder, valves are threaded into the top portion of the tank during tank construction. Turning the valve counterclockwise will allow gas to flow from the cylinder; turning the valve clockwise will prevent gas from escaping from the cylinder. The valves also can be opened to allow the cylinders to be refilled at the manufacturing plant. The valve for smaller cylinders (i.e., A–E) is located on the top portion of the cylinder yoke. The yoke is the small stem that protrudes from the cylinder. It is rectangular and has four sides. A small hand wrench is needed to turn the valve, which opens and closes the flow of oxygen from the cylinder. The regulator is placed over and secured to the cylinder yoke. It is important to note that a small plastic washer is needed to seal the connection and prevent gas leaks between the regulator and the cylinder yoke. For larger tanks (i.e., H cylinders), a permanent hand wheel is used to control the valve and the regulator is attached to

the cylinder by a threaded connection. Identical to the small cylinders, a clockwise turn will close the valve and a counterclockwise turn will open the valve. Cylinder valves are constructed of materials that resist the mechanical, chemical, and thermal effects of the gas(es) contained within the cylinder. Typically they are made from brass and are chrome plated. There are two types of valves, direct acting and indirect acting (**Figure 1-11**).

Direct Acting

Direct-acting valves have two fiber washers and a Teflon packing. Direct acting refers to the action the stem has on the seat. As the stem is turned, so does the seat. As the seat rises, gas is allowed to escape from the cylinder through the yoke. The valve must also be in the open position to allow the cylinder to be filled by the gas manufacturing plant. When the seat is lowered, the gas flow to the yoke is closed off. These valves are manufactured to withstand pressures in excess of 1,500 psi.

Indirect Acting

Indirect-acting valves are also known as diaphragm valves. A diaphragm is positioned between the stem and the seat of this type of valve and is controlled by turning the stem. As the stem is turned the diaphragm raises and lowers, which opens and closes the valve, respectively. A spring around the seat opposes the pressure applied to the diaphragm. This type of cylinder valve is more expensive to manufacture, but is less prone to leaks and easier to open. Indirect-acting valves only need a half turn to open the flow of gas from the cylinder, compared to direct-acting valves, which need three quarters of a turn. This type of valve is typically used in tanks where the pressure is less than 1,500 psi. They are more commonly used for cylinders containing anesthetic gases, which are flammable, meaning gas leaks cause a high risk of fire.

Pressure Relief Valves

A pressure relief valve is a safety feature required on every gas cylinder. This safety feature is based on Gay-Lussac's law, which states that pressure in a closed container is directly proportional to the temperature of the gas. Pressure relief valves are designed to vent gas and prevent the accumulation of excess pressure within the cylinder and reduce the risk of explosion when the cylinder is exposed to extreme or high temperatures. Excess pressure may also result from overfilling the cylinder.

There are three types of pressure relief valves: rupture disks, fusible plugs, and spring-loaded devices. A **rupture disk**, also known as a frangible disk, is a thin metal disk that will either break apart or buckle under the increased pressure. These disks are rated for certain pressures. When that pressure is exceeded, the disk will buckle or rupture and allow gas to escape to the atmosphere. A **fusible plug** is made of a special metal alloy. This metal will melt when the temperature of the gas reaches between 208°F and 220°F (97.8–104°C). As the plug melts, gas is permitted to escape. Typically, **Wood's metal** is used to construct this type of valve. Wood's metal is a fusible alloy composed of bismuth, lead, cadmium, and tin. This alloy is also used to allow water to escape from automatic sprinklers. **Spring-loaded devices** are designed to maintain a certain pressure within the cylinder. As the pressure exceeds the predetermined level, the pressure pushes up on a spring, which will cause a valve to be unseated and the gas is allowed to escape. Once the pressure falls below the set pressure, the valve is allowed to reseat. This type of pressure relief valve will conserve the gas that is escaping, whereas rupture disks and fusible plugs release all of the cylinder's contents once the pressure relief valve is broken. Unfortunately, spring-loaded pressure relief valves are more susceptible to leaks and are affected by environmental changes. For example, should the cylinder be exposed to extreme cold, the spring-loaded pressure relief valve may freeze and not function properly. This type of pressure relief valve is more commonly found on larger cylinders. Rupture disks and fusible plugs are used more with smaller cylinders (**Figure 1-12**).

Index Safety Connections

The outlets on high pressure cylinders are manufactured to ensure the regulator or connector attached to the gas delivery system is the one appropriate for its use. For example, an oxygen regulator cannot attach to a cylinder containing a heliox mixture. There are three indexed safety systems specific for medical gases:

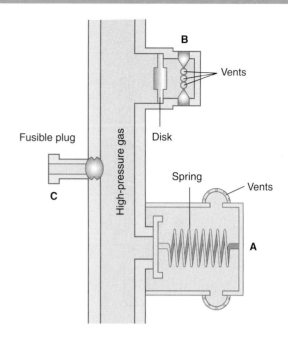

FIGURE 1-12 Pressure relief valves. A. Spring loaded device. When gas pressure exceeds the spring tension, the spring is compressed to the top, allowing gas to escape through the vents. When gas pressure is reduced to normal, the spring tension re-seats the valve. B. Frangible disk. When gas pressure exceeds safe limits, the disk ruptures, allowing all of the contents of the cylinder to escape into the atmosphere through the vents. C. Fusible plug. If the temperature inside or outside the cylinder exceeds safe limits, the plug melts, allowing all of the gas in the cylinder to safely escape.

Adapted from Branson RD, Hess DR, Chatburn RL. *Respiratory care equipment*. 2nd ed. Philadelphia: Lippincott Williams & Wilkins; 1999.

the **American Standard Safety System (ASSS)**, the **Pin Index Safety System (PISS)**, and the Diameter Index Safety System (DISS). The ASSS is used for large capacity cylinders, above 2,000 psig, though typically it is seen more often in the large cylinders such as H and K sizes. This safety system sets the specifications for threaded high pressure connections between compressed gas cylinders and their attachments, including the thread characteristics (right or left handed, number of threads per inch, use of internal or external threads). The diameter of the outlet and the shape of the mating nipple on the corresponding regulator are unique to each type of specialty gas or gas mixture. The combination of the previously mentioned factors reduces error by making it very difficult for clinicians to place a regulator intended for one gas (e.g., air) on a cylinder containing a different type of gas or gas mixture (e.g., heliox) (**Figure 1-13**).

The numbers used in this system help with the identification process. A large cylinder containing oxygen will have a series of numbers to describe the characteristics of the threaded outlet, specifically 0.903-14-RH-Ext. The first number (0.903) describes

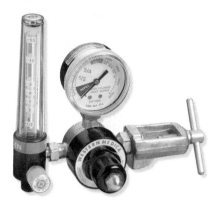

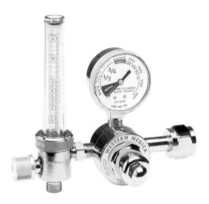

FIGURE 1-13 Pin Index Safety System for small cylinders (top) and American Standard Safety System for large cylinders (bottom).

Photos courtesy of Western Enterprises, a Scott Fetzer Company.

TABLE 1-2
Pin Index Safety System Pin and Hole Positions for Medical Gases

Medical Gas	Index Pins
Oxygen	2, 5
Helium and oxygen (He:O_2) He $\leq$ 80%	2, 4
Air	1, 5
Ethylene	1, 3
Nitrous oxide	3, 5
Cyclopropane	3, 6
CO_2/O_2 (Carbogen) CO_2 $\leq$ 7%	2, 6
CO_2/O_2 (Carbogen) CO_2 > 7%	1, 6

the diameter of the cylinder's outlet in inches. The number of threads per inch on the connect is described by the next sequence. In the alphanumeric series above, the oxygen connection has 14 threads per square inch. The letters that follow next also refer to thread characteristics. In the example for oxygen, RH stands for right hand, the direction in which the threads are located. The letters that follow (Ext or Int) refer to whether the threads are internal or external. In the previous example, oxygen has external threads, designated by the letters *Ext*.

Smaller cylinders (A through E) use the Pin Index Safety System. This system uses a specific combination of two holes on the post valve of the cylinder. Any device that connects to the yoke of the cylinder will have pins that correspond to the holes on the post valve. This system uses a series of pins in six different locations. Each type of gas or gas mixture has a specific pin sequence (**Table 1-2**); for example, the pin sequence for oxygen is 2, 5. That means that only a regulator with pins in the 2 and 5 positions will sit correctly on an oxygen tank. The pin sequence for air is 1, 5. Therefore, it would be difficult to get a regulator or connector intended for an oxygen cylinder onto a cylinder containing air (**Figure 1-14**).

The DISS is designed by the CGA for low pressure (less than 200-psi) connections and fittings. With this

system a female nut and nipple mate with a specifically diameter-threaded male outlet. Gases (e.g., oxygen, nitrogen) and gas mixtures (e.g., HE:O_2, CO_2:O_2) have connections that differ with respect to the diameter, pitch thread, and nipple configuration.

The DISS connection for the outlet of a flowmeter and the 50-psi working gas pressure connection have the same DISS-threaded connection. Respiratory therapists must use caution to avoid connecting low-flow devices, such as the humidifier for a nasal cannula, to the 50-psi working gas pressure connection. The excessive pressure delivered through this connection will cause the humidifier to rupture and delay delivery of medical gas to the patient. Equipment failure can also transpire as the high pressure gas line (e.g., the high pressure oxygen line for an air–oxygen blender) is attached to the threaded connection of a flowmeter. Equipment failure will result from the delivery of inadequate working pressure (15–20 psi with the flowmeter vs. 50 psi from the high pressure connection).

Cylinder Duration

It is important to determine the volume of gas remaining in a cylinder and the duration of cylinder use. This skill is useful for intra- and interhospital transports as well as when educating patients and families on the use of their portable home oxygen equipment. Failure to calculate tank duration may cause equipment malfunction and compromise patient safety by inducing hypoxemia and/or hypoventilation. Calculating how much volume a cylinder may have is done by measuring either the weight of the cylinder, for gases stored partially in liquid form, or the pressure in the cylinder for nonliquefied gases. For nonliquefied gases, it is important to know the conversion factor for the

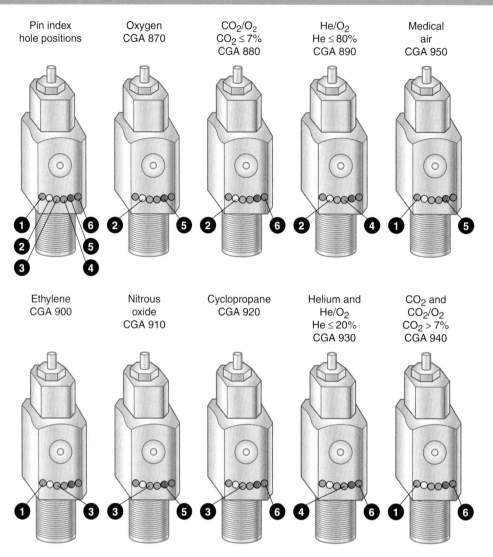

FIGURE 1-14 Pin Index Safety System.

size tank. Each cylinder size has its own specific conversion factor (**Table 1-3**).

The duration of flow for gas cylinders is calculated by dividing the product of the cylinder's pressure and the tank conversion factor by the set flow (L/min).

$$\text{Cylinder duration (minutes)} = \frac{\text{Cylinder pressure (psig)} \times \text{Conversion factor}}{\text{Flow (L / minute)}}$$

For example, a patient ordered a nasal cannula at 4 L/min is transferred from the emergency department to the general care ward. An oxygen e-cylinder is available for transport. The cylinder pressure is 1,100 psig. To calculate the duration of oxygen flow:

1,100 psig (cylinder pressure) × 0.28 L/psig (conversion factor for an e-cylinder) = 308 L

308 L/4 L/min (ordered flow of oxygen) = 77 minutes

= 1 hour 17 minutes

Common Problems and Troubleshooting

An easily followed list of rules and regulation can be found in the Compressed Gas Association's *Handbook of Compressed Gas*. The Joint Commission and state and local regulatory agencies may have additional regulations that respiratory care departments should be aware of and comply with to minimize errors from reaching the patient and causing harm.[47] Despite all the care given and precautions taken, there still may

TABLE 1-3
Volume–Pressure Conversion Factors

Cylinder Size	Conversion Factor
D	0.16
E	0.28
G	2.39
H or K	3.14

TABLE 1-4
Common Problems Encountered with High Pressure Gas Cylinders

Problem	Actions Leading to Potential Solutions
Hissing noise and gas escaping at the yoke of the cylinder	1. For an e-cylinder, assess the regulator to determine whether the plastic or Teflon washer is missing or damaged. a. Replace missing or damaged plastic or Teflon washer. b. Reseat the regulator. c. Release the flow of gas from the tank. 2. If the plastic or Teflon washer is present and intact on the regulator of an e-cylinder, or a larger cylinder (M or H) is in use: a. Reseat/reposition the regulator and tighten the connection with a wrench.
No gas flow from the flowmeter	1. Ensure the cylinder valve is turned fully to the on position. a. Cylinder valve may be damaged. Obtain another cylinder and appropriately label the cylinder for assessment by the gas supplier. 2. Assess the tank pressure to determine if gas is present in the tank.

be isolated errors, most of which come from human error. Common problems respiratory therapists may encounter with gas cylinders and potential solutions are provided in **Table 1-4**.

Liquid Oxygen Systems

Bulk liquid oxygen systems were discussed earlier in this chapter. This type of system has very large reservoirs containing up to 10,000 gallons of liquid oxygen and are housed adjacent to the healthcare facility. Large capacity liquid oxygen systems are expensive to maintain and are not practical for long-term facility or home use; however, liquid oxygen is available in smaller vessels that can be stored within a long-term care facility or patient home. Portable liquid oxygen units can be transfilled from the larger base unit to allow residents of long-term care facilities or patients at home a viable means of oxygen delivery for ambulation. (The NFPA Recommendations and Regulations for Portable Liquid Oxygen Systems can be found in **Appendix 1-C**.) Liquid home units generally consist of two parts, a larger stationary or reservoir unit and a smaller portable unit.

The stationary reservoir base is very similar in construction to large bulk oxygen systems used in hospitals. There is an insulated bottle that holds the liquid oxygen, a vaporizing coil to allow the liquefied gas to become nonliquefied, and a series of pressure relief valves to deliver the gas at a working pressure of approximately 20 psig. Typically, liquid stationary units for use outside an acute care facility have a capacity of 12–60 liters of liquefied oxygen.

The systems operate when the flow control valve is open for gas flow to be delivered to the patient. A pressure gradient develops between the gas-filled upper section of the container, sometimes called the head pressure, and atmospheric pressure. Gas will then flow through the economizer valve through warming coils and then out the flow control valve to the patient. The warming coils will help increase the temperature before

it reaches the patient. As gas flow continues, the head pressure will drop slowly until it falls below 0.5 psig. At that point the economizer valve will close and liquid oxygen is drawn up through the coils. The economizer valve ensures a constant flow of oxygen to the patient.

When the contents of the stationary unit are low, the system needs to be refilled properly. The manufacturer's specifications must be followed when transfilling stationary units. Transfilling must take place in a well-ventilated, non-patient-care area. Each transfilling station should have its own pressure relief valves and connectors from the manufacturer. Stationary units also can be equipped to fill smaller portable units that allow the patients to be more mobile. These units are constructed as smaller versions of the stationary units and must be carried in an upright position. Generally, the portable units are equipped with a shoulder strap for ease of use.

When filling the smaller portable units from the stationary base, it is essential to follow the manufacturer's recommendations. Connections between the stationary unit and portable unit must be dry prior to seating the portable unit onto its stationary base. Moisture will cause the pressure valves to freeze in the open position and impair the filling process. The portable units must then remain out of service until the valve thaws and can close properly. Once the portable unit is filled, care should be taken not to touch the connections the unit was seated upon. Liquid oxygen is stored at very low temperatures, so touching the frosty connections with bare skin may result in frostbite and skin damage.

Liquid oxygen systems are a fire hazard if the connections or equipment become contaminated with a combustible material, such as oil or grease. Vaporization of spilled liquid oxygen can cause an oxygen-enriched environment and may increase the risk for fire. Failure to maintain the units in accordance with manufacturer recommendations increases the risk for improperly functioning pressure relief valves.

Should the pressure relief valve fail, overpressure accidents may cause harm to patients or staff.

In order to determine the length of time a portable liquid system will last, the unit of measure of the liquid gas in the portable container must be converted from pounds to liters. There are two conversion factors that are essential to remember: (1) 1 liter of liquid oxygen weighs 2.5 pounds or 1.1 kilograms, and (2) 1 liter of liquid oxygen produces 860 liters of gaseous oxygen. To calculate the duration of flow for liquid oxygen, the respiratory therapist must know the weight of the liquid vessel and the flow of gas the patient is receiving. The therapist must first calculate the amount of gas remaining in the liquid reservoir:

$$\text{Gas remaining} = \frac{\begin{array}{c}\text{Liquid weight (lb)} \times \text{Gas volume that}\\ \text{1 L of liquid oxygen produces (860 L)}\end{array}}{\text{Weight of 1 L of liquid oxygen (2.5 lb)}}$$

The therapist then calculates the duration of the contents by dividing the gas remaining by the flow of oxygen the patient is receiving:

$$\text{Duration of contents (min)} = \frac{\text{Gas remaining (L)}}{\text{Flow (L/min)}}$$

For example, a portable liquid oxygen unit containing 3 pounds of liquid oxygen is used by a patient receiving oxygen by nasal cannula at 3 L/min. To calculate the amount of time the flow of gas from the liquid oxygen will last, use the following equation:

$$\begin{aligned}\text{Gas remaining} &= \frac{3\,\text{lb} \times 860}{2.5\,\text{lb/L}}\\ &= \frac{2{,}580\,\text{lb}}{2.5\,\text{lb/L}}\\ &= 1{,}032\,\text{L}\\ \text{Duration of contents} &= \frac{1{,}032\,\text{L}}{3\,\text{L/min}}\\ &= 344\text{ minutes or}\\ &\quad 5\text{ hours, }44\text{ minutes}\end{aligned}$$

Oxygen Concentrators

Oxygen concentrators entrain ambient air and separate oxygen from other gases through the use of special filters, and then store it for delivery to the patient. Oxygen concentrators are predominately used in non-acute-care settings. This type of oxygen delivery system is commonly found in extended care facilities (nursing homes) or in the home. There are two types of oxygen concentrator designs: those using a molecular sieve and those using a semipermeable plastic membrane.

Molecular Sieve

This type of concentrator gained popularity because of its simplicity of operation. An air compressor within the unit draws in ambient air. As air enters the unit, it passes through a series of filters and a heat exchanger where any moisture or heat is dissipated. It then passes through a solenoid valve where it is directed to pass through at least one molecular sieve bed where the oxygen becomes concentrated. The sieve beds contain zeolite crystals, which separate gases according to their sizes and polarity. The zeolite traps nitrogen, water, and other gases, allowing oxygen to pass through. These beds work well if they are pressurized.

The two sieve beds are alternately pressurized (to generate oxygen) and depressurized (to release nitrogen). As air is first pressurized in one sieve bed to help with the increase of nitrogen absorption, the oxygen it generates is diverted to a product tank where some of the oxygen is stored. The rest of the oxygen is used to purge the sieve to get rid of the nitrogen. This process is called pressure swing absorption. Pressure cycles occur every 10–30 seconds and make enough oxygen for the product tank as well as to purge the beds of nitrogen.

The oxygen in the tank is typically less than 10 psig and is delivered to the patient after passing through a bacterial filter and then out the flowmeter. Oxygen delivery to the patient is inversely proportional to the flow. The lower the flow, the higher the concentration of oxygen. Gas flows of less than 6 L/min will generally deliver around 93% oxygen. It should be noted that the flowmeters on oxygen concentrators are not back-pressure compensated.

Semipermeable Membranes

Oxygen concentrators using membranes pass air through a 1-micrometer-thick membrane that separates the gases according to their diffusion rates. Gas diffusion depends on several factors: diffusion constant, solubility of the membrane, and pressure gradient across the membrane. The oxygen then passes through a condensing coil where excess water vapor is removed. This type of concentrator can deliver approximately 40% oxygen at a flow of 1–10 L/min.

Stationary concentrators are good for home use or use in long-term care facilities. Unlike cylinders or liquid oxygen units, concentrators do not need to be refilled and only yearly maintenance service is needed. Some concentrators are equipped with alarms that signal a loss of power, high and low pressures, as well as low oxygen concentration. Many are nearly silent, which makes them ideal for home living because the noise will not interfere with the TV, radio, or sleeping. These are electrically powered and can be plugged into an existing wall outlet.

Portable oxygen concentrators (POCs) are for home care patients and give them the ability to travel and in general to be more mobile. They are battery powered or

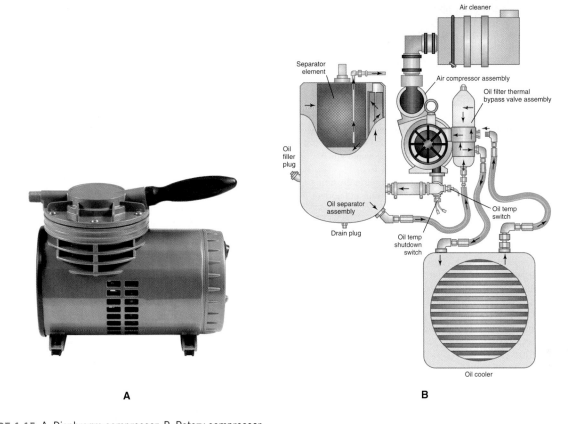

FIGURE 1-15 A. Diaphragm compressor. B. Rotary compressor.

Photo © Yanas/Shutterstock, Inc. Art reproduced from the U.S. Army Technical Manual, TM 5-4310-354-14-HR , Compressor, Rotary; Air, Skid Mounted; Diesel Engine Driven , 125 CFM, 100 PSIG (Davey Model 6M125), Fig. 5-2.

can be operated via an AC or DC power supply. Some have the option of an external battery for longer life. Many of the batteries will last up to 10 hours. Note, however, that there is a large variability in performance among POCs.[48]

Portable Air Compressors

Air compressors are used to power many things in respiratory care, from delivery of 50 psi of air to a mechanical ventilator to running a small volume nebulizer. Many institutions may have piped-in air from an onsite compressor. If a building does not have piped-in gases, portable compressors will come in handy. There are three types: piston, diaphragm, and rotary (**Figure 1-15**).

Piston compressors use a motor that drives a piston that will compress the air. Air is pulled in through a one-way valve into a chamber as the piston moves down (down stroke). Once that chamber is filled or the piston has drawn back as far as it will go, the piston then starts to move up (up stroke). The one-way valve will close, and as the air gets pressurized another one-way valve will open allowing the pressurized gas to go out the valve. Because air cannot come in contact with contaminants, Teflon is used to seal the ring so that no air escapes. The air then goes through a coiled tube to allow the gas, which was heated, to cool to room temperature. This tube will also remove moisture from the gas. This water can be drained. Because this does not

completely remove all water from the compressed air, there should be a filter/water trap prior to the inlet of any device that has electronics. Some piston compressors can generate the high pressures and flows needed to run a mechanical ventilator.

Diaphragm compressors simply substitute a flexible diaphragm for the piston. As the diaphragm is pulled back, air is allowed to enter the chamber through a one-way intake valve and then is compressed and pushed out a one-way outflow valve. Diaphragm compressors can only generate low pressures and moderate flows. They are typically used for running small volume nebulizers at the home or in facilities where there is no piped-in gas.

Rotary compressors use a vane that rotates at high speeds to entrain the air through a one-way valve. The air is compressed as the vane rotates and then is forced out a one-way outflow valve. Many ventilator companies use this type of compressor on their ventilators. Rotary compressors can generate a pressure between 45 and 55 psi with flow rates of 60–80 L/min.

References

1. Compressed Gas Association. *Handbook of compressed gases.* 4th ed. Norwell, MA: Kluwer Academic; 1999.
2. National Fire Protection Agency. *Health care facilities handbook.* 8th ed. Quincy, MA: National Fire Protection Agency; 2005.
3. Yardley IE, Donaldson LJ. Surgical fires, a clear and present danger. *Surgeon.* 2010;8(2):87-92.

4. Rinder CS. Fire safety in the operating room. *Curr Opin Anaesthesiol.* 2008;21(6):790-795.

5. Fulmer JD, Snider GL. ACCP-NHLBI National Conference on Oxygen Therapy. *Chest.* 1984;86(2):234-247.

6. Blue Cross Blue Shield Association. *Medical policy 01.01.12 oxygen.* http://mcgs.bcbsfl.com/?doc=Oxygen. Accessed June 1, 2014.

7. Berg RA, Hemphill R, Abella BS, et al. Part 5: Adult basic life support: 2010 American Heart Association guidelines for cardiopulmonary resuscitation and emergency cardiovascular care. *Circulation.* 2010;122(18 Suppl 3):S685-S705.

8. Kallstrom TJ. AARC clinical practice guideline: Oxygen therapy for adults in the acute care facility—2002 revision and update. *Respir Care.* 2002;47(6):717-720.

9. AARC clinical practice guideline. Oxygen therapy in the home or alternate site health care facility—2007 revision and update. *Respir Care.* 2007;52(8):1063-1068.

10. Short JA, van der Walt JH. Oxygen in neonatal and infant anesthesia—current practice in the UK. *Paediatr Anaesth.* 2008;18(5):378-387.

11. Jensen K, Kehlet H, Lund CM. Post-operative recovery profile after laparoscopic cholecystectomy: A prospective, observational study of a multimodal anaesthetic regime. *Acta Anaesthesiol Scand.* 2007;51(4):464-471.

12. Petty TL, Bliss PL. Ambulatory oxygen therapy, exercise, and survival with advanced chronic obstructive pulmonary disease (the Nocturnal Oxygen Therapy Trial revisited). *Respir Care.* 2000;45(2):204-211.

13. Stoll BJ, Hansen NI, Bell EF, et al., Eunice Kennedy Shriver National Institute of Child Health and Human Development Neonatal Research Network. Neonatal outcomes of extremely preterm infants from the NICHD Neonatal Research Network. *Pediatrics.* 2010;126(3):443-456.

14. SUPPORT Study Group of the Eunice Kennedy Shriver NICHD Neonatal Research Network, Carlo WA, Finer NN, Walsh MC, et al. Target ranges of oxygen saturation in extremely preterm infants. *N Engl J Med.* 2010;362(21):1959-1969.

15. Lodato RF. Oxygen toxicity. *Crit Care Clin.* 1990;6(3):749-765.

16. Benditt JO. Adverse effects of low-flow oxygen therapy. *Respir Care.* 2000;45(1):54-61.

17. Ranjit S. Acute respiratory failure and oxygen therapy. *Indian J Pediatr.* 2001;68(3):249-255.

18. Bailey JE, Argyropoulos SV, Kendrick AH, Nutt DJ. Behavioral and cardiovascular effects of 7.5% CO_2 in human volunteers. *Depress Anxiety.* 2005;21(1):18-25.

19. Seddon K, Morris K, Bailey J, et al. Effects of 7.5% CO_2 challenge in generalized anxiety disorder. *J Psychopharmacol.* 2011;25(1):43-51.

20. Environmental Protection Agency. Carbon dioxide as a fire suppressant: Examining the risks. Report no. EPA430-R-00-002. http://www.epa.gov/ozone/snap/fire/co2/co2report.html. Accessed June 1, 2014.

21. Ashkanian M, Gjedde A, Mouridsen K, Vafaee M, Hansen KV, Ostergaard L, Andersen G. Carbogen inhalation increases oxygen transport to hypoperfused brain tissue in patients with occlusive carotid artery disease: Increased oxygen transport to hypoperfused brain. *Brain Res.* 2009;22(12):90-95.

22. Chatburn RL, Anderson SM. Controlling carbon dioxide delivery during mechanical ventilation. *Respir Care.* 1994;39(11):1039-1046.

23. Hooshang B. *Clinical application of the intra-aortic balloon pump.* 3rd ed. Armonk, NY: Wiley-Blackwell; 1998.

24. Frazier MD, Cheifetz IM. The role of heliox in pediatric respiratory disease. *Paediatr Respir Rev.* 2010;11(1):46-53.

25. Fleming MD, Weigelt JA, Brewer V, McIntire D. Effect of helium and oxygen on airflow in a narrowed airway. *Arch Surg.* 1992;127(8):956-959.

26. Kneyber MC, van Heerde M, Twisk JW, Plötz FB, Markhors DG. Heliox reduces respiratory system resistance in respiratory syncytial virus induced respiratory failure. *Crit Care.* 2009;13(3):R71.

27. Gluck EH, Onoranto DJ, Castriotta R. Helium-oxygen mixtures in intubated patients with status asthmaticus and respiratory acidosis. *Chest.* 1990;98(3):693-698.

28. Anderson M, Svartengren M, Bylin G, Philipson K, Camner P. Deposition in asthmatics of particles inhaled in air or in helium-oxygen. *Am Rev Respir Dis.* 1993;147(3):524-528.

29. Kim IK, Phrampus E, Venkataraman S, et al. Helium/oxygen-driven albuterol nebulization in the treatment of children with moderate to severe asthma exacerbations: A randomized, controlled trial. *Pediatrics.* 2005;116(5):1127-1133.

30. O'Callaghan C, White J, Jackson J, Crosby D, Dougill B, Bland H. The effects of heliox on the output and particle-size distribution of salbutamol using jet and vibrating mesh nebulizers. *J Aerosol Med.* 2007;20(4):434-444.

31. Habib DM, Garner SS, Brandeberg S. Effect of helium-oxygen on delivery of albuterol in a pediatric, volume-cycled, ventilated lung model. *Pharmacotherapy.* 1999;19(2):143-149.

32. Berkenbosch JW, Grueber RE, Dabbagh O, McKibben AW. Effect of helium-oxygen (heliox) gas mixtures on the function of four pediatric ventilators. *Crit Care Med.* 2003;31(7):2052-2058.

33. Brown MK, Willms DC. A laboratory evaluation of two mechanical ventilators in the presence of helium-oxygen mixtures. *Respir Care.* 2005;50(3):354-360.

34. Waseda M, Murakami M, Kato T, Kusano M. Helium gas pneumoperitoneum can improve the recovery of gastrointestinal motility after a laparoscopic operation. *Minim Invasive Ther Allied Technol.* 2005;14(1):14.

35. Day RW, Barton AJ, Pysher TJ, Shaddy RE. Pulmonary vascular resistance of children treated with nitrogen during early infancy. *Ann Thorac Surg.* 1998;65:1400-1404.

36. Stayer S, Gouvion J, Evey L, Andropoulos D. Subambient gas delivery. *Anesth Analg.* 2002;94(6):1674-1675.

37. Myers TR, Chatburn RL. Accuracy of oxygen analyzers at subatmospheric concentrations used in treatment of hypoplastic left heart syndrome. *Respir Care.* 2002;47(10):1168-1172.

38. DiBlasi RM, Myers TR, Hess DR. Evidence-based clinical practice guideline: Inhaled nitric oxide for neonates with acute hypoxic respiratory failure. *Respir Care.* 2010;55(12):1717.

39. Pal K, Gupta DK. Serial perfusion study depicts pulmonary vascular growth in the survivors of non-extracorporeal membrane oxygenation-treated congenital diaphragmatic hernia. *Neonatology.* 2010;98(3):254-259.

40. Gladwin MT, Kato GJ, Weiner D, et al., for the DeNOVO Investigators. Nitric oxide for inhalation in the acute treatment of sickle cell pain crisis: A randomized controlled trial. *JAMA.* 2011;305(9):893.

41. Rieger-Fackeldey E, Hentschel R. Bronchopulmonary dysplasia and early prophylactic inhaled nitric oxide in preterm infants: Current concepts and future research strategies in animal models. *J Perinat Med.* 2008;36(5):442-447.

42. Donohue PK, Gilmore MM, Cristofalo E, et al. Inhaled nitric oxide in preterm infants: A systematic review. *Pediatrics.* 2011;127(2):414-422.

43. Cole FS, Alleyne C, Barks JD, et al. NIH consensus development conference statement: Inhaled nitric-oxide therapy for premature infants. *Pediatrics.* 2011;127(2):363.

44. Ritz RH, Previtera JE. Oxygen supplies during a mass casualty situation. *Respir Care.* 2008;53(2):215-225.

45. Stoller JK, Stefanak M, Orens D, Burkhart J. The hospital oxygen supply: an "O_2K" problem. *Respir Care.* 2000;45(3):300-305.

46. Safdar N, Dezfulian C, Collard HR, Saint S. Clinical and economic consequences of ventilator-associated pneumonia: A systematic review. *Crit Care Med.* 2005;33(10):2184-2193.

47. The Joint Commission. *About our standards.* http://www.jointcommission.org/standards_information/standards.aspx. Accessed May 1, 2011.

48. Chatburn RL, Williams TJ. Performance comparison of 4 portable oxygen concentrators. *Respir Care.* 2010;55(4):433-442.

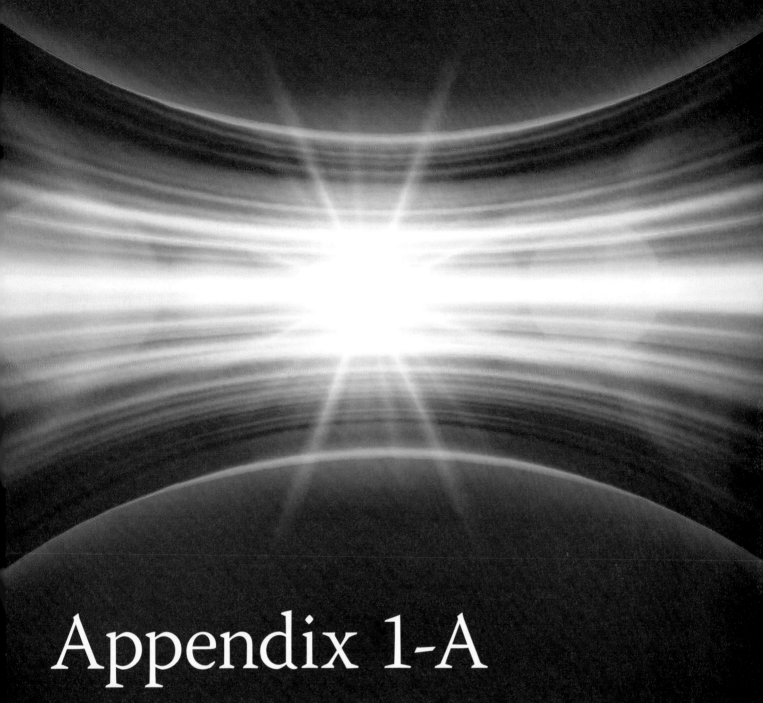

Appendix 1-A

National Fire Protection Association (NFPA) and Compressed Gas Association (CGA) Recommendations for Compressed-Gas Cylinders

Storage

1. Storage rooms must be dry, cool, and well ventilated. Cylinders should not be stored in an area where the temperature exceeds 125°F (51.7°C).
2. No flames should have the potential of coming in contact with the cylinders.
3. The storage facility should be fire resistant where practical.
4. Cylinders must not be stored near flammable or combustible substances.
5. Gases that support combustion must be stored in a separate location from those that are combustible.
6. The storage area must be permanently posted.
7. Cylinders must be grouped by content.
8. Full and empty cylinders must be segregated in the storage area.
9. Below-ground storage should be avoided.
10. Cylinders should never be stored in the operating room.
11. Large cylinders must be stored upright.
12. Cylinders must be protected from being cut or abraded.
13. Cylinders must be protected from extreme weather to prevent rusting, excessive temperatures, and accumulations of snow and ice.
14. Cylinders should not be exposed to continuous dampness or corrosive substances that could promote rusting of the cylinder and its valve.
15. Cylinders should be protected from tampering.
16. Valves on empty cylinders should be kept closed at all times.
17. Cylinders must be stored with protective caps in place.
18. Cylinders must not be stored in a confined space, such as a closet or the trunk of a car.

Transportation

1. If protective valve caps are supplied, they should be used whenever cylinders are in transport and until they are ready for use.
2. Cylinders must not be dropped, dragged, slid, or allowed to strike each other violently.
3. Cylinders must be transported on an appropriate cart secured by a chain or strap.

Use

1. Before connecting equipment to a cylinder, make sure that connections are free of foreign materials.
2. Turn the valve outlet away from personnel and crack the cylinder valve to remove any dust or debris from the outlet.
3. Cylinder valve outlet connections must be American Standard or CGA pin indexed; low-pressure connections must be CGA diameter indexed.
4. Cylinders must be secured at the administration site and not to any moveable objects or heat radiators.
5. Outlets and connections must be tightened only with appropriate wrenches and must never be forced.
6. Equipment designed to use for one gas should not be used with another.
7. Never use medical cylinder gases when contamination by backflow of other gases may occur.
8. Regulators should be off when the cylinder is turned on, and the cylinder valve should be opened slowly.
9. Before equipment is disconnected from a cylinder, the cylinder valve should be closed and the pressure released from the device.
10. Cylinder valves should be closed at all times except when in use.
11. Do not transfill cylinders; this is hazardous.
12. Cylinders may be refilled only if permission is secured from the owner.
13. Cylinders must not be lifted by the cap.
14. Equipment connected to oxygen cylinders containing gaseous oxygen should be labeled: OXYGEN—USE NO OIL.
15. Enclosures intended to contain patients must have the minimum text regarding No Smoking, and the labels must be located (1) in a position to be read by the patients and (2) on two or more opposing sides visible from the exterior. It should be noted that oxygen hoods fall under the classification of oxygen enclosure and require these labels as well. In addition, another label is required that instructs visitors to get approval from hospital personnel before placing toys in an oxygen enclosure.
16. High pressure oxygen equipment must not be sterilized with flammable agents (e.g., alcohol and ethylene oxide), and the agents used must be oil free and nondamaging.
17. Polyethylene bags must not be used to wrap sterilized, high pressure oxygen equipment because when flexed polyethylene releases pure hydrocarbons that are highly flammable.
18. Oxygen equipment exposed to pressure of less than 60 psi may be sterilized either with a nonflammable mixture of ethylene oxide and carbon dioxide or with fluorocarbons.
19. Cylinders must not be handled with oily or greasy hands, gloves, or clothing.
20. Never lubricate valve outlets or connecting equipment. (Oxygen and oil under pressure cause an explosive oxidation reaction.)
21. Do not flame test for leaks. (Usually a soap solution is used.)
22. When a cylinder is in use, open the valve fully and then turn it back a quarter to a half turn.
23. Replace the cap on an empty cylinder.
24. Position the cylinder so that the label is clearly visible. The label must not be defaced, altered, or removed.
25. Check the label before use; it should always match the color code.
26. No sources of open flames should be permitted in the area of administration. A No Smoking sign must be posted in the area of administration. It must be legible from a distance of 5 feet and displayed in a conspicuous location.
27. Inform all area occupants of the hazards of smoking and of the regulations.

28. Equipment designated for use with a specific gas must be clearly and permanently labeled accordingly. The name of the manufacturer should be clearly marked on the device. If calibration or accuracy depends on gas density, the device must be labeled with the proper supply pressure.
29. Cylinder carts must be of a self-supporting design with appropriate casters and wheels, and those intended for use in surgery where flammable anesthetics are used must be grounded.
30. Cold cylinders must be handled with care to avoid hand injury resulting from tissue freezing caused by rapid gas expansion.
31. Safety-relief mechanisms, uninterchangeable connections, and other safety features must not be removed or altered.
32. Control valves on equipment must be closed both before connection and when not in use.

Repair and Maintenance

1. Use only the service manuals, operator manuals, instructions, procedures, and repair parts that are provided or recommended by the manufacturer.
2. Allow only qualified personnel to maintain the equipment.
3. Designate and set aside an area that is clean and free from oil and grease for the maintenance of oxygen equipment. Do not use this area for the repair and maintenance of other types of equipment.
4. Follow a scheduled preventative maintenance program.

Appendix 1-B

National Fire Protection Association (NFPA) Recommendations and Regulations for Bulk Oxygen Systems

1. Containers that are permanently installed should be mounted on noncombustible supports and foundations.
2. Liquid oxygen containers should be constructed from materials that meet the impact test requirements of paragraph UG-48 of the ASME Boiler and Pressure Vessel Codes, Section VII, and must be in accordance with DOT specifications and regulations for 4L liquid oxygen containers. Containers operating above 15 psi must be designed and tested in accordance with the ASME Boiler and Pressure Vessel Code, Section VII, and the insulation of the liquid oxygen container must be of noncombustible material.
3. All high pressure nongaseous oxygen containers must comply with the construction and test requirements of ASME Boiler and Pressure Vessel Code, Section VIII.
4. Bulk oxygen storage containers must be equipped with safety-release devices as required by ASME Code IV and the provisions of ASME-1.3 or DOT specifications for both container and safety releases.
5. Isolation castings on liquid oxygen containers shall be equipped with suitable safety-release devices. These devices must be designed or located so that moisture cannot either freeze the unit or interfere in any manner with its proper operation.
6. The vaporizing columns and connecting pipes shall be anchored or sufficiently flexible to provide for expansion and contraction as a result of temperature changes. The column must also have a safety-release device to properly protect it.
7. Any heat supplied to oxygen vaporizers must be done in an indirect fashion, such as with steam, air, water, or water solutions that do not react with oxygen. If liquid heaters are used to provide the primary source of heat, the vaporizers must be electrically grounded.
8. All equipment composing the bulk system must be cleaned to remove oxidizable material before the system is placed into service.
9. All joins and connections in the tubing should be made by welding or using flanged, threaded slip or compressed fittings, and any gaskets or thread seals must be of a suitable substance for oxygen service. Any valves, gauges, or regulators placed into the system must be designed for oxygen service. The piping must conform to ANSI B 31.3 piping that operates below $-20°F$ ($-28.0°C$) and must be composed of materials meeting ASME Code, Section VIII.
10. Storage containers, piping valves, and regulating equipment must be protected from physical damage and tampering.
11. Any enclosure containing oxygen-control or operating equipment must be adequately ventilated.
12. The location shall be permanently posted to indicate OXYGEN—NO SMOKING—NO OPEN FLAMES or an equivalent warning.
13. All bulk systems must be regularly inspected by a qualified representative of the oxygen supplier.
14. Weeds and tall grass must be kept to a minimum of 15 feet from any bulk oxygen container. The bulk oxygen system must be located so that its distance provides maximum safety for the other areas surrounding it. The maximum distances for location of a bulk oxygen system near the following structures are as follows:
    a. 25 feet from any combustible structure.
    b. 25 feet from any structure that consists of fire-resistant exterior walls or buildings of other construction that have sprinklers.
    c. 10 feet from any opening in the adjacent walls of fire-resistant structures.
    d. 25 feet from flammable liquid storage above ground that is less than 1,000 gallons in capacity, or 50 feet from these storage areas if the quantity is in excess of 1,000 gallons.
    e. 15 feet from an underground flammable liquid storage that is less than 1,000 gallons, or 30 feet from one in excess of 1,000 gallons. The distance from the oxygen storage containers to connections used for filling and venting of flammable liquid must be at least 25 feet.
    f. 25 feet from combustible gas storage above ground that is less than 1,000 gallons capacity, or 50 feet from the storage of over 1,000 gallons capacity.
    g. 15 feet from combustible liquid storage underground and 25 feet from the vent or filling connections.
    h. 50 feet from flammable gas storage less than 5,000 ft^3; 90 feet from flammable gas in excess of 5,000 ft^3 normal temperature and pressure (NTP).
    i. 25 feet from solid materials that burn slowly (e.g., coal and heavy timber).
    j. 75 feet away in one direction and 35 feet away at an approximately 90-degree angle from confining walls unless they are made from a fire-resistant material and are less than 20 feet high. (This is to provide adequate ventilation in the area in case venting occurs.)
    k. 50 feet from places of public assembly.
    l. 50 feet from nonambulatory patients.
    m. 10 feet from public sidewalks.
    n. 5 feet from any adjoining properly line.
    o. Must be accessible by a mobile transport unit that fills the supply system.
15. The permanent installation of a liquid oxygen system must be supervised by personnel familiar with the proper installation and construction as outlined in NFPA 50.
16. The oxygen supply must have an inlet for the connection of a temporary supply in emergency and maintenance situations. The inlet must be physically protected to prevent tapering or unauthorized use and must be labeled EMERGENCY LOW-PRESSURE GASEOUS OXYGEN INLET. The inlet is to be installed downstream from the main supply line shutoff valve and must have the necessary valves to provide the emergency supply of oxygen as well as isolate the pipeline to the normal source of supply. There must be a check valve in the main line between the inlet connection and the main shutoff valve and another check valve between the inlet connection and the emergency supply shutoff valve. The inlet connection must have a pressure relief valve of adequate size

to protect the downstream piping from pressures in excess of 50% above normal pipeline operating pressure.

17. The bulk oxygen system must be mounted on noncombustible supports and foundations.

18. A surface of noncombustible material must extend at least 3 feet beyond the reach of liquid oxygen leaks during system operation or filling. Asphalt or bitumastic paving is prohibited. The slope of the area must be considered in sizing of the surface.

19. The same type of surface must extend at least the full width of the vehicle that fills the bulk unit and at least 8 feet in the transverse direction.

20. No part of the bulk system should be underneath electrical power lines or within reach of a downed power line.

21. No part of the system can be exposed to flammable gases or to piping containing any class of flammable or combustible liquids.

22. The system must be located so as to be readily accessible to mobile supply equipment at ground level, as well as to authorized personnel.

23. Warning and alarm systems are required to monitor the operation and condition of the supply system. Alarms and gauges are to be located for the best possible surveillance, and each alarm and gauge must be appropriately labeled.

24. The master alarm system must monitor the source of supply, the reserve (if any), and the mainline pressure of the gas system. The power source for warning systems must meet the essentials of NFPA 76A.

25. All alarm conditions must be evaluated and necessary measures taken to establish or ensure the proper function of the supply system.

26. Two master alarm panels, with alarms that cannot be cancelled, are to be located in separate locations to ensure continuous observation. One signal must alert the user to a changeover from one operating supply to another, and an additional signal must provide notification that the reserve is supplying the system.

27. If check valves are not installed in the cylinder leads and headers, another alarm signal should be initiated when the reserve reaches a 1-day supply.

28. All piping systems must have both audible and visible signals that cannot be cancelled to indicate when the mainline pressure increases or decreases 20% from the normal supply pressure. A pressure gauge must be installed and appropriately labeled adjacent to the switch that generates the pressure alarm conditions.

29. All warning systems must be tested before being placed in service or being added to existing service. Periodic retesting and appropriate recordkeeping are required.

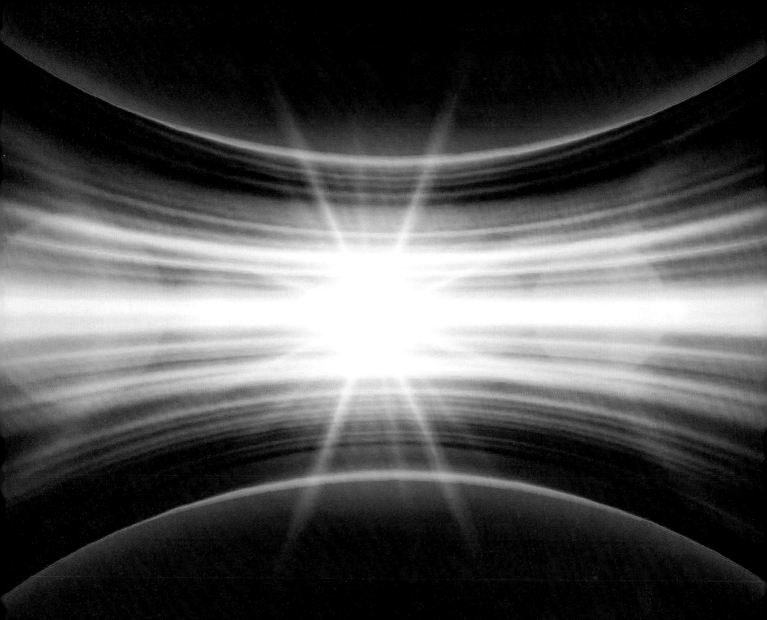

Appendix 1-C

National Fire Protection Association (NFPA) Recommendations and Regulations for Portable Liquid Oxygen Systems

1. Liquid oxygen units will vent gas when not in use, creating an oxygen-enriched environment. This can be particularly hazardous in the following situations:
   a. When the unit is stored in a closed space
   b. When the unit is tipped over
   c. When the oxygen is transferred to another container
2. Liquid oxygen units should not be located adjacent to heat sources, which can accelerate the venting of oxygen.
3. The unit surface should not be contaminated with oil or grease.
4. Verify the contents of liquid containers when setting up the equipment, changing the containers, or refilling the containers at home.
5. Connections for the containers are to be made with the manufacturer's operating instructions.
6. The patient and family must be familiar with the proper operation of the liquid devices, along with all precautions, safeguards, and troubleshooting methods.
7. Transfill one unit for another in compliance with CGA pamphlet P-26, "Transfilling of Low Pressure Liquid Oxygen to Be Used for Respiration," and in accordance with the manufacturer's operating instructions.
8. All connections for filling must conform to CGA V-1, and the hose assembly must have a pressure release set no higher than the container's related pressure.
9. Liquid containers must have a pressure release to limit the container pressure to the rated level, and a device must be incorporated to limit the amount of oxygen introduced into a container to the manufacturer's specified capacity.
10. Delivery vehicles should be well vented to prevent the buildup of high oxygen levels, and transfilling should take place with the delivery vehicle doors wide open.
11. No Smoking signs must be posted, and there can be no sources of ignition within 5 feet.
12. The transfiller must affix the labels required by DOT and FDA regulations, and all records must be kept stating the content and purity. Instructions must be on the container, and the color coding and labeling must meet CGA and NFPA standards.
13. All devices used with liquid oxygen containers must be moisture free, and pressure releases must be positioned correctly to prevent freezing and the buildup of high pressures.
14. When liquid oxygen is spilled, both the liquid and gas that escape are very cold and will cause frostbite or eye injury. When filling liquid oxygen containers, wear safety goggles with side shields, along with loose-fitting, properly insulated gloves. High-top boots with cuffless pants worn outside the boots are recommended.
15. Items exposed to liquid oxygen should not be touched because they can not only cause frostbite, but also stick to the skin. Materials that are pliable at room temperature become brittle at the extreme temperatures of liquid oxygen.
16. If a liquid oxygen spill occurs, the cold liquid and resulting gas condense the moisture in the air, creating a fog. Normally the fog will extend over an area larger than the area of contact danger, except in extremely dry climates.
17. In the event of a spill, measures should be taken to prevent anyone from walking on the surface or wheeling equipment across the area for at least 15 minutes. All sources of ignition must be kept away from the area.
18. Liquid oxygen spilled onto asphalt or oil-soaked concrete constitutes an extreme hazard because an explosive reaction can occur.
19. If the liquid oxygen comes in contact with the skin, remove any clothing that may constrict blood flow to the frozen area. Warm the affected area with water at about body temperature until medical personnel arrive. Seek immediate medical attention for eye contact or blistering of the skin.
20. Immediately remove contaminated clothing and air it away from sources of ignition for at least 1 hour.

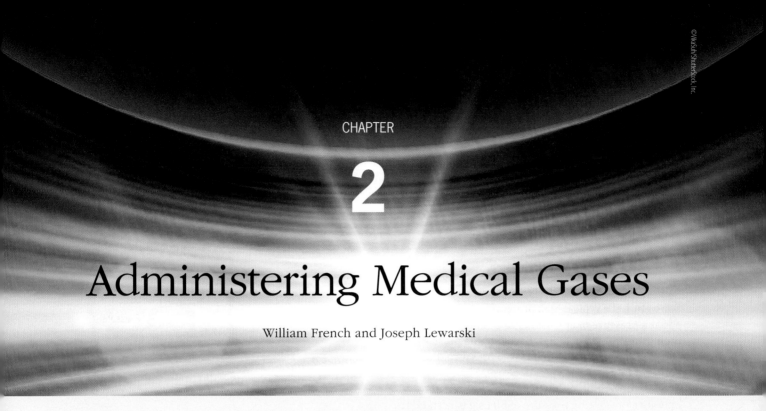

CHAPTER

2

Administering Medical Gases

William French and Joseph Lewarski

OBJECTIVES

1. Describe the basic operation of single-stage and multistage regulators.
2. Describe the basic operation of a Thorpe tube flowmeter.
3. Compare pressure-compensated devices to non-pressure-compensated devices.
4. Describe the basic operation of a Bourdon gauge.
5. Discuss the operation and uses of oxygen blenders.
6. List the indications for and hazards of oxygen therapy.
7. Define low flow oxygen therapy, list the devices that provide low flow therapy, and state the flow and F_IO_2 specifications for these devices.
8. Discuss how the F_IO_2 from a low flow device is determined.
9. Describe the basic operation of oxygen-conserving devices.
10. Define high flow oxygen therapy and list the specifications for each device.
11. Explain the operation and uses of reservoir delivery devices.
12. Describe the operation and uses of helium–oxygen therapy.
13. Describe the operation and uses of nitric oxide.
14. Describe the operation and uses of carbon dioxide–oxygen therapy.
15. Describe the basic function of an oxygen concentrator.

KEY TERMS

Air entrainment mask	Nonrebreathing mask
Air/oxygen blender	Oxygen concentrator
Bourdon gauge	Oxygen-conserving device (OCD)
Carbogen	Oxygen tent
Flowmeter	Reducing valve
Flow restrictor	Reservoir cannula
Heliox	Simple mask
High flow	Thorpe tube
High flow nasal cannula	Transtracheal oxygen catheter
Low flow	
Nasal cannula	
Nitric oxide	

Introduction

When Joseph Priestly discovered "dephlogisticated air" (later renamed oxygen) in 1774, he unknowingly introduced two problems into the practice of medicine. The first was when to use this purified air therapeutically. The second was how to deliver it to the patient. Oxygen therapy has particular significance for the profession of respiratory care because the first respiratory care practitioners were typically hospital orderlies who specialized in the application of oxygen.[1] From those days, in the 1940s, when oxygen technicians mostly set up oxygen tents and moved large gas cylinders, a profession began to form. Currently, although the general indications for oxygen therapy are well established, there is still some ongoing debate as to the best methods for safely delivering medical gases.

This chapter is primarily concerned with the equipment necessary to provide precise doses of oxygen to patients. This equipment includes the devices (**flowmeters**, regulators) that allow precise flows from bulk oxygen sources (e.g., cylinders, wall outlets, etc.), as well as the specific interfaces that are attached to the patient (e.g., nasal cannulas, nonrebreathing masks, etc.). The chapter will also explore other therapeutic gases, such as helium–oxygen mixtures (heliox), nitric oxide, and carbon dioxide–oxygen mixtures (carbogen).

Pressure-Regulating Devices

Once the decision has been made to administer a prescribed amount of oxygen to a patient, the next logical step is to determine the best way to do it.

Typically, the patient care setting will determine what oxygen source is available. Hospitals use large bulk liquid oxygen reservoirs and complex piping systems connected to outlets at the patient's bedside. Oxygen concentrators, portable liquid oxygen units, and high pressure tanks are commonly used to provide oxygen to patients cared for at home or in long-term care facilities. Once the oxygen source has been identified, the clinician must determine if there is a need to obtain equipment to regulate the flow from the oxygen source and select the appropriate patient interface.

Reducing Valves/Regulators

When full, the typical high pressure cylinder stores its gas at a pressure of at least 2,000 pounds per square inch gauge pressure (psig). Because this pressure is so high, it must be reduced to a pressure that is considerably lower for practical use. Most oxygen delivery devices and flowmeters are designed to operate at a working pressure of 50 psig (the standard pressure in hospital medical gas delivery systems). Thus, in order for the cylinder to be clinically useful, it must have a valve that will lower and maintain the pressure at the necessary level. Essentially, *regulator* and *reducing valve* refer to the same type of device, with the principal difference being that a regulator combines a reducing valve with some type of flowmeter (usually a Bourdon gauge—see later in this chapter).

Reducing valves can be either preset by the manufacturer (fixed) or adjustable. Fixed reducing valves are set to reduce the pressure to a single level (usually 50 psig). On the other hand, an adjustable regulator can reduce the pressure down to levels selected by the operator. Because the great majority of oxygen delivery devices and pneumatic-powered equipment are designed to operate at 50 psig, adjustable regulators are uncommon.

Reducing valves can be either single-stage or multistage. As the names suggest, a single-stage reducing valve drops the pressure to its working level in one stage, whereas a multistage reducing valve drops the pressure in two or more stages, with each stage connected in series. Multistage reducing valves are relatively uncommon in clinical practice because they are larger and more expensive, and provide a level of precision that is generally unnecessary in typical clinical applications.

As can be seen in **Figure 2-1**, a single-stage reducing valve contains the following components: inlet port, pressure gauge, high pressure chamber, pressure relief valve, outlet port, flexible diaphragm, ambient pressure chamber, spring, and valve stem. Once the valve on the cylinder is opened, gas enters through the inlet port into the high pressure chamber. The pressure exerted by the gas pushes against the flexible diaphragm. This would cause the valve stem to seal the valve inlet;

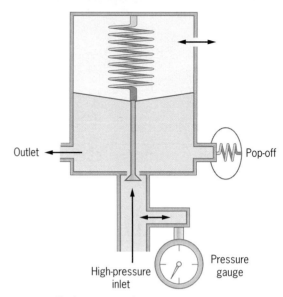

FIGURE 2-1 Single stage regulator.

Reproduced from *Egan's Fundamentals of Respiratory Care*. 7th ed. Scanlan CL, Wilkins RL, Stoller JK. Copyright Elsevier (Mosby) 1999.

however, the pressure is countered by the tension of the spring. As long as the outlet is open, the two pressures will equilibrate and remain at the preset level. Thus, the pressure is reduced to whatever tension the spring is set for (usually 50 psig). The pressure gauge provides a visual indicator of the contents of the cylinder.

A multistage reducing valve reduces pressure by connecting two or more single-stage regulators in a series. This type of regulator is larger and much heavier than a single-stage regulator. In a multistage regulator, the first stage reduces pressure to a preset intermediate pressure (500–700 psig), after which each of the following stages further reduces the pressure until it reaches 50 psig. The more regulators connected in series, the more precisely the pressure being reduced is controlled. For example, in a two-stage reducing valve, the working pressure is lowered to 200 psig in the first stage and then to 50 psig in the second stage (**Figure 2-2**). In a valve with more stages, the pressure within the cylinder is reduced more gradually. Therefore, multistage regulators provide smoother flow and more precise control of pressure when compared to single-stage regulators.

Flow Regulating Devices

In order for oxygen delivery devices to accomplish their intended purpose, they generally require a well-regulated flow of gas. This is achieved through one of three types of devices: flow restrictor, Thorpe tube, or Bourdon gauge. Each will provide a precise and measurable flow to an attached delivery device (e.g., nasal cannula or simple mask).

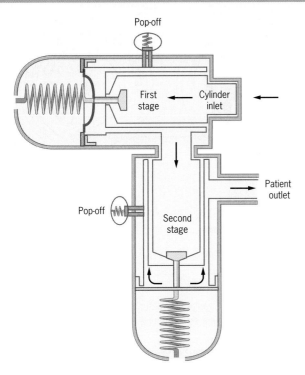

FIGURE 2-2 Multiple stage regulator.

Modified from Cairo JM, Pilbeam SP. *Mosby's respiratory care equipment.* 6th ed. St. Louis, MO: Mosby; 1999. Reprinted with permission.

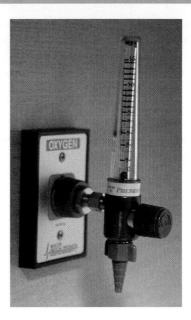

FIGURE 2-3 Thorpe tube flow meter

© Jones & Bartlett Learning. Courtesy of MIEMSS.

Thorpe Tube

The flowmeter most typically found in hospitals and other clinical venues is the **Thorpe tube** (see **Figure 2-3**). The Thorpe tube is a true flowmeter, in the sense that it "meters" or measures gas flow. The device can be either pressure compensated or pressure uncompensated (see **Figure 2-4**). If the flowmeter is pressure uncompensated, its accuracy is affected by changes in back pressure caused by downstream flow resistance. Also, as can be seen in Figure 2-4, the needle valve controlling the intake of gas is proximal to the tube. Virtually all Thorpe tube flowmeters produced at this time are pressure compensated. They are calibrated to produce an accurate flow rate at 50 psig.

The Thorpe is a clear tube that is tapered so that the diameter increases from the bottom to the top. Inside this clear tapered tube is a float (usually a steel ball). When the flowmeter is turned on, the force of the flowing gas pushes against the float, causing it to rise in opposition to gravity. As the float rises higher in the tube, the flow increases around it because the diameter of the tube is larger. Flow is indicated by the position of the float against the calibrated markings on the outside of the tube. The calibration is specific for both the type of gas (e.g., oxygen, air, or helium) and the pressure at which the gas is assumed to flow.

A Thorpe tube is designed to be pressure compensated by placing the needle valve downstream of the float (Figure 2-4). With this arrangement, the gas

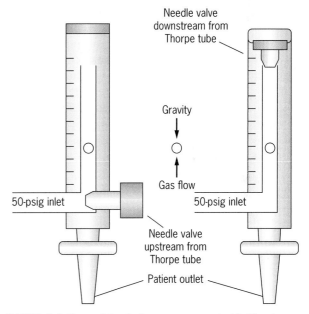

FIGURE 2-4 Thorpe tube designs; uncompensated (left) and compensated (right).

Modified from Cairo JM, Pilbeam SP. *Mosby's respiratory care equipment.* 6th ed. St. Louis, MO: Mosby; 1999. Reprinted with permission.

moving the float is at the supply pressure (e.g., 50 psig) so its density remains constant regardless of any back pressure after the needle valve (such as what may be produced by supply tubing kinks or large volume nebulizers). The float on a pressure-compensated Thorpe tube will jump when the flowmeter is connected to a 50-psig pressure source. One occasionally encounters uncompensated Thorpe tubes, often called "rotameters," that are used for calibrating laboratory equipment. They are uncompensated because the needle valve is located upstream of the float. The tube is calibrated with the assumption that the float is at essentially barometric pressure. Hence, any back pressure will change the density of the gas flowing around the float and invalidate the flow scale, making the reading less than actual flow.

The typical Thorpe tube has a flow range of 1 to 15 L/min. Some Thorpe tubes are calibrated to flows as low as 0.025 L/min for neonatal uses. The flowmeter will also produce flows much greater than 15 L/min when the dial is turned as far as it will turn (called the "flush" setting, perhaps as much as 40–60 L/min).

The principal disadvantage of the Thorpe tube is that it is very sensitive to gravity—it must remain straight vertically in order to operate.

Bourdon Gauge

The **Bourdon gauge** is a pressure gauge that is often configured as a flowmetering device (see **Figure 2-5**). In terms of function, it is generally described as a fixed orifice, variable-pressure flowmeter device.

The Bourdon gauge flowmeter contains a precision orifice; a connector; and a curved, hollow, closed tube that changes shape when exposed to pressure (**Figure 2-6**). Although the needle on the indicator is responding to pressure changes, the scale is calibrated to read flow (usually L/min). Turning the dial on the regulator adjusts the pressure in the reducing valve. This adjustment changes the pressure gradient between the valve and the fixed orifice. Changes in the pressure gradient cause changes in flow, because the output flow is directly proportional to the driving pressure.

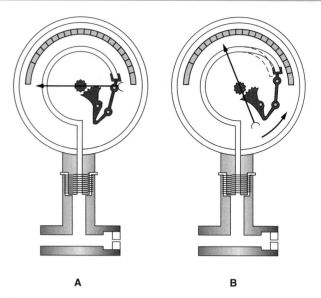

A　　　　　　　**B**

FIGURE 2-6 Bourdon gauge flowmeter. A. Unpressurized state. B. Pressurized state causing straightening of the tube and movement of the indicator needle.

Modified from Ward JJ. Equipment for mixed gas and oxygen therapy. In: Barnes TA, ed. *Core textbook of respiratory care practice.* 2nd ed. St. Louis, MO: Mosby; 1994.

This relationship will hold as long as there are no restrictions distal to the orifice. However, if any restrictions do occur (such as a kink in the supply tubing), the increase in back pressure will cause the indicator to read a flow that is higher than what is actually coming out of the device. In fact, even if the outlet is completely occluded, the indicator will still register or indicate a flow (**Figure 2-7**).

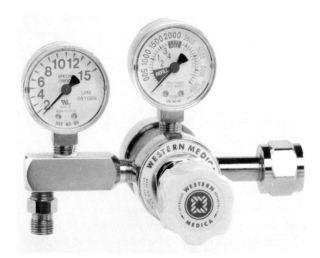

FIGURE 2-5 Single-stage adjustable pressure regulator with two Bourdon gauges. The gauge on the right, closest to the connection to the gas source, is calibrated in psi, indicating the contents of the cylinder. The Bourdon gauge on the left, closest to the outlet containing a small-diameter fixed orifice, is calibrated in L/min. Flow is adjusted by turning the regulator knob, which sets the pressure, causing flow through the orifice.

Courtesy of Western Enterprises, a Scott Fetzer Company.

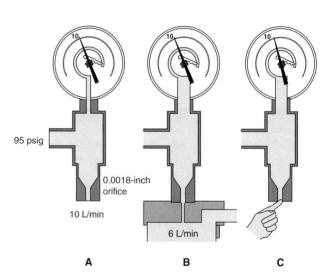

A　　　　　　**B**　　　　　　**C**

FIGURE 2-7 Bourdon gauge. A. The gauge displays a predictable outlet flow, assuming a constant known inlet pressure and known orifice size. B. Adding downstream resistance (e.g., attaching a large volume nebulizer) causes flow to decrease, but the reading may not be changed or may increase. C. Even with a complete obstruction, the Bourdon gauge indicates flow because it measures pressure, not flow.

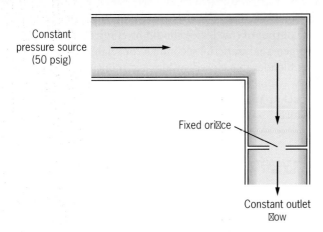

Constant pressure source (50 psig)

Fixed orifice

Constant outlet flow

FIGURE 2-8 Schematic of a fixed orifice flow restrictor. Flow through the orifice is proportional to the pressure difference across it.

This article was published in *Egan's Fundamentals of Respiratory Care.* 7th ed. Scanlan CL, Wilkins RL, Stoller JK. Copyright Elsevier (Mosby) 1999.

Flow Restrictors

The **flow restrictor** is a very simple flowmetering device. As can be seen in **Figure 2-8**, the device is basically a tube with a fixed orifice placed distal to the oxygen source. It is calibrated to deliver a specific flow at a specific pressure (usually 50 psig).

Flow restrictors are generally available in flows ranging from 0.5 L/min to 3 L/min. There are also flow restrictors that allow the user to vary the orifice size, thus rendering the device capable of producing a variety of flows.

Advantages of flow restrictors include low cost, reliability, gravity independence, and flow specificity. Their disadvantage is that they are not back pressure compensated. Downstream resistance makes flow less than expected because the meter is calibrated with the assumption that the only resistance is the internal orifice. Flow restrictors are relatively uncommon in clinical practice, generally giving way to Bourdon gauges and Thorpe tubes.

Air/Oxygen Blenders

Some clinical applications of oxygen therapy require that air and oxygen be combined in precise amounts in order to create a stable F_IO_2. The simplest way to accomplish this would be to combine the flow from an air flowmeter with the flow from an oxygen flowmeter. The ratio of the two flows creates the F_IO_2. For example, if a clinician wanted a patient to receive 60% oxygen, she would set each flowmeter so that the ratio of air to oxygen would equal 1:1 (e.g., set the air flowmeter at 10 L/min and the oxygen flowmeter at 10 L/min). This ratio is derived from a simple mass balance equation:

Mass oxygen in total flow = Mass oxygen in oxygen flow + Mass oxygen in air flow

which can be expressed as:

$$F_TO_2 \times \text{Total flow} = 1.0 \times \text{Oxygen flow} + 0.21 \times \text{Air flow}$$

where F_TO_2 is the fraction of oxygen in the total flow and *total flow* is the sum of the air and oxygen flows. From this basic equation we can derive the equation for estimating the ratio of oxygen and air flow for a desired F_IO_2:

$$\text{Air flow:Oxygen flow} = (1.0 - 0.21)/(F_IO_2 - 0.21)$$

Table 2-1 gives some approximate air/oxygen ratios for various desired F_IO_2 values.

Although combining the flows as described may be the simplest method of creating a stable F_IO_2, the number of possible applications this method can serve is limited. Thus, occasionally it may be desirable to use a dedicated **air/oxygen blender** (sometimes also referred to as a proportioner).

As can be seen in **Figure 2-9**, the air/oxygen blender is connected to a high pressure (usually 50 psig) air source and a high pressure oxygen source. The two pressures must be equal in order for the device to be accurate. When activated, both air and oxygen flow into the blender and then through dual pressure regulators that cause the pressure of the two gases to equalize.

TABLE 2-1
Air:Oxygen Flow Ratios for Desired Values of Inspired Oxygen

Desired F_IO_2	Mix Ratio Air:Oxygen
0.24	25:1
0.28	10:1
0.3	8:1
0.35	5:1
0.4	3:1
0.45	2.3:1
0.5	1.7:1
0.55	1.3:1
0.6	1:1
0.65	0.8:1
0.7	0.6:1
0.75	0.5:1
0.8	0.3:1

Reproduced from Branson RD. Gas delivery systems: Regulators, flowmeters, and therapy devices. In Branson RD, Hess DR, Chatburn RL, eds. *Respiratory care equipment.* 2nd ed. Philadelphia: Lippincott Williams and Wilkins; 1999.

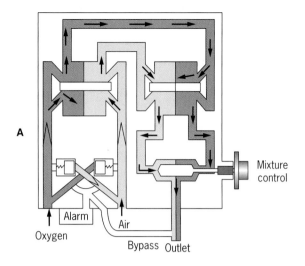

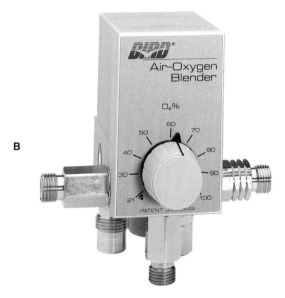

FIGURE 2-9 A. Schematic of an air/oxygen blender. B. Photo of an oxygen blender.

Art modified from Ward JJ. Equipment for mixed gas and oxygen therapy. In: Barnes TA, ed. *Core textbook of respiratory care practice.* 2nd ed. St. Louis, MO: Mosby; 1994:365–439. Photo reproduced with permission from CareFusion.

The gases then move to a precision proportioning valve. At this point, because the pressure of the two gases is equal, the concentration of oxygen (F_IO_2) is controlled by varying the size of the air and oxygen inlets. The blended gas then flows out of the outlet port to the delivery device, with a small amount of the gas being shunted to an alarm.

The alarm on the blender functions to provide an audible warning whenever the pressure of one of the source gases drops below a certain prespecified level. Should such failure occur, the alarm system has a bypass feature built in that will cause the blender to switch to the remaining source gas (e.g., should the pressure of compressed air drop, the blender will switch to provide 100% oxygen).

Two key factors need to be considered whenever an air/oxygen blender is in use. The first is that the blender may not be entirely accurate. Thus, the F_IO_2 of the output of the device should be confirmed with an oxygen analyzer. The second factor relates to the use of the blender in a closed system (e.g., continuous positive airway pressure [CPAP]). Such a system should have a backup inspiratory valve in place in case of gas flow failure.

Oxygen Concentrators

Outside of the acute hospital setting, oxygen therapy is commonly provided by a variety of systems including liquid oxygen vessels, compressed gas cylinders, and **oxygen concentrators**. In North America, it is estimated that oxygen concentrators represent more than 95% of all stationary home oxygen therapy delivery systems. Around the world, oxygen concentrators represent a critical tool for the provision of oxygen therapy and are particularly important in many developing countries, where oxygen concentrators have been identified as the most consistent and lowest cost source of oxygen available.[2,3]

Oxygen concentrators are used in both medical and industrial applications and have been available commercially in some parts of the world for medical applications for over 30 years. Modern stationary oxygen concentrators are electromechanical devices that generally operate from an AC power source, weigh approximately 30 to 50 pounds, and have sound pressure levels of 39 to 55 decibels. (Specifications vary by manufacturer, make, and model.)

Oxygen concentrators separate the oxygen in the air from the other gases using a chemical sieve gas-separation technology. The most common method of separating the gases employed in oxygen concentrators is known as pressure-swing adsorption (PSA). Oxygen PSA systems pump air under specific pressure through a molecular sieve bed, normally composed of a ceramic zeolite that preferentially adsorbs the nitrogen molecules in the air, while allowing the oxygen molecules to pass through the bed. At the end of the first pressurization cycle, the sieve bed is left saturated with the adsorbed nitrogen and must be regenerated before the next adsorption cycle. During the sieve bed regeneration phase, a lower pressure and a small volume of oxygen is routed to the saturated bed to help "wash" the nitrogen off the sieve molecules in a depressurization process referred to as desorption. This cyclic "swinging" of pressures from higher (adsorption) to lower (desorption) is what gives the PSA process its name. Most oxygen concentrators operate using a two-bed system, with one bed adsorbing nitrogen while the other bed is desorbing. Because the sieve beds only adsorb nitrogen, a small amount of argon passes through with the oxygen. As a result of the presence of argon, the maximum output purity of modern

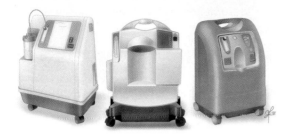

FIGURE 2-10 Stationary oxygen concentrators.

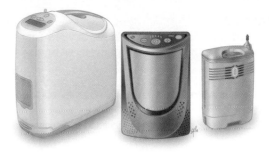

FIGURE 2-11 Portable oxygen concentrators.

oxygen concentrators is about 95%. Once separated, the output oxygen is typically collected in a small storage (product) tank, pressurized, and delivered at the prescribed setting to the user.

There are various types, makes, and models of stationary oxygen concentrators commercially available (**Figure 2-10**); the most common are capable of delivering a range of continuous flows up to 5 L/min, with an oxygen purity of ≥ 87%, although many modern devices routinely exceed 93%. Due to advancements in sieve material efficiency and compressor technologies, there are now a number of commercially available medical concentrators capable of providing a continuous flow of oxygen up to 10 L/min. Continuous flow devices supply oxygen at a fixed rate, generally measured in liters per minute. As a patient breathes using a continuous flow device, they simply draw in oxygen from the available, fixed flow of gas. The flowmeters used with oxygen concentrators are similar in specifications and performance and operate in the same way to those commonly used in institutional healthcare settings.

In recent years, a new class of smaller, lightweight (some under 5 pounds) oxygen concentrators has been introduced to the market. This new category of oxygen concentrators, commonly referred to as portable oxygen concentrators (POCs), also operate using the PSA system (**Figure 2-11**). This group of devices is classified by the oxygen delivery methodology: (1) conserving (pulse dose) only or (2) continuous flow and pulse dose. The latter may deliver up to 3 L/min of continuous flow and can vary greatly in the available pulse dose range (setting) and output volumes. Unlike continuous flow systems, pulse dose devices deliver oxygen in response to the patient's inspiratory demand (see the section Oxygen-Conserving Systems later in this chapter).

Technical characteristics common to all oxygen concentrators for home medical use include low operating pressures, small volumes of oxygen stored and delivered under low pressures, and no significant alteration of the surrounding ambient gas mixture or oxygen concentration. Contrary to some common misperceptions, oxygen concentrators do not produce large volumes of oxygen, they do not store such gases at high pressures, and they do not vent high levels of oxygen into the ambient atmosphere, all characteristics that make them ideal and safe for home use. Oxygen pressures within the concentrator system are typically < 25 psig and the output delivery pressures often are quite low, with an operating range of about 5–8 psig. The safety and efficacy profile of oxygen concentrators is well documented, as is evidenced by the Federal Aviation Administration (FAA) approval of POC use on commercial aircraft. In contrast, other traditional home oxygen systems, such as stationary liquid vessels or compressed gas cylinders, can store large volumes of oxygen at very high pressures (2,000–3,000 psi) with output delivery pressures of 20–50 psi.

Oxygen concentrators are the current standard of care for the provision of low flow oxygen in the home and other nonhospital settings. They are designed for laypersons to operate; are relatively easy to use, safe, and quiet; and generally require little maintenance and servicing. Modern oxygen concentrators have been demonstrated to be quite reliable and cost effective.

Oxygen Delivery Devices

Oxygen therapy is very commonly applied in both acute care and long-term care. The principal indications for oxygen therapy are hypoxemia and cardiopulmonary distress. The principal goal of oxygen therapy is to treat or prevent hypoxemia and to minimize the effects of hypoxemia.[4]

In order for medical gas therapy to be effective therapeutically, it must be administered to the patient using some type of interface. Traditionally, these interface devices can be classified as **low flow, high flow**, reservoir, and enclosure devices. Device selection for a particular patient will depend on how much oxygen the patient needs (i.e., F_IO_2), how much flow the patient needs, the patient's need for comfort and mobility, and the need for precise delivery of desired oxygen concentrations (**Table 2-2**).

TABLE 2-2
Comparison of Interfaces Used for Oxygen Therapy

F_IO_2 Characteristics	Performance Characteristics/F_IO_2 Stability	
	Fixed	Variable
Low < 0.35	Air entrainment mask Mask attached to an air entrainment nebulizer Isolette Oxyhood	Nasal cannula Nasal catheter Transtracheal oxygen catheter
Moderate 0.35–0.60	Air entrainment mask Mask attached to an air entrainment nebulizer Oxyhood	Simple mask
High > 0.60	Oxyhood Mask attached to an air entrainment nebulizer	Partial rebreathing mask Nonrebreathing mask

Low Flow Oxygen Delivery Devices

A low flow oxygen delivery device provides a portion of the total flow of gas a patient inhales per breath. These are sometimes also referred to as variable performance devices because the actual tracheal F_IO_2 can vary from breath to breath. The following situation will serve to demonstrate how this works (simplified):

> Patient inspiratory volume (tidal volume) = 500 mL
> Inspiratory time = 1 second
> Oxygen flow (nasal cannula) = 2 L/min (33.3 mL/ second)

In this situation, the patient is receiving 33.3 mL of 100% oxygen per breath. The remainder of the inspiratory volume (500 mL – 33.3 mL = 466.7 mL) comes from room air (21% oxygen). Some textbooks give gross approximations of the F_IO_2 delivered by low flow systems (e.g., nasal cannulas) based on a mathematical model that takes into account the factors (breath rate and ratio of inspiratory time to expiratory time, I:E) that affect inspiratory time and the small amount of oxygen possibly stored in the anatomic reservoir (i.e., nose and upper airway) during the latter portion of exhalation when flow is zero for patients with normal lungs. Interestingly, patients with chronic obstructive pulmonary disease (COPD) often do not have a period of zero flow at end expiration; therefore, the anatomic reservoir may not provide any extra oxygen and hence the equation overestimates the F_IO_2.[5]

As can be seen by the previous example, two factors go into defining a low flow oxygen delivery system: (1) only a relatively small portion of the patient's inspiratory volume comes from the device, and (2) the patient's tracheal F_IO_2 while wearing the device is highly variable and dependent on such factors as tidal volume, respiratory rate, and inspiratory time. In clinical practice, the variability of the F_IO_2 is critical for the clinician to understand. As will be seen later in this chapter, there are guidelines for equating oxygen liter flows with specific F_IO_2s (e.g., 2 L/min = 28%). However, these are *only rough approximations*.

In actual practice, the patient's tracheal F_IO_2 could possibly vary from one breath to the next, especially if the patient's respiratory pattern is relatively unstable. As a general rule, the tracheal F_IO_2 will vary as the inspiratory volume varies, such that there is an inverse correlation between tidal volume and F_IO_2 (i.e., the higher the tidal volume, the lower the F_IO_2, and vice versa).

The most common low flow device in use today is the nasal cannula. (The high flow nasal cannula will be addressed in the section on high flow delivery devices.) Patients requiring continuous oxygen in the home may use a **reservoir cannula** that has been designed to conserve oxygen (e.g., pendant or mustache). The transtracheal catheter is a low flow device used most commonly for long-term oxygen therapy. The nasal catheter is a low flow device that is rarely used clinically.

Nasal Cannula

The **nasal cannula** is by far the most common type of oxygen delivery device in use today. It generally consists of at least 7 feet of small-bore oxygen delivery tubing connected to two short prongs that are inserted into the nose with the prongs angled down (see **Figure 2-12**). There are cannulas manufactured for home and long-term care use that provide 25 feet of small-bore tubing before the connection to the two prongs. The longer supply tubing enables patients to ambulate and remain connected to a stationary oxygen source, such as oxygen concentrators.

Obviously, for the cannula to be an effective delivery device, the nares and nasal passages must be patent. Although the cannula may be worn for extensive periods of time, the prongs and continuous flow of gas may irritate the inner lining of the nose or cause skin irritation or breakdown around the ears, face, and/ or nares opening. Gauze or foam pads can be used to protect areas where the plastic cannula may rub

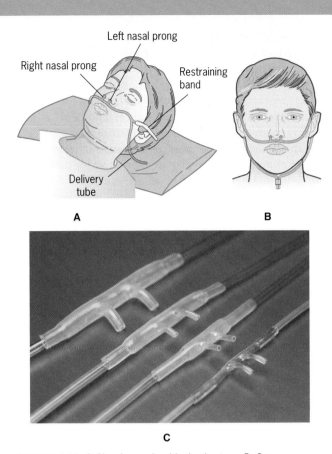

FIGURE 2-12 A. Nasal cannula with elastic strap. B. Over-the-ear style nasal cannula. C. Various styles of nasal prongs.

Photo courtesy of Teleflex.

the skin. Padding pressure points, such as behind the ears or over the cheekbones, may be especially helpful to prevent skin breakdown. The prongs of the nasal cannula should occlude more than 50% of the nares. Tightly fitting prongs may cause breakdown around or within the nares.

Because this is a low flow device, it does not provide the total flow needed to meet all of the inspiratory demands of the patient, and should not be used on patients for whom a precise F_IO_2 is necessary. For adults, the standard flow range is 1 L/min to 6 L/min. Although some sources cite the maximum flow as 8 L/min, this is not common in actual practice, primarily because there is very little F_IO_2 gain with flow rates above 6 L/min. Additionally, flows greater than 6 L/min may irritate the nasal mucosa causing patient discomfort. The standard F_IO_2 range is 0.24 to 0.40 at these flow rates. However, recent studies have shown a significant degree of variability in correlating flow to tracheal or pharyngeal F_IO_2.[6–9] A very general rule for determining F_IO_2 at a specific flow rate is the "rule of fours," which states that the F_IO_2 will change 4% for every L/min above 1 (e.g., 1 L/min ≈ 24%, 2 L/min ≈ 28%, etc.). This is only a crude approximation; actual tracheal F_IO_2 is subject to the variables indicated previously for low flow oxygen delivery systems. Owing to the variability of the F_IO_2, it is generally recommended

that the clinician titrate the flow of this low flow device to an objective measure of the patient's oxygenation status. Pulse oximetry is often used to noninvasively monitor a patient's oxygenation status. An example of a common physician order would be: Oxygen at 2 L/min by nasal cannula. Titrate oxygen flow to maintain an SpO_2 of 93–95%.

For pediatric and neonatal patients, the flow range is much lower due to the patients' anatomical features and lower tidal volume. Two liters per minute is considered the maximum flow rate for a nasal cannula used for infants.[10] The flow rate appropriate for this population ranges from 25 mL/min to 2 L/min.[11] The maximum flow for pediatric patients is 3 L/min.

In the past, it was common practice to attach the nasal cannula to a bubble humidifier. However, studies showed that this practice did not provide benefit to the patient. Based on this research, clinical practice guidelines suggest using a bubble humidifier with flow rates that are greater than or equal to 4 L/min or if the patient complains of nasal dryness.[6]

Nasal Catheter

The nasal catheter is a long, narrow tube with a series of holes on the distal end; the approximate outside diameter is usually between 3 and 4 mm. It is generally made of soft, flexible plastic. This device is inserted through the nose to a level just above and behind the uvula (see **Figure 2-13**). The proximal end is connected to oxygen delivery tubing. The catheter should be lubricated with a water-soluble gel just prior to insertion. Insertion itself should be slow and careful, with the catheter being advanced along the floor of the nasal passage. The catheter should be secured with tape

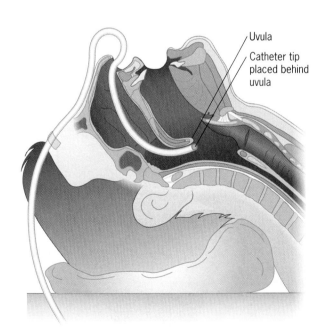

FIGURE 2-13 Nasal catheter for oxygen administration.

after it is inserted. Generally, the catheter is withdrawn and inserted into the other nare approximately every 8 hours.

Historically, the nasal catheter was used as an oxygen delivery device similar to the way the nasal cannula is used today. Although the nasal catheter is still commercially available, it is rarely used in day-to-day clinical practice because the nasal cannula is equally efficacious, more comfortable, and easier to use. The flow range for the nasal catheter is 1 to 6 L/min. The F_IO_2 range is about the same as that for the nasal cannula: 24% to 44%. As with the nasal cannula, the tracheal F_IO_2 is highly variable and dependent on the patient's respiratory rate and tidal volume.

The use of the nasal catheter may be problematic. First, at least one nare and nasal passage must be entirely patent. Second, the presence of the catheter within the nose is irritating and may cause inflammation and bleeding. There is also a chance that mucus can clog the small holes at the distal end, reducing the flow of gas through the device. Additionally, tape used to secure the catheter may irritate the facial skin.

Transtracheal Catheter

The **transtracheal oxygen catheter** is a flexible, small diameter tube (about 3.3 mm), generally made of soft plastic or Teflon. It is inserted directly into the trachea through a small incision through the tracheal wall, usually between the second and third ring. When properly positioned, the tip of the catheter is 2 to 4 cm above the carina (see **Figure 2-14**). It is then secured with a bead chain necklace. Once inserted, it is removed only for cleaning or replacement.

The transtracheal catheter was first described in 1982 and became commercially available in 1986, at which time it was inserted via the modified Seldinger technique. It is meant as a replacement for the nasal cannula for patients who are on long-term oxygen

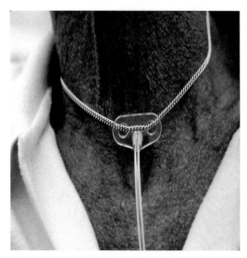

FIGURE 2-14 Transtracheal oxygen catheter in place.
Courtesy of TransTracheal Systems.

therapy. In 1996, Lipkin's surgical approach was introduced as an alternative. Regardless of the insertion technique, the process is composed of four clinically defined phases:[12] (1) patient selection and evaluation, (2) tract creation, (3) beginning of therapy in an immature tract (removal of the catheter requires a guide wire), and (4) regular therapy through a mature tract.

The principal advantages of the transtracheal catheter are that it provides an alternative for patients who do not tolerate a nasal cannula, provides relief to patients experiencing nasal irritation and bleeding with nasal cannula use, and is easy to conceal under clothing—an advantage for those oxygen-dependent patients who are self-conscious about wearing their oxygen device in public.

Because the catheter is placed directly in the trachea, bypassing the upper airway, the patient generally requires less oxygen flow to produce like effects. Christopher[12] estimates that oxygen flow can be reduced by over 50% at rest and about 30% during exercise.

However, there are limitations to its use. A surgical procedure is necessary to initially place the catheter. Because the catheter resides in the trachea, there is risk for tracheal irritation and/or infection. Mucus may clog the distal end, reducing or completely obstructing the flow of oxygen to the patient. Therefore, patients must remove the catheter and clean it on a regular basis.

The flow range for the transtracheal catheter is 0.25 to 4 L/min, producing an F_IO_2 range of 0.22 to 0.35.

Reservoir Delivery Devices

Reservoir delivery devices allow the continuous flow of oxygen from the source to accumulate within that interface and thus to increase the amount of oxygen available to the patient just prior to each inhalation. Reservoir devices are generally made of plastic and can be masks (simple mask, partial rebreathing mask, or nonrebreathing mask) or cannulas (mustache or pendent).

Simple Mask

The **simple mask** is a single unit that fits over the mouth and the bridge of the nose. An adjustable elastic strap, attached to the periphery of the mask, wraps around the back of the patient's head, securing it in place. A flexible thin metal strip molds the mask to the contours of the bridge of the nose, preventing gas from escaping and irritating the patient's eyes. There are small holes on either sides of the mask that serve as outlet ports for exhaled gas. A long, small diameter tubing connects the mask to the oxygen source (see **Figure 2-15**). The inside of the mask has a reservoir of approximately 100 to 200 mL. Although the F_IO_2 from the device is highly variable, the reservoir helps to increase the F_IO_2 potential.

Because the F_IO_2 is variable and not much higher than that for the nasal cannula (maximum of

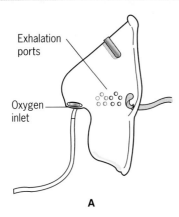

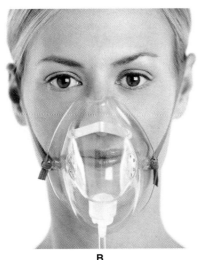

FIGURE 2-15 A. Schematic of a simple oxygen mask. B. Oxygen mask in place on a patient.

Art modified from Scanlan CL, et al. *Egan's fundamentals of respiratory care*. 7th ed. Mosby; 1999. Photo © Corbis/age fotostock

approximately 0.50 within the accepted flow range of the mask), the use of the simple mask is essentially limited to those clinical situations in which a nasal cannula is unavailable (in an emergency oxygen kit) or when the use of a nasal cannula is contraindicated (skin breakdown around or within the nares). It may also be useful in patients who need a moderate amount of oxygen over a short period of time because its design makes it easier to place on a patient's face than a nasal cannula. It is not recommended for patients who require a precise concentration of oxygen.[4]

There are limitations to the use of the simple mask. The reservoir could collect CO_2 exhaled at the end of a breath. If the flow of oxygen to the mask is not sufficient to flush out this CO_2, the patient could then rebreathe the CO_2 on the next inhalation. For this reason it is important for the clinician to ensure the flow of oxygen to the mask is at least 5 L/min. Precautions should be taken to avoid or quickly detect any interruptions in the flow of oxygen to the device (i.e., disconnections).[6,11] Long-term use of the mask can potentially result in skin irritation and skin breakdown,

interferes with communication by muffling speech, and limits the patient's ability to eat, drink, and expectorate.

The generally acceptable flow range for the simple mask is 5–10 L/min. The F_IO_2 range is approximately 0.35 to 0.50. Again, remember that the F_IO_2 is variable, largely determined by the patient's respiratory rate and tidal volume.

Partial Rebreathing Mask

The partial rebreathing mask is a tight-fitting face mask usually made of disposable plastic. It has small holes on both sides that serve as exit ports for exhaled gas. The primary feature of the mask is a reservoir bag attached to the bottom (see **Figure 2-16**). Seven feet of small-bore tubing connects the oxygen flowmeter to a port just above the reservoir bag.

The name *partial rebreathing mask* is derived from the fact that a portion of the patient's exhaled gas (generally the first third) flows into the reservoir bag and is then subsequently rebreathed during the next inhalation. The original idea behind the creation of this mask was to conserve oxygen in situations where the supply of oxygen was limited (e.g., using a high pressure oxygen tank). Because the first third of the patient's exhaled gas comes from the anatomic deadspace, the assumption is that the patient will not rebreathe CO_2. Therefore, this type of mask may not be the interface of choice in clinical situations where it is desirable for the patient to rebreathe CO_2 (e.g., hyperventilation syndrome).

Generally, the partial rebreathing mask is used when a patient requires a moderate F_IO_2 (e.g., 0.50 to 0.60) for a short period of time. Because this mask may not provide the total flow needed by the patient, it is unable to guarantee precise F_IO_2 delivery.

Similar to a simple mask, a partial rebreathing mask is relatively easy to assemble and apply. Once the flow of oxygen to the device has filled the reservoir bag, the

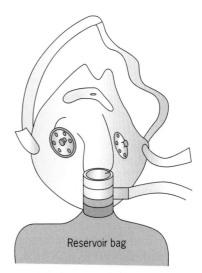

FIGURE 2-16 Schematic of a partial rebreathing oxygen mask.

Modified from Scanlan CL, et al. *Egan's fundamentals of respiratory care*. 7th ed. St. Louis, MO: Mosby; 1999.

mask can be applied to the patient's face and secured with an adjustable elastic strap. The oxygen flow is then adjusted so the bag does not deflate to more than one half of its volume during inspiration. Failure to provide adequate flow will result in the delivery of lower oxygen concentrations to the patient. When operated properly, this device delivers moderate to high concentrations of oxygen.

As with any mask, the partial rebreathing mask restricts the patient's access to atmospheric gas. The same precautions taken with a simple mask apply with this device as well. The clinician must ensure that the minimum oxygen flow is adequate (at least 5 L/min) to prevent rebreathing of CO_2, as well as prevent or readily detect any disruptions to the flow of oxygen to the device.

As with any face mask, the patient's ability to eat, drink, or expectorate is severely limited. Because the mask must fit snuggly against the skin of the patient's face, there is potential risk for skin irritation and breakdown. It is important to note the integrity of the skin prior to the application of the mask. The skin should then be assessed at scheduled intervals. Any redness, irritation, or breakdown should be noted and communicated to the physician.

The generally accepted flow range for the partial rebreathing mask is 8–15 L/min. This results in an F_IO_2 range of about 0.40 to 0.70. It should be remembered that, like the low flow devices described previously, the F_IO_2 is variable and will be partially influenced by the patient's respiratory rate and tidal volume.

Nonrebreathing Mask

The **nonrebreathing mask** has the same basic design as the partial rebreathing mask with the addition of three one-way valves (usually circular flaps made of soft rubber). Two of the valves cover the holes on both sides of the mask. These are designed to open to the atmosphere when the patient exhales and close when the patient inhales, reducing access to room air. The third valve is between the reservoir bag and the mask. This valve is designed to open when the patient inhales and close when the patient exhales to prevent the patient's exhaled gas from entering the reservoir (see **Figure 2-17**). The design minimizes any dilution of oxygen with room air or the patient's exhaled breath, so the nonrebreathing mask can provide high concentrations of oxygen.

The nonrebreathing mask is most useful for patients who have high oxygen requirements for relatively short periods of time. These might include patients with acute heart failure, trauma, carbon monoxide poisoning, and transient severe hypoxemic failure.

Similar to the partial rebreathing mask, it is important to have oxygen flowing to the mask and filling the reservoir before fitting it to the patient's face. The adjustable elastic band secures the mask in place. A snug fit restricts the air entrainment, thus maintaining a high F_IO_2. Once the mask is in place, the oxygen flow

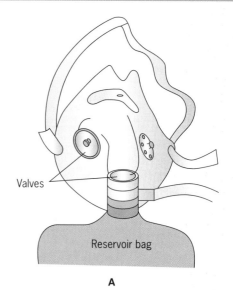

Valves

Reservoir bag

A

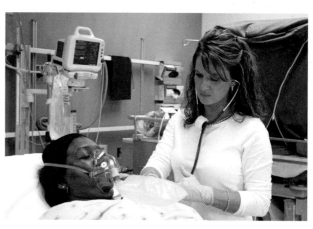

B

FIGURE 2-17 A. Schematic of a nonrebreathing mask. B. Nonrebreathing mask in use on a patient.

Art modified from Scanlan CL, et al. *Egan's fundamentals of respiratory care.* 7th ed. Mosby; 1999. Photo © Andrew Gentry/ShutterStock, Inc.

is adjusted to ensure that the reservoir does not fully collapse during inspiration. Generally, this requires minimum flows of 10 L/min to 15 L/min.[4,9]

The limitations and precautions for this mask are identical to those of the partial rebreathing mask. However, if the flow of oxygen were to stop, the risk of harm is greater with the nonrebreathing mask. The presence of the one-way valves covering the side ports on the sides of the mask interferes with the patient's ability to entrain room air. Although it is less common, some manufacturers produce nonrebreathing masks with one-way valves covering both side ports. If you remove one of the valves the risk of harm is reduced if flow is interrupted.

The generally reported flow range for the nonrebreathing mask is 10–15 L/min; however, depending on the patient's inspiratory effort, flows greater than 15 L/min may be necessary to keep the reservoir bag partially inflated during inspiration. Theoretically, the concentration of oxygen should approach 100%; however, published reports indicate an F_1O_2 range of 0.60 to 0.80.[2,7] The actual F_1O_2 is variable and dependent on the seal of the mask, the oxygen flow, and the patient's respiratory rate and tidal volume.

Oxygen-Conserving Systems

The term **oxygen-conserving device (OCD)** has been used to describe a variety of oxygen technologies that are intended to increase the duration of use of a portable low flow oxygen system by limiting or conserving the flow of oxygen to only the inspiratory portion of the breathing cycle. OCDs are also referred to in the scientific literature as intermittent flow devices (IFDs), demand oxygen delivery devices (DODDs), and pulsed dose oxygen conservers (PDOCs). In this text we will use OCD to represent the broad category of conserving devices.

OCDs intended for use in the management of patients receiving long-term oxygen therapy (LTOT) were first introduced commercially in the early 1980s. Reservoir nasal cannula systems were introduced around 1983 and mechanical oxygen-conserving devices followed in 1984.[13] Although OCD technology has been around for more than 30 years, widespread acceptance and the dramatic rise in use have been observed in the United States only over the last 10 to 15 years. Today, nearly every modern portable oxygen device incorporates some form of oxygen-conserving technology. OCDs are routinely used with ambulatory LTOT patients to a level that is arguably the standard of care in the United States.

Pulsed Dose Oxygen-Conserving Devices

Pulsed dose oxygen-conserving devices (PDOCs) are a logical technological extension of continuous, low flow oxygen delivery devices. Although low flow oxygen therapy prescriptions are typically written in liters per minute (L/min), these devices actually deliver an unpredictable volume of oxygen to the patient. For example, a patient prescribed 2 L/min of oxygen via nasal cannula does not actually inspire 2 full liters of oxygen; the 2 liters of gas flowing per minute is available to draw from only during inspiration and the rest is wasted during expiration. PDOCs were designed to conserve oxygen by delivering pulses of gas only during inspiration, thus avoiding the waste typically seen with a nasal cannula.

Modern PDOCs are either electronically or pneumatically operated devices and typically deliver oxygen on demand (**Figure 2-18**). The patient's demand is sensed as the pressure drop caused by inspiratory flow past the sensor (typically a nasal cannula). Once triggered, the device delivers a predetermined flow of gas over a preset time interval, which produces a certain dose or bolus of oxygen. The clinical foundation of PDOCs relies on the assumption that the oxygen participating in gas exchange in the lungs enters the

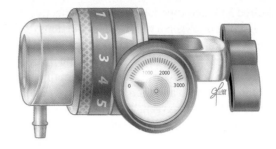

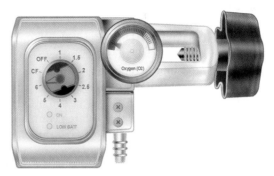

FIGURE 2-18 Examples of commercially available pulsed dose oxygen-conserving devices that fit on E cylinders of oxygen. (Top) Pneumatically controlled device. (Bottom) Electronically controlled device.

airways quickly, during the first two thirds of the inspiratory cycle. Oxygen flowing at the end of the inspiration, during exhalation and during the pause prior to the next inspiration, is essentially wasted because it plays no role in gas exchange and blood oxygenation. The physiology of breathing suggests that approximately one third of a person's inspiratory volume remains in the larger airways, sinuses, nose, and mouth (anatomical dead space). Gas held in the anatomical dead space does not participate in alveolar gas exchange and represents the first volume of exhaled gas. Early work by Tiep and Lewis noted that the efficiency of pulsed oxygen therapy can be improved by focusing the oxygen delivery on early inspiration.[14]

In the United States and in many other countries, PDOCs are currently accepted as a standard of practice for stable, ambulatory LTOT users. PDOC technology is incorporated into nearly all modern ambulatory oxygen systems, including small cylinders, lightweight liquid oxygen vessels, and portable oxygen concentrators. There are a few key elements associated with efficient PDOC technology, including bolus size, trigger sensitivity, and bolus flow/speed. A common assumption with PDOCs is that the earlier the oxygen bolus is delivered into the inspiratory cycle, the more efficient the oxygen delivery will be, which correlates to F_1O_2. To respond and deliver oxygen effectively in this relatively small window of time requires excellent trigger sensitivity and a very quick bolus response. Oxygen boluses delivered late in inspiration may not produce the desired F_IO_2 and therefore will be less effective in improving blood oxygen levels, because portions of the bolus may fall into the anatomical dead space.

OCDs operate using precision valves and orifices to sense breathing by measuring extremely small pressure changes in the tubing and then responding (triggering) rapidly to deliver the oxygen. The valve systems may be pneumatic, electronic, or a combination of systems. The outlet pressures, flow rates, and patterns are precise and calculated to deliver a specific volume of oxygen. The trigger sensitivity, flow rate, bolus size, and waveform characteristics per setting are generally specific to each make/model of OCD and are not uniform across all devices (**Figure 2-19**). That is to say, the setting of 1, 2, 3, and so on for a given device may deliver a different net amount of oxygen per breath than another make/model of OCD at the same setting. This is a very important point that is often confusing to clinicians and a frequent source of debate among engineers, researchers, healthcare practitioners, and patients.

PDOCs are low flow oxygen delivery devices that are modeled after low, continuous flow nasal cannula oxygen therapy. In theory, they are designed to deliver a volume of oxygen consistent with what would be delivered using a traditional, continuous flow nasal cannula system (i.e., settings of 1, 2, etc. are often claimed in the operator's manuals to be equivalent to 1 L/min, 2 L/min, etc. of continuous flow). However, continuous flow oxygen delivery via nasal cannula results in high breath-to-breath F_IO_2 variability. Therefore, the setting number on a PDOC is based on simplifying assumptions including typical values for physiologic variables include tidal volume, respiratory rate, I:E ratio, inspiratory flow rate, and anatomic dead space. However, these values rarely, if ever, match the actual parameters of a real patient at any moment during oxygen therapy. This means that proper use of a PDOC requires some type of titration procedure (e.g., a 6-minute walk with pulse oximetry) to determine the setting on a particular device that satisfies the patient's oxygenation needs.

High Flow Devices

A high flow device is generally defined as one that can deliver a precise F_IO_2 at a flow rate that meets or exceeds the patient's inspiratory demand. Such devices are also classified as fixed-performance oxygen delivery systems. The three main types of high flow delivery devices are high flow nasal cannulas, **air entrainment masks**, and air entrainment (large volume) nebulizers.

High Flow Nasal Cannula

As indicated earlier, the generally accepted upper limit for the nasal cannula is 6 L/min in adults. One of the primary reasons for setting this upper limit is that flows greater than 6 L/min are cool and dry the nasal mucosa, causing irritation and patient discomfort. In early 2002, Vapotherm introduced a **high flow nasal cannula** that could provide flow rates up to 40 L/min through a nasal cannula with heated humidification.

The Vapotherm 2000i (no longer in production) was capable of producing flows from 1 to 40 L/min at temperatures between 91.4°F (33°C) and 109.4°F (43°C) and a relative humidity of at least 95%. F_IO_2 was controlled by an air/oxygen blender located proximal to the device and adjustable from 0.21 to 1.0. Flow rate was controlled by a flowmeter attached to the blender. Warming and humidification of the gas going to the patient occurs in a vapor transfer cartridge, where air and water are separated by a membrane permeable to water vapor. The membrane consisted of microtubules constructed of polysulfone material.[15]

Vapotherm's current product, the Precision Flow (**Figure 2-20A**), incorporates an internal electronic blender and flow controller to deliver heated, humidified high flow gas therapy. As with the Vapotherm 2000i, water and gas pathways are incorporated into a disposable high or low flow patient circuit. Circuits are also available for administration of specialty gas, such as heliox and nitric oxide. Because the blender and flow controller are electronic, an internal battery is incorporated into the unit for emergency backup in the event of an AC power failure. The battery life is limited to 15 minutes and requires 2 hours to recharge.

The specific interface is a special nasal cannula that comes in different sizes, depending on the age of the patient (see **Figure 2-20B, C**).

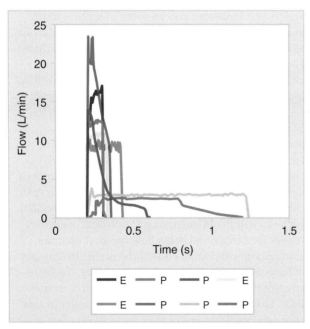

FIGURE 2-19 Oxygen pulse flow waveforms for PDOCs: (E) electronically controlled, (P) pneumatically controlled.

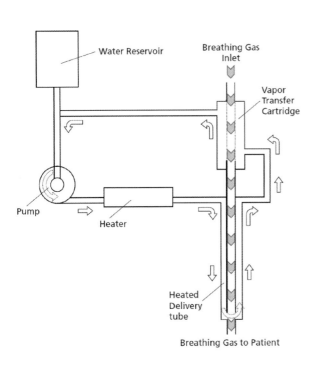

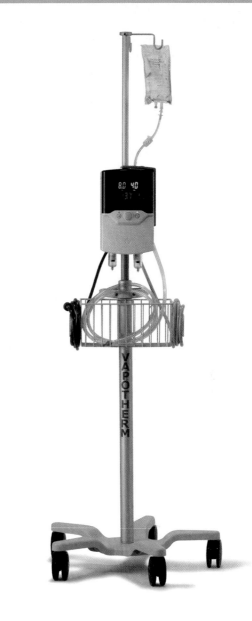

A

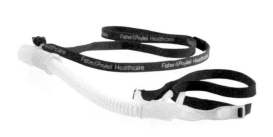

B

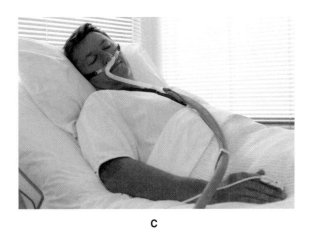

C

FIGURE 2-20 A. Examples of a device providing heated high flow gas for nasal oxygen therapy. B, C. Example of the interface used for heated high flow nasal oxygen. The cannula prongs are larger compared to a standard nasal cannula.

Art and photo A courtesy of Vapotherm. Photos B and C courtesy of Fisher & Paykel Healthcare.

Salter Labs produces a nonheated high flow system consisting of a special nasal cannula (1600HF) and bubble humidifier (#7900). This system is designed to provide flows of up to 15 L/min. It is capable of delivering oxygen concentrations of up to 75% and a relative humidity of up to 79%.[6,16]

As a relatively new modality, clinicians are still determining the best uses for the high flow nasal cannula. Several studies have shown that the high flow nasal cannula is a viable alternative to reservoir masks for patients requiring high concentrations of oxygen.[17–19] In a systematic review, Kernick and Magarey[20] reported the high flow nasal cannula "may be used as an intermediate therapy to improve oxygenation in adult critical care patients."

Several studies addressed the debate regarding the potential for a high flow nasal cannula to produce a CPAP effect and to serve as a viable alternative to nasal or mask CPAP. In a systematic review of nine studies in preterm infants, Dani et al.[21] concluded that the high flow nasal cannula should be limited to patients requiring oxygen therapy. Parke et al.[22], using the Fisher-Paykel Optiflow system, examined the amount of positive pressure generated in the airways of post–cardiac surgery patients. The Fisher-Paykel Optiflow system is capable of delivering oxygen concentrations from 21% to 100% and flow rates up to 50 L/min. Pressures of about 3 cm H_2O were generated at a flow of 50 L/min. The investigators concluded that the pressure generated by the high flow nasal cannula was of questionable clinical significance.

In a bench study of pressures generated in an infant model, Volsko et al.,[23] using flow rates of 2–6 L/min, determined that the high flows did not generate clinically important continuous airway pressure. Urbano et al.[24] studied the amount of positive pressure generated at various flows in a pediatric model. They also concluded that the high flows produced a low-level CPAP.

Based on the previous data, high flow nasal oxygen systems should be considered oxygen delivery systems, not nasal CPAP systems. High flow oxygen systems appear to be a viable alternative to reservoir masks in patients requiring moderate concentrations of oxygen. Roca et al.[19] compared the high flow nasal cannula with oxygen administration by face mask in patients experiencing acute respiratory failure and concluded the high flow nasal cannula was well tolerated and associated with improved oxygenation.

Gas heated to body temperature at 95–100% relative humidity may have the added benefit of increasing ciliary activity and decreasing the viscosity of airway secretions. Regardless of its intended use, because it is delivered directly into the nose rather than over the face, high flow oxygen therapy is generally viewed as more comfortable and less confining for the patient than a mask. Oxygen is delivered in a manner that does not disrupt the patient's ability to communicate, eat, drink, or expectorate.

The prongs of the high flow nasal cannula are a wider bore when compared to the traditional low flow nasal cannula. The prongs are placed inside the patient's nares, and the cannula unit secured to the patient's face by an adjustable elastic band. Stiff, smooth lumen tubing at the end of the cannula connects to the special high flow humidifier.

Therapeutic benefits are improved when the patient's nares and nasal passages are patent. The larger bore prongs may be uncomfortable for some patients. Skin integrity must be assessed, and any irritation or breakdown addressed. As a precaution, the temperature of the humidified gas flow is monitored to reduce the risk of thermal injury. There is also a potential for gastric distension, because a relatively high flow of gas is administered intranasally. As a further precaution, because of the increased heat and humidity, microbial contamination can be a risk.

Air-Entrainment Masks

The air-entrainment mask is a high flow oxygen delivery device that can provide a variety of precise F_iO_2s at flows that can greatly exceed the patient's inspiratory demand. Although these masks are often referred to erroneously as "Venturi" masks, they operate on the principle of jet mixing, not the Venturi principle.[25] A 7-foot hose connects the oxygen flowmeter to a jet that is placed just below the reservoir of the mask. Small holes (or entrainment ports) surround the jet (see **Figure 2-21**). As the oxygen flows through the jet, it accelerates. Fast-moving oxygen molecules collide with the stationary molecules in the room air and drag them through the ports. The mixture of room air and oxygen then flows to the patient.

The specific F_iO_2 is determined by the ratio of room air to oxygen in the gas mixture (every F_iO_2 between 0.22 and 0.99 has a unique ratio, see later in this section). The ratio of room air to oxygen is controlled by varying either the diameter of the jet or the diameter of the entrainment ports, depending on the manufacturer. Generally, the smaller the diameter of the jet, the more room air will be entrained, thus resulting in a decreased F_iO_2. Conversely, the smaller the entrainment ports, the less room air will be entrained, thus resulting in an increased F_iO_2. Studies have shown that these masks are reasonably accurate, especially at an F_iO_2 of 0.30 or less and in patients with relatively low inspiratory demand (< 200 L/min).[26–29]

Some air-entrainment masks include an optional collar that goes around the entrainment ports. A large-diameter hose connects the collar to a large volume nebulizer. This provides additional humidification, should that be desired.

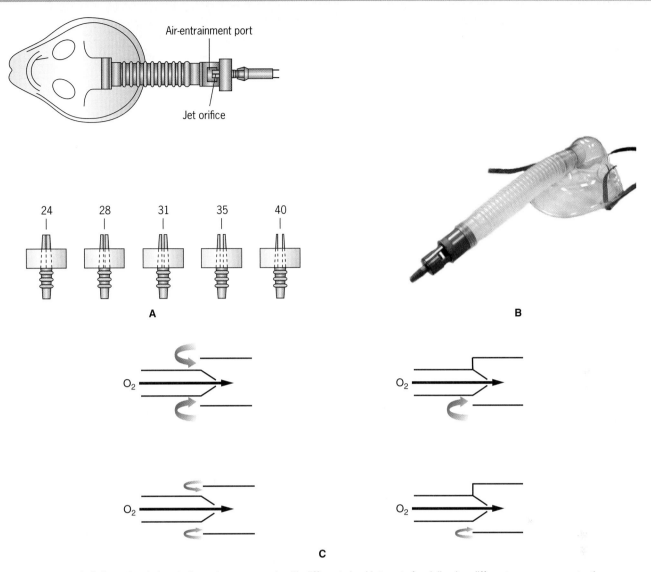

FIGURE 2-21 A. Schematic of air entrainment oxygen mask with different sized jet ports for delivering different oxygen concentrations. B. Photo of entrainment mask. C. Changes in oxygen concentration can also be achieved by changing the size of the air entrainment ports. The less entrainment of room air, the higher the oxygen concentration delivered by the mask. F_IO_2 is lowest in upper left diagram (most air entrainment) and highest in lower right diagram (least air entrainment).

Art A adapted from Kacmarek RM. Methods of oxygen delivery in the hospital. *Prob Respir Care*. 1990; 3:536–574. Photo courtesy of Dr. Dean Hess.

Air-entrainment masks are mostly used in patients who require precise concentrations of oxygen in the low to moderate range (e.g., patients with COPD who chronically retain CO_2) or in patients who have a highly variable respiratory pattern. They might also be useful for conditions requiring low concentrations of oxygen in which a nasal cannula may not be well tolerated (i.e., cleft palate, nasal septal defects, etc.).

Air-entrainment masks are confining and may interfere with a patient's ability to communicate, eat, drink, or expectorate. Especially while eating, the patient may frequently remove the mask, disrupting the oxygen therapy. In such cases, a nasal cannula may be used to provide oxygen therapy for short durations (i.e.,

during meals). The clinician should take care that the entrainment ports remain free of obstruction.

Traditionally, air-entrainment masks provide six to seven F_IO_2 settings, ranging from 0.24 to 0.50 (e.g., 0.24, 0.28, 0.31, 0.35, 0.40, 0.50). The oxygen flow should be set so that the combined flow of air and oxygen always exceeds the patient's inspiratory demand. Woolner and Larkin[28] recommend that the total flow exceed 30% of the patient's peak inspiratory flow at settings of 0.30 or less. Other sources recommend that the total flow should be at least 3 times the patient's minute volume. Mask manufacturers traditionally publish recommended flowmeter settings for each F_IO_2. These range from 4 L/min for 0.24 to 12–15 L/min for 0.50.

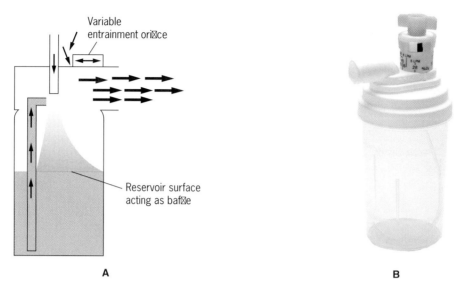

Variable
entrainment orifice

Reservoir surface
acting as baffle

A

B

FIGURE 2-22 Air entrainment large volume nebulizer.

Art modified from Cohen N, Fink J. Humidity and aerosols. In: Eubanks DH, Bone RC, eds. *Principles and applications of cardiorespiratory care equipment.* St. Louis, MO: Mosby; 1994. Photo courtesy of Teleflex.

Air-Entrainment Nebulizer

The air-entrainment nebulizer or large volume nebulizer (**Figure 2-22**) is a device that provides both a precise F_IO_2 and particulate water or saline (i.e., aerosol). It is used in conjunction with face masks (generally aerosol masks), face tents, tracheostomy masks, and T-pieces (Brigg's adaptors) (see **Figure 2-23**). These devices work

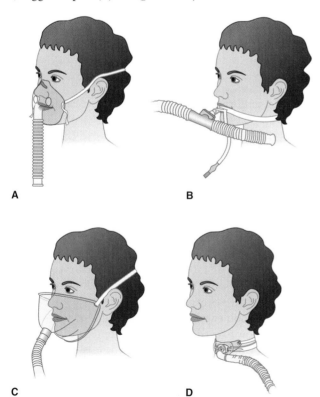

A   B

C   D

FIGURE 2-23 A. Aerosol mask. B. Briggs T-piece. C. Face tent. D. Tracheostomy collar.

Art adapted from Fink JR, Hunt GE. *Clinical practice of respiratory care.* Philadelphia, PA: Lippincott Williams & Wilkins; 1999.

on the same principle as entrainment masks. Oxygen from a flowmeter flows through a jet nozzle surrounded by an entrainment port. The acceleration of the gas molecules through the jet causes room air to be drawn in through the port in such an amount as to produce a specific ratio of air to oxygen. The device is designed so that the diameter of the jet is fixed but the size of the entrainment port is variable, controlled by a labeled dial at the top.

Because the air-entrainment nebulizer combines high gas flow with aerosol particles, it is especially useful for patients with artificial airways (endotracheal or tracheostomy tube). A patient whose upper airway is bypassed generally requires that the inspiratory gas be heated and humidified in order to minimize the drying of the airway mucosa. Because some patients with tracheostomy tubes might not require supplemental oxygen, the device can be attached to a compressed air flowmeter or an air compressor and used strictly to provide humidified gas to the lower airway.

The air-entrainment nebulizer is filled with sterile water or normal saline and attached to the appropriate gas source (usually an oxygen flowmeter). The entrainment dial is set to the prescribed F_IO_2 and the flowmeter is set at the appropriate liter flow (see later in this chapter). The device is connected to the appropriate patient interface (face mask, T-piece, face tent, or tracheostomy mask) via large-bore corrugated tubing.

The air-entrainment nebulizer is a high flow device. Thus, the clinician must ensure that the total flow of gas (air plus oxygen) going to the patient always exceeds the patient's inspiratory demand. This concern for sufficient total flow is especially significant when the F_IO_2 is 0.50 or above. Under these circumstances, it is recommended that two air-entrainment nebulizers be used in parallel in order to double the flow going to the patient. Based on the data presented in Foust et al.,[30] it is further recommended that these devices not be used at all for patients who require an F_IO_2 of 0.80 or greater.

Because the device generates an aerosol, there is always the potential for microbial contamination. This is especially important to monitor because, in the case of artificial airways, the upper airway defense mechanisms have been bypassed. Also, as the aerosol particles flow through the corrugated tubing, some of the particles will rain out and accumulate in the gravity-dependent portion of the tubing. The presence of water in the tubing could potentially create back pressure that will decrease the amount of air being entrained, thus increasing the F_IO_2. A drainage bag should be placed in the circuit so as to minimize this accumulation. As a final precaution, the clinician should ensure that the fluid in the nebulizer reservoir does not fall below recommended levels.

The air-entrainment nebulizers commercially available are disposable and offer 6 to 8 F_IO_2 settings, generally ranging from 0.28 to 1.0. The flow rates are adjusted so as to ensure a total flow that always exceeds inspiratory demand. Often, in actual practice, the clinician will use a flowmeter setting of 15 L/min.

Calculation of Required Flow to Meet Patient Inspiratory Demand

A high flow device is only high flow if the total flow delivered to the patient at least meets the patient's peak inspiratory flow. The patient's peak inspiratory flow can be approximated by first assuming the flow waveform is sinusoidal and estimating the inspiratory time based on the spontaneous breathing frequency and the tidal volume based on the patient's ideal body weight. Then we calculate the air and oxygen flows necessary to meet this peak flow from the entrainment ratio:

1. *Calculate the ventilatory period:* This is equal to 60 seconds divided by the patient's breathing frequency (e.g., if the patient is breathing 20 times a minute the ventilatory period is 3 seconds).
2. *Calculate the inspiratory time:* A sine wave has an inspiratory to expiratory time ratio of 1:1, so the inspiratory time is half the ventilatory period (e.g., 3 seconds divided by 2 = 1.5 seconds).
3. *Estimate the patient's tidal volume:* This is roughly 7 mL per kilogram of ideal body weight. Ideal body weight is estimated using one of these equations:

> Male ideal body weight (kg) = 50 + [0.91 × (Height in cm − 152.4)]

> Female ideal body weight (kg) = 45.5 + [0.91 × (Height in cm − 152.4)]

For example, a male with a height of 5'10" (178 cm) has an ideal body weight of about 73 kg. The estimated tidal volume is thus 7 mL/kg × 73 kg = 511 mL.

4. *Calculate the peak inspiratory flow:* Average inspiratory flow is tidal volume divided by inspiratory time (e.g., 511 mL/1.5 s = 341 mL/s). Convert mL/s to L/min using a factor of 0.06. For example, (341 mL/s) × (60 s/min) × (1 L / 1,000 mL) = 20 L/min. Peak inspiratory flow is calculated by using the fact that the peak value of a sine wave is 1.6 times the mean value. Rounding up for safety, we get: Peak flow = 2 × Mean flow (e.g., Peak flow = 2 × 20 L/min = 40 L/min).
5. *Determine the entrainment ratio from the desired F_IO_2 (see also **Table 2-1**):* Air flow/Oxygen flow = (1.0 − 0.21)/(F_IO_2 − 0.21). For example, if we want to deliver 40% oxygen, then air flow:oxygen flow = (1.0 − 0.40)/(0.40 − 0.21) ≈ 3.
6. *Determine the oxygen flow to an entrainment mask that will make the total flow delivered to the patient at least equal to the patient's peak inspiratory flow:* The entrainment ratio gives the number of parts air per part oxygen per minute. The total parts are the entrainment ratio plus 1. Divide the estimated peak inspiratory flow by the number of parts to get the oxygen flow setting. For example, the entrainment ratio for 40% oxygen is 3. Total parts are 3 + 1 = 4. Oxygen flow required to make a total flow equal to the estimated peak inspiratory flow = 40 L/min divided by 4 = 10 L/min. Note that this is a conservative estimate because if the patient really does have a sinusoidal inspiratory flow waveform, the peak flow exists for only a fraction of a second and the flow during most of the inspiration is well below this value. Therefore, providing 40 L/min of total flow to our example patient should be more than enough to meet his flow demands and assure a stable F_IO_2.

Note that the higher the F_IO_2, the lower the total flow for any given oxygen flowmeter setting. If the patient requires a high F_IO_2 and also has a high estimated peak inspiratory flow (e.g., is breathing rapidly) the total flow can be doubled by attaching two nebulizers in tandem (**Figure 2-24**).

Enclosure Devices

As the name would suggest, these are devices in which all or part of the patient's body is placed. Oxygen then flows into the device, increasing the F_IO_2 inside the enclosure. Currently, enclosure devices are used almost exclusively with neonates and infants. Examples of enclosures include oxygen hoods, incubators (often called isolettes after the name of a very popular early brand of infant incubator), and oxygen tents.

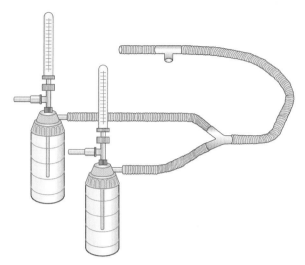

FIGURE 2-24 Total flow to the patient can be increased by joining two nebulizers.

Oxygen Hoods

Oxygen hoods are devices that fit around the head of a neonate or infant. Oxygen then flows into the hood from a heated humidifier attached to an air/oxygen blender or from an air entrainment nebulizer (see **Figure 2-25**). The hoods are typically made of transparent plastic.

The oxygen hood is best used for neonates who require a moderately high F_IO_2 but cannot tolerate other delivery devices.[31] It may also be used as an alternative for infants and neonates who cannot tolerate nasal oxygen. Although only the patient's head is within the hood, there is still potential for disruption of therapy in the case of feeding or routine nursing care. In these cases, an alternative form of oxygen delivery should be available.

Because infants and neonates are particularly sensitive to temperature changes, the temperature in the hood should be such as to preserve a neutral thermal environment.[9] Thus, the oxygen going into the hood should be heated and the temperature inside the hood should be monitored.

The baby's oxygen level should be monitored in order to minimize hypoxia or hyperoxia. Also, oxygen concentrations may vary within the hood, so the F_IO_2 should be monitored with an oxygen analyzer whose sensor is placed as near the mouth and nose as possible.[9] Another concern is the increased noise level produced by the flow of oxygen in the hood.[32] This should be considered and monitored, as well. One method that has been suggested to reduce noise levels when using a heated air entrainment nebulizer is to power the nebulizer with compressed air and bleed in the oxygen.[33]

Flow rates into the hood should be >7 L/min in order to flush out CO_2.[11,31] Generally, flows in the 10–15 L/min range should be sufficient for infants.[11] Because the flow is generated through either an air/oxygen blender or an air entrainment nebulizer, the F_IO_2 can theoretically range from 0.21 to 1.0. However, although patients requiring high oxygen concentrations can be managed in the oxygen hood, it is difficult to maintain an F_IO_2 greater than 0.5 because of the neck opening and the need to open the hood for nursing care.[31]

Incubator

The incubator (also called an isolette) is an enclosure device designed to contain the entire body of the neonate at a temperature that will facilitate thermal stability. It is usually made of transparent plexiglass (see **Figure 2-26**).

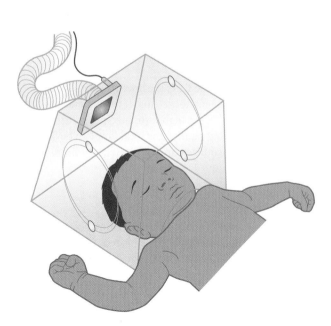

FIGURE 2-25 Oxygen hood.

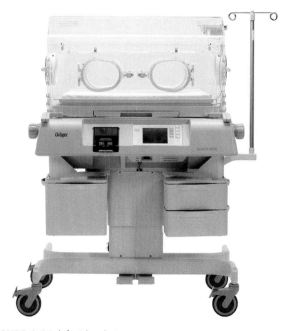

FIGURE 2-26 Infant incubator.

Although it can be used as an oxygen delivery device, it is most often used to provide a temperature-controlled environment to small infants and neonates. To accomplish this, temperature is regulated via a servo-control mechanism and a sensor attached to the patient. As with the oxygen hood, the patient should be maintained in a neutral thermal environment. Humidity can be provided via a blow-over humidifier built into the unit or via an external humidifier.

Oxygen delivery is achieved by connecting small-bore tubing from a flowmeter to a nipple connector on the unit. Some incubators have two oxygen connections, one for an F_IO_2 of around 0.40 and one for high concentrations of oxygen. This is accomplished by opening or closing an air entrainment port. Although some units have solenoids that can control the inward flow of oxygen, it is still difficult to regulate the oxygen concentration within the enclosure because the incubator is frequently opened to provide care and it has a large inside volume, making it less than ideal as an oxygen delivery device. For this reason, hoods are sometimes used inside the incubator. Clearly, the internal F_IO_2 should be monitored intermittently and the patient's oxygenation status should be checked, especially if a high concentration is needed to prevent or minimize hyperoxia. At least one manufacturer, Dräger Medical, makes an incubator with automatic control of oxygen from 21% to 65%.

Oxygen Tent

As the name would suggest, the **oxygen tent** is a clear plastic enclosure that fits over the entire bed. The patient remains within the enclosure. Oxygen flows into the device usually from an air-entrainment nebulizer or a high-output aerosol generator, producing a relatively dense mist. The mist is cooled by a refrigeration unit or by flowing over ice. The oxygen tent was one of the first oxygen delivery devices used; however, it is seldom used today, especially for oxygen delivery.

The primary use of the tent is to provide a cool, moist, oxygenated environment for patients experiencing severe laryngotracheobronchitis.[34] In this situation, the cool mist might facilitate vasoconstriction and, thus, help to relieve the upper airway obstruction associated with the condition. Also, it could potentially be useful in pediatric patients who are too large for an oxygen hood. However, the value of this therapy is questionable and informal communication among respiratory care managers (i.e., from professional organization listservs) suggests that many hospitals have eliminated tent therapy altogether.

There are many problems associated with oxygen tents. The first is the risk of electric shock. This could result from sparks generated by any electronic or friction device (e.g., call light or friction toy) contained in the enclosure. Second, it is very difficult to control F_IO_2 within the enclosure because of the enormous volume and because the tent is frequently opened to observe

the child or provide care. The F_IO_2 should be monitored periodically with an oxygen analyzer, with the sensor placed near the patient's face.[34] A third problem is that the dense mist can make it difficult to observe the patient from outside; thus, it becomes necessary to open the enclosure often. Also, with the enclosure, there is a slight risk of asphyxiation. Finally, should the refrigeration unit fail or the flow of gas into the tent be disrupted, there is a loss of the cooling effect along with loss of oxygen.

There are no recommended flow ranges for the oxygen tent available in the peer-reviewed literature. Clearly, the flow needs to be relatively high (i.e., > 10 L/min) in order to flush any exhaled carbon dioxide out of the large volume of the enclosure. The oxygen concentration is highly variable, regardless of the device used to generate the oxygen flow. This is again because of the large volume and the frequent opening of the tent. It is highly unlikely that F_IO_2s greater than 0.40 can be achieved consistently. Because of this variability, the patient's oxygenation should be monitored periodically.

Heliox

Helium is a gas that is less dense than either air or oxygen (**Table 2-3**). It is also an inert gas, meaning that it does not take part in biochemical reactions in the body. The low density is the property that makes it useful as a medical gas because it decreases the effective flow resistance in patients with upper airway obstruction (e.g., foreign body aspiration, postextubation stridor, or croup). This can be appreciated by recalling that airway obstruction causes turbulent flow when breathing air or oxygen. Turbulent flow requires a higher pressure drop across the airway for a given flow than normal laminar flow and hence increases the effort to inspire. Whether turbulence develops depends on the density of the gas; the lower the density, the less high the flow can be without turbulence (Reynolds number[35]). Thus, breathing helium decreases turbulence around an airway obstruction and decreases the work of breathing. On the other hand, for laminar flow (typical in the lower airways) the pressure drop across the airway is dependent on the viscosity of the gas (Poiseuille's law[35]); the higher the viscosity, the higher the pressure drop across the airways for a given flow and the higher the effort to inspire. Because helium has a higher viscosity than air and only

TABLE 2-3
Physical Properties of Medical Gases

Gas	Density (g/L)	Viscosity (μ poise)	Thermoconductivity (μ cal × cm × 5 × °K)
Air	1.293	170.8	58.0
Oxygen	1.429	192.6	58.5
Helium	0.179	188.7	352.0

Courtesy of Dr. Dean Hess.

slightly less viscosity than oxygen, breathing helium may have limited value for diseases affecting the small airways (e.g., emphysema and asthma). Nevertheless, there is some evidence of benefit in the management of pediatric and adult respiratory disease.[36,37]

Because helium is inert, it must be mixed with oxygen to support life. The mixture is called **heliox**. Heliox is available in standard mixtures in large compressed gas cylinders (80% oxygen/20% helium or 70% oxygen/30% helium). A heliox mixture may be diluted with oxygen to increase the F_IO_2, but this decreases the concentration of helium. An $F_IO_2 > 0.40$ has a low concentration of helium and probably no clinical benefit.

Nonintubated patients may receive heliox therapy using a nonrebreathing oxygen mask (**Figure 2-27**). If you use a flowmeter calibrated for oxygen to deliver heliox, the lower density of an 80% helium/20% oxygen mixture will cause the actual flow of heliox to be 1.8 times greater than the indicated flow. However, accurate flow measurement is not necessary for mask administration, because the only requirement is that flow is sufficient to keep the reservoir bag from deflating on inspiration.

Heliox can be administered through a mechanical ventilator with caution. Some ventilators (e.g., the CareFusion Avea ventilator) are designed to deliver accurate ventilation with heliox. Ventilators not designed for heliox use may be adversely affected by the density, viscosity, and thermal conductivity differences of the gas compared to air or oxygen.[38]

Ventilation with helium–oxygen in place of air–oxygen mixtures can influence both the droplet size distribution and the mass of nebulized aerosol delivered to patients.[39] Compared to the usual aerosol delivery technique, heliox-driven salbutamol nebulization may shorten the stay in the emergency department.[40] A recent bench study also suggests that heliox may improve aerosol delivered to pediatric patients through a high flow nasal cannula.[41]

Carbon Dioxide

At one time physicians thought that rebreathing carbon dioxide from a paper bag could relieve anxiety attacks. Ironically, today it is well known that inhalation of carbon dioxide can induce in humans an emotion closely replicating spontaneous panic attacks, as defined by current psychiatry nosology.[42] Carbon dioxide/oxygen mixtures, called **carbogen**, have been used to terminate seizures (petit mal), to improve regional blood flow by dilating vessels in the brain of stroke victims, and to encourage ophthalmic artery blood flow.[43] Introducing small amounts of carbon dioxide into inspired gas before and after cardiac surgery on infants with hypoplastic left heart syndrome can help limit pulmonary blood flow by increasing pulmonary vascular resistance. A system to do this has been described by Chatburn and Anderson.[44]

Nitric Oxide

Inhaled **nitric oxide** has been used as a selective (i.e., affecting the lung rather than the systemic vasculature) pulmonary vasodilator. It has been approved by the FDA for use in conjunction with ventilatory support where it is indicated for the treatment of term and near-term (> 34 weeks) neonates with hypoxic respiratory failure associated with clinical or echocardiographic evidence of pulmonary hypertension where it improves oxygenation and reduces the need for extracorporeal membrane oxygenation. When delivered along with oxygen, nitric oxide (NO) forms small amounts of nitrogen dioxide (NO_2), a toxic gas. The levels of NO_2 generated are dependent on F_IO_2, NO dose, and contact time between NO and oxygen. Therefore, delivery methods designed to minimize NO_2 generation and

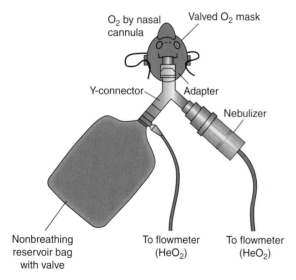

FIGURE 2-27 Mask setup for administration of heliox.

O₂ by nasal cannula
Valved O₂ mask
Y-connector
Adapter
Nebulizer
Nonbreathing reservoir bag with valve
To flowmeter (HeO₂)
To flowmeter (HeO₂)

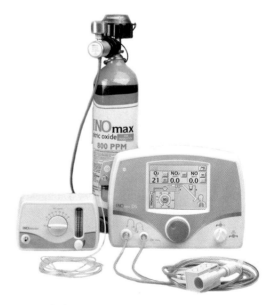

FIGURE 2-28 INOmax DSIR delivery system.
© Ikaria, Inc.

careful dosing of nitric oxide and monitoring of nitrogen dioxide are important.

Currently, the only commercially available device for delivering inhaled nitric oxide that is compatible with most ventilators in the United States is the INOmax DSIR system from IKARIA (**Figure 2-28**). This device can be used with or without a mechanical ventilator (e.g., noninvasive devices such as cannulas and nasal CPAP systems) and delivers nitric oxide from an 88 or a D-size compressed gas cylinder containing 800 parts per million (ppm) of nitric oxide (balance gas is nitrogen). During mechanical ventilation, the gas is introduced into the inspiratory limb on the dry side of the patient circuit through a port on an injector module that also contains a hot-film flow sensor, which measures ventilator gas flow. As flow in the ventilator circuit is measured, the nitric oxide is injected in a constant proportion to inspiratory flow to deliver a precise dose from 0.1 to 80 ppm. The delivery system monitors inspired gas concentrations for oxygen, nitric oxide, and nitrogen dioxide, with an alarm setting for each. The system also has a number of other alarms for delivery designed to minimize interruption of therapy. In the event of a system malfunction, the system also has two pneumatically powered systems to provide continuous delivery of nitric oxide.

References

1. Glover DW. *The history of respiratory therapy*. Bloomington, IN: AuthorHouse; 2010.
2. Duke T, Peel D, Graham S, et al. Oxygen concentrators: A practical guide for clinicians and technicians in developing countries. *Ann Top Paediatr.* 2010;30(2):87–101.
3. Dobson MB. Oxygen concentrators and cylinders. *Int J Tuberc Lung Dis.* 2001;5(6):520–523.
4. American Association for Respiratory Care. AARC guideline: Oxygen therapy for adults in the acute care facility. *Respir Care.* 2002;47(6):717–720.
5. Zhou S, Chatburn RL. Effect of the anatomic reservoir on low-flow oxygen delivery via nasal cannula: Constant flow versus pulse flow with portable oxygen concentrator. *Respir Care.* 2014;59(8):1199-1209. doi:10.4187/respcare.02878.
6. Wettstein R, Shelledy D, Peters J. Delivered oxygen concentrations using low-flow and high-flow nasal cannulas. *Respir Care.* 2005;50(5):604–609.
7. Casaburi R. Assessing the dose of supplemental oxygen: Let us compare methodologies. *Respir Care.* 2005;50(5):594–595.
8. Markovitz G, Colthurst J, Sorer T, Cooper C. Effective inspired oxygen concentration measured via transtracheal and oral gas analysis. *Respir Care.* 2010;55(4):453–459.
9. Branson R. The nuts and bolts of increasing arterial oxygenation: Devices and techniques. *Respir Care.* 1995;40(6):672–685.
10. Kuluz JW, McLaughlin GE, Gelman B, et al. The fraction of inspired oxygen in infants receiving oxygen via nasal cannula often exceeds safe levels. *Respir Care.* 2001;46(9):897–901.
11. American Association for Respiratory Care. AARC guideline: Neonatal and pediatric O2 delivery. *Respir Care.* 2002;47(6):707-716.
12. Christopher KL. Transtracheal oxygen catheters. *Clin Chest Med.* 2003;24(3):489–510.
13. McCoy R. Oxygen conserving techniques and devices. *Respir Care.* 2000;45(1):95–103.
14. Tiep BL, Lewis MI. Oxygen conservation and oxygen conserving devices in chronic lung disease: A review. *Chest.* 1987;92(2):263–272.
15. Vapotherm. *Operating manual for the 2000i.* Rev. E. Stevensville, MD: Vapotherm.
16. Waugh JB, Granger WM. An evaluation of 2 new devices for nasal high-flow gas therapy. *Respir Care.* 2004;49(8):902–906.
17. Price AM, Plowright C, Makowski A, Misztal B. Using a high-flow respiratory system (Vapotherm) within a high dependency setting. *Nurs Crit Care.* 2008;13(6):298–304.
18. Turnbull B. High-flow humidified oxygen therapy used to alleviate respiratory distress. *Br J Nurs.* 2008;17(19):1226–1230.
19. Roca O, Riera J, Torres F, Masclans J. High flow oxygen therapy in acute respiratory failure. *Respir Care.* 2010;55(4):408–413.
20. Kernick J, Magarey J. What is the evidence for the use of high flow nasal cannula oxygen in adult patients admitted to critical care units? A systematic review. *Aust Crit Care.* 2010;23(12):53–70.
21. Dani C, Pratesi S, Migliori C, Bertini G. High flow nasal cannula therapy as respiratory support in the preterm infant. *Pediatr Pulmonol.* 2009;44(7):629–634.
22. Parke RL, Eccleston ML, MacGuinness SP. The effects of flow on airway pressure during nasal high-flow oxygen therapy. *Respir Care.* 2011;56(8):1151–1155.
23. Volsko TA, Fedor K, Amadei J, Chatburn RL. High flow through a nasal cannula and CPAP effect in a simulated infant model. *Respir Care.* 2011;56(12):1893–1900.
24. Urbano J, del Castillo J, López-Herce J, Gallardo J, Solana MJ, Carillo A. High-flow oxygen therapy: Pressure analysis in a pediatric airway model. *Respir Care.* 2012;57(5):721–726.
25. Scacci R. Air entrainment masks: Jet mixing is how they work; the Bernoulli and Venturi principles are how they don't. *Respir Care.* 1977;24(7):928–931.
26. Hill SL, Barnes PK, Hollway T, Tennant R. Fixed performance masks: An evaluation. *Br Med J.* 1984;288(4):1261–1264.
27. Wagstaff TA, Soni N. Performance of six types of oxygen delivery devices at varying respiratory rates. *Anesthesia.* 2007;62(5):492–503.
28. Woolner DF, Larkin J. An analysis of the performance of a variable Venturi-type oxygen mask. *Anaesth Intensive Care.* 1980;8(1):44–51.
29. Fracchia G, Torda TA. Performance of Venturi oxygen delivery devices. *Anaesth Intensive Care.* 1980;8(4):426–430.
30. Foust GN, Potter WA, Wilons MD, Golden EB. Shortcomings of using two jet nebulizers in tandem with an aerosol face mask for optimal oxygen therapy. *Chest.* 1991;99(6):1346–1351.
31. Walsh BK, Brooks TM, Grenier BM. Oxygen therapy in the neonatal environment. *Respir Care.* 2009;54(9):1193–1202.
32. Mishoe SC, Brooks CW, Dennison FX. Octave waveband analysis to determine sound frequencies and intensities produced by nebulizers and humidifiers used with hoods. *Respir Care.* 1995;40(11):1120–1124.
33. Beckham RW, Mishoe SC. Sound levels inside incubators and oxygen hoods used with nebulizers and humidifiers. *Respir Care.* 1982;27(1):33–40.
34. Barnhart SL. Oxygen administration. In Walsh BK, Czervinske MP, DiBlasi RM, eds. *Perinatal and pediatric respiratory care.* St. Louis: Saunders; 2010:147–164.
35. Chatburn RL, Mireles-Cabodevila E. *Handbook of respiratory care.* 3rd ed. Sudbury, MA: Jones & Bartlett Learning; 2011.
36. Frazier MD, Cheifetz IM. The role of heliox in paediatric respiratory disease. *Paediatr Respir Rev.* 2010;11(1):46–53.
37. Adams JY, Sutter ME, Albertson TE. The patient with asthma in the emergency department. *Clin Rev Allergy Immunol.* 2012;43(1–2):14–29.
38. Venkataraman ST. Heliox during mechanical ventilation. *Respir Care.* 2006;51(6):632–639.

39. Martin AR, Ang A, Katz IM, Häussermann S, Caillibotte G, Texereau J. An in vitro assessment of aerosol delivery through patient breathing circuits used with medical air or a helium-oxygen mixture. *J Aerosol Med Pulm Drug Deliv.* 2011;24(5):225–234.

40. Braun Filho LR, Amantéa SL, Becker A, Vitola L, Marta VF, Krumenauer R. Use of helium-oxygen mixture (Heliox˚) in the treatment of obstructive lower airway disease in a pediatric emergency department. *J Pediatr (Rio J).* 2010;86(5):424–428.

41. Ari A, Harwood R, Sheard M, Dailey P, Fink JB. In vitro comparison of heliox and oxygen in aerosol delivery using pediatric high flow nasal cannula. *Pediatr Pulmonol.* 2011;46(8):795–801.

42. Colasanti A, Esquivel G, Schruers KJ, Griez EJ. On the psychotropic effects of carbon dioxide [published online ahead of print May 24, 2012]. *Curr Pharm Des.* 2012;18(35):5627–5637.

43. Hess DR, MacIntyer NR, Mishoe SC, Galvin WF, Adams AB. *Respiratory care. Principles and practice.* Sudbury, MA: Jones & Bartlett Learning; 2012:289.

44. Chatburn RL, Anderson SM. Controlling carbon dioxide delivery during mechanical ventilation. *Respir Care.* 1994;39(11):1039–1046.

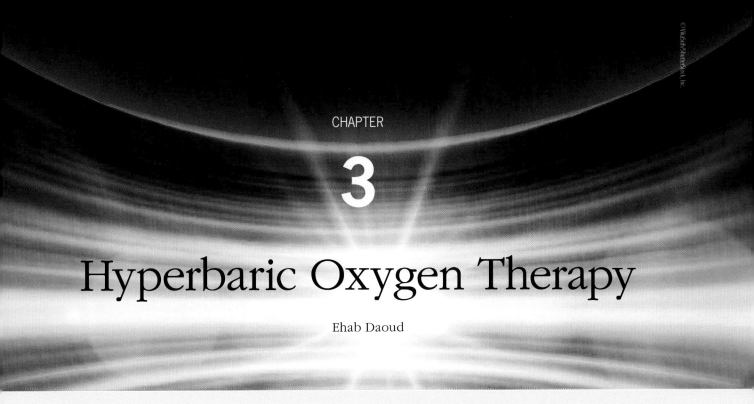

CHAPTER

3

Hyperbaric Oxygen Therapy

Ehab Daoud

CHAPTER OBJECTIVES

1. Discuss the physiology of hyperbaric oxygen.
2. Explain the mechanisms of action of hyperbaric oxygen.
3. Describe the indications and contraindications of hyperbaric oxygen.
4. List the side effects of hyperbaric oxygen.
5. Identify the hazards of hyperbaric oxygen.
6. Explain the concurrent use of mechanical ventilation and hyperbaric oxygen.
7. Describe the current available devices for hyperbaric oxygen.

KEY TERMS

Angiogenesis
Atmosphere absolute (ATA)
European Committee for
  Hyperbaric Medicine
  (ECHM)
Hyperbaric oxygen (HBO$_2$)
  therapy

Partial pressure
Reperfusion injury
Undersea and Hyperbaric
  Medical Society (UHMS)

Introduction

Hyperbaric oxygen (HBO$_2$) therapy is a fascinating, fast-growing field of medicine with many benefits and indications, and even more areas of growing research opportunities. This field requires knowledge of the physics of gases, gas laws, and the different oxygen delivery systems, thus making the respiratory care practitioner obviously suited to participate in and contribute to this field.

HBO$_2$ therapy is inhalation of oxygen at a pressure greater than atmospheric pressure at sea level. It can be viewed as a new application for an old, established technology that has emerged as either a primary or an adjunctive therapy to a multitude of medical and surgical conditions.[1,2]

This chapter will discuss the physiological principles of hyperbaric oxygen, as well as its indications, contraindications, complications, and hazards. A discussion of the different chambers, equipment, and monitoring used to evaluate oxygenation and ventilation as well as the use of concurrent mechanical ventilation is presented.

History

The first hyperbaric chamber was built by Henshaw in London in 1662 using manual bellows to compress room air. In 1791, Smeaton, an English engineer, had the first chamber built in cast steel and fed it with compressed air from a pump on a boat. The therapeutic use of hyperbaric oxygen grew in France between the middle of the 19th and the beginning of the 20th centuries. This was followed by multiple chambers opening in Europe and North America. The first chamber built in the United States was in 1861 in Rochester, New York, and the largest was built in 1927 in Cleveland, Ohio, by Cunningham. The largest chamber was 6 stories high and comprised 72 rooms. Among many people with an influence on the history of hyperbaric medicine, the most famous is certainly Paul Bert. His work *La Pression Barométrique* (1878) is universally known and is one of the foundations of hyperbaric medicine. His studies led to the discovery of the toxic effects HBO_2 has on living organisms.

Currently more than 500 centers in the United States offer hyperbaric oxygen therapy.[3] The recent advances in hyperbaric medicine started in 1955, which began the era of its scientific use. The Undersea Medical Society (UMS) was founded in 1967 by a group of physicians largely from the military. The society's name was changed in 1987 to the **Undersea and Hyperbaric Medical Society (UHMS)**, and the group now acts as the primary scientific body for hyperbaric medicine. Its published guidelines are adopted by the Centers for Medicare and Medicaid Services (CMS) as well as third-party payers to evaluate reimbursement for this therapy.

Description

Hyperbaric oxygen therapy is defined as a treatment in which a patient intermittently breathes 100% oxygen in a chamber pressurized higher than atmospheric pressure at sea level. Pressure is defined as force per unit surface. It can be measured in **atmosphere absolute (ATA)**, pounds per square inch (psi), millimeters of mercury (mm Hg or Torr), centimeters of water (cm H_2O), or feet of sea water (FSW) (**Table 3-1**).[2]

One way to classify a pressurized chamber is according to the number of occupants placed within it. A monoplace chamber is a single chamber accommodating one patient; a multiplace chamber is a larger chamber accommodating multiple patients. The monoplace chambers are directly pressurized with oxygen, whereas multiplace chambers are pressurized with air, and the oxygen is supplied by face mask, hood tent, or endotracheal tube. Monoplace chambers are usually used for treatment of chronic conditions, whereas multiplace

chambers are usually used to treat acute conditions to allow closer monitoring, especially of critically ill patients.[4] Mobile monoplace and multiplace chambers are available; however, portable chambers are only available as monoplace chambers.

Chamber pressure is usually maintained between 2.5 and 3 ATA. Acute conditions may require a small number of sessions (one or two), whereas chronic conditions may require multiple sessions (20 or more). Treatment sessions usually last between 45 and 300 minutes.[5] Detailed descriptions of the chambers and their equipment will follow in this chapter.

Principles of Operation/ Physiologic Principles

The principles of hyperbaric oxygen depend on many physical principles of gases and gas laws (e.g., Boyle's law, Henry's law, Dalton's law, Fick's law, Amontons' law). A very important mechanism of action of this therapy is its effects on the blood oxygen content and the oxygen tension in various tissues.

A pressure gradient called the *oxygen cascade* aids in the delivery of oxygen from the air to the tissues and the mitochondrial cellular level (**Figure 3-1**). At room air, the **partial pressure** of oxygen (PO_2) is around 160 mm

TABLE 3-1
Units of Pressure for Medical Gases and Their Equivalency at and Above Atmospheric Pressure at Sea Level

ATA	psi	mm Hg	cm H_2O	FSW
1	14.7	760	1,033	0
2	29.4	1,520	2,066	33
4	44.1	2,280	3,099	66
5	73.5	3,800	5,165	132
6	88.2	4,560	6,198	165

ATA: atmosphere absolute, psi: pounds per square inch, mm Hg: millimeters of mercury, cm H_2O: centimeters of water, FSW: feet of sea water

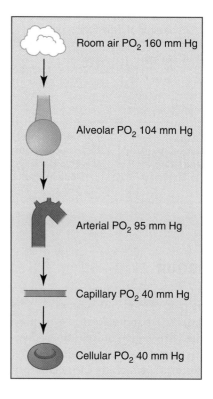

FIGURE 3-1 Oxygen cascade, with the partial pressure of oxygen at room air, alveolar level, arterial level, capillary level, and cellular level.

Data from Tibbles RM, Edelsberg JS. Hyperbaric-oxygen therapy. *N Engl J Med.* 1996;334:1642; Lumb AB. *Nunn's applied respiratory physiology.* 5th ed. Edinburgh, UK: Butterworth-Heinemann; 2003; Auerbach PS. *Wilderness medicine.* 5th ed. Philadelphia, PA: Elsevier Health Sciences; 2007.

TABLE 3-2
Partial Pressures of Gases (mm Hg) in Various Body Locations

	Inspired Gas	Alveolar Gas	Arterial Blood	Body Tissues	Venous Blood	Expired Gas
PO_2	160	100	95	40	40	115
PCO_2	0.28	39	40	45	45	33
PN_2	594	574	574	574	574	565
PH_2O	6	47	47	47	47	47

Hg; this drops to 100 mm Hg at the alveolar level, further dropping to 95 mm Hg at the arterial level. The pressure gradient continues at the capillary and interstitial spaces, where the PO_2 is about 40 mm Hg. The cells have a PO_2 of 3–4 mm Hg.[6,7] The partial pressures of gases at different levels in the body is summarized in **Table 3-2**.

The oxygen-carrying capacity of the blood depends on two factors: the amount of oxygen saturating the hemoglobin and the amount of oxygen dissolved in the plasma. This is illustrated in the following equation describing the arterial oxygen content (CaO_2):

$$CaO_2 = (1.34 \times Hgb \times SaO_2) + (0.003 \times PaO_2)$$

Where:

1.34 is the amount of oxygen carried by hemoglobin (mL standard temperature and pressure dry per g of hemoglobin).
Hgb is the hemoglobin concentration (g/100 mL).
SaO_2 is the arterial oxygen saturation (%).
0.003 is the amount of oxygen dissolved in plasma (mL/mm Hg).
PaO_2 is the arterial partial pressure of oxygen (mm Hg).

The amount of oxygen dissolved in plasma (0.3 mL/dL) is usually very small and mostly negligible at sea level with normal PaO_2, SaO_2, and Hgb.[8] Increasing the pressure from 1 ATA to 2.5 ATA results in increasing the oxygen dissolved in plasma 3 to 5 times; increasing the oxygen inspired to 100% increases the oxygen dissolved in plasma 17 to 20 times (6 mL/dL) (**Figure 3-2**). This can increase the PaO_2 to 2,000 mm Hg and oxygen tension in tissues to 400 mm Hg.[5,7,9] The PaO_2, oxygen dissolved in plasma (**Figure 3-3**), and CaO_2 continue to rise exponentially as the ATA increases (**Figure 3-4**). This increase in arterial oxygen content can meet the resting tissue requirements without any contribution from the oxygen bound to hemoglobin.[10]

Gas Laws

The gas laws explain the physical relationships of gas under changing pressure, volume, and temperature within fluids.[2,11] These physical relationships explain

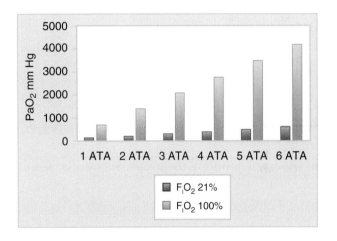

FIGURE 3-2 Partial pressure of oxygen (PaO_2) at different atmospheric pressures from 1 to 6 at F_iO_2 of 21% (room air) compared to 100% at the same ATA.

Data from Tibbles RM, Edelsberg JS. Hyperbaric-oxygen therapy. *N Engl J Med*. 1996;334:1642; Lumb AB. *Nunn's applied respiratory physiology*. 5th ed. Edinburgh, UK: Butterworth-Heinemann; 2003; Auerbach PS. *Wilderness medicine*. 5th ed. Philadelphia, PA: Elsevier Health Sciences; 2007.

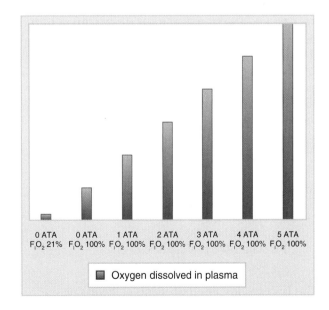

FIGURE 3-3 Oxygen dissolved in plasma increases exponentially as the F_iO_2 and ATA increase.

Data from Tibbles RM, Edelsberg JS. Hyperbaric-oxygen therapy. *N Engl J Med*. 1996;334:1642; Lumb AB. *Nunn's applied respiratory physiology*. 5th ed. Edinburgh, UK: Butterworth-Heinemann; 2003; Auerbach PS. *Wilderness medicine*. 5th ed. Philadelphia, PA: Elsevier Health Sciences; 2007.

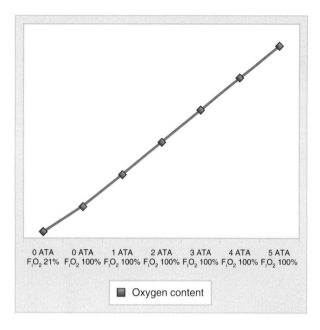

0 ATA	0 ATA	1 ATA	2 ATA	3 ATA	4 ATA	5 ATA
F_iO_2 21%	F_iO_2 100%	F_iO_2 100%	F_iO_2 100%	F_iO_2 100%	F_iO_2 100%	F_iO_2 100%

■ Oxygen content

FIGURE 3-4 Oxygen content (CaO_2) increases exponentially as the F_iO_2 and ATA increase.

Data from Tibbles RM, Edelsberg JS. Hyperbaric-oxygen therapy. *N Engl J Med.* 1996;334:1642; Lumb AB. *Nunn's applied respiratory physiology.* 5th ed. Edinburgh, UK: Butterworth-Heinemann; 2003; Auerbach PS. *Wilderness medicine.* 5th ed. Philadelphia, PA: Elsevier Health Sciences; 2007.

the beneficial physiologic effects of hyperbaric oxygen therapy on intravascular and tissue gas bubble reduction, improved oxygen delivery, vasoconstriction, modulation of inflammation, **angiogenesis,** and antimicrobial activity.[9,12]

Boyle's Law

First described by Sir Robert Boyle (1627–1691) in 1662, this law states: The product of pressure (P) and volume (V) in a confined amount of gas at equal temperature (T) remains constant. It describes how the volume of gas in a fluid is related to the pressure exerted on it. The volume is inversely proportionate to pressure; that is, if the pressure increases, the volume of gas decreases and vice versa.

$$P_1 \times V_1 = P_2 \times V_2$$

Where:

P is pressure applied to the gas.
V is the volume of the gas.
1 is state 1 of a confined amount of gas.
2 is state 2 of a confined amount of gas.

This law explains how the benefits of increasing the pressure will lead to the reduction of gas bubbles in air embolism. It also explains some of the side effects of this therapy; during decompression of pressure, any trapped gas in a body cavity (e.g., ear or thorax) can expand and cause barotraumas.

Henry's Law

First described by William Henry (1774–1836) in 1803, this gas law states: The mass of a gas (C) that dissolves in a defined volume of liquid is directly proportional to the pressure of the gas (P). It describes the effect of pressure on the concentration of a gas in a fluid depending on the solubility coefficient (α) of that gas. The amount of gas dissolved in a liquid is proportional to the partial pressure of that gas.

$$C = P \times \alpha$$

Where:

C is the concentration (mass).
P is the pressure applied to the gas.
α is the solubility coefficient of the gas in mL of gas/atmosphere/L of fluid.

In Celsius, the solubility coefficient (α) of air is 14.8; oxygen, 24.4; nitrogen, 12.6; helium, 8.3; and carbon dioxide, 18.8.

This law explains the benefit of hyperbaric oxygen therapy in increasing the tissue oxygen tension. It also explains how the pressure-dependent solubility of inert gases (e.g., nitrogen) in body liquids and tissues is crucial for the development of decompression sickness.

Dalton's Law

First described by John Dalton (1766–1844) in 1801, this gas law states: The total pressure exerted by a gaseous mixture is equal to the sum of the pressures that would be exerted by the gases if they alone were present and occupied the total volume. The partial pressure of a gas (P) equals the product of total pressure of the gaseous mixture (P_{tot}) and the fraction of the gas (F).

$$P = P_{tot} \times F$$

Where:

P is the partial pressure of the gas.
P_{tot} is the total pressure of the whole gaseous mixture.
F is the fraction of the gas in the whole volume (e.g., FO_2 in air is 0.21).

This law can explain the oxygen toxicity that may occur with hyperbaric oxygen, because both the partial pressure and the fraction percentages are markedly elevated.

Fick's Law of Diffusion

First described by Adolf Fick (1829–1901) in 1855, this gas law states: The diffusion of a gas across a membrane is proportional to the surface area of the membrane, the concentration gradient of the gas (partial pressure difference across the membrane), and the diffusion coefficient of the gas but is inversely related to the distance.

$$R = D \times A \times \frac{(\Delta P)}{d}$$

Where:

  R is the rate of diffusion.
  D is the diffusion coefficient of the gas (proportional to the solubility of the gas but inversely proportional to the molecular weight of the gas).
  A is the surface area of the membrane.
  ΔP is the partial pressure difference across the membrane.
  d is the distance across the membrane.

This law explains the increased oxygen diffusion to tissues when using hyperbaric oxygen therapy through increasing the partial pressure difference across tissue membranes.

Amontons' Law

First described by Guillaume Amontons (1663–1705) in 1699, this law states: The quotient of pressure (P) and temperature (T) in a confined amount of gas at equal volume (V) remains constant. As the pressure of a gas increases, the temperature of the gas increases, too.

$$P/T = \text{constant or } P_1/T_1 = P_2/T_2$$

Where:

  P is the pressure of the gas.
  T is the temperature of the gas.

This law explains the correction of the pressure made to the chamber as the temperature of the gas cools off.

Application

Hyperbaric oxygen therapy has been proposed as a primary or an adjunctive therapy for a multitude of medical and surgical conditions. There are thousands of citations in the literature regarding its use. It has been described as a "therapy in a search of disease."[13] Most of the reported indications are derived from the theoretical cellular and biochemical benefits of this therapy. [4,11,12] Table 3-3 lists a summary of those benefits.

Many of the accepted indications for its use are based on experimental animal studies, case reports, or small human studies.[14] The UHMS publishes a list of indications for acute or chronic conditions approved by the society where the literature for its use is convincing (Table 3-4).[13] In the United States, CMS publishes a list of acute and chronic conditions that are approved for reimbursement (Table 3-5).[15] A list of clinical conditions that are considered research conditions and

TABLE 3-3
Benefits of Hyperbaric Oxygen Therapy

Improves oxygenation in hypoxic tissues
Mechanical decrease in gas bubble volume
Vasoconstriction and reduction of edema
Stimulation of angiogenesis and promotion of wound healing
Decreases ischemic reperfusion injury and decreases release of toxic oxygen radicals
Antimicrobial activity
  Reduces production of clostridial alpha toxin
  Direct bactericidal effect on certain anaerobic bacteria
  Direct bacteriostatic effect on some aerobic bacterial species
  Enhances transport and augments antibiotic efficacy
  Improves neutrophil-mediated bacterial killing
Inflammation and immune modulation
  Decreases leukocyte endothelial adherence
  Modulates neutrophil and macrophage function
  Stimulates platelet derived growth factor (PDGF) receptor appearance
  Increase in nitric oxide (NO) generation
  Enhanced interleukin 10 (IL-10) expression by macrophages
  Decreases the serum concentration of tumor necrosis factor-α (TNF-α)
  Attenuates disease severity in experimental models of autoimmune disease
  Improves graft tolerance through histocompatibility protein changes

TABLE 3-4
Indications for Hyperbaric Oxygen Therapy Published by the UHMS in 2008

Acute Conditions
Air or gas embolism
Carbon monoxide poisoning
Carbon monoxide poisoning complicated by cyanide poisoning
Central retinal artery occlusion
Clostridial myositis and myonecrosis (gas gangrene)
Crush injury, compartment syndrome, and other acute traumatic ischemias
Decompression sickness
Exceptional blood loss (anemia)
Intracranial abscess
Necrotizing soft tissue infections (necrotizing fasciitis)
Thermal burns

Chronic Conditions
Delayed radiation injury (soft tissue and bony necrosis)
Enhancement of healing in selected problem wounds
Refractory osteomyelitis
Skin grafts and flaps (compromised)

nonreimbursable by Medicare and Medicaid are listed in Table 3-6.[15]

Indications
Gas Embolism (GE)

Gas embolism (GE) refers to all pathological events related to the entry or the occurrence of gas bubbles in the vascular system. It can occur while scuba diving,[16] though in current practice GE is largely an iatrogenic

TABLE 3-5
Indications for Hyperbaric Oxygen Therapy Covered for Reimbursement by Medicare and Medicaid

Acute Conditions

Acute carbon monoxide poisoning
Acute peripheral arterial insufficiency
Crush injuries and suturing of severed limbs
Cyanide poisoning
Decompression sickness
Gas embolism
Gas gangrene
Osteoradionecrosis
Progressive necrotizing infections (necrotizing fasciitis)

Chronic Conditions

Actinomycosis (refractory)
Preparation and preservation of compromised skin grafts
Diabetic wounds meeting select criteria
Chronic refractory osteomyelitis

TABLE 3-6
Clinical Conditions Considered Research Conditions and Nonreimbursable by Medicare and Medicaid

Acute cerebral edema
Acute or chronic cerebral vascular insufficiency
Acute frostbite
Acute thermal and chemical pulmonary damage
Aerobic and anerobic septicemia
Arthritic disease
Brown recluse spider bites
Cancer
Cardiogenic shock
Chronic peripheral vascular insufficiency
Chronic neurological conditions (cerebral palsy, multiple sclerosis)
Cutaneous, decubitus, and stress ulcers
Chronic headaches
Hearing loss
Hepatic necrosis
Myocardial infarctions
Nonvascular cases of chronic brain syndrome including
  Alzheimer's disease
Organ storage
Organ transplantation
Pulmonary emphysema
Sickle cell anemia
Sports and athletic performance
Tetanus

problem that can result in serious morbidity and even death.[11,17] It can be caused by procedures performed in almost all clinical specialties, such as cardiac surgery,[18] neurosurgery,[19] endoscopy,[20] hemodialysis,[21] central venous catheterization,[22] penetrating chest trauma,[23] mechanical ventilation,[24] and bronchoscopy,[25] and is even associated with childbirth.[26] Upon entering the vascular system, gas bubbles follow the bloodstream until they obstruct small vessels. Depending on the access route, gas embolism may be classified as a venous or an arterial gas embolism. Neurological and hemodynamic deterioration are among the most common initial presentations. The development of symptoms depends on the gas type, embolus volume, rate of injection, patient position, and hemodynamic condition of the patient.[17]

A high level of suspicion is required to make the diagnosis. The diagnosis can be made by hearing a millwheel murmur or observing a decrease in the end tidal carbon dioxide by capnometry. Doppler ultrasonography, transesophageal echocardiography, or computerized tomography of the brain can confirm the diagnosis.[17]

Treatment with HBO_2 should be started early. This therapy reduces the volume of gas bubbles, improves oxygen delivery to ischemic tissues, reduces cerebral edema, and decreases ischemic **reperfusion injury**. The current recommendations are 100% oxygen at 2.8 ATA for 2 to 4 hours, and repeated treatments until no further improvements are seen.[27,28]

Carbon Monoxide (CO) Poisoning

Carbon monoxide (CO) poisoning primarily caused by smoke inhalation (e.g., fire smoke, exhaust from internal combusting engines, and faulty heating appliances); suicide is the most common cause of death by CO poisoning in the United States.[29] CO has a 200 times greater affinity to bind to hemoglobin than does oxygen, resulting in a shift of the oxyhemoglobin dissociation curve to the left and causing tissue hypoxia. Additionally, CO binds to myoglobin and cytochrome oxidase, resulting in decreased intracellular respiration and increased oxidative stress, both of which contribute to cell death.[30] Mild cases present with symptoms of headaches, nausea, and flu-like symptoms; severe cases present with severe neurological conditions (e.g., syncopy, seizures, coma), pulmonary edema, myocardial ischemia, and severe metabolic acidosis. Additionally, victims of CO poisoning are prone to delayed neuropsychological sequelae.[11,30] Carboxyhemoglobin levels do not correlate well with the severity of the intoxication.

HBO_2 accelerates the rate of CO dissociation from hemoglobin, decreasing the carboxyhemoglobin half-life from 5.5 hours on room air to 23 minutes breathing 100% oxygen at 3 ATA. Studies concerning HBO_2 therapy for CO poisoning have yielded conflicting results, but some studies have shown benefits in both the acute and delayed effects.[31,32] Other studies showed no significant benefit from hyperbaric therapy.[33,34] The current recommendation for severe cases is 2.5–3 ATA for 90–120 minutes for a single session;[11,35] repetitive sessions may be required for residual neurologic symptoms.

Cyanide poisoning may accompany CO poisoning, and their toxic effects may be synergistic.[36] HBO_2 may have brain-protective effects against cyanide and may protect against methemoglobin induced by treatment with sodium and amyl nitrates.[37]

Central Retinal Artery Occlusion (CRAO)

Retinal artery occlusion leads to a sudden severe and painless vision loss in the affected eye; it can affect the central artery or one of its branches. The leading cause of CRAO is emboli deriving from arteriosclerotic plaques in the aorta or from the carotids. Other sources of emboli include calcified heart valves, thrombi originating from areas of restricted heart movements, or in patients with atrial arrhythmias. The retina is very sensitive to ischemia. Experimental data have shown that a total occlusion of the central retinal artery causes irreversible damage to the inner retina if occlusion time exceeds 100 minutes.[38] The aim of HBO_2 is to maintain an oxygen supply to the retina through the choroidal vasculature until spontaneous recanalization occurs. The bradytrophic vitreous could serve as an oxygen deposit after HBO_2 therapy, and a local release of tissue plasminogen activator under HBO_2 could help to further accelerate reperfusion.[39] The current recommendations suggest 2.4 ATA for three 30 minute sessions in the first day, followed by twice daily for the next 2 days.[39]

Clostridial Myositis and Myonecrosis (Gas Gangrene)

Invasive clostridial infection usually results from injury or wound contamination. It is classically associated with traumatic war wounds, but may occur after abdominal surgeries.[40] Clostridium is an anaerobic, spore-forming, gram-positive encapsulated bacillus. *Clostridium perfringens* is a facultative anaerobe that is isolated in 80% to 90% of cases. Although more than 20 toxins are produced, the most lethal is the alpha toxin.[41] The patient presents with pain out of proportion to the apparent severity of his or her wounds and often has evidence of tissue destruction with gas in the tissues that can be evident on x-ray films or computerized scan. Toxemia and shock are usually evident.[5] The beneficial effects of HBO_2 include improved tissue oxygenation, decreased production of the toxins, bacteriostatic effect on the bacteria, and augmented antibiotic activity. Treatment consists of antibiotics, usually penicillin; surgical debridement; and early initiation of HBO_2.[42] There are multiple studies reporting improved survival, as well as limb and tissue saving.[43,44] The current recommendation for treatment of this condition with HBO_2 is 90-minute sessions every 8 hours at 3 ATA, followed by twice daily sessions for 2 to 5 days or until clinical improvement is seen.[45]

Crush Injuries, Compartment Syndrome, and Acute Traumatic Ischemia

Crush injury and other acute traumatic ischemia are characterized by a vicious circle of ischemia, hypoxia, edema, and disturbed microcirculation. HBO_2 therapy ameliorates the effects of acute traumatic ischemia through hyperoxygenation, vasoconstriction with edema reduction, angiogenesis, and tissue protection from reperfusion injury. Surgical treatment is the cornerstone of therapy. A randomized, double-blinded trial in crush injuries showed that concomitant HBO_2 improved healing in 94% of the cases compared to 59% of cases who did not undergo therapy.[46] The current recommendation calls for early application of HBO_2 therapy within 4 to 6 hours. Therapy is administered at 2 to 2.5 ATA for 90 to 120 minutes. Sessions are given three times daily for the first 2 days, followed by twice daily for the next 2 days, and then daily for the following 2 days.[45]

Decompression Sickness (DCS)

This condition is mostly related to recreational diving. The rapid ascent to the surface causes an increase in the partial pressure of nitrogen, leading to gas bubble formation in tissues, blood vessels, and lymphatics, which causes obstruction. Symptoms range from self-limited rash to severe neurologic conditions like seizures and paralysis. HBO_2 therapy reduces the gas bubble size, reverses the tissue ischemia, and reduces the cerebral edema. HBO_2 therapy is the only established lifesaving treatment for DCS. The outcome is more likely to be successful if started within 6 hours. The current recommendation calls for an initial session of 2 to 4 hours at ATA 2.8. This can be repeated up to 10 times if symptoms persist.[47]

Exceptional Blood Loss Anemia

Severe anemia can markedly decrease oxygen delivery, leading to tissue ischemia. In cases where blood transfusion is not possible (e.g., religious beliefs or unavailability of blood), HBO_2 therapy can increase the dissolved plasma oxygen to meet tissue oxygen requirements. Hart[48] has described 70% survival in 26 patients with HBO_2 therapy after losing more than 50% of their circulating blood volume. The UHMS recommends three or four sessions daily, each for 2–4 hours at 3 ATA, until anemia is corrected.[45]

Intracranial Abscess (ICA)

Intracranial abscesses (i.e., cerebral abscess, epidural and subdural empyema) is the most recent addition to the approved indications for HBO_2 therapy. Mortality described in the literature is about 20%. Reports of adjunctive HBO_2 therapy shows reduced mortality to 3%.[49] The proposed beneficial mechanisms of HBO_2 therapy in ICA include reduction of brain swelling, inhibition of anaerobic flora, enhancement of host defense, and improvement in concomitant skull osteomyelitis. HBO_2 therapy is approved in ICA if at least one of the following criteria is met: multiple abscesses, abscess in a deep or dominant location, compromised host, surgery is contraindicated or the patient is a poor surgical risk, or no response or further deterioration in spite of standard surgical (e.g., one or two needle aspirates) and antibiotic treatment.[50] The current recommendation calls for once or twice daily sessions at 2–2.5 ATA for 60–90 minutes. The number of sessions needed is not clear, but averaged 13 in the literature. Utilization review is recommended after 20 sessions.[50]

Necrotizing Fasciitis (NF)

Necrotizing fasciitis is a rapidly progressive infection of the skin and underlying tissue without muscle invasion. Hemolytic streptococci are a typical causative organism, though mixed anaerobic and aerobic polymicrobial infections are common. The benefits of HBO_2 therapy are similar to the ones outlined previously for gas gangrene. Treatment conventionally consists of antibiotics and surgical debridement. Mortality for this condition is high (30–60%); the addition of HBO_2 therapy may reduce mortality by up to two thirds.[43] The current recommendation calls for twice daily sessions of 2–2.5 ATA for 90–120 minutes until the infection is controlled. If the infection is severe, three treatments of 3 ATA on the first day are recommended.[45]

Thermal Burns

Thermal burns activate the coagulation cascade and inflammation causing edema, tissue hypoxia, and necrosis. They also can compromise the respiratory system and affect the host defense. There is evidence that HBO_2 therapy reduces coagulability, decreases edema, and enhances collagen formation and angiogenesis. It also decreases leukocyte endothelial adherence, lessens healing time, enhances bacterial killing, and reduces infection.[51] Some studies have translated those beneficial effects to a reduction in surgical procedures, costs, hospitalization, and mortality.[52,53] A Cochrane review found insufficient evidence to support the use of HBO_2 therapy for thermal burns.[54] Currently, HBO_2 therapy is recommended for serious burns greater than 20% of total body surface area; involvement of the hands, feet, face, or perineum; and either partial or full thickness injuries. Treatment should be started early. The UHMS recommends three initial treatments at 2–2.5 ATA for 90 minutes, followed by twice daily sessions for 10–14 days.[45]

Delayed Radiation Injuries (Soft Tissue and Bony Necrosis)

Delayed radiation complications are seen after a latent period of 6 months to years after radiation therapy. Radiation therapy leads to progressive obliterative endarteritis, which results in hypocellular, hypovascular, and hypoxic tissues. These effects are seen clinically as tissue edema, ulceration, bony necrosis, and poor wound healing.[2] HBO_2 therapy increases vascular density, oxygenation, leukocyte bactericidal activity, and angiogenesis in the radiation-damaged tissues.[55] HBO_2 therapy was studied extensively in mandibular osteoradionecrosis, and more recently for radiation injuries at other sites (proctitis, enteritis, cystitis, and head and neck radiation injuries).[9] A cost-effectiveness analysis for HBO_2 therapy in osteoradionecrosis found that it is six times more expensive to not use this therapy.[56] The UHMS recommends daily 90- to 120-minute sessions at 2–2.5 ATA for about 40 days.[45]

Problem Wounds

A chronic nonhealing wound or the so-called "problem wound" is defined as any wound that fails to heal within a reasonable period of time through the use of conventional medical or surgical techniques. Chronic wounds are often categorized as diabetic wounds, venous stasis ulcers, arterial ulcers, or pressure ulcers. Hypoperfusion, ischemia, and infection impair wound healing by decreasing fibroblast proliferation, collagen production, and angiogenesis. The beneficial effects of HBO_2 therapy include fibroblast proliferation and collagen synthesis. In addition, this therapy likely stimulates growth factors involving angiogenesis and other mediators of the wound healing process, plus it has direct and indirect antimicrobial activity and kills intracellular leukocytes.[57] In an effort to select patients appropriately for HBO_2 therapy, various objective vascular evaluation methods have been used, including transcutaneous oximetry, capillary perfusion pressure, laser Doppler, and other types of vascular studies. HBO_2 therapy in conjunction with appropriate general and local wound care have shown improved outcomes including lower amputation rates.[58,59] The UHMS recommends once or twice daily sessions of 90–120 minutes at 2–2.5 ATA for 30 sessions.[45]

Refractory Osteomyelitis

Refractory osteomyelitis is defined as acute or chronic osteomyelitis that is not cured or recurs after appropriate antibiotics, removal of foreign materials, or surgical debridement. The beneficial effects of HBO_2 therapy include increased oxygenation, vascularity, collagen deposition, angiogenesis, antibiotics effectiveness, and leukocyte killing. A unique mechanism by which HBO_2 therapy is beneficial in osteomyelitis is in promoting the osteoclast function, improving resorption of necrotic bone by osteoclasts.[60] Human reports have shown improved long-term success rates of 63% to 86% with the addition of HBO_2 therapy.[61] The current

UHMS recommendation calls for daily sessions for 90–120 minutes at 2–2.5 ATA for 20–40 sessions.[45]

Compromised Skin Grafts and Flaps

Skin grafts are quite different from flaps because they are avascular. Conversely, flaps have an innate vascular support. The transplanted tissue placed on the host survives primarily because oxygen diffuses into it from the underlying wound bed; later it relies on the promoted angiogenesis of the wound margins. HBO_2 therapy reduces leukocyte endothelial adherence, prevents vasoconstriction, and prevents reperfusion injury.[62] Other benefits include fibroblast stimulation, collagen synthesis, and angiogenesis. Flap survival with HBO_2 therapy averaged 90% compared to 67% without it.[63] The UHMS recommends twice daily treatment at 2–2.5 ATA for 90–120 minutes,

followed by once daily when the graft has stabilized.[45] The average number of treatments is usually 10–20 sessions.

Table 3-7 summarizes the treatment algorithms for each condition. Note that different algorithms for each condition may exist at different centers; we present a sample of those algorithms.

Complications

Oxygen Toxicity

Tissue injury from oxygen is mediated by reactive oxygen species, including superoxide anion, hydroxyl radial, and hydrogen peroxide. Those species can cause cell membrane disruption, cell injury, and cell death.[64] Pulmonary oxygen toxicity secondary to inspiring a high fraction of oxygen for extended periods is well recognized.

TABLE 3-7
Summary of Clinical Conditions and Sample of Treatment Algorithm

Acute Conditions	Pressure (ATA)	Recommended Number of Treatment Sessions	Length of Sessions (hours)
Air or gas embolism	2.5–3.0	1–2 sessions initially; continue treatment sessions until no further improvement	2.0–4.0
Carbon monoxide poisoning Carbon monoxide poisoning complicated by cyanide poisoning	2.5–3.0	1–2 initially; continue treatment sessions as needed for residual neurological symptoms or until no further improvement	1.5–2.0
Central retinal artery occlusion	2.4	3 sessions on first day of therapy, then 2 sessions per day for the next 2 days	0.5
Clostridial myositis and myonecrosis (gas gangrene)	3.0	3 sessions on first day, then twice daily sessions for an additional 5 days	1.5
Crush injury, compartment syndrome, and other acute traumatic ischemias	2.0–2.5	3 times daily for the first 2 days, then 2 times per day for days 3 and 4, and daily for treatment days 5 and 6	1.5–2.0
Decompression sickness	2.5–3.0	1 session initially; may need to repeat up to 10 sessions	2.0–4.0
Exceptional blood loss (anemia)	3.0	3–4 sessions daily until anemia is corrected	2.0–4.0
Intracranial abscess	2.0–2.5	1–2 sessions daily for 10–20 days	1.0–1.5
Necrotizing soft tissue infections (necrotizing fasciitis)	2.0–2.5	3 sessions first day, then 2 sessions per day until improvement is noted	1.5–2.0

Chronic Conditions	Pressure (ATA)	Recommended Number of Treatment Sessions	Length of Sessions (hours)
Delayed radiation injury (soft tissue and bony necrosis)	2.0–2.5	1 session per day for 40 days	1.5–2.0
Enhancement of healing in selected problem wounds	2.0–2.5	1–2 sessions daily for 30 days	1.5–2.0
Osteomyelitis (refractory)	2.0–2.5	1 session daily for 20–40 days	1.5–2.0
Skin grafts and flaps (compromised)	2.0–2.5	2 sessions per day until stabilized, then 1 session per day for 10–20 days	1.5–2.0

High levels of oxygen given for short duration (90–120 minutes) under hyperbaric conditions at 2–3 ATA have not been shown to cause pulmonary oxygen toxicity.[65]

Central and Peripheral Nervous System Toxicity

Symptoms of central and peripheral nervous system toxicity may include dizziness, irritability, tinnitus, nausea, paresthesias, and seizures. The incidence of tonic-clonic seizures during HBO_2 therapy is estimated at 0.3% at 2.4 ATA, and up to 2.5% at 3 ATA. Factors increasing susceptibility to seizures include exertion, fever, thyrotoxicosis, hypoglycemia, elevated $PaCO_2$, acidosis, brain trauma, preexisting seizure conditions, and some medications (catecholamines, steroids, aspirin, and insulin). Oxygen-induced seizures are self-limiting and resolve quickly after discontinuing oxygen, and are generally not associated with neurologic sequelae. Anticonvulsant prophylaxis or treatment is not indicated.[9,47]

Barotrauma

Barotrauma may affect the middle ear, sinuses, or pulmonary system. Middle ear trauma develops in 2% of cases. It can present with edema, hemorrhage, mucosal congestion, and rarely rupture of the tympanic membrane. This type of trauma usually resolves spontaneously, but may need decongestants, tympanotomies, or myringotomies.[66] Pulmonary barotrauma in the form of pneumothorax is a dangerous complication that should be recognized and treated immediately.[67]

Ophthalmologic

The most common ophthalmologic side effect is progressive myopia that may develop in patients who undergo more than 20 treatment sessions. Fortunately this is temporary and reverses completely within 6 weeks after discontinuing treatment.[68]

Claustrophobia

Some patients may experience anxiety, especially in small monoplace chambers. Pretreatment with anxiolytics may be required.[69]

Contraindications

HBO_2 therapy is usually a safe therapy, with very few contraindications.[69]

Absolute Contraindications

Absolute contraindications to HBO_2 therapy include the following:

- Untreated pneumothorax is an absolute contraindication for HBO_2 therapy because it can progress to tension pneumothorax during decompression. Once chest tube relief of the pneumothorax is achieved, the patient can safely undergo therapy.

- Concurrent treatment with some medications (e.g., bleomycin, cisplatin, doxorubicin, disulfiram) is considered a contraindication to use of HBO_2.

Relative Contraindications

Relative contraindications to HBO_2 therapy include the following:

- Pulmonary lesions
- Obstructive lung disease
- Seizure disorder
- Acute viral illness
- Fever
- Acute or chronic sinusitis
- Reconstructive ear surgery
- Optic neuritis
- Congestive heart failure
- Acidosis
- Certain medications (narcotics, insulin, steroids, nicotine, nitroprusside, hydrocarbon-based ointments or gels)

Hazards

A hazard is a potential source of harm that relates to physical injury or damage to the health of people, or damage to property or the environment. Due to its nature, HBO_2 therapy has some unique hazards.[11,70] Identification of the hazards and the resulting risks connected with the HBO_2 therapy is the first step in safety management.

The **European Committee for Hyperbaric Medicine (ECHM)** classifies hazards associated with HBO_2 therapy into generic and specific hazards (**Table 3-8**).[71]

Fire and Safety Requirements

Fire is the single most dangerous event leading to fatal accidents in any hyperbaric chamber. This type of accident is rare, but is almost always fatal. Extreme precautions must be taken to avoid this disaster. There are two types of fire hazards in a hyperbaric center (i.e., outside and inside the chamber). The potential for accidental ignition of flammable materials is increased in the hyperbaric environment and their burning rate is markedly enhanced by a raised percentage or raised partial pressure of oxygen. Care must be taken to exclude various flammable substances and equipment that could be sources of ignition because many different types of equipment may not be appropriate for the hyperbaric environment.[70,71] A list of equipment that can and cannot be used in hyperbaric chambers is found in **Table 3-9**.[9]

Electrical and heating equipment should be protected to prevent spark generation and overheating during normal operation and in case of a single fault condition. A study evaluating the causes of fires inside hyperbaric chambers (between 1923 and 1997) showed

TABLE 3-8
Hazards of Hyperbaric Oxygen Therapy

Generic Hazards

Energy hazards and contributory factors
Biological hazards and contributory factors
Environmental hazards and contributory factors
Hazards resulting from incorrect output of energy and substances
Hazards related to the use of the medical device and contributory factors
Inappropriate, inadequate, or overcomplicated user interface
Hazards arising from function failure, maintenance, aging, and contributory factors

Specific Hazards

Pressures (risk of explosion, loss of pressure, vessel integrity)
Adequacy and integrity of pressurized gas supplies
Pressure differentials (catheter/cannula cuffs, seals, vascular lines, drainage)
Oxygen (risk of ignition, cerebral and pulmonary toxicity)
Quality and quantity of breathing gas supplies
Electricity (electrical safety within the pressure vessel)
Prohibited materials within the chamber
Fire (procedures for prevention, suppression, and evacuation)
Suitability of medical devices used inside the chamber
Staff health and safety, including medical surveillance and precautions against dysbaric injuries in staff
Hygiene and infection control (disinfection of masks, hoods, ventilators, and associated equipment; alert pathogens policy; chamber disinfection)
Management of body fluids, waste, sharps, and infected materials
Manual handling of patients on entry, exit from chamber and during treatment (use of slides, hoists, and patient handling aids)
Noise hazards and control measures (both for internal occupants of chambers and external staff)
Thermal stress
Any other hazards (display screen equipment, slip, trip, bump, and fall hazards)

TABLE 3-9
Permitted Equipment and Equipment That Should Be Avoided in Hyperbaric Chambers

Equipment Allowed in the Hyperbaric Chamber

Approved IV pump
Approved ventilator
Arterial line
Central venous catheter
Doppler
Echocardiography
Electrocardiogram (ECG)
Foley catheter
Glass bottles
Nasogastric tube
Permanent pacemaker
Pressure bag
Pulmonary artery catheter
Pulse oximetry devices
Noninvasive blood pressure machines (nonmercury)
Transcranial Doppler

Equipment Not Allowed in the Hyperbaric Chamber

Batteries and equipment supplied by >12 volts
Defibrillator
Pneumatic stockings
Patient-controlled anesthesia (PCA) pumps
Transport ventilator
Telemetry device

that many fires are caused by objects introduced by patients.[72] The confined environment of the hyperbaric chamber increases the dangers of high pressure and oxygen concentration in the case of fire. The two major factors that lead to death in confined spaces are failure to recognize and control the hazards associated with confined spaces and inadequate or incorrect emergency responses.[73] Fire prevention can be achieved by creating a safe environment and removing unsafe materials, providing patient and personnel education, and having policies and procedures for fire prevention.[74]

The American Society of Mechanical Engineers (ASME) publishes standards for the design, fabrication, inspection, testing, marking, and stamping of pressure vessels for human occupancy that have an internal or external pressure differential exceeding 2 psi. These standards also provide requirements for the design, fabrication, inspection, testing, cleaning, and certification of piping systems for pressure vessels for human occupancy (PVHO).[75] A list of those publications can be found on the web at http://www. asme.org/kb/standards. The National Fire Protection Association (NFPA) also publishes codes and standards to establish criteria to minimize the hazards of fire,

explosion, and electricity in healthcare facilities providing services to human beings (NFPA 99, Chapter 20). A list of those publications can be found on the web at http://www.nfpa.org/aboutthecodes/list_of_codes_and_standards.asp. A detailed description of those standards are beyond the scope of this chapter, but they should be reviewed carefully by all personnel involved in operating a hyperbaric facility.

Facilities providing HBO_2 therapy should have a written emergency policy detailing procedures for in-chamber fire prevention and general actions in the event of fire in the chamber and/or the facility buildings. All personnel must be familiar with those policies. Staff training should be two-fold and include education regarding fire prevention as well as the actions to be taken in case of a fire. Policies and procedures should also address evacuation procedures should a fire occur within the facility offering HBO_2 therapy and include a detailed description of how to safely remove patients from the chamber and proper documentation of the evacuation event.[11]

Monitoring: General Considerations

HBO_2 therapy exposes the patient to an environment that is potentially hazardous due to the increased ambient pressure and increased partial pressure of oxygen. Before starting HBO_2 therapy for the first time, a history and medical examination must be performed to make sure no contraindications for therapy exist.[11]

Hyperbaric oxygen is an important therapeutic modality for critically ill patients. Critically ill patients requiring transfer from the intensive care unit (ICU) to a hyperbaric chamber within the hospital or outside the hospital require additional extensive monitoring. The Society of Critical Care Medicine (SCCM) published detailed guidelines for critically ill patients requiring transfer outside the ICU.[76] Continuous three-lead electrocardiogram (ECG) monitoring can be used to monitor any arrhythmias in the critically ill patient. Additional monitoring may be needed for some patients. Continuous EEG monitoring is also possible to monitor any seizure activity. This is not used routinely for every patient, only for those deemed necessary. Blood pressure monitoring, either manually or through automated devices, is possible, but care must be taken because these devices can pose a fire hazard. Invasive arterial, central venous, and pulmonary artery catheter monitoring is plausible during therapy. Monitors are usually located outside the chamber, with the cables penetrating to inside the chamber. If the monitor is contained within the chamber, some adjustment in the pressure bagging is needed because of the different ambient pressure exerted within the chamber.

Monitoring Oxygenation

It is possible to monitor tissue oxygenation and perfusion during HBO_2 therapy using devices that measure transcutaneous partial pressure of oxygen ($TcPO_2$). $TcPO_2$ has been shown to correlate with tissue perfusion.[77] Repetitive monitoring of $TcPO_2$ during the course of therapy may help to evaluate progress in the healing process.[78]

Systemic oxygenation can be assessed using pulse oximetry devices or arterial blood gas (ABG) sampling. ABG sampling for analysis needs meticulous attention to avoid air bubbles during fast decompression to ambient pressure, which will falsely lower the partial pressure of oxygen, rendering the results difficult to interpret.[79,80] PaO_2 may initially drop in the first hour of therapy, but increases again within the second or third hour.[81]

Monitoring Ventilation

Ventilation can be assessed using ABG analysis. It is important to consider that hyperbaric pressure has less effect on pH and $PaCO_2$ than on PaO_2. End tidal carbon dioxide partial pressure ($P_{ET}CO_2$) in expiration gas can be used to monitor ventilation noninvasively. Transcutaneous partial pressure of carbon dioxide ($TcPCO_2$) monitoring can be used to indirectly assess the ventilation status of the patient, and may be superior to $P_{ET}CO_2$.[82]

HBO_2 with Mechanical Ventilation

Mechanical ventilators used in hyperbaric chambers should ensure the same modes and parameters as modern ICU ventilators.[83] Note that not all

mechanical ventilator devices are approved for use in hyperbaric chambers. Most ventilators have a tendency to change operating characteristics as the ambient pressure and gas density changes.[83] The literature does include reports regarding the safe operation of various ventilators under hyperbaric condition (e.g., RCH-LAMA, Monaghan 225, Emerson pneumatic, IMV Bird).[84–88]

The mode of ventilation may not act the same in a hyperbaric environment compared to a normobaric one. Stahl and colleagues found that the volumes delivered with pressure control ventilation (PCV) remained stable compared to volume control ventilation (VCV).[89] Use of the VCV mode inside the hyperbaric chamber requires constant adaptation of settings depending on the environmental pressure to assure proper ventilation because the tidal volume delivered to the patient will usually decrease with increasing ambient pressure. HBO_2 therapy has been used safely with high frequency oscillatory ventilation in an experimental study.[90] Manual ventilation can be used during transport or even during therapy. Resuscitation bags must be equipped with a regulating system ensuring appropriate gas delivery at higher pressures. Care has to be taken that the manual resuscitator is equipped with a device that ensures the oxygen-enriched exhalation gas is vented out of the chamber, to avoid a potential fire hazard.[11]

Tracheal tubes also need attention prior to the initiation of HBO_2 therapy. The endotracheal tube cuff is usually inflated with air. During compression and decompression, the volume of air within the cuff will change according to the laws of physics. Thus the air in the cuff must be emptied before therapy and the cuff filled with distilled water to achieve an adequate seal. Foam-cuffed tubes or an automatic cuff blocking device that keeps the cuff pressure constant in relation to the ambient pressure could be used as an alternative. If tracheal tube suctioning is necessary, pressure-regulated suction devices are recommended.[11]

Currently Available Devices

There are multiple requirements for a hyperbaric chamber to operate and be accredited:[11,91]

- *Pressure requirement:* The minimum operational pressure for hyperbaric chambers should be at least 2 ATA. No maximum pressure has been identified.
- *Structure, size, and dimensions requirements:* For a multiplace chamber, the pressure chambers should contain at least two compartments, one as a main chamber used for treatment and one as an antechamber used for transferring people or equipment. The chamber should offer enough space for the patient and an attendant.

- *Breathing systems requirements:* A breathing unit is needed, including a demand system, free flow system, and/or mechanical ventilator.
- *Pressure control requirements:* Each chamber should have its own pressure control system.
- *Environmental control requirements:* This is needed to control the environment's atmosphere.
- *Electrical installation requirements:* Specific requirements for the amount of voltage of the electric installation are required to reduce fire hazards.
- *Fire protection requirements:* Specific strict requirements are needed to reduce the risk of fire hazards.
- *Firefighting systems requirements:* These are crucial given the high risk of fire.
- *Control console requirements:* Most equipment should be controlled from a central observation point.
- *Communication requirements:* These are necessary to allow communication between staff and between staff and patients.
- *Emergency power supply requirements:* These allow for operational safety and uninterrupted treatments.

Specifications

There are multiple designs for both monoplace and multiplace chambers with different dimensions and capabilities. Common features required for both types of chambers include:

- Air pressurization and ventilation (**Figure 3-5**)
- Gas delivery system (**Figures 3-6** and **3-7**)
- Oxygen tanks (**Figure 3-8**)
- Oxygen generators (**Figure 3-9**)
- Fire suppression tanks (**Figure 3-10**)
- Compressors (**Figure 3-11**)
- Potable water
- Communications (**Figure 3-12**)
- Atmospheric conditioning
- Gas analysis (**Figure 3-13**)
- Patient entertainment (**Figure 3-14**)
- Video monitoring consoles

Monoplace Chambers

Monoplace chambers (**Figures 3-12** and **3-15**) are able to treat only one patient at a time, usually in the supine position, sometimes sitting. The maximum working pressure for most monoplace chambers is 3 ATA (6 ATA for a few exceptions), limiting their usage to medium-pressure treatment schedules. During the session the patient can breathe oxygen directly from the internal atmosphere or through a mask. Monoplace chambers can support patients that require intensive care during the session.[92] All devices are located outside the chamber; tubes, lines, and wires are transferred to the chamber through ports in the bulkhead.

Monoplace chambers have some advantages over multiplace chambers, mainly related to relatively low cost of operation, small space requirements, limited number of personnel for operation and maintenance, no occupational hazard for the attendant, and no special decompression required. The disadvantage of such chambers is the difficulty to directly assist the patient contained within the chamber should an emergency arise. Portable inflatable monoplace chambers are commercially available to deliver on-the-scene treatments and are also used by athletes to enhance recovery after tissue injury.

Multiplace Chambers

Multiplace chambers (**Figures 3-14, 3-16,** and **3-17**) are manufactured with capabilities to manage multiple patients at the same time, including critically ill patients. The chambers are usually divided into two compartments, the entry compartment and the treatment chamber. The entry compartment allows personnel and equipment to enter the treatment chamber without loss of pressure (**Figure 3-18**). Generally a nurse or another observer who monitors the patients and assists with equipment manipulation or emergencies is inside the chamber. Other personnel sit outside

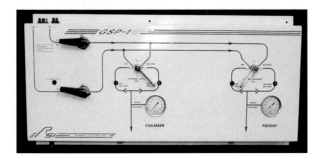

FIGURE 3-5 Gas pressurization control for hyperbaric chamber.
Courtesy of Reimers Systems, Inc.

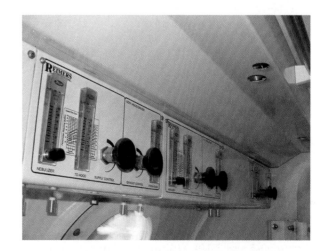

FIGURE 3-6 Gas delivery panel inside a multiplace chamber.
Courtesy of Reimers Systems, Inc.

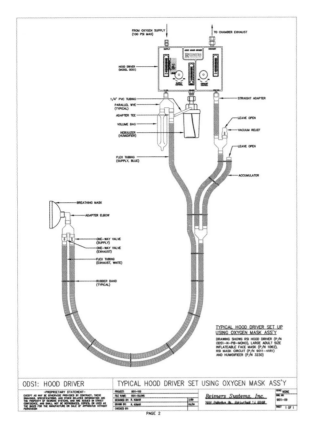
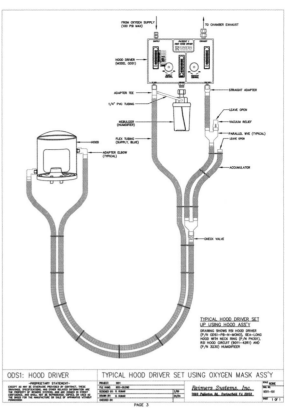

FIGURE 3-7 Gas delivery connection from and to the panel to a mask and hood.
Courtesy of Reimers Systems, Inc.

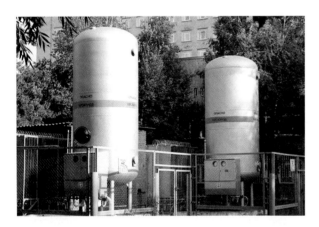

FIGURE 3-8 Liquid oxygen tanks.
© HGalina/Shutterstock, Inc.

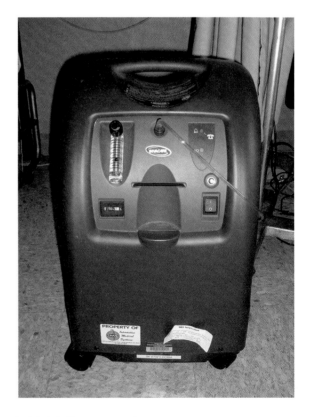

FIGURE 3-9 Oxygen generators.
© BrokenSphere/Wikimedia Commons

in the control room to monitor pressure, oxygen, temperature, and the like, as displayed in **Figure 3-16**.

Patients in a multiplace chamber breathe 100% oxygen via a mask or close-fitting plastic hood (**Figures 3-7** and **3-19**). Multiplace chambers can usually be pressurized to the equivalent of about 6 ATA of pressure. Advantages of multiplace chambers

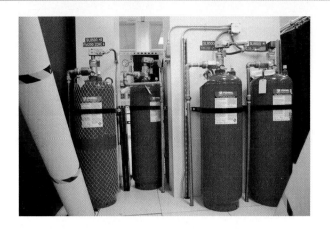

FIGURE 3-10 Fire suppression tanks.
Courtesy of Derrick Coetzee/Flickr under Creative Commons Attribution 2.0 Generic license.

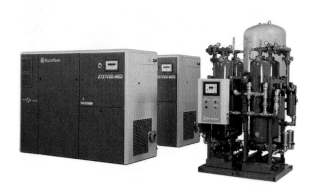

FIGURE 3-11 Air compressors.
Courtesy of Atlas Copco.

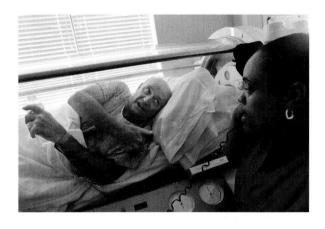

FIGURE 3-12 Communication within monoplace chambers.
© Chris Hondros, Getty Images News/Thinkstock

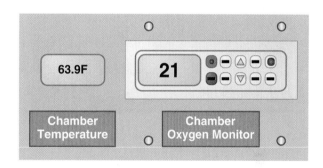

FIGURE 3-13 Oxygen and temperature monitors.

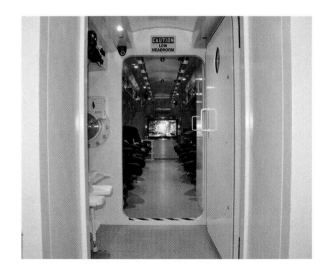

FIGURE 3-14 Entertainment in multiplace chambers.
Courtesy of Reimers Systems, Inc.

include the ability to treat multiple patients at the same time, availability of personnel inside the chamber for monitoring patients, and ability to better attend to the needs of critically ill patients. Disadvantages of these chambers are their limited availability, relative expense, and fire hazards inside the hospital environment.

Oxygen Delivery System in Multiplace Chambers

The oxygen supply for the session comes from a separate gas delivery system capable of delivering high flow oxygen up to 100 L/min; the usual flow rate is about 20–60 L/min depending on the ATA used and patient size (**Figure 3-20**). Multiplace chambers are pressurized with air. Supplemental oxygen may be

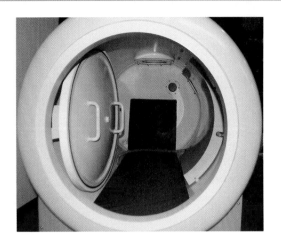

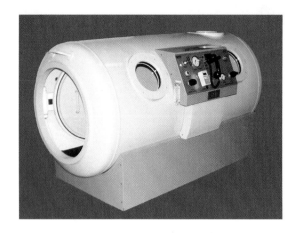

FIGURE 3-15 Monoplace chamber.

Photos courtesy of Reimers Systems, Inc.

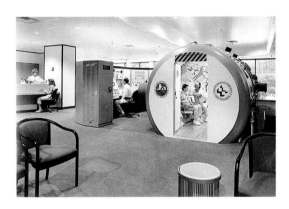

FIGURE 3-16 Multiplace chamber showing an assistant with a patient and monitoring personnel.

Courtesy of Reimers Systems, Inc.

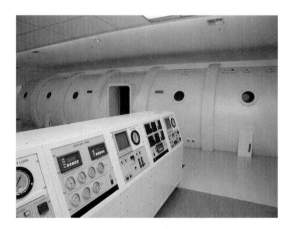

FIGURE 3-17 Multiplace chamber showing the outside of the chamber and attached monitoring console.

Courtesy of Reimers Systems, Inc.

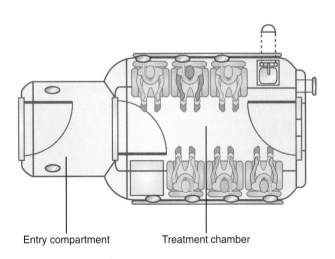

Entry compartment   Treatment chamber

FIGURE 3-18 Diagram of a multiplace chamber showing the entry compartment and the treatment chamber.

Courtesy of Reimers Systems, Inc.

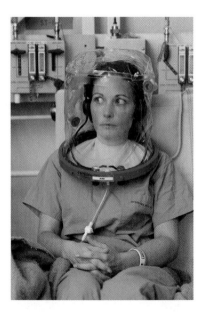

FIGURE 3-19 Patient inside a multiplace chamber getting the hyperbaric oxygen through a hood.

Courtesy of U.S. Air Force Photo/Ken Wright.

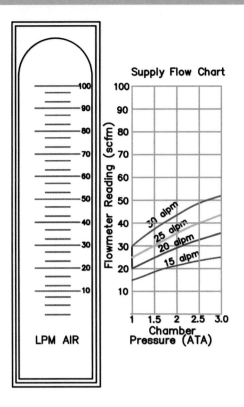

FIGURE 3-20 Diagram showing an oxygen flow meter and the respective ATA.

Courtesy of Reimers Systems, Inc.

administered through a tight-fitting mask, a head tent, or a mechanical ventilator. The exhaust gas may be either vented outside the chamber or recirculated through a CO_2 scrubber. The sample line attached to the exhaust hose allows monitoring of the patient breathing gas. **Figure 3-21** shows details of connections from the gas delivery system to the patient's mask or tent and vice versa.

Chamber Compression Gas Supply

To ensure adequate compression and ventilation of the hyperbaric chamber, especially at high pressures (> 3 ATA), a large volume of gas may be required. This necessitates large air compressors and large gas cylinders (**Figures 3-8** and **3-9**).

Mobile Chambers

A mobile chamber can be either monoplace (**Figure 3-22**) or multiplace (**Figure 3-23**).

Acknowledgment

We would like to thank Reimers Systems, Inc. for supplying many of the figures in this chapter.

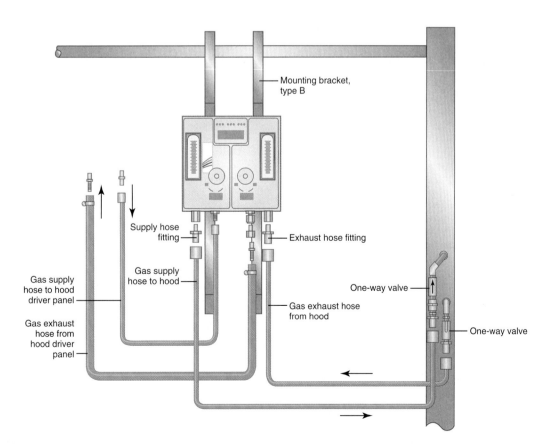

FIGURE 3-21 Diagram showing the oxygen entry and exhaust connections from the gas delivery panel from and to the patient's hood or mask.

Courtesy of Reimers Systems, Inc.

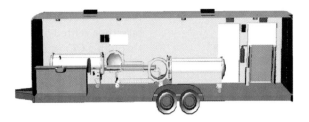

FIGURE 3-22 Mobile monoplace chambers in a trailer.
Courtesy of Reimers Systems, Inc.

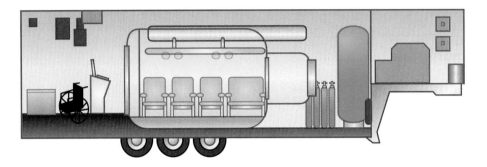

FIGURE 3-23 Mobile multiplace chamber in a trailer.
Courtesy of Reimers Systems, Inc.

References

1. Undersea and Hyperbaric Medicine Society. Available at www.uhms.org.
2. Gill AL, Bell CN. Hyperbaric oxygen: Its uses, mechanisms of action and outcomes. *QJM.* 2004;97:385.
3. Edwards ML. Hyperbaric oxygen therapy. Part 1: History and principles. *J Vet Emerg Crit Care.* 2010;20(3):284-288.
4. Lech RM, Rees PJ, Wilmshurst P. Hyperbaric oxygen therapy. *BMJ.* 1998;317:1140.
5. Tibbles RM, Edelsberg JS. Hyperbaric-oxygen therapy. *N Engl J Med.* 1996;334:1642.
6. Guyton AC, Hall JE. *Textbook of medical physiology.* 10th ed. Philadelphia, PA: WB Saunders; 2000.
7. Lumb AB. *Nunn's applied respiratory physiology.* 5th ed. Edinburgh, UK: Butterworth-Heinemann; 2003.
8. Lambertsen CJ, Kough RH, Cooper DY, Emmel GL, Loeschcke HH, Schmidt CF. Oxygen toxicity: Effects in man of oxygen inhalation at 1 and 3.5 atmospheres upon blood gas transport, cerebral circulation and cerebral metabolism. *J Appl Physiol.* 1953;5:471-486.
9. Auerbach PS. *Wilderness medicine.* 5th ed. Philadelphia, PA: Elsevier Health Sciences; 2007.
10. Boerema I, Meyne NG, Brummelkamp WK, et al. Life without blood (a study of the influence of high atmospheric pressure and hypothermia on dilution of the blood). *J Cardiovasc Surg.* 1960; 1:133-146.
11. Mathieu D. *Handbook on hyperbaric medicine.* 1st ed. Berlin: Springer; 2006.
12. Edwards ML. Hyperbaric oxygen therapy. Part 2: Application in disease. *J Vet Emerg Crit Care.* 2010;20(3):289-297.
13. Gabb G, Robin ED. Hyperbaric oxygen—a therapy in search of disease. *Chest.* 1987;92:1074-1082.
14. Gesell LB. *Hyperbaric oxygen therapy indications. The Hyperbaric Oxygen Therapy Committee Report.* 12th ed. Durham, NC: Undersea and Hyperbaric Medical Society; 2008:7-196.
15. Centers for Medicare and Medicaid Services. Manual section number 20.29: Hyperbaric oxygen therapy. In: *Medicare national coverage determinations manual.* Version number 3. Washington, DC: U.S. Department of Health and Human Services; 2006.
16. Undersea and Hyperbaric Medical Society. Air or gas embolism. http://membership.uhms.org/?page=AGE&hhSearchTerms=%22air+or+gas+embolism%22. Accessed May 19, 2008.
17. Muth C, Shank E. Gas embolism. *N Engl J Med.* 2000;342: 476-482.
18. Ziser A, Adir Y, Lavon H, Shupak A. Hyperbaric oxygen therapy for massive arterial air embolism during cardiac operations. *J Thorac Cardiovasc Surg.* 1999;117:818-821.
19. Mammoto T, Hayashi Y, Ohnishi Y, Kuro M. Incidence of venous and paradoxical air embolism in neurosurgical patients in the sitting position: Detection by transesophageal echocardiography. *Acta Anaesthesiol Scand.* 1998;42:643-647.
20. García BA, Blanco AG, Martínez AM, Blanco JC. Cerebral artery air embolism secondary to endoscopic retrograde cholangiopancreatography. *Gastroenterol Hepatol.* 2009; 32(9):614-617.
21. Yu AS, Levy E. Paradoxical cerebral air embolism from a hemodialysis catheter. *Am J Kidney Dis.* 1997;29:453-455.
22. Halliday P, Anderson DN, Davidson AT, Page JG. Management of cerebral air embolism secondary to a disconnected central venous catheter. *Br J Surg.* 1994;81:71.
23. Halpern P, Greenstein A, Melamed Y, Taitelman U, Sznajder I, Zveibil F. Arterial air embolism after penetrating lung injury. *Crit Care Med.* 1983;11:392-393.

24. Mahmud F. Air embolism from mechanical ventilation in respiratory distress syndrome. *South Med J.* 1979;72(7):783-785.

25. Wherrett CG, Mehran RJ, Beaulieu MA. Cerebral arterial gas embolism following diagnostic bronchoscopy: Delayed treatment with hyperbaric oxygen. *Can J Anaesth.* 2002;49(1):96-99.

26. Weissman A, Kol S, Peretz BA. Gas embolism in obstetrics and gynecology: A review. *J Reprod Med.* 1996;41:103-111.

27. Moon RE, de Lisle Dear G, Stolp BW. Treatment of decompression illness and iatrogenic gas embolism. *Respir Care Clin N Am.* 1999;5:93-135.

28. McDermott J, Dutka A, Koller W, Pearson R, Flynn E. Comparison of two recompression profiles in treating experimental cerebral air embolism. *Undersea Biomed Res.* 1992;19:171-185.

29. National Center of Health Statistics. *Vital statistics of the United States, 1990.* Vol. II. Mortality. Part A. DHHS pub. no. (PHS) 95-1101. Washington, DC: Government Printing Office; 1994.

30. Piantadosi, CA. Carbon monoxide poisoning. *N Engl J Med.* 2002;347:1054-1055.

31. Weaver LK, Hopkins RO, Chan KJ, et al. Hyperbaric oxygen for acute carbon monoxide poisoning. *N Engl J Med.* 2002; 347:1057-1067.

32. Tibbles PM, Perrotta PL. Treatment of carbon monoxide poisoning: A critical review of human outcome studies comparing normobaric oxygen with hyperbaric oxygen. *Ann Emerg Med.* 1994;24:269-276.

33. Raphael J-C, Elkharrat D, Jars-Guincestre MC, et al. Trial of normobaric and hyperbaric oxygen for acute carbon monoxide intoxication. *Lancet.* 1989;2:414-419.

34. Thom SR, Taber RL, Mendiguren II, et al. Delayed neuropsychologic sequelae after carbon monoxide poisoning: Prevention by treatment with hyperbaric oxygen. *Ann Emerg Med.* 1995; 25:474-480.

35. Piantadosi CA. Carbon monoxide poisoning. *Undersea Hyperb Med.* 2004;31(1):167-177.

36. Norris JC, Moore SJ, Hume AS. Synergistic lethality induced by the combination of carbon monoxide and cyanide. *Toxicology.* 1986;40:121.

37. Scolnick CD, Hamel D, Woolf AD. Successful treatment of life-threatening propionitrile exposure with sodium nitrite/sodium thiosulfate followed by hyperbaric oxygen. *J Occup Med.* 1993;35(6):577.

38. Haymore JG, Mejico LJ. Retinal vascular occlusion syndromes. *Int Ophthalmol Clin.* 2009;49(3):63-79.

39. Butler FK, Hagan C, Murphy-Lavoie H. Hyperbaric oxygen therapy and the eye. *Undersea Hyperb Med.* 2008;35(5):333-387.

40. Finsterer J, Hess B. Neuromuscular and central nervous system manifestations of *Clostridium perfringens* infections. *Infection.* 2007;35(6):396-405.

41. Morris WE, Fernández-Miyakawa ME. Toxins of *Clostridium perfringens.* *Rev Argent Microbiol.* 2009;41(4):251-260.

42. Brummelkamp WH, Hogenijk J, Boerema I. Treatment of anaerobic infections (clostridial myositis) by drenching the tissue with oxygen under high atmospheric pressure. *Surgery.* 1961;49:299-302.

43. Riseman JA, Zamboni WA, Curtis A, et al. Hyperbaric oxygen therapy for necrotizing fasciitis reduces mortality and the need for debridements. *Surgery.* 1990;108(5):847-850.

44. Korhonen K. Hyperbaric oxygen therapy in acute necrotizing infections. With a special reference to the effects on tissue gas tensions. *Ann Chir Gynaecol.* 2000;89(Suppl 214):7-36.

45. Hampson NB, ed. *Hyperbaric oxygen therapy: 1999. Committee report.* Kensington, MD: Undersea and Hyperbaric Medical Society; 1999.

46. Bouachour G, Cronier P, Gouello JP, et al. Hyperbaric oxygen therapy in the management of crush injuries: A randomized double-blind placebo-controlled clinical trial. *J Trauma.* 1996; 41(2):333-339.

47. Moon RE, Sheffield PJ. Guidelines for the treatment of decompression illness. *Aviat Space Environ Med.* 1997; 68:234-243.

48. Hart GB. HBO and exceptional blood loss. In: Kindwall EP, ed. *Hyperbaric medicine practice.* Flagstaff, AZ: Best; 1994: 517-524.

49. Mathieu D, Wattel F, Neviere R, et al. Intracranial infections and hyperbaric oxygen therapy: A five year experience. *Undersea Hyperb Med.* 1999;26(Suppl):67.

50. Feldmeier J. *Hyperbaric oxygen 2003: Indications and results. The Hyperbaric Oxygen Therapy Committee Report.* Kensington, MD: Undersea and Hyperbaric Medical Society; 2003.

51. Grossman AR, Grossman AJ. Update on hyperbaric oxygen and treatment of burns. *Burns.* 1982;8:176-179.

52. Cianci P, Sato R, Green B. Adjunctive hyperbaric oxygen reduces length of hospital stay, surgery, and the cost of care in severe burns. *Undersea Biomed Res.* 1991;18(Suppl):108.

53. Pritchard J, Anand P, Broome J, et al. Double-blind randomized phase II study of hyperbaric oxygen in patients with radiation-induced brachial plexopathy. *Radiother Oncol.* 2001;58:279-286.

54. Villanueva E, Bennett MH, Wasiak J, et al. Hyperbaric oxygen therapy for thermal burns. *Cochrane Database Syst Rev.* 2004(3):CD004727.

55. Marx RE, Ehler WJ, Tayapongsak P, et al. Relationship of oxygen dose to angiogenesis induction in irradiated tissue. *Am J Surg.* 1973;160:519-524.

56. Dempsey J, Haynes N, Smith T, et al. Cost-effectiveness analysis of hyperbaric therapy in osteoradionecrosis. *Can J Plast Surg.* 1997;5:221-229.

57. Ladizinsky D, Roe D. New insights into oxygen therapy for wound healing. *Wounds.* 2010;22(12):294-300.

58. Abidia A, Laden G, Kuhan G, et al. The role of hyperbaric oxygen therapy in ischemic diabetic lower extremity ulcers: A double-blind randomized-controlled trial. *Eur J Vasc Endovasc Surg.* 2003;25(6):513.

59. Wang C, Swaitzberg S, Berliner E, et al. Hyperbaric oxygen for treating wounds: A systemic review of the literature. *Arch Surg.* 2003;138:272-279.

60. Strauss MB, Malluche HH, Faugere MC. Effect of hyperbaric oxygen on bone resorption in rabbits. *Seventh Annual Conference on Clinical Application of HBO,* Anaheim, CA. June 1982:8-18.

61. Chen CE, Shih ST, Fu TH, et al. Hyperbaric oxygen therapy in the treatment of chronic refractory osteomyelitis: A preliminary report. *Chang Gung Med J.* 2003;26(2):114.

62. Zamboni WA, Roth AC, Russell RC, et al. Morphological analysis of the microcirculation during reperfusion of ischemic skeletal muscle and the effect of hyperbaric oxygen. *Plastic Reconstr Surg.* 1993;91:1110-1123.

63. Waterhouse MA, Zamboni WA, Brown RE, et al. The use of HBO in compromised free tissue transfer and replantation, a clinical review. *Undersea Hyperb Med.* 1993;20(Suppl):64.

64. Fife CE, Piantadosi CA. Oxygen toxicity. In: Moon RE, Camporesi EM, eds. *Clinical application of hyperbaric oxygen: Problems in respiratory care.* Philadelphia, PA: JB Lippincott; 1991.

65. Clark J. Side effects and complications. In: Gesell LB, ed. *Hyperbaric oxygen therapy indications.* Durham, NC: Undersea and Hyperbaric Medical Society; 2003.

66. Blanshard J, Toma A, Bryson P, Williamson P. Middle ear barotrauma in patients undergoing hyperbaric oxygen therapy. *Clin Otolaryngol Allied Sci.* 1996;21(5):400-403.

67. Plafki C, Peters P, Almeling M, et al. Complications and side effects of hyperbaric oxygen therapy. *Aviat Space Environ Med.* 2000;71:119-124.

68. Lyne AJ. Ocular effects of hyperbaric oxygen. *Trans Ophthalmol Soc.* 1978;98(1):66.

69. Kindwall EP. Contraindications and side effects to hyperbaric oxygen treatment. In: Kindwall EP, Whelan HT, eds. *Hyperbaric medicine practice.* 2nd ed. rev. Flagstaff, AZ: Best; 2002.

70. European Committee for Hyperbaric Medicine. *Recommendations for safety in multiplace medical hyperbaric chambers.* 1998. Available at: http://www.echm.org/documents/ECHM%20Recommendations%20for%20Safety%201998.pdf. Accessed June 23, 2014.

71. Working Group of the COST Action B14. A European code of good practice in hyperbaric oxygen therapy. May 2004. Available at: http://www.mnof.cz/data/files/user/centrum_hyperbaricke_mediciny/ecgp_for_hbo_-_may_2004.pdf. Accessed June 23, 2014.

72. Sheffield PJ, Desautels DA. Hyperbaric and hypobaric chamber fires: A 73-year analysis. *Undersea Hyperb Med.* 1997;24(3):153-164.

73. Occupational Safety and Health Administration. Standard for confined space entry 29 CFR 1910.146. Available at: https://www.osha.gov/pls/oshaweb/owadisp.show_document?p_xml:id=9797&p_table=STANDARDS. Accessed June 23, 2014.

74. National Fire Protection Association. *NFPA 99, Standards for health care facilities, Ch. 19, Hyperbaric facilities.* Boston, MA: National Fire Protection Association; 1996.

75. American Society of Mechanical Engineers (ASME). Safety standard for pressure vessels for human occupancy (PVHO-1). 2007. Available at: https://law.resource.org/pub/us/code/ibr/asme.pvho-1.2007.pdf. Accessed June 23, 2014.

76. SCCM guidelines. Guidelines for the transfer of critically ill patients. *Crit Care Med.* 1993;21:931-937.

77. Shoemaker WC. Tissue perfusion and oxygenation: A primary problem in acute circulatory failure and shock states. *Crit Care Med.* 1991;19(5):595-596.

78. Wattel F, Mathieu D, Coget JM, Billard V. Hyperbaric oxygen therapy in chronic vascular wound management. *Angiology.* 1990;41:59-65.

79. Radermacher P, Frey G, Berger R. Hyperbaric oxygen therapy—intensive care in a hostile environment? In: Vincent JL, ed. *Yearbook of intensive care and emergency medicine 1997.* New York, NY: Springer; 1997:821-835.

80. Weaver LK, Howe S. Normobaric measurement of arterial oxygen tension in subjects exposed to hyperbaric oxygen. *Chest.* 1992;102:1175-1181.

81. Ratzenhofer-Komenda B, Offner A, Ofner P, et al. Arterial oxygen tension increase 2-3 h after hyperbaric oxygen therapy: A prospective observational study. *Acta Anaesthesiol Scand.* 2007;51(1):68-73.

82. Casati A, Squicciarini G, Malagutti G, et al. Transcutaneous monitoring of partial pressure of carbon dioxide in the elderly patient: A prospective, clinical comparison with end-tidal monitoring. *J Clin Anesth.* 2006;18(6):436-440.

83. Vezzani G. Characteristics of an ideal ventilator for use in hyperbaric environment. In: Wattel F, Mathieu D, eds. *Proceedings of the First European Consensus Conference on Hyperbaric Medicine.* Lille, France: CRAM Nord-Picardie; 1994:337-342.

84. Bouachour G, Lemasson Y, Varache N, et al. Evaluation du respirateur pour chamber hyperbare. *MEDSUBHYP.* 1989;8:178-187.

85. Longoni C, Marchesi G. Adapting the hyperbaric chamber to the health care environment: History and future trends. In: Oriani G, Marroni A, Wattel F, eds. *Handbook on hyperbaric medicine.* Berlin: Springer-Verlag; 1996:741-764.

86. Moon RE, Bergquist LV, Conklin B, et al. Monaghan 225 ventilator use under hyperbaric conditions. *Chest.* 1986;89(6):846-851.

87. Gallagher TJ, Smith RA, Bell GC. Evaluation of mechanical ventilators in a hyperbaric environment. *Aviat Space Environ Med.* 1978;49(2):375-376.

88. Gallagher TJ, Smith RA, Bell GC. Evaluation of the IMV bird and the modified Mark 2 bird in a hyperbaric environment. *Respir Care.* 1977;22(5):501-504.

89. Stahl W, Radermacher P, Calzia E. Functioning of ICU ventilators under hyperbaric conditions: Comparison of volume- and pressure-controlled modes. *Intensive Care Med.* 2000;26(4):442-448.

90. Van Baren R, Heij HA, Van Vugt JM, et al. Hyperbaric oxygen and high-frequency oscillator ventilation in experimental diaphragmatic hernia. *Undersea Hyperb Med.* 1995;22(3):315-316.

91. European Committee for Standardisation. *prEN14931: Pressure Vessels for Human Occupancy (PVHO)—Multi-Place Pressure Chamber Systems for Hyperbaric Therapy—Performance, Safety Requirements and Testing.* Brussels: European Committee for Standardisation (CEN); 2004.

92. Weaver LK. Management of critically ill patients in the monoplace hyperbaric chamber. In Kindwall EP, ed. *Hyperbaric medicine practice.* Flagstaff, AZ: Best; 1995:174-246.

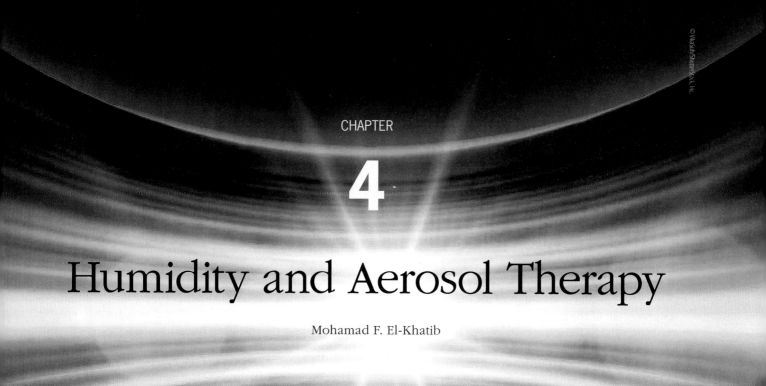

4

Humidity and Aerosol Therapy

Mohamad F. El-Khatib

CHAPTER OBJECTIVES

1. Describe the natural physiologic humidification process.
2. Identify indications and contraindications for humidity therapy.
3. Understand the principle of operation of different types of humidifiers used in clinical practices.
4. Recognize the consequences of inadequate humidification.
5. Compare the different types of humidifiers. Compare and contrast the different types of humidifiers in terms of their functions, applications, and characteristics.

KEY TERMS

Aerosol therapy
Bubble humidifier
Heat and moisture exchangers (HMEs)
Heated humidifier
Humidification

Large volume jet nebulizer
Passover humidifier
Relative humidity
Vibrating mesh nebulizer (VMN)

Introduction

Providing humidity and aerosol therapies are common practices in the field of respiratory care. Respiratory care practitioners are often in charge of the tasks to provide optimal humidity and efficient aerosol therapies to patients who are either spontaneously breathing or receiving invasive ventilatory support with mechanical ventilation.

It is essential that respiratory care practitioners not only have a firm understanding of the rationale, physiological basis, indications, and contraindications for humidity and aerosol therapies, but also have a good grasp of the different technical considerations

regarding the multitude of devices available for such use in the clinical arena. The respiratory therapist's understanding of the classifications, principles of operation, range of applications, specifications, and hazards of these devices is as important as the therapies these devices are intended to provide.

This chapter describes the various devices currently used in the clinical practice of providing humidity and aerosol therapies in spontaneously breathing and mechanically ventilated patients.

Before proceeding any further, it is important that some terms are defined:

- *Humidity:* The presence of moisture in its molecular form in a gas or gas mixture
- *Absolute humidity:* The weight of water in a volume of gas or gas mixture expressed as milligrams per liter (mg/L)
- **Relative humidity:** The absolute humidity of a volume of gas expressed as a percentage of the water vapor capacity of the gas (i.e., capacity is absolute humidity when saturated with water vapor).

Physiologic Control of Heat and Moisture

The upper respiratory tract system, and in particular the nose, has the essential function of conditioning inspired gases for optimal heat and moisture before they flow through the bronchial tree and expand the lung parenchyma. It is crucial for the proper functioning of the lower airways and alveoli that inspired gases are fully saturated with water vapor and warmed to body temperature upon reaching just below the carina. This point in the upper airways is called the isothermic saturation boundary (ISB). At this boundary, the inspired gas should have 100% relative humidity and a temperature of 98.6°F (37°C).

During inspiration, the induced turbulence in the flow of the inspired gas as it passes through the nasal turbinates increases the contact between the molecules of inspired gas and the nasal mucosa and results in efficient warming of the inspired gas. This is called turbulent convection. With the efficient warming of the inspired gas, water is then transferred and added to the inspired gas by evaporation from the mucosa. Evaporation results in cooling and decreasing the water content of the tracheal and nasal mucosa. During expiration and as the gas is exhaled, the tracheal and nasal mucosa cools the exhaled gas and reclaims part of its water content. This is called condensation.

Below the isothermic saturation boundary, temperature and relative humidity remain constant with body temperature and pressure, saturated (BTPS) conditions (i.e., 98.6°F [37°C] body temperature, barometric pressure, and 100% relative humidity). When the ISB is not achieved just below the carina, there will be a further distal downshift in the ISB. Several clinical and technical conditions can lead to such displacement of the ISB.[1] These include situations when patients breathe cold and dry air, as when breathing medical gases provided by hospitals' medical gas supply systems; when patients breathe through their mouths at higher minute ventilation, which is mostly the case during respiratory distress situations; or when patients' natural anatomical **humidification** and heating structures are bypassed by artificial airways or endotracheal tubes during mechanical ventilation. With the distal shift of the ISB, additional surfaces from the lower airways will be required to provide humidity and heat. This can negatively impact the epithelial integrity of these airways, make them susceptible to infection and inflammation, and lead to the narrowing of their cross-sectional areas.[2] As such, whenever the body's capability for humidifying and heating inspired gas is compromised, external measures for humidifying and heating of these inspired

medical gases are indicated and needed to prevent a negative impact on a patient's health. The recommended humidity and heat levels are shown in **Table 4-1**.

Effects of Inadequate Humidification

The objective of humidity therapy is to condition medical gases to approximate normal inspiratory conditions. With proper humidification, the ISB remains just below the carina with no downward shift toward the small airways. Extrinsic humidification and heating of inspired dry medical gases should be ensured (whether the nose and upper airways are bypassed or not) during different modalities of respiratory support using either medical gas therapies or invasive and noninvasive ventilator support. Inadequate humidification can result in substantial water and heat loss from the airways that can lead to the disruption of the mucociliary transport system and an increase in mucus production with thickening of the pulmonary secretions, an increase in the airway irritability, and ultimately structural damage to the lung.[2]

There are several signs and symptoms of inadequate humidification.[3] These are more evident and significant during invasive mechanical ventilation when the normal water and heat exchange capabilities of upper airways are bypassed with the use of endotracheal tubes. The clinical signs and symptoms usually include thick, dehydrated, and encrusted secretions; dry and nonproductive cough; patient complaint of substernal pain; atelectasis; increased incidence of infection; bacterial infiltration of mucosa; increased airway resistance; and increased work of breathing.

Application

Indications for Humidity Therapy

Humidity and heat therapy is administered during numerous respiratory care therapeutic modalities to a wide variety of patients under different clinical scenarios and medical conditions. This can be provided in both the hospital and home setting. The generally accepted indication for this type of therapy is

TABLE 4-1
Recommended Heat and Humidity Levels

Site	Temperature Range (°C)	Relative Humidity (%)	Absolute Humidity (mg/L)
Nose/mouth	20–22	50	10
Hypopharynx	29–32	95	28–34
Trachea	32–35	100	36–40
Carina	37	100	44

Reproduced with permission from Chatburn R, Primiano F. A rational basis for humidity therapy. *Respir Care.* 32:249, 1987; permission conveyed through Copyright Clearance Center, Inc.

TABLE 4-2
Indications for Humidity Therapy

1. Delivering adequate humidity when spontaneously breathing medical gases for therapeutic purposes
2. Providing adequate humidification in the presence of artificial airway during invasive mechanical ventilation
3. Providing adequate humidification in the presence of high gas flows during noninvasive ventilation and high flow nasal cannula oxygen therapy
4. Thinning dried and/or thick secretions
5. Promoting bronchial hygiene
6. Managing hypothermia in intubated and mechanically ventilated patients
7. Treating bronchospasm caused by cold air in spontaneously breathing patients

conditioning the dry inspired mix of medical gases, particularly when the normal and anatomical structures of the body (nose and upper airways) are either compromised or bypassed.[4] The different indications for humidity therapy are summarized in **Table 4-2**.

Contraindications for Humidity Therapy

In general, there are no contraindications to providing humidification of inspired gas during spontaneous breathing or mechanical ventilation. However, there might be some contraindications for using certain humidification devices during specific clinical conditions.[5] A heat and moisture exchanger (HME) is contraindicated in patients with thick, copious, or bloody secretions. A minute ventilation greater than 10 L/min is a contraindication for the use of an HME as the means for providing humidification during ventilator support. Also, HMEs are contraindicated in patients with expired tidal volume less than 70% of the delivered tidal volume, such as in patients with large bronchopleural fistulas, severe tracheomalasia, or uncuffed endotracheal tubes. The use of heat and moisture might also be contraindicated in patients with body temperature of less than 89.6°F (32°C). Unless it is bypassed, the HME has to be removed from the patient's breathing circuits when he or she is receiving in-line aerosol drug treatments.

Hazards of Humidity Therapy

Hazards and complications encountered during humidification therapy are infrequent and mainly associated with the use of the humidification devices rather than the therapy itself.[6] With the use of **heated humidifiers**, there are potentials of electrical shock, hyperthermia, thermal injury to the airways, tubing meltdown if circuits and heated humidifiers are incompatible, burns to caregivers from the humidifier's hot metal, and pooled condensation in the patient's breathing circuits. With excessive pooled condensation, there will be risks for patient–ventilator dysynchrony and improper ventilator performance, elevated airway pressures, inadvertent tracheal lavage from pooled condensation or overfilling of humidifier, and nosocomial infection for both patients and clinicians when pooled condensates are aerosolized into the patient's

environment when breathing circuits are disconnected while the ventilator is generating high flows.[7]

With HMEs, there are risks for hypothermia; possible increase in the resistive work of breathing through the HME, particularly after long use (> 24 hours); and possible hypoventilation due to increased mechanical dead space.[8]

Monitoring Therapeutic Effectiveness

The primary goal for humidity therapy is to condition medical gases to achieve normal inspiratory conditions of 100% relative humidity and 98.6°F (37°C) just below the carina and before the medical gases enter the airways. Ideal measurement and monitoring of the therapeutic effectiveness of humidity therapy requires the placement of a hygrometer (a device that measures humidity) and a thermometer at the level of the carina. Currently this is not available; the closest point for measurement of these parameters is at the patient Y for mechanically ventilated patients and the mouth opening for spontaneously breathing patients. However, hygrometers are not widely used in clinical practice; most of the time the temperature is measured and monitored at the patient's Y during mechanical ventilation. Therefore, monitoring therapeutic effectiveness of humidity therapy is not direct and remains mainly subjective and widely dependent on the careful qualitative assessment of the patient and patient's breath sounds, patient's cough along with the characteristics of the sputum expectorated, and secretions and formation of mucus plugs as surrogates for effective humidification therapy.[9] In general, the absence of underhydration, thick secretions, mucus plugging of airways, obstruction of the endotracheal or tracheostomy tube, and mechanical ventilation–induced inflammatory responses, along with normal breath sounds can be considered as signs of effective humidity therapy.

Active Humidifiers

Active humidification can be accomplished using either bubble, passover, or heated humidifiers. The levels of humidification achieved with these humidifiers depend greatly on the design and principle of operation of each of these devices.

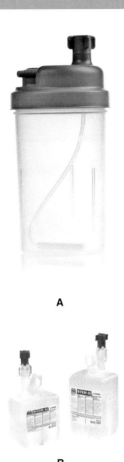

A

B

FIGURE 4-1 Simple bubble jet humidifiers: A. Disposable. B. Prefilled.

Photo A courtesy of Teleflex. Photo B courtesy of Smiths Medical.

Bubble Humidifiers

A **bubble humidifier** consists of a bottle or reservoir partially filled with water attached to a conduction system that allows the inspired medical gases to be introduced below the water surface. A diffuser that is usually either a foam or a metallic mesh is attached to the end of the conduction system. Bubble humidifiers are either reusable or single patient use humidifiers.[10] Furthermore, single patient use humidifiers are either dry or prefilled. Bubble humidifiers incorporate a pressure relief valve that releases pressure from inside the humidifier bottle to prevent bursting of the bubble in the event there is an obstruction to the flow path out of the humidifier bottle. Usually these pressure relief valves function at a pressure of greater than 2 psi. Bubble humidifiers are also known as bubble diffuser humidifiers or just diffusers (**Figure 4-1**).

> *Indications:* The bubble humidifier is used to humidify the inspired medical gases delivered to patients via a cannula or face mask.
> *Contraindications:* This type of humidifier is contraindicated for patients with an endotracheal tube, a tracheostomy, or tenacious secretions.

> *Hazards:* If heated, bubble humidifiers result in excessive condensate that tends to obstruct the small bore delivery tubing that connects between the humidifier output and the patient's interface. With prolonged use, there is a risk that the pressure relief valve becomes dysfunctional, which can lead to the build-up of excessive pressures and burst the humidifier bottle whenever a flow obstruction occurs. Whenever high flow rates (usually in excess of 10 L/min) are used, bubble humidifiers can produce aerosols. These water droplets can transmit pathogenic bacteria from the humidifier reservoir to the patient.
> *Principles of operation:* As inspired medical gases leave the diffuser and enter the water, gas bubbles are formed that flow through the liquid. This allows for greater exposure time and contact area, thereby increasing the capability of the flowing dry medical gases to extract humidity from the water. With these types of unheated bubble humidifiers, an absolute humidity level between approximately 15 and 20 mg/L is usually achieved. Bubble humidifier units function at a flow rate of 2 L/min and should not be operated at greater than 6 L/min because they start to lose their efficiency in providing humidity. The higher the flow rate, the less exposure time in the water medium and the higher risk for cooling the reservoir.[11] These humidifiers are not recommended for use at flow rates greater than 10 L/min. In the event of a flow obstruction out of the humidifier bottle, the pressure relief valve opens and releases pressure from inside the bottle while giving an audible alarm. Once the flow obstruction is eliminated, the pressure relief valve automatically resumes its normal position.
> *Currently available devices:* Bubble humidifiers remain widely used in the practice of respiratory care. Almost every single patient using low flow oxygen therapy via a nasal cannula or a face mask will need a bubble humidifier. There are many commercially available bubble humidifiers with different specifications, as presented in **Table 4-3**.

Passover Humidifiers

These are mainly of three types: the simple passover, the wick, and the membrane device (**Figure 4-2**). The simple **passover humidifier** is just a reservoir/jar containing water over which the dry inspired gas will flow and increase its water content. The wick humidifier consists of a reservoir in addition to a porous material (wick) that absorbs water and provides a larger area for air-water mix for better evaporation. Some of these wick humidifiers include a fan to aid in the evaporation of the water.

TABLE 4-3
Types and Specifications of Bubble Humidifiers

Manufacturer	Product Name/ Number	Type	Sterile/ Closed System	Volume (mL)	Audible Safety Pressure- Relief Valve	Pressure- Relief Level (psi)	Min/Max Indicators	Lid	Nut	Diffuser	Heater
Afton Medical	80300	Dry-disposable	No	300	Yes	3	Yes	Plastic	Plastic	NS	No
	80400	Dry-disposable	No	400	Yes	4	Yes	Plastic	Plastic	NS	No
	80600	Dry-disposable	No	400	Yes	6	Yes	Plastic	Plastic	NS	No
Allied Health Care Products, Inc.	64375	Dry-disposable	No	300	Yes	3	Yes	Plastic	Plastic	Foam	No
	64376	Dry-disposable	No	300	Yes	3	Yes	Plastic	Metal	Foam	No
	64377	Dry-disposable	No	300	Yes	6	Yes	Plastic	Plastic	Foam	No
	64378	Dry-disposable	No	300	Yes	6	Yes	Plastic	Metal	Fcam	No
	61350S	Prefilled-disposable	Yes	350	Yes	6	N/A	Plastic	Plastic	Foam	No
	61550S	Prefilled-disposable	Yes	350	Yes	6	N/A	Plastic	Plastic	Foam	No
	34-10-0001	Dry-reusable	No	NS	NS	NS	Yes	Plastic	Plastic	Metal	No
	34-10-0005	Dry-reusable	No	NS	Yes	NS	Yes	Plastic	Plastic	Metal	No
	34-10-0025	Dry-reusable	No	NS	Yes	NS	Yes	Plastic	Plastic	Metal	No
Besmed	HB-1130	Dry-disposable	No	300	Yes	3	Yes	Plastic	Plastic	PVC or ceramic	No
	HB-1132	Dry-disposable	No	500	Yes	4	Yes	Plastic	Plastic	PVC or ceramic	No
	HB-2401	Dry-disposable	No	400	Yes	6	Yes	Plastic	Plastic	PVC or ceramic	No
	HB-2411	Dry-disposable	No	400	Yes	4	Yes	Plastic	Plastic	PVC or ceramic	No
	HB-2601	Dry-disposable	No	400	Yes	6	Yes	Plastic	Plastic	PVC or ceramic	No
	HB-2611	Dry-disposable	No	400	Yes	4	Yes	Plastic	Plastic	PVC or ceramic	No

(continues)

TABLE 4-3
Types and Specifications of Bubble Humidifiers (Continued)

Manufacturer	Product Name/ Number	Type	Sterile/ Closed System	Volume (mL)	Audible Safety Pressure-Relief Valve	Pressure-Relief Level (psi)	Min/Max Indicators	Lid	Nut	Diffuser	Heater
CareFusion	AirLife 2620	Prefilled-disposable	Yes	500	Yes	4	N/A	Plastic	Plastic	NS	No
	AirLife 2702	Prefilled-disposable	Yes	750	Yes	4	N/A	Plastic	Plastic	NS	No
	AirLife 2003	Dry-disposable	No	370	Yes	3	Yes	Plastic	Plastic	Foam	No
	AirLife 2006	Dry-disposable	No	370	Yes	6	Yes	Plastic	Plastic	Foam	No
Galemed	BH-1	Dry-disposable	No	NS	Yes	2, 4, or 6	Yes	Plastic	Plastic	NS	No
	BH-2	Dry-disposable	No	NS	Yes	2	Yes	Plastic	Plastic	NS	Yes
	BH-3	Dry-disposable	No	NS	Yes	4	Yes	Plastic	Plastic	NS	No
	ECO	Dry-disposable	No	NS	Yes	4	Yes	Plastic	Plastic	NS	No
Genstar Technologies, Inc.	7100R	Dry-reusable	No	300	Yes	NS	Yes	Plastic	Plastic	NS	No
	7200R	Dry-reusable	No	140	No	NS	Yes	Metal	Metal	NS	No
	638-001	Dry-disposable	No	250	Yes	NS	Yes	Plastic	Plastic	NS	No
	638-002	Dry-disposable	No	400	Yes	NS	Yes	Plastic	Plastic	NS	No
	638-003	Dry-disposable	No	400	Yes	NS	Yes	Plastic	Plastic	NS	No
GF Health Products, Inc.	BF61550S	Prefilled-disposable	Yes	550	Yes	6	N/A	Plastic	Plastic	NS	No
	GF64375	Dry-disposable	No	250	Yes	6	Yes	Plastic	Plastic	NS	No

TABLE 4-3
Types and Specifications of Bubble Humidifiers

Manufacturer	Product Name/ Number	Type	Sterile/ Closed System	Volume (mL)	Audible Safety Pressure- Relief Valve	Pressure- Relief Level (psi)	Min/Max Indicators	Lid	Nut	Diffuser	Heater
Intersurgical	AquaFlow 1507	Dry-disposable	No	120 & 500	Yes	NS	Yes	Plastic	Plastic	NS	No
	AquaFlow 1521	Dry-disposable	No	120	Yes	NS	Yes	Plastic	Plastic	NS	No
Ohio Medical Corp.	6700-0338-800	Dry-reusable	No	300	Yes	2	Yes	Plastic	Plastic	Chrome-plated brass	No
Salter Labs	7100	Dry-disposable	No	350	Yes	3	Yes	Plastic	Plastic	PVC	No
	7600	Dry-disposable	No	350	Yes	6	Yes	Plastic	Plastic	PVC	No
	7900	Dry-disposable	No	350	Yes	NS	Yes	Plastic	Plastic	PVC	No
Teleflex	003-40	Prefilled-disposable	Yes	340	Yes	NS	N/A	Plastic	Plastic	NS	No
	005-40	Prefilled-disposable	Yes	540	Yes	NS	N/A	Plastic	Plastic	NS	No
	006-40	Prefilled-disposable	Yes	650	Yes	NS	N/A	Plastic	Plastic	NS	No
	3230	Dry-disposable	No	500	Yes	4	Yes	Plastic	Plastic	NS	No
	3260	Dry-disposable	No	500	Yes	6	Yes	Plastic	Plastic	NS	No
Ventlab Corp.	VTB6900	Dry-disposable	No	350	NS	NS	Yes	Plastic	Plastic	NS	NS
Westmed	0480	Dry-disposable	No	NS	Yes	NS	Yes	Plastic	Plastic	PVC	No
	0795	Dry-disposable	No	NS	Yes	NS	Yes	Plastic	Plastic	PVC	No

N/A: Not applicable, NS: Not specified, PVC: Polyvinylchloride

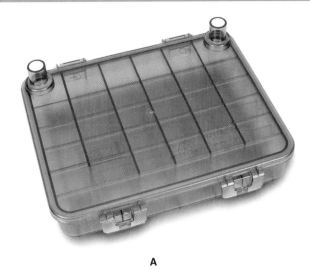

A

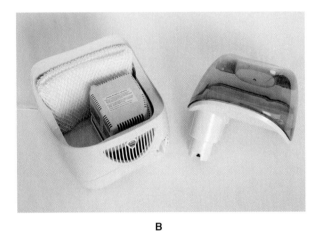

B

FIGURE 4-2 Different types of passover humidifiers: A. Simple. B. Wick type.

Photo A reproduced with permission from Philips Healthcare.

Membrane Devices

Membrane passover humidifiers consist of a jar that can be filled with water with no conduction system for the inspired gas inside the jar. A hydrophobic membrane separates the gas stream from the water. Inspired gases flow in one side, pass over the water surface and membrane, and exit from another side of the humidifier. There is no bubbling of water inside the humidifier. The efficiency of this unit is rather low, because exposure area and time of contact are limited and the water is usually not heated. Membrane passover humidifiers can maintain saturation at high flow rates with no or little resistance to spontaneous breathing circuits.[12] Additionally they do not generate aerosols, leading to minimal risk for spreading infection.

> *Indications:* Passover humidifiers are usually used with invasive and noninvasive ventilator support (e.g., nasal continuous positive airway pressure or bilevel positive airway pressure support).[13]

> *Contraindications:* There are no contraindications for using passover humidification to provide physiologic conditioning of inspired gas during invasive and noninvasive mechanical ventilation.[14]

> *Hazards:* Passover humidifiers have minimal hazards. However, if a heat element is used, then there will be the risk of electrical shock. Hypo- or hyperthermia can result from inadequate adjustment of the temperature. Excessive heating and evaporation can result in accumulation of condensate in the breathing circuit with the risk of contamination, patient–ventilator asynchrony, and condensate aerosolization whenever the patient is disconnected from the ventilator. In addition, if the compressible volume losses from the humidifier reservoir are not compensated for, there is a risk for inaccurate tidal volume measurement.

> *Principles of operation:* As the inspired gases pass over the water surface and hydrophobic membrane, the water vapor can easily pass through the wick or membrane, mix with the dry inspired gas, and increase its water content. Liquid water will not cross the hydrophobic membrane.

> *Currently available devices:* Passover humidifiers are very common during invasive and noninvasive mechanical ventilation. There are several commercially available passover humidifiers with different specifications and features, as presented in **Table 4-4**.

Heated Humidifiers

A heated humidifier consists of a reservoir and a heating element. Some heated humidifiers include a wick element. The wick is usually surrounded by the heating element to maintain adequate saturation of the wick during the operation of the device.[15] The heating element improves water output and usually has a controller that regulates the element's heating power and subsequently maintains a set temperature of inspired gas at the patient airway. These systems incorporate alarms and alarm-activated heater shutdown.

There are four different types of heating systems:

- A hot plate located at the base of the humidifier chamber
- A wraparound that surrounds the humidifier chamber
- A collar that sits between the water reservoir and the gas outlet
- An immersion type where the heating element is placed in the water

All modern heated humidifiers are equipped with automatic feed systems with a flotation valve control for adequate and continuous control of the water level inside the humidifier chamber (**Figure 4-3**).

TABLE 4-4
Types and Specifications of Passover Humidifiers

Manufacturer	Product Name/Number	Type	Sterile/Closed System	Volume (mL)	Audible Safety Pressure-Relief Valve	Pressure-Relief Level (psi)	Min/Max Indicators	Lid	Nut	Diffuser	Heater Interface
Afton Medical	80300	Dry-disposable	No	300	Yes	3	Yes	Plastic	Plastic	NS	No
	80400	Dry-disposable	No	400	Yes	4	Yes	Plastic	Plastic	NS	No
	80600	Dry-disposable	No	400	Yes	6	Yes	Plastic	Plastic	NS	No
Allied Health Care Products, Inc.	64375	Dry-disposable	No	300	Yes	3	Yes	Plastic	Plastic	Foam	No
	64376	Dry-disposable	No	300	Yes	3	Yes	Plastic	Metal	Foam	No
	64377	Dry-disposable	No	300	Yes	6	Yes	Plastic	Plastic	Foam	No
	64378	Dry-disposable	No	300	Yes	6	Yes	Plastic	Metal	Foam	No
	61350S	Prefilled-disposable	Yes	350	Yes	6	N/A	Plastic	Plastic	Foam	No
	61550S	Prefilled-disposable	Yes	350	Yes	6	N/A	Plastic	Plastic	Foam	No
	34-10-0001	Dry-reusable	No	NS	NS	NS	Yes	Plastic	Plastic	Metal	No
	34-10-0005	Dry-reusable	No	NS	Yes	NS	Yes	Plastic	Plastic	Metal	No
	34-10-0025	Dry-reusable	No	NS	Yes	NS	Yes	Plastic	Plastic	Metal	No
Besmed	HB-1130	Dry-disposable	No	300	Yes	3	Yes	Plastic	Plastic	PVC or Ceramic	No
	HB-1132	Dry-disposable	No	500	Yes	4	Yes	Plastic	Plastic	PVC or Ceramic	No
	HB-2401	Dry-disposable	No	400	Yes	6	Yes	Plastic	Plastic	PVC or Ceramic	No
	HB-2411	Dry-disposable	No	400	Yes	4	Yes	Plastic	Plastic	PVC or Ceramic	No
	HB-2601	Dry-disposable	No	400	Yes	6	Yes	Plastic	Plastic	PVC or Ceramic	No
	HB-2611	Dry-disposable	No	400	Yes	4	Yes	Plastic	Plastic	PVC or Ceramic	No
CareFusion	AirLife 2620	Prefilled-disposable	Yes	500	Yes	4	N/A	Plastic	Plastic	NS	No
	AirLife 2702	Prefilled-disposable	Yes	750	Yes	4	N/A	Plastic	Plastic	NS	No
	AirLife 2003	Dry-disposable	No	370	Yes	3	Yes	Plastic	Plastic	Foam	No
	AirLife 2006	Dry-disposable	No	370	Yes	6	Yes	Plastic	Plastic	Foam	No

(continues)

TABLE 4-4
Types and Specifications of Passover Humidifiers (Continued)

Manufacturer	Product Name/ Number	Type	Sterile/ Closed System	Volume (mL)	Audible Safety Pressure- Relief Valve	Pressure- Relief Level (psi)	Min/Max Indicators	Lid	Nut	Diffuser	Heater Interface
Galemed	BH-1	Dry-Disposable	No	NS	Yes	2, 4, or 6	Yes	Plastic	Plastic	NS	No
	BH-2	Dry-Disposable	No	NS	Yes	2	Yes	Plastic	Plastic	NS	Yes
	BH-3	Dry-Disposable	No	NS	Yes	4	Yes	Plastic	Plastic	NS	No
	ECO	Dry-Disposable	No	NS	Yes	4	Yes	Plastic	Plastic	NS	No
Genstar Technologies, Inc	7100R	Dry-Reusable	No	300	Yes	NS	Yes	Plastic	Plastic	NS	No
	7200R	Dry-Reusable	No	140	No	NS	Yes	Metal	Metal	NS	No
	638-001	Dry-Disposable	No	250	Yes	NS	Yes	Plastic	Plastic	NS	No
	638-002	Dry-Disposable	No	400	Yes	NS	Yes	Plastic	Plastic	NS	No
	638-003	Dry-Disposable	No	400	Yes	NS	Yes	Plastic	Plastic	NS	No
GF Health Products, Inc.	BF61550S	Prefilled-Disposable	Yes	550	Yes	6	N/A	Plastic	Plastic	NS	No
	GF64375	Dry-Disposable	No	250	Yes	6	Yes	Plastic	Plastic	NS	No
Ohio Medical Corp.	6700-0338-800	Dry-Reusable	No	300	Yes	2	Yes	Plastic	Plastic	Chrome-plated brass	No
Salter Labs	7100	Dry-Disposable	No	350	Yes	3	Yes	Plastic	Plastic	PVC	No
	7600	Dry-Disposable	No	350	Yes	6	Yes	Plastic	Plastic	PVC	No
	7900	Dry-Disposable	No	350	Yes	NS	Yes	Plastic	Plastic	PVC	No
Teleflex	003-40	Prefilled-Disposable	Yes	340	Yes	NS	N/A	Plastic	Plastic	NS	No
	005-40	Prefilled-Disposable	Yes	540	Yes	NS	N/A	Plastic	Plastic	NS	No
	006-40	Prefilled-Disposable	Yes	650	Yes	NS	N/A	Plastic	Plastic	NS	No
	3230	Dry-Disposable	No	500	Yes	4	Yes	Plastic	Plastic	NS	No
	3260	Dry-Disposable	No	500	Yes	6	Yes	Plastic	Plastic	NS	No
Ventlab Corp.	VTB6900	Dry-Disposable	No	350	NS	NS	Yes	Plastic	Plastic	NS	No
Westmed	0480	Dry-Disposable	No	NS	Yes	NS	Yes	Plastic	Plastic	PVC	No
	0795	Dry-Disposable	No	NS	Yes	NS	Yes	Plastic	Plastic	PVC	No

N/A: Not applicable, NS: Not specified, PVC: Polyvinylchloride

Similar to membrane device passover humidifiers, no bubbling occurs and subsequently no aerosol is produced.

Indications: Heated humidifiers provide a high level of humidity and heat, and for that reason are mainly used with intubated and mechanically ventilated patients.[16] In these patients, the upper airways are bypassed by the endotracheal tubes and the patients are fully dependent on external sources that provide the highest possible levels of humidity and heat for optimal conditioning of the inspired gases.

Contraindications: There are no contraindications for using heated humidifiers in order to provide physiologic conditioning of inspired gas during invasive mechanical ventilation.

Hazards: Like with any other electrical devices, there will always be a risk of electrical shock. If the temperature is not adequately set, heated humidifiers can result in hypo- or hyperthermia. Thermal injury to the airway can occur from heated humidifiers; in addition, burns to the patient and to the caregiver and tubing meltdown can result if heated-wire circuits are covered or circuits and heated humidifiers are incompatible. Pooled contaminated condensate in the breathing circuit can result in patient–ventilator asynchrony or unintentional tracheal lavage or can be aerosolized when disconnecting the patient from the mechanical ventilator, which can put the patient and the caregiver at risk for nosocomial infection. Because the chambers of these humidifiers can be of substantial volume, the compressible volume losses should be compensated for; otherwise, inaccurate tidal volume is measured with a decrease in the ventilator response.[17]

Principles of operation: During operation, the heating element, which is usually either a plate or a rod, increases and maintains the water temperature in the reservoir at 37–38°C via a servo controlled closed system. The dry and cold gas passes over the heated and warm water before being expelled out of the water reservoir during inspiration and more humidification takes place. This device can deliver 100% relative humidity.

Currently available devices: The currently available commercial devices do not include wick elements. The systems are passover humidifiers with either a heated plate chamber or a heated wire chamber. The specifications of commercially available heated humidifiers are presented in **Table 4-5**.

Aerosol Generators

Aerosol generators are required for the delivery of sterile water or hypotonic, isotonic, or hypertonic saline aerosols. During bland **aerosol therapy**, liquid particles are generated and delivered to the patient's airway suspended in the inspired gas.[18] Several devices can be used for aerosol generation during bland aerosol therapy. The most common are the large volume jet nebulizers and vibrating mesh or "ultrasonic" nebulizers.

Large Volume Jet Nebulizer

The use of **large volume jet nebulizers** is very common in respiratory care practice. Large volume jet nebulizers are pneumatically powered with direct attachment to a flowmeter and compressed gas source. These devices deliver cool or heated aerosols with the possibility for precisely regulating inspired oxygen concentrations by using a variable oxygen diluter (**Figure 4-4**). When using these units, the flow selected should always match or exceed the patient's peak inspiratory flow rates.[18,19] Similar to heated humidifiers, a hot plate or immersion element can be added if active heating of the inspired gas is required. These devices rarely have automatic servo-controlled systems to control delivered inspired gas temperature. Depending on the design, flow, and air entrainment setting, the total water output of unheated large volume jet nebulizers varies between 26 mg H_2O/L and 35 mg H_2O/L. However, when heated, output can be

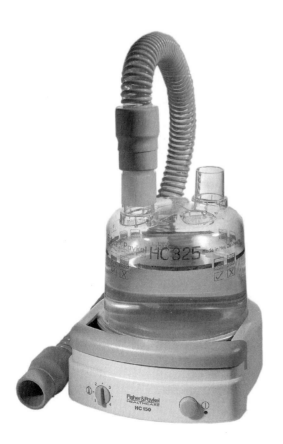

FIGURE 4-3 Heated humidifier.
Courtesy of Fisher & Paykel Healthcare.

TABLE 4-5
Types and Specifications of Heated Humidifiers

Manufacturer	Product Name/ Number	Integrated Flow Generator	Patients	O₂ Range	Flow Range	Disinfection Kit	Temperature Range	Relative Humidity Indicator	Overheat Protection	Dimensions	Weight (lb)
Fisher & Paykel Healthcare	AIRVO 2	Yes	Spontaneously breathing—in hospital	21–80%	5–50 L/min	Yes	37°C	No	No	11.6" x 6.7" x 6.9"	4.6
	myAIRVO2	Yes	Spontaneously breathing—home	No precise control	5–50 L/min	Yes	37°C	No	No	11.6" x 6.7" x 6.9"	4.8
	HC150	N/A	Spontaneously breathing—CPAP/ BiPAP	N/A	N/A	N/A	30°C–65°C	No	No	2.1" x 5.2" x 5.7"	1.8
	MR850	N/A	All groups	N/A	N/A	N/A	10°C–70°C	No	Yes	5.6" x 6.9" x 5.4"	6.3
Galemed	HumiAIDE 7	N/A	All groups	N/A	N/A	N/A	10°C–40°C	Yes	Yes	5.8" x 5.6" x 7.2"	2.9
	HumiAIDE 5	Yes	Spontaneously breathing—home	N/A	NS	NS	10°C–40°C	Yes	Yes	5.8" x 5.6" x 7.2"	0.55
	64377										
Smiths-Medical	Thera-Heat	N/A	All groups	N/A	N/A	N/A	NS	Yes	NS	NS	NS
Vapotherm, Inc.	Vapotherm	Yes	Spontaneously breathing—in hospital	21–100%	1–40 L/min	NS	33°C–43°C	N/A	Yes	11.5" x 8" x 7"	12

N/A: Not applicable, NS: Not specified

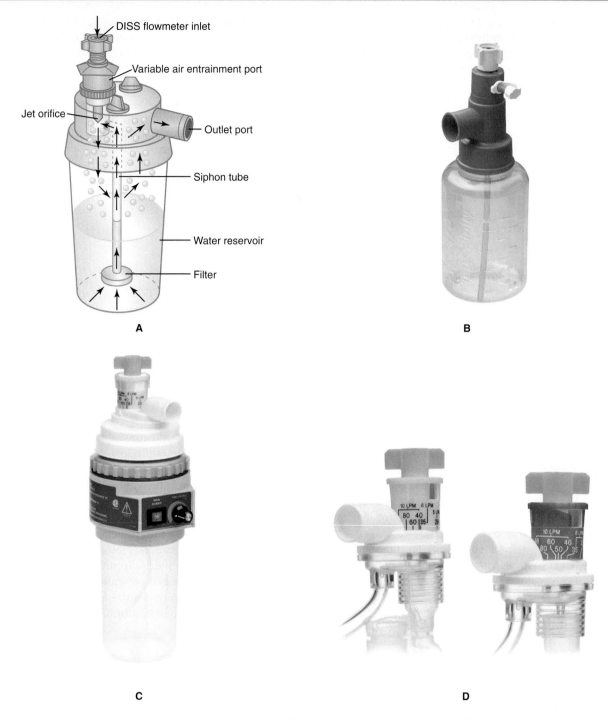

FIGURE 4-4 Large volume jet nebulizer: A. Schematic. B. Dry disposable. C. Heated disposable. D. Prefilled heated disposable.
Photo B reproduced with permission from CareFusion. Photo C courtesy of Teleflex. Photo D courtesy of Teleflex.

increased to between 33 mg H_2O/L and 55 mg H_2O/L. If aerosols are delivered into mist tents, volume jet nebulizers with reservoirs of 2–3 liters are used.

> *Indications:* There are several clinical conditions that warrant the use of large volume jet nebulizers.[18,20] Cool bland aerosol is indicated in the presence of upper airway edema, subglottic edema, and postextubation edema. Furthermore, bland aerosol

with large volume jet nebulizers is indicated in patients with laryngotracheobronchitis and whenever mobilization of secretions and sputum specimens are needed.

> *Contraindications:* In patients with a history of upper airway hyper-responsiveness and those who are at risk for bronchorestriction, bland aerosol generation with a large volume jet nebulizer is contraindicated.

Hazards: The hazards and complications associated with bland aerosol therapy are not related to the large volume jet nebulizer per se, but rather to the therapy itself.[18,21] Patients might be at risk for wheezing or bronchospasm during bland aerosol therapy. Also there is a risk for edema associated with decreased compliance and gas exchange and with increased airway resistance. During coughing and sputum induction, the caregivers will be exposed to airborne contagions, and those patients with common respiratory diseases (e.g., chronic obstructive pulmonary disease [COPD], asthma, or cystic fibrosis) will be at risk for bronchoconstriction.

When inadequate flow is used, when the siphon tube is obstructed, or when the jet orifices are misaligned, large volume jet nebulizers will produce inadequate mist. Also many systems of large volume jet nebulizers do not shut down when the reservoir is empty, resulting in the delivery of dry inspired gas to the patient. Finally, some of these systems tend to be noisy.

Principles of operation: A large volume jet nebulizer works by directing a high flow of gas (usually a mixture of room air and oxygen) through a small jet orifice. The low pressure generated at the jet orifice draws fluid up a siphon tube. Once the water level reaches the top, it is removed by shear forces. This is a continuous process, and the water removed forms a dense aerosol.[18,22] Generated aerosolized particles are of different sizes. Downstream a short distance from the jet is a baffle that serves to stabilize particle size. When the aerosolized particles meet the baffle, larger unstable particles with higher inertia are rained out and fall back into the reservoir to minimize waste. The remaining small and stable particles leave through the outlet port and get carried in the gas stream provided to the patient. Many nebulizers have an air intake or Venturi to allow the entrainment of room air for dilution of the primary gas, usually oxygen, to be able to provide precise concentration of inspired oxygen.

Currently available devices: Large volume jet nebulizers used to be very common in the practice of respiratory care; however, recent technical developments have led to a decrease in the dependence on these devices. Some of the currently available devices are described in **Table 4-6**.

Vibrating Mesh Nebulizer

Vibrating mesh nebulizers (VMNs) are exceptionally good at producing very fine aerosols (up to a mass median aerodynamic diameter of 4.5 µm) with higher respirable fraction (RF) at slower velocities and within a short time (2–30 minutes) depending on the fill volume and the type of drug being nebulized. VMNs are capable of producing consistently high, efficient aerosol outcomes.[23] The integral component of VMNs is a vibrating mesh plate, or aperture plate, with high-precision-formed holes that control the size and flow of the aerosolized particles (**Figure 4-5**). Vibrating mesh nebulizers operate around 128 KHz. A separate or attached power supply provides electricity (via batteries or AC power supply) to the vibrating piezo-electric element. VMNs have medication reservoirs and a patient interface (a mouthpiece for spontaneously breathing patients and a T-piece adapter that fits in-line with the ventilator circuit for intubated and mechanically ventilated patients). Because vibrating mesh nebulizers do not require an external gas source for nebulization, no additional external flow

TABLE 4-6
Types and Specifications of Large Volume Jet Nebulizers

Manufacturer	Product Name/ Number	Type	Sterile/ Closed System	Volume (mL)	Inspired Oxygen Range (%)	Oxygen Flow (L/ min)	MMAD (µm)	Min/Max Indicators	Heater Interface
CareFusion	AitLife 5007p	Disposable	No	350	28–98	5–11	2.8	Yes	No
Galemed	Neb-3 Large Volume Nebulizer	Disposable	No	500	35–100	NS	5	Yes	Yes
Intersurgical	AquaMist 1509	Disposable	No	500	28–60	5–11	NS	Yes	No
Teleflex	Large Volume Neb 1770	Disposable	No	500	28–98	5–10	NS	Yes	Yes

MMAD: Mass median aerodynamic diameter, NS: Not specified

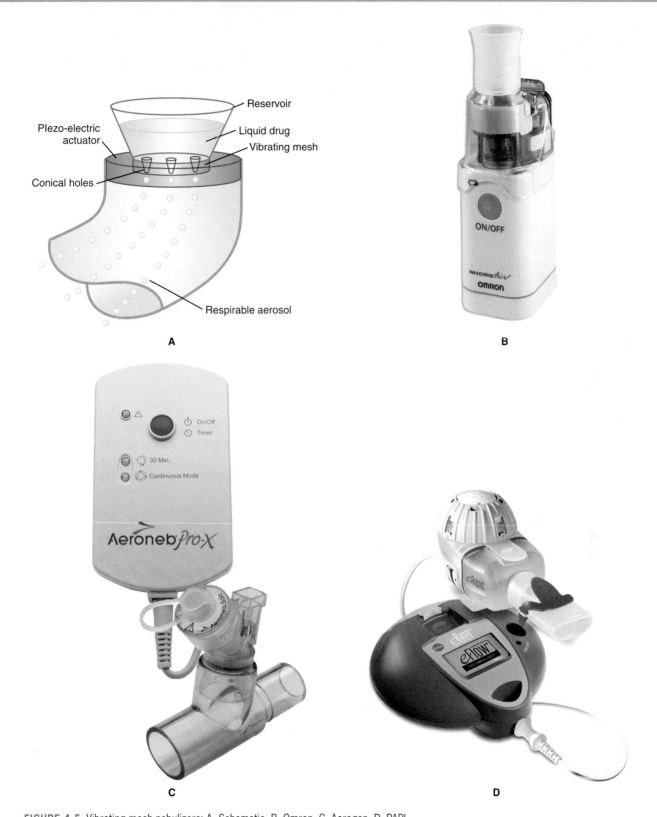

FIGURE 4-5 Vibrating mesh nebulizers: A. Schematic. B. Omron. C. Aerogen. D. PARI.

Photo B courtesy of Omron Healthcare. Photo C courtesy of Aerogen. Photo D courtesy of PARI Respiratory Equipment. "eFlow® Technology" are registered trademarks of PARI GmbH.

will be added to the total inspiratory flow provided by the ventilator; subsequently, the nebulization process will not interfere with the performance of mechanical ventilators. Due to their high efficiency, the residual drug volumes left in vibrating mesh nebulizers are very minimal (0.01 to 0.4 mL depending on reservoir design), ensuring adequate doses delivered to patients during treatments. VMNs are more expensive and

TABLE 4-7
Technical Features and Specifications of Vibrating Mesh Nebulizers

Manufacturer	Product Name/ Number	Patients	Medication Cup Capacity (mL)	MMAD (µm)	Residual Volume	Calculated Respirable Dose Delivered via Endotracheal Tube	Mode
Aerogen	Aeroneb Go	Spontaneously breathing	6	3.6	< 0.3 ml	N/A	Intermittent
	Aeroneb Pro	Mechanically ventilated	10	2.1	0.3 ml	13%	Intermittent
	Aeroneb Solo	Mechanically ventilated	6	3.4	< 0.1 mL for 3 mL dose	13–17%	Intermittent & continuous
Omron	Micro Air NE-U22	Spontaneously breathing	7	4.2	0.1	N/A	Intermittent
Pari	eRapid	Spontaneously breathing	NS	4.1	NS	N/A	Intermittent

MMAD: Mass median aerodynamic diameter

generally more costly to repair than pneumatically powered devices, though they are sometimes replaceable under a limited warranty by the manufacturer.

> *Indications:* Vibrating mesh nebulizers are useful for the treatment of thick secretions that are difficult to expectorate, and they can help to stimulate a cough and sputum induction. In addition to the classical bronchodilators, current evidence suggests that vibrating mesh nebulizers can play a role in nebulizing and delivering directly to the lung parenchyma a wide range of medications previously known to be delivered only intravenously,[24] such as antibiotics (e.g., aztronam, colistin, tobramycin), pulmonary vasodilators (e.g., ilioprost), insulin, other proteins and peptides, and fragments of DNA.
>
> *Contraindications:* In patients with a history of upper airway hyper-responsiveness and those who are at risk for bronchorestriction, bland aerosol generation with vibrating mesh nebulizers might be contraindicated.
>
> *Hazards:* Vibrating mesh nebulizers are limited in that they cannot aerosolize viscous solutions. (Sterile water and normal saline are preferred.) Blockage of the minute apertures with drug particles can result if these devices are not cleaned well. As with any other nebulizer, the reservoirs of these devices can easily become contaminated, resulting in airborne transmission of pathogens. Care should be taken to ensure that these units

are cleaned according to the manufacturer's recommendations and that residual volumes of solutions are discarded from the reservoir periodically between cleanings.

> *Principles of operation:* Vibrating mesh nebulizers work on the principle of high frequency sound waves that can break water into aerosol particles.[23,25] When the power supply is turned on, the piezoelectric transducer emits vibrations forcing the liquid solution to pass through the holes and thus producing a dense aerosol at extremely low flow rates. Most currently available vibrating mesh nebulizers are powered by a preset controller; clinicians need only select the duration of the nebulization process.
>
> *Currently available devices:* Among the new generation of nebulizers are several devices that employ a vibrating mesh or plate with multiple apertures to generate a liquid aerosol. The characteristics and specifications of these devices are presented in **Table 4-7**.

Passive Humidifiers

Passive humidifiers are mainly retainers of water vapor expelled with the exhaled gas from the lungs during the expiratory phase of a breath. During the inspiratory phase of a breath, previously retained water vapor is released into the gas flowing to the patient's lungs. The main type of passive humidifier is the heat and moisture exchanger.

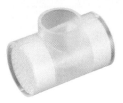

FIGURE 4-6 One type of commercially available heat and moisture exchanger.

Courtesy of Smiths Medical.

TABLE 4-8
Contraindications for Heat and Moisture Exchangers (HMEs)

Thick, copious, or bloody secretions
Expired tidal volume less than 70% of the delivered tidal volume
When using low tidal volume
Body temperature less than 89.6°F (32°C)
High minute ventilation (≥ 10 L/min)
Patients on noninvasive ventilation with large mask leaks
Patient receiving in-line aerosol drug treatments

Heat and Moisture Exchangers

Heat and moisture exchangers (HMEs), also referred to as artificial noses, are simple, small, and passive humidifiers. They are of three main types: (1) simple condenser, (2) hygroscopic condenser, or (3) hydrophobic condenser.[26] All HMEs contain a condenser element with low thermal conductivity. The condensers are either impregnated with hygroscopic salt or composed of a water-repellent element (hydrophobic) with large surface area for more efficient humidification (**Figure 4-6**). HMEs are typically used for short-term ventilatory support and for humidification during anesthesia. Whenever filtration capability is added to these humidifiers, they are called heat and moisture exchangers/filters (HMEFs).[27] The efficiency of the HMEs is quite variable, depending on the HME design, tidal volume, patient's characteristics, and atmospheric conditions.[28] While in use, HMEs are usually connected between the endotracheal tube adaptor and the Y of the breathing circuit. A small corrugated tube approximately 10 cm long is usually used to connect the HME to the endotracheal tube in order to decrease the weight effect of the HME and decrease the risk of endotracheal tube displacement. As such, HMEs are the main source of mechanical dead space during mechanical ventilation. All types of HMEs are for single patient use, and almost all of them are fitted with a Luer port for measurement of the end tidal carbon dioxide tension.

> *Indications:* HMEs are typically used for short-term mechanical ventilation (< 72 hours), during patient transport, and during anesthesia.[29]
> *Contraindications:* There are no contraindications to providing physiologic conditioning of inspired medical gases and optimal humidification during mechanical ventilation. However, because of their nature, HMEs are contraindicated under some circumstances (see **Table 4-8**).
> *Hazards:* There are several hazards associated with the use of HMEs.[30] HMEs with low humidity outputs (< 25 mg/L) can result in hypothermia because the patient needs to add a significant

amount of humidity to achieve an isothermic saturation condition of 44 mg H_2O/L (100% humidity). The moisture output can decrease significantly as the minute volume increases, and usually HMEs are contraindicated when minute ventilation is ≥ 10 L/min. Trapping water vapor on the condenser elements has the possibility of increasing the HME resistance causing increased work of breathing through the HME. This is seen mainly after prolonged used of the HME (> 24–48 hours). Also the increase of the HME resistance as the water saturates the condenser can lead to an ineffective low-pressure alarm during disconnection of the patient from the ventilator. HMEs remain the main source of mechanical dead space during mechanical ventilation and can lead to increases in minute ventilation. Finally, unless calculated and accounted for during mechanical ventilation, HMEs can cause significant compressible volume loss that can lead to inaccurate effective tidal volume delivery and reduction in the ventilator performance.

> *Principles of operation:* Unless a heating element is added, HMEs do not actively add heat or water vapor to the system.[31] Exhaled heat and moisture in expired gas during a breath are captured by the condenser element of the HME and on the next inspiration, cool and dry inspired gas is warmed and humidified as it flows through the condenser element of the HME. A good heat and moisture exchanger should be at least 70% efficient with humidity output ≥ 30 mg/L water vapor, with standard connections, minimal dead space volume, and minimal flow resistance.
> *Currently available devices:* HMEs are widely used in critical care areas during mechanical ventilation and in operating rooms during anesthesia. Most of these devices have an additional filtration component aimed at protecting the patient from hospital-acquired infections. Several commercial products are available, and their general specifications and characteristics are presented in **Table 4-9**.

TABLE 4-9
Types and Specifications of Heat and Moisture Exchangers

Manufacturer	Product Name/ Number	Recommended Tidal Volume (ml)	Moisture Output (mg H₂O/L)							Resistance in cm H₂O						Filtration Efficiency		Dead Space Volume (mL)	Weight (g)
			VT = 25 mL	VT = 50 mL	VT = 100 mL	VT = 250 mL	VT = 500 mL	VT = 750 mL	VT = 1000 mL	Flow = 5 L/min	Flow = 15 L/min	Flow = 20 L/min	Flow = 30 L/min	Flow = 60 L/min	Flow = 90 L/min	Bacterial	Viral		
ARC Medical, Inc.	ThermoFlo	250–1500	N/A	N/A	N/A	N/A	33	N/A	31	N/A	N/A	N/A	0.4	N/A	N/A	N/A	N/A	75	32
	ThermoFlo Filter	250–1500	N/A	N/A	N/A	N/A	33	N/A	31	N/A	N/A	N/A	1.2	N/A	N/A	> 99.9%	> 99.9%	75	33
	ThermoFlo Filter S	250–1500	N/A	N/A	N/A	N/A	32	N/A	30	N/A	N/A	N/A	1/2	N/A	N/A	> 99.9%	> 99.9%	75	33
	ThermoFlo Midi	150–1200	N/A	N/A	N/A	N/A	32	N/A	30	N/A	N/A	N/A	1.5	N/A	N/A	> 99.9%	> 99.9%	47	29
Covidien	DAR 352U5805	300–1500	N/A	N/A	N/A	33.9	33.3	N/A	32.4	N/A	N/A	N/A	0.9	2.1	3.6	≥ 99.999%	99.999%	90	50
	DAR 352U5877	150–1200	N/A	N/A	N/A	34.4	33.6	N/A	32.9	N/A	N/A	N/A	1	2.8	4.7	≥ 99.99%	> 99.99%	51	28
	DAR 352U5996	150–1200	N/A	N/A	N/A	34.4	33.6	N/A	32.9	N/A	N/A	N/A	1.2	2.9	5.2	≥ 99.99%	> 99.99%	61	29
	DAR 354U5876	300–1500	N/A	N/A	N/A	34.7	34.1	N/A	33.4	N/A	N/A	N/A	0.8	2.5	4.2	≥ 99.999999%	≥ 99.999%	96	49
	DAR 354U19028	200–1500	N/A	N/A	N/A	33	31.5	N/A	29.6	N/A	N/A	N/A	1.2	2.7	4.6	≥ 99.999%	≥ 99.999%	66	36
	DAR 355U5430	75–300	N/A	N/A	N/A	32.3	N/A	N/A	N/A	N/A	N/A	1.6	2.6	N/A	N/A	99.999%	> 99.99%	31	21
	DAR 355U5427	30–100	N/A	30	N/A	N/A	N/A	N/A	N/A	0.6	N/A	N/A	N/A	N/A	N/A	99.999%	> 99.99%	10	9
Galemed	HMEF 39012	N/A	N/A	N/A	N/A	N/A	N/A	N/A	N/A	N/A	N/A	N/A	N/A	N/A	N/A	99.99%	99.99%	N/A	N/A
	HME Compact 3485	N/A	N/A	N/A	N/A	N/A	N/A	N/A	N/A	N/A	N/A	N/A	N/A	N/A	N/A	99.99%	99.99%	N/A	N/A
Smiths Medical	PORTEX 002812	120–1500	N/A	N/A	N/A	N/A	31	N/A	N/A	N/A	0.22	N/A	N/A	N/A	N/A	N/A	N/A	42	21

TABLE 4-9
Types and Specifications of Heat and Moisture Exchangers

Manufacturer	Product Name/ Number	Recommended Tidal Volume (ml)	Moisture Output (mg H₂O/L)							Resistance in cm H₂O						Filtration Efficiency		Dead Space Volume (mL)	Weight (g)
			VT = 25 mL	VT = 50 mL	VT = 100 mL	VT = 250 mL	VT = 500 mL	VT = 750 mL	VT = 1000 mL	Flow = 5 L/min	Flow = 15 L/min	Flow = 20 L/min	Flow = 30 L/min	Flow = 60 L/min	Flow = 90 L/min	Bacterial	Viral		
Smiths Medical	PORTEX 002813	900–1500	N/A	N/A	N/A	31	N/A	N/A	N/A	N/A	1	N/A	N/A	N/A	N/A	N/A	N/A	26	18
	PORTEX 002814P	400–1500	N/A	N/A	N/A	N/A	30	N/A	27	N/A	N/A	N/A	1	3	5	N/A	N/A	70	27
	PORTEX 002815	>10	32	N/A	N/A	N/A	N/A	N/A	N/A	0.9	N/A	N/A	N/A	N/A	N/A	N/A	N/A	3	3
	PORTEX 002816	200–1500	N/A	N/A	N/A	N/A	31	N/A	N/A	N/A	N/A	N/A	0.3	N/A	N/A	N/A	N/A	66	30
	PORTEX 002817P	150–1500	N/A	N/A	N/A	31	N/A	N/A	N/A	N/A	N/A	N/A	N/A	1.8	N/A	N/A	N/A	31	27
	PORTEX 002818P	90–1500	N/A	N/A	N/A	31	31	N/A	N/A	N/A	0.1	N/A	N/A	N/A	N/A	N/A	N/A	31	19
	PORTEX 002821	200–1500	N/A	N/A	N/A	N/A	31	N/A	N/A	N/A	N/A	N/A	1	N/A	N/A	99.9999%	99.9999%	66	31
	PORTEX 002822	90–1500	N/A	N/A	N/A	N/A	32	N/A	N/A	N/A	N/A	N/A	0.98	N/A	N/A	99.9999%	99.9999%	76	38
	PORTEX 002823P	150–1500	N/A	N/A	N/A	N/A	31	N/A	N/A	N/A	N/A	N/A	1.4	N/A	N/A	99.9999%	99.9999%	55	40
	PORTEX 002825	90–1500	N/A	N/A	N/A	31	N/A	N/A	N/A	N/A	1.1	N/A	N/A	N/A	N/A	99.9999%	99.9999%	32	18
	PORTEX 002841	400–1500	N/A	N/A	N/A	N/A	31	N/A	28	N/A	N/A	N/A	1	2	4	N/A	N/A	70	27
	PORTEX 002851P	N/A	N/A	N/A	N/A	N/A	33	N/A	26	N/A	N/A	N/A	1	2.2	4	> 99.9%	> 99.9%	103	52
	PORTEX 002865	N/A	N/A	N/A	N/A	N/A	25	N/A	17	N/A	N/A	N/A	1	2.2	4	> 99.9%	> 99.9%	32	20

(continues)

TABLE 4-9
Types and Specifications of Heat and Moisture Exchangers (Continued)

Manufacturer	Product Name/ Number	Recommended Tidal Volume (ml)	Moisture Output (mg H₂O/L)							Resistance in cm H₂O						Filtration Efficiency		Dead Space Volume (mL)	Weight (g)
			VT = 25 mL	VT = 50 mL	VT = 100 mL	VT = 250 mL	VT = 500 mL	VT = 750 mL	VT = 1000 mL	Flow = 5 L/min	Flow = 15 L/min	Flow = 20 L/min	Flow = 30 L/min	Flow = 60 L/min	Flow = 90 L/min	Bacterial	Viral		
Smiths Medical	PORTEX 002866	N/A	N/A	N/A	N/A	N/A	27	N/A	24	N/A	N/A	N/A	1	2.2	4	> 99.9%	> 99.9%	67	46
	PORTEX 580021	N/A	N/A	N/A	N/A	N/A	N/A	N/A	25	N/A	N/A	N/A	N/A	1.2	N/A	N/A	N/A	32	18.6
Teleflex	Gibeck 19912	250–1500	N/A	N/A	N/A	N/A	N/A	N/A	30.4	N/A	N/A	N/A	N/A	1.5	N/A	N/A	N/A	57	43
	Gibeck 10011	15–50	30	N/A	N/A	N/A	N/A	N/A	N/A	N/A	1	N/A	N/A	N/A	N/A	N/A	N/A	2.4	4.5
	Gibeck 11112	50–600	N/A	N/A	30	N/A	N/A	N/A	N/A	N/A	N/A	0.3	N/A	N/A	N/A	N/A	N/A	14	11.6
	Gibeck 13312	150–1500	N/A	N/A	N/A	N/A	27	N/A	N/A	N/A	N/A	N/A	N/A	0.8	N/A	N/A	N/A	29	20.9
	Gibeck 17731	250–1500	N/A	N/A	N/A	N/A	27	N/A	N/A	N/A	N/A	N/A	N/A	0.8	N/A	N/A	N/A	54	26.4
	Gibeck 11012	50–250	N/A	N/A	30	N/A	N/A	N/A	N/A	N/A	N/A	1.4	N/A	N/A	N/A	N/A	N/A	13	14.5
	Gibeck 18502	150–1000	N/A	N/A	N/A	N/A	N/A	N/A	N/A	N/A	N/A	N/A	2.1	N/A	N/A	N/A	N/A	27	22
	Gibeck 18402	150–1000	N/A	N/A	N/A	N/A	30	N/A	30	N/A	N/A	N/A	N/A	1.8	N/A	N/A	N/A	38	32.3
	Gibeck 18832	250–1500	N/A	N/A	N/A	N/A	N/A	N/A	31	N/A	N/A	N/A	N/A	2	N/A	N/A	N/A	60	30
Vital Signs (GE)	HMEF 1000	300–1000	N/A	N/A	N/A	N/A	33	32	30	N/A	N/A	N/A	1	2.3	N/A	99.9999%	99.99%	77	24
	HMEF 750	120–750	N/A	N/A	N/A	32	30	27	N/A	N/A	N/A	N/A	0.9	2.2	N/A	99.9999%	99.998%	34	17
	HMEF 500	120–500	N/A	N/A	N/A	31	30	N/A	N/A	N/A	N/A	N/A	1.5	3.3	N/A	99.999%	99.98%	30	15
	HMEF Mini	60–500	N/A	N/A	N/A	31	27	N/A	N/A	N/A	N/A	N/A	1.4	3.2	N/A	99.999%	99.98%	21	14
Westmed	6218	150–1000	N/A	N/A	N/A	N/A	28.4	N/A	N/A	0.48	N/A	N/A	2.7	N/A	N/A	99.99%	99.99%	21.3	N/A
	6219	150–1000	N/A	N/A	N/A	N/A	28.8	N/A	N/A	N/A	N/A	N/A	0.22	N/A	N/A	99.99%		19.7	N/A
	6220	150–1000	N/A	N/A	N/A	N/A	29.2	N/A	N/A	N/A	N/A	N/A	2.5	N/A	N/A	99.99%	99.99%	19.7	N/A
	6221	350–1500	N/A	N/A	N/A	N/A	32.1	N/A	N/A	N/A	N/A	N/A	1.3	N/A	N/A	99.99%	99.99%	69	N/A
	6229	150–1000	N/A	N/A	N/A	N/A	28.4	N/A	N/A	0.35	N/A	N/A	N/A	N/A	N/A		99.99%	21.3	N/A
	6379	350–1500	N/A	N/A	N/A	N/A	32.1	N/A	N/A	N/A	N/A	N/A	1.3	N/A	N/A	99.99%	99.99%	69	N/A

References

1. Tabka Z, Ben Jebria A, Guénard H. Effect of breathing dry warm air on respiratory water loss at rest and during exercise. *Respir Physiol.* 1987;67(2):115-125.
2. Sottiaux TM. Consequences of under- and over-humidification. *Respir Care Clin N Am.* 2006;12(2):233-252.
3. Branson RD. The effects of inadequate humidity. *Respir Care Clin N Am.* 1998;4(2):199-214.
4. Graff TD. Humidification: Indications and hazards in respiratory therapy. *Anesth Analg.* 1975;54(4):444-448.
5. Kola A, Eckmanns T, Gastmeier P. Efficacy of heat and moisture exchangers in preventing ventilator-associated pneumonia: Meta-analysis of randomized controlled trials. *Intensive Care Med.* 2005;31(1):5-11.
6. Jackson C. Humidification in the upper respiratory tract: A physiological overview. *Intensive Crit Care Nurs.* 1996;12(1):27-32.
7. Sassoon CS, Foster GT. Patient-ventilator asynchrony. *Curr Opin Crit Care.* 2001;7(1):28-33.
8. Branson RD. Secretion management in the mechanically ventilated patient. *Respir Care.* 2007;52(10):1328-1342.
9. Robinson BR, Athota KP, Branson RD. Inhalational therapies for the ICU. *Curr Opin Crit Care.* 2009;15(1):1-9.
10. Klein E. Performance characteristics of conventional prototype humidifiers and nebulizers. *Chest.* 1993;64:690.
11. Darin J, Broadwell J, MacDonell R. An evaluation of water-vapor output from four brands of unheated, prefilled bubble humidifiers. *Respir Care.* 1982;27(1):41-50.
12. Randerath WJ, Meier J, Genger H, Domanski U, Rühle KH. Efficiency of cold passover and heated humidification under continuous positive airway pressure. *Eur Respir J.* 2002;20(1):183-186.
13. Holland AE, Denehy L, Buchan CA, Wilson JW. Efficacy of a heated passover humidifier during noninvasive ventilation: A bench study. *Respir Care.* 2007;52(1):38-44.
14. Randerath WJ, Meier J, Genger H, Domanski U, Rühle KH. Efficiency of cold passover and heated humidification under continuous positive airway pressure. *Eur Respir J.* 2002;20(1):183-186.
15. Peterson BD. Heated humidifiers. Structure and function. *Respir Care Clin N Am.* 1998;4(2):243-259.
16. Bench S. Humidification in the long-term ventilated patient; a systematic review. *Intensive Crit Care Nurs.* 2003;19(2):75-84.
17. Kelly M, Gillies D, Todd DA, Lockwood C. Heated humidification versus heat and moisture exchangers for ventilated adults and children. *Anesth Analg.* 2010;111(4):1072.
18. Ari A, Fink JB. Guidelines for aerosol devices in infants, children and adults: Which to choose, why and how to achieve effective aerosol therapy. *Expert Rev Respir Med.* 2011;5(4):561-572.
19. Berger W. Aerosol devices and asthma therapy. *Curr Drug Deliv.* 2009;6(1):38-49.
20. Huang A, Govindaraj S. Topical therapy in the management of chronic rhinosinusitis. *Curr Opin Otolaryngol Head Neck Surg.* 2013;21(1):31-38.
21. Gonda I. Systemic delivery of drugs to humans via inhalation. *J Aerosol Med.* 2006;19(1):47-53.
22. Rodrigo GJ. Inhaled therapy for acute adult asthma. *Curr Opin Allergy Clin Immunol.* 2003;3(3):169-175.
23. Denyer J, Dyche T. The adaptive aerosol delivery (AAD) technology: Past, present, and future. *J Aerosol Med Pulm Drug Deliv.* 2010;23(Suppl 1):S1-S10.
24. Luyt CE, Combes A, Nieszkowska A, Trouillet JL, Chastre J. Aerosolized antibiotics to treat ventilator-associated pneumonia. *Curr Opin Infect Dis.* 2009;22(2):154-158.
25. Dhand R, Guntur VP. How best to deliver aerosol medications to mechanically ventilated patients. *Clin Chest Med.* 2008;29(2):277-296.
26. Wilkes AR. Heat and moisture exchangers. Structure and function. *Respir Care Clin N Am.* 1998;4(2):261-279.
27. Rathgeber J, Kietzmann D, Mergeryan H, Hub R, Züchner K, Kettler D. Prevention of patient bacterial contamination of anaesthesia-circle-systems: A clinical study of the contamination risk and performance of different heat and moisture exchangers with electret filter (HMEF). *Eur J Anaesthesiol.* 1997;14(4):368-373.
28. Lellouche F, Taillé S, Lefrançois F, et al.; Groupe de travail sur les Respirateurs de l'AP-HP. Humidification performance of 48 passive airway humidifiers: comparison with manufacturer data. *Chest.* 2009;135(2):276-286.
29. Hedley RM, Allt-Graham J. Heat and moisture exchangers and breathing filters. *Br J Anaesth.* 1994;73(2):227-236.
30. Wilkes AR. Heat and moisture exchangers and breathing system filters: Their use in anaesthesia and intensive care. Part 2—practical use, including problems, and their use with paediatric patients. *Anaesthesia.* 2011;66(1):40-51.
31. Wilkes AR. Heat and moisture exchangers and breathing system filters: Their use in anaesthesia and intensive care. Part 1—history, principles and efficiency. *Anaesthesia.* 2011;66(1):31-39.

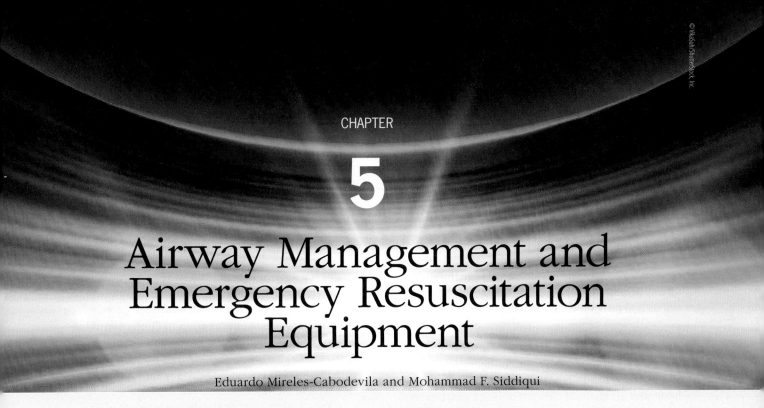

CHAPTER

5

Airway Management and Emergency Resuscitation Equipment

Eduardo Mireles-Cabodevila and Mohammad F. Siddiqui

CHAPTER OBJECTIVES

1. Describe the indications and contraindications of equipment used in respiratory care for airway management and emergency resuscitation.
2. Recognize the differences in equipment available.
3. Describe the hazards and contraindications of each device.

KEY TERMS

Endotracheal tube
Esophageal/tracheal tube
Laryngeal mask airway (LMA)
Laryngoscope
Nasopharyngeal

Oropharyngeal
Suction
Supraglottic device
Tracheostomy tube

Introduction

A patient's airway patency being compromised is a frequent clinical scenario. Management of the airway (access and maintenance) is of essential importance in the care of any patient. Airway patency may be affected due to a loss of consciousness, which can be medically induced (e.g., anesthesia) or disease-related (e.g., cardiac arrest). The airway patency can also be affected in conscious patients, in conditions such as neuromuscular disorders or drug anaphylaxis.

The respiratory practitioner has a wide selection of equipment he or she can use to secure and maintain airway patency. The practitioner needs to be familiar with the indications, proper use, and limitations of airway management equipment, because all of these devices have the potential to harm as well as help. This chapter presents equipment used in the routine and emergency care of the airway.

Upper Airway Devices

The upper airway is the first contact with the environment of the respiratory system. Both the nasal and oral cavities conduct air to the lower airway or trachea and conducting airways. With an intact airway, the conduction of air in a conscious patient is rarely affected; however, when consciousness is altered (e.g., sleep, sedation), the relaxation of the tongue and neck muscles may cause obstruction in the hypopharynx.[1] A simple maneuver, such as head positioning, may be used to alleviate this type of airway obstruction. The *jaw thrust* or the *head-tilt/chin-lift maneuver* are commonly used in cardiopulmonary resuscitation and anesthesia to relieve most cases of airway obstruction.[2] In prolonged resuscitations or in patients with a crowded oropharynx it may become a challenge to maintain the airway. In such instances, airway support devices are routinely used as an adjuvant or in lieu of head positioning.[2] In conscious patients, or in patients in whom the oral cavity cannot be accessed (e.g., those with trismus), the nasal cavity can be made more patent and accessible (for suctioning) with the use of a **nasopharyngeal** airway.[3] However, these devices do not provide lower airway protection, because the trachea and conducting airways are not isolated from the esophagus.

Pharyngeal Airways

There have been multiple designs of **oropharyngeal** and nasopharyngeal airways through history.[4,5] Currently, most of these devices are single use and plastic-based.

Polyvinyl chloride (PVC), silicone, or soft rubber are the most commonly used materials. These devices are used to maintain upper airway patency and/or to provide ready access to the larynx during procedures.

Oropharyngeal Airways

An oropharyngeal airway is a device to maintain or increase patency of the upper airway by creating a conduit from the lips to the hypopharynx, allowing free movement of air or passage of devices, such as a **suction** catheter. When positioned properly, the tongue is displaced and positioned away from the posterior pharyngeal wall. These devices are used to maintain upper airway access and patency in patients who are unconscious and have no cough or gag reflex.[3]

Description

An oropharyngeal device is usually made of hard plastic molded to resemble the configuration of the airway (**Figure 5-1**). It has three portions: the flange, body, and air channel. The *flange* is the proximal end of the device; it prevents displacement deeper than the lips/teeth. It takes the form of a ridge or "lip" and sits at the mouth opening resting against the patient's lips/teeth. The *body* is the curved portion that follows along the hard palate, soft palate, and pharynx. It displaces the tongue away from the palate and the posterior wall of the pharynx. The distal opening rests just above the larynx. A bite area is located on the body just after the flange. The front teeth or gums rest against this portion. It is hard enough to maintain the patency of the airway when the patient bites. The *air channel* is the passage in the device through which air can travel. There are two types of channel design: (1) a Guedel airway has a single opening from the flange to the distal tip of the body, and (2) a Berman airway has two channels, one on either side of an *I*-shaped body.

Application

Oropharyngeal airways are used to maintain airway patency in patients with altered mental status. They allow the passage of equipment such as bronchoscopes or suction catheters into the airway, and facilitate bag-valve-mask ventilation.[6] In addition to maintaining a patent airway, these devices may also be used as bite blocks to keep patients from biting and occluding oral **endotracheal tubes**. Oropharyngeal airways should be used only on unconscious patients.[3] They should not be used on patients with abnormal oropharyngeal/facial anatomy; trauma to the oral cavity, mandible, or maxilla; or when a foreign body/lesion obstructs the upper airway.

There are two main techniques for insertion.

- *Technique 1:* The patient's mouth is opened with the dominant hand. A tongue depressor held by the nondominant hand is used to depress the tongue. The dominant hand advances the oropharyngeal airway over the tongue and tongue depressor until the flange is in contact with the lips.
- *Technique 2:* The patient's mouth is opened with the nondominant hand. The dominant hand inserts the oropharyngeal airway upside down into the oral cavity. The oropharyngeal airway tip is advanced in contact with the hard palate as the curved portion displaces the tongue caudally. When the oropharyngeal airway is halfway in, or it reaches the soft palate, it is turned 180 degrees. The oropharyngeal airway is advanced until the flange is in contact with the lips.

Placing an oropharyngeal airway may stimulate the pharyngeal structures (soft palate, base of tongue, uvula, and posterior pharynx), leading to emesis. If the oropharyngeal airway comes in contact with the larynx, or the patient is awake, it may cause laryngospasm. Coughing or gagging indicates that the patient's level of consciousness is inappropriate for this type of airway.

Careless placement of the device may cause lip, teeth, tongue, mucosal, epiglottal, and/or laryngeal injury. When left in place for a long time it may result in pressure-induced injury of mucosa, nerves, and oropharyngeal structures. Inappropriate insertion, sizing, posterior tongue displacement, or secretion blockage may cause obstruction and hypoventilation. Patency of the airway should be assessed after insertion and while the airway is in place.[7]

The oropharyngeal airways have standard sizing and are color coded according to type (see **Table 5-1**); however, there is variation among manufacturers and models.[8] In order to choose the correct size, the oropharyngeal airway is placed on the side of the patient's face with the flange resting at the lip commissure.[9] The distal tip of the airway should reach (not pass) the angle of the jaw.

Currently Available Devices

The most commonly used devices for routine and emergent airway care are the Guedel and Berman airways. Other devices are used to assist with endotracheal intubation or endoscopic procedures.

- *Berman:* The Berman oropharyngeal airway was described by Robert A. Berman in 1949.[10] It has two parallel lateral air channels that are open to the oral cavity, creating a passage from the flange to the distal opening.
- *Guedel:* The Guedel oropharyngeal airway was designed by Arthur Guedel in 1922.[11] It has one air channel that is surrounded by plastic (i.e., it is not in contact with the oral structures), creating a passage from the flange to the distal opening.
- *Berman Intubating Pharyngeal Airway (Vital Signs):* Designed as an aid to help blind orotracheal intubation,[12] this is now mainly used for

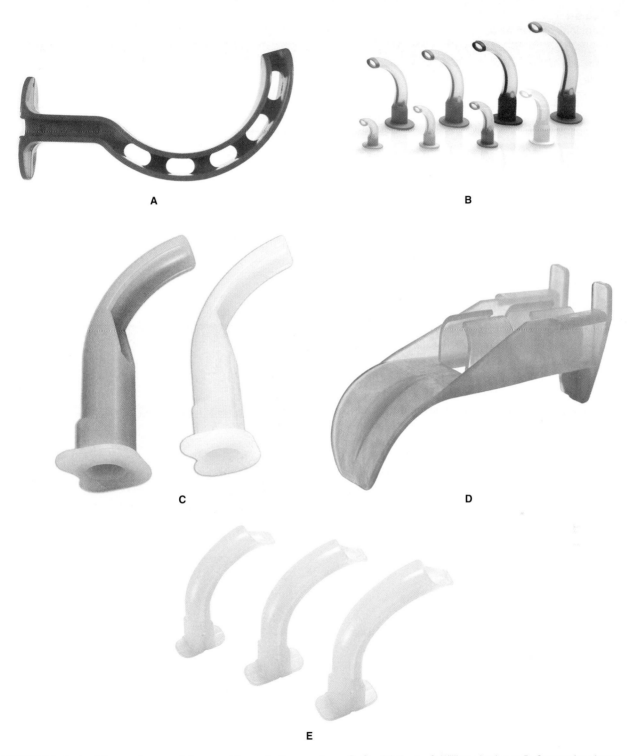

FIGURE 5-1 Parts of the oropharyngeal airway and types. A. Berman airway. B. Guedel airway. C. Williams intubator. D. Ovassapian airway. E. Berman Intubating Pharyngeal Airway.

Photo A © deepspacedave/Shutterstock, Inc. Photo B courtesy of Intersurgical Ltd/Wikimedia Commons. Photo C courtesy of SunMed. Photo D courtesy of Teleflex. Photo E reproduced with permission from CareFusion.

fiber-optic intubation and as an airway to protect bronchoscopic equipment.[13] The device has a large air channel in the center. The right border has a slot and the left border is hinged to allow opening such that it can be removed over the endotracheal tube. It has a distal lip to help lift the epiglottis. There are three available sizes: Small #8, Medium #9, and Large #10.

- *Ovassapian airway (Hudson RCI):* This was designed as an aid to help with fiber-optic intubation or bronchoscopic procedures. It has a flat lingual surface that widens distally. The dorsal or

TABLE 5-1
Dimensions of Oral Airways

Age	Guedel	Berman	ISO Size	Length (mm)
Neonate	Pink	Pink	4	40
Infant	Blue	Turquoise	5	50
Child: small	Black	Black	6	60
Child	White	White	7	70
Adult: small	Green	Green	8	80
Adult: medium	Yellow	Yellow	9	90
Adult	Red	Purple	10	100
Adult: large	Orange	Orange	11	110

ISO: International Organization for Standardization

palatal surface is open. There are two vertical side-walls and two pairs of curved walls at the proximal section. The curved walls create a large central air channel that fits an endotracheal tube or bronchoscope. The inner curved walls are open in the dorsal surface to facilitate removal of the endotracheal tube (ETT).[13,14] One (adult) size is available.

- *Williams Airway Intubator (SunMed):* This was designed for blind oral intubation in awake patients.[15] This airway resembles a Guedel airway with the distal half open to the lingual surface. The device cannot be removed unless the 15-mm connector from the ETT is removed. It is now used as an aid during fiber-optic intubation or endoscopic procedures. There are two available sizes, 9 and 10.[13,14]

Nasopharyngeal Airways

A nasopharyngeal airway is a device to maintain or increase patency of the upper airway by creating a conduit from the tip of the nose to the hypopharynx allowing movement of air or devices.[3] It is sometimes referred to as a nasal trumpet.

Description

A nasopharyngeal device is usually made of soft rubber (latex) or plastic (PVC). It is a hollow structure and has two portions: the flange and the body. The flange is at the proximal end. It is a ridge or lip that sits at the nose opening. It prevents the nasopharyngeal airway from being displaced deeper into the nasal cavity. The body is a curved and flexible tube (**Figure 5-2**). When inserted, it follows along the hard palate, below the turbinates, and reaching the hypopharynx. The distal opening of the body has a beveled edge (which typically aims to the right) to facilitate insertion. The tip should rest above the larynx.[16]

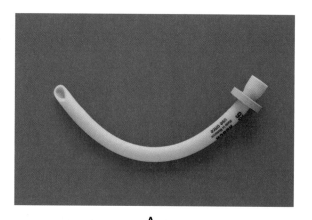

A

B

FIGURE 5-2 Parts of the nasopharyngeal airway and types. A. Adjustable nasopharyngeal airway. B. Robertazzi nasopharyngeal airway.
Photos courtesy of Teleflex.

Application

Nasopharyngeal airways are most often used with patients who need frequent nasotracheal suctioning. The purpose is to minimize damage to the nasal mucosa by the suction catheter. This type of airway is sometimes used to prevent airway obstruction due to swelling after facial surgery. Nasopharyngeal airways may be used in conscious or unconscious patients when an oropharyngeal airway cannot be placed (e.g., due to trauma or trismus). It may facilitate bag-valve-mask ventilation and allow passage of equipment into the airway.[6] These airways should not be used on patients with trauma of the nose or base of the skull.[17] Insertion should be avoided in the presence of epistaxis or predisposition for severe epistaxis (e.g., coagulopathy).[18] Nasal airways should not be used in patients with nasal foreign objects or lesions in the pharynx.

When placing a nasopharyngeal airway, the most patent nare should be selected. The tip and body of the nasopharyngeal airway is lubricated with a water-based jelly. The tip is advanced through the nare horizontally, aiming straight to the pharynx and along the roof of the hard palate until the tip rests about 1 cm above the epiglottis. The device may be dislodged or inserted beyond the flange; some come with a safety pin that serves as a flange and securing device. Patency of the airway should be assessed after insertion and while the airway is in place.

There are hazards in the insertion and placement of a nasopharyngeal airway. Inappropriate insertion, sizing, displacement, or secretion blockage may cause obstruction.[18,19] During insertion, mucosal damage, structure displacement, or abnormal structures may be encountered and even in the absence of force lead to epistaxis. Insertion may cause coughing, gagging, and emesis, a sign that insertion may be too deep. The nasopharyngeal airway creates a passage that bypasses the nasal turbinates, decreasing the humidity in the air, potentially leading to thick and tenacious secretions. Finally, when the airway is left in place for prolonged periods of time, the drainage of nose and sinus mucus will be impaired. There is a risk of pressure-induced injury of the nostril, septum, mucosa, turbinates, and epiglottis.

Nasopharyngeal airways have standard external diameter sizing in French units. However, some manufacturers state the size in mm, referring to the *inner* diameter (Table 5-2). It is essential to remember that the most important feature of sizing nasopharyngeal airways is the length, because a short device will not separate the soft palate from the posterior pharynx, and one that is too long may penetrate the larynx, worsen cough, or cause paradoxical obstruction by displacing the epiglottis.

The French gauge system (abbreviated as Fr, FR, or F) is commonly used to measure the size of an airway or catheter according to the *outside* diameter (essentially the circumference of the device). One Fr equals 0.33 mm; thus, the outer diameter of the catheter in millimeters can be determined by dividing the French size by 3. For example, if the French size is 9, the outside diameter is 3 mm. It follows that an increasing French size corresponds to a larger diameter catheter.

TABLE 5-2
Nasopharyngeal Airway Sizing

Approximate Age Group for Use	Size (Fr)*	Size (mm)*	Internal Diameter (mm)	External Diameter (mm)	Length (mm)
	12	3	3	4	NA
	14	3.5	3.5	4.7	NA
	16	4	4	5.3	NA
	18	4.5	4.5	6	NA
Pediatric	20	5	5	6.7	115
	22	5.5	5.5	7.3	125
Small adult, adult female	24	6	6	8	130
Small adult	26	6.5	6.5	8.7	140
Adult male	28	7	7	9.3	155
	30	7.5	7.5	10	165
Large adult	32	8	8	10.7	170
	34	8.5	8.5	11.3	175
	36	9	9	12	180

*The size of a nasopharyngeal airway can be found in two ways. If French units are used (Rusch airways), it refers to the external diameter. If it is in millimeters (Portex), it refers to the internal diameter.

Traditionally it has been suggested that the diameter should be chosen by approximately matching the size of the fifth finger or the nostril opening to the diameter of the nasopharyngeal cannula. Similarly, to choose the correct length, the nasopharyngeal airway is placed on the side of the patient's face with the flange resting at the side of the nostril or nose tip. The distal orifice of the airway should reach the earlobe (some authors state it should reach the tragus and then add 2 cm). A review of available literature on nasopharyngeal airway sizing based the recommendations on anthropomorphic measurements.[16] These are: (1) Forget about the diameter measurements based on the nostril or little finger because they are inaccurate; (2) for an average height adult female use a size 6 (24 Fr) nasopharyngeal airway, and for an average height adult male use a size 7 (28 Fr); (3) in children, the insertion length should be shorter (approximately 1 cm) than the distance between the nose tip and the earlobe.

Currently Available Devices

- *Nasopharyngeal adjustable:* The flange of these devices can be adjusted to allow proper positioning of the airway to prevent deep insertions. Others have a safety pin that can be passed through the nasopharyngeal airway to adjust the insertion depth and prevent migration. Multiple brands are available.
- *Robertazzi:* The flange is not adjustable; it is part of the device. Multiple brands are available.

Supraglottic Airway Devices

Supraglottic devices are designed to maintain the airway (elective or emergent), allow administration of anesthetic gases, allow airway instrumentation, and permit the administration of manual or mechanical ventilation.[4,20-22] These are used both in the controlled setting as an alternative to endotracheal intubation and in the emergency setting when endotracheal intubation cannot be done.[6] There are different devices; each has specific characteristics that make it unique in function, insertion, and management. In general they consist of passages, usually tubes, that end in a mask (pneumatic or gel) or a chamber. The device is inserted orally and the distal opening rests in front of, inside, or by the glottis (laryngeal opening). The mask or chamber allows gas to travel to the lungs and attempts to maintain the esophagus occluded. No laryngoscopy is required, which means that it is a blind insertion procedure.

Because there are several designs of supraglottic devices and no standard definitions, we arbitrarily grouped them as follows:

> *Supraglottic airways* are used to create and maintain the upper airway by isolating the larynx or directing a flow of air to the larynx.
> **Laryngeal mask airways (LMAs)** are devices that have an inflatable mask that fits over the larynx.

Esophageal/tracheal tubes are devices that may be inserted blindly in the esophagus or trachea.

Supraglottic Airways

Supraglottic airways are designed for blind insertion in the upper airway in case of failed traditional endotracheal intubation or as an alternative to intubation or mask ventilation.[23–27]

Description

The designs of each device are provided later in this section. The devices differ in insertion techniques and usage. The user must read the instruction manual and have training before using them. All have standard 15-mm adapters to allow the use of any bag-valve device for ventilation. There are no other standard features among them.

Application

Supraglottic devices provide an artificial airway to deliver bag-valve ventilation. The goal is to obtain an airway while obstructing the esophagus to allow spontaneous breathing and/or the administration of bag-valve or mechanical ventilation. These are temporal airways (i.e., for procedures or while an endotracheal tube is placed). These devices should not be used in conscious patients or those with an intact gag reflex, esophageal disease (e.g., varices, strictures), or those who have ingested caustic chemicals. They should not be used if there is abnormal anatomy. Hazards of use include aspiration, hypoventilation, oropharyngeal mucosa injury, and structural injury of larynx, esophagus, or related structures (i.e., nerves, vascular structures). Mechanical obstruction of the airway may occur if there is displacement of the epiglottis or penetration into the glottis. Changes in the position of the head and neck may cause problems in the performance of the devices.[28,29]

Currently Available Devices
Laryngeal Tubes

There are two manufacturers of laryngeal tubes (King Systems and VBM Medizintechnik) and two models (the LT/LT-D and the LTS [laryngeal tube suction]). The laryngeal tube is used mainly in lieu of endotracheal intubation in emergencies and for short procedural anesthesia.[26] The Advanced Cardiac Life Support guidelines give the laryngeal tube a class IIb recommendation as an alternative to bag-mask ventilation or endotracheal intubation in cardiac arrest.[6] A meta-analysis of alternative airways used in prehospital care reported a 96.7% success rate for insertion in all patients and by all clinicians.[30] When compared to LMAs for a procedural airway its performance seems to be similar.[31,32]

The LT and LT-D supraglottic airways consist of a single-lumen tube with two cuffs and a single valve/pilot balloon (**Figure 5-3**). (The *D* stands for disposable.) The proximal cuff stabilizes the device and seals

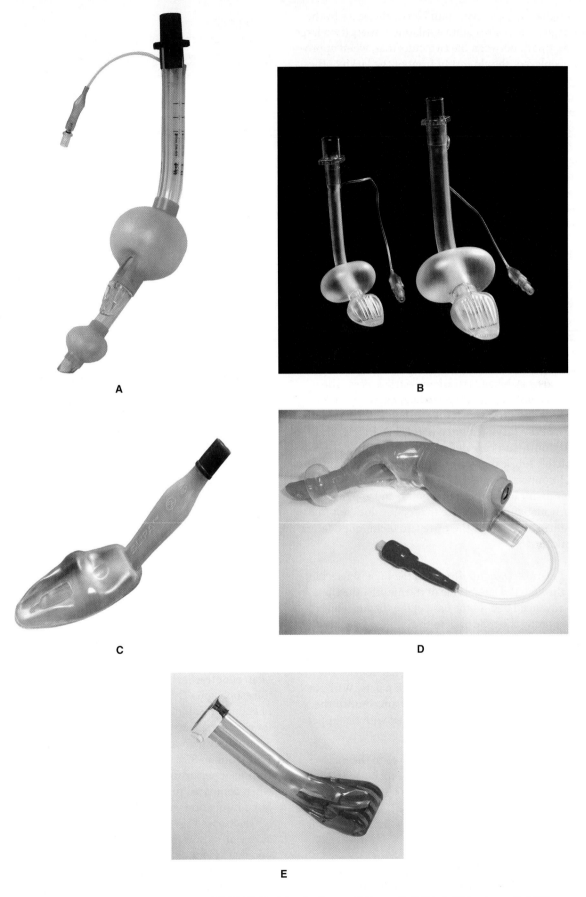

FIGURE 5-3 Supraglottic airways. A. Laryngeal tube (KING LTS). B. Cobra Perilaryngeal Airway. C. SLIPA. D. Elisha airway. E. SALT.

Photo A courtesy of King Systems. Photo B courtesy of Pulmodyne. Photo C courtesy of Donald Miller, MD. Photo D courtesy of Luis Gaitini, MD. Photo E courtesy of Ecolab.

the oropharynx; the distal cuff blocks the entry to the esophagus. There are eight ventilation outlets (two large and six small) between the two cuffs that, when appropriately placed, should rest in front of the larynx. The King LT is reusable up to 50 times. The airway outer diameter is 18 mm and the inner diameter is 10 mm. The ventilation lumen is not round. Maximum size for a bronchoscope is 7 mm, an endotracheal tube is 6 mm, and a tube exchanger is 19 Fr. The King LT-D is a single patient use device. As with the LT, the airway outer diameter is 18 mm and the inner diameter is 10 mm. The ventilation lumen is not round. Maximum size for a bronchoscope is 6 mm, an endotracheal tube cannot be passed though the device, a gastric tube maximum size is 18 Fr, and a tube exchanger maximum is 19 Fr.

The LTS, LTS II (VBM), and LTS-D have an esophageal port, so instead of one lumen (LT model) they have a double-lumen tube with two cuffs and a single valve/pilot balloon. The proximal cuff stabilizes the device and seals the oropharynx; the distal cuff seals the esophagus. There are several ventilation outlets between the two cuffs that, when appropriately placed, should rest in front of the larynx. The second lumen opens to the esophagus to allow gastric access. The sizes and color-coding vary between manufacturers. Sizes are shown in Tables 5-3 and 5-4.

To insert a laryngeal tube (LT, LT-D, LTS II, and LTS-D), both cuffs are deflated and the tubes are completely lubricated with water-soluble lubricant. The LT connector is held with the dominant hand. The nondominant hand opens the mouth and applies the chin-lift maneuver to ensure the tongue does not fold back during insertion. There are two techniques, lateral and midline:

- *Lateral technique:* The tip of the tube is inserted through the lateral side of the mouth. The tip is advanced behind the base of the tongue while rotating the tube back to the midline. The blue orientation line should face the chin of the patient.
- *Midline technique:* The tip is introduced through the midline of the mouth. The flat edge of the LT tip is placed against the hard palate. Without excessive force, the tube is advanced until the thick black marker line is aligned with the upper incisors or gums.

After insertion, the cuffs are inflated to the maximum volume indicated in the syringe included in the kit. Recommended pressure is 60 cm H_2O. If resistance is felt during bag ventilation, the tube is withdrawn until ventilation becomes easy and the air seal is adjusted as necessary.

Cobra Perilaryngeal Airway (PLA)

The Cobra Perilaryngeal Airway (PLA; Pulmodyne) consists of a breathing tube, a circumferential pharyngeal cuff, and a laryngeal opening head. The Cobra PLA

TABLE 5-3
Laryngeal Tubes KING LT and LT-D

Patient Height	Color	Size	Cuff Volume
90–115 cm 35–45 inches	Green	2	25–35 mL
105–130 cm 41–51 inches	Orange	2.5	30–40 mL
122–155 cm 4–5 feet	Yellow	3	45–60 mL
155–180 cm 5–6 feet	Red	4	60–80 mL
> 180 cm > 6 feet	Purple	5	70–90 mL

Data from http://www.kingsystems.com. Accessed May 10, 2011.

TABLE 5-4
Laryngeal Tube VBM LT, LTS II, and LT-D

Patient Weight/Height	Connector Color	Size
< 5 kg	Transparent	0
5–12 kg	White	1
12–25 kg	Green	2
125–150 cm	Orange	2.5
< 155 cm	Yellow	3
155–180 cm	Red	4
> 180 cm	Purple	5

Data from http://vbm-medical.de. Accessed May 28, 2011.

head displaces the pharyngeal tissues and allows ventilation through slotted openings that are directed to the laryngeal opening. These openings allow the passage of an endotracheal tube. The device does not occlude the esophagus. This device is intended for use in lieu of endotracheal intubation (emergent or elective) and for short procedural anesthesia. A prehospital cardiac arrest study demonstrated successful insertion and ventilation in 82% of the patients.[33] In the anesthesia setting, it performs similarly to an LMA;[34,35] however, when compared to an intubating LMA the success for blind intubation was 47–87%.[36,37]

The Cobra PLA is a disposable device. Positive pressure ventilation (mechanical or with bag- valve) is possible as long as peak pressures are below 20–25 cm H_2O. When the cuff is inflated (60 cm H_2O) it seals the hypopharynx. The CobraPLUS has an integrated thermistor on the cuff for measurement of core temperature. The three smallest sizes of the CobraPLUS have a distal

TABLE 5-5
Cobra PLA Sizes

Patient Weight (kg)	Patient Size	Device Size	ID (mm)	Cuff Volume (mL)	ETT Max Size (mm)
> 2.5	Neonate	$\frac{1}{2}$	5	< 8	≤ 3*
> 5	Infant	1	6	< 10	≤ 4.5*
> 10	Child	$1\frac{1}{2}$	6	< 25	≤ 4.5*
> 15	Child	2	10.5	< 40	≤ 6.5
> 35	Adult	3	10.5	< 65	≤ 6.5
> 70	Adult	4	12.5	< 70	≤ 8
> 100	Large Adult	5	12.5	< 85	≤ 8
> 130	Large adult	6	12.5	< 85	≤ 8

*Uncuffed

Data from http://www.pulmodyne.com. Accessed May 10, 2011.

$ETCO_2$ sampling port. Cobra PLA sizes are shown in **Table 5-5**. The manufacturer recommends smaller sizes are usually better than larger sizes: #3 for women and #4 for men.

To insert the Cobra Perilaryngeal Airway, the cuff is deflated and folded back over the tube. All sides of the Cobra PLA head and cuff are lubricated. The patient is placed in sniffing position (head flexion, neck extension) and the position is maintained with the nondominant hand. The dominant hand advances the device to the hypopharynx until moderate resistance is felt. Performing a jaw-lift maneuver may help insertion. The cuff should not be visible once the device is inserted. The cuff is inflated to achieve enough seal to minimize air leak.

i-gel

The i-gel (Intersurgical Ltd.) is a device with similar construction to an LMA. It is disposable and consists of a breathing tube that has an integrated bite block, a separate gastric channel, and a larger body to help stabilize the device in the airway. At the distal end it has a gel cuff that resembles an LMA; however, in contrast to an LMA it is not inflatable. The supraglottic mask that covers the larynx is made of medical-grade thermoplastic elastomer gel (styrene ethylene butadiene styrene). The distal tip of the cuff contains the opening of the gastric channel. Another difference from a conventional LMA is that there are no aperture bars, meaning that the laryngeal opening is wide open. There is a lip on the proximal end of the cuff to allow the epiglottis to "rest." Once inserted, the patient's head should remain in a neutral position to avoid affecting ventilation.[29] This device is intended for emergent and procedural airway management. It performs similarly to the LMAs,[38-40] and also allows for intubation.

To insert, the i-gel is removed from the protective cradle, lubricated on *all* external surfaces, and then placed back in the cradle until the patient is positioned. The patient is placed in sniffing position (head flexion, neck extension) and the position is maintained with the nondominant hand. The device is removed from the protective cradle with the dominant hand holding the integrated bite block. The cuff is placed facing the chin of the patient. The chin is pressed down gently by the nondominant hand and the tip of the device is introduced into the mouth toward the hard palate. The device is advanced downward and backward along the hard palate until definitive resistance is felt. Performing a jaw-lift maneuver may help insertion. The ideal position is to have the incisors aligned with the horizontal line marker in the bite block. Sizes are shown in **Table 5-6**.

Streamlined Liner of the Pharynx Airway (SLIPA)

The Streamlined Liner of the Pharynx Airway (SLIPA, CurveAir Ltd.) is a disposable thermoplastic device contoured to resemble the space in the hypopharynx. The device is designed to soften as it heats up to body temperature, which should improve the seal. It is a hollow structure and has no inflatable chambers. The distal tip is designed to block the esophagus. There is one airway opening shaped like an inverted bottle. The manufacturer states that the hollow structure allows the collection of stomach regurgitation or secretions, preventing aspiration. The SLIPA can be suctioned if

TABLE 5-6
i-gel Sizes

Patient Weight (kg)	Patient Size	Device Size	ID (mm)	Gastric Tube Max Size (Fr)	ETT Max Size (mm)
2–5	Neonate	1	5	N/A	3
5–12	Infant	1.5	6	10	4
10–25	Small child	2	6	12	5
25–35	Large child	2.5	10.5	12	5
30–60	Small adult	3	10.5	12	6
50–90	Medium adult	4	12.5	12	7
> 90	Large adult	5	12.5	14	8

Data from http://www.i-gel.com. Accessed May 10, 2011.

TABLE 5-7
SLIPA Sizes

Patient Height	Patient Size	Color-Coded Connector	Size
4′9″–5′3″	Very small female	Green	47
5′–5′6″	Small female	Blue	49
5′3″–5′9″	Medium female	Yellow	51
5′4″–6′	Large female or small male	White	53
5′8″–6′4″	Medium male	Red	55
5′11″–6′7″	Large male	Orange	57

Data from http://www.slipa.com. Accessed May 10, 2011.

secretions pool in the chamber. The device is fairly recent, and some studies have shown it yields similar performance in procedural sedation compared to the laryngeal mask airway, although it may lead to gastric insufflation.[41]

The device is inserted by first lubricating all sides except the plastic stem. *Do not use the LMA insertion technique because this can result in injury.* The patient is placed in sniffing position (head flexion, neck extension) and the position is maintained with the nondominant hand. An assistant or the nondominant hand performs a jaw-lift maneuver. The SLIPA is inserted into the mouth, directing the tip downward and caudally in the direction of the esophagus. Lifting the jaw and tongue may help with insertion. Once the device starts sliding through the posterior pharynx and past the teeth, it is pushed down and then caudally until definite resistance is felt. An inflation pressure of at least 14 cm H_2O confirms correct size and position. The head is kept in a neutral position. Sizes are shown in **Table 5-7**.

Elisha Airway Device (EAD)

The Elisha Airway Device (EAD, Elisha Medical Technologies, Ltd.) is based on spiral computed tomography of the airway cavity. It is made of silicone and has three separate channels (ventilation, intubation, and gastric tube insertion). It allows blind or fiber-optic intubation with an 8-mm ETT. Two high volume–low pressure balloons seal the oropharynx and the esophagus. In a preliminary study in patients undergoing anesthesia, the EAD was placed on the first attempt in 76% of patients, and up to 96% after the second attempt. Intubation was successful in 85% of patients. There were no comparative trials.[42]

Supraglottic Airway Laryngopharyngeal Tube (SALT)

The Supraglottic Airway Laryngopharyngeal Tube (SALT, Microtek Medical, Inc.) is a rigid airway that is measured and inserted in a similar way to the oropharyngeal airway (tongue depressor technique). It comes with a specially designed tongue blade to aid with insertion. It is used mainly in the emergency pre-hospital setting. An endotracheal tube can be passed through the SALT for a blind or fiber-optic intubation. It then serves as the tube's securing device.[43]

Laryngeal Mask Airway (LMA)

The LMA is a device that has evolved over the last 20 years.[4] It was designed by Dr. Archie Brain in the 1980s[44] as a device to allow positive pressure ventilation without penetration of the larynx or esophagus. The ease of use, lack of need for instrumentation, and improved performance (when compared with routine bag-valve-mask ventilation) have made it almost universally available and frequently used.[45–48] It is an essential part of the difficult airway algorithm as recommended by the American Society of Anesthesiologists.[49] The Advanced Cardiac Life Support guidelines give it a class IIa recommendation as an alternative to bag-mask ventilation or endotracheal intubation for airway management.[6]

Description

An LMA consists of a tube that ends in an inflatable cuff. The cuff is designed (from imprints of the pharyngeal area)[50] as a laryngeal mask; that is, the mask, using air pressure to seal the area around the larynx, directs the airflow to the glottis. The device has evolved rapidly; several variations are now available, each with specific characteristics and indications.[51] The *airway tube* is a hollow tube connecting the LMA with the equipment connector (15-mm connector). The tube material varies according to function; rigid plastic or metal in the intubating LMA, wire-reinforced for ear, nose, and throat (ENT) procedures, or preformed to facilitate insertion. The *laryngeal mask* is an inflatable oval cuff with a semi-rigid body (**Figure 5-4**). *Epiglottic or aperture bars* have various designs, but the goal is to prevent the epiglottis from obstructing the LMA's distal lumen. In some models the epiglottic bar is mobile in order to allow passage of an endotracheal tube. A *pilot balloon and inflation tube* allow inflating the laryngeal mask as well as monitoring the inflating pressure.

Application

There are different types and manufacturers of LMA. Each may have specific details regarding the insertion procedure. The operator must read this information for each product he or she uses.[52,53] A spare device should always be available. The purpose of an LMA is to provide an artificial airway to deliver bag-valve ventilation in an unconscious patient with no gag or cough reflex. It can be used as a rescue airway when endotracheal intubation is difficult, hazardous, or unsuccessful and is commonly used in the prehospital setting[48] (where endotracheal intubation proficiency may be lower due to decreased experience and practice). An LMA is also used to deliver anesthesia without intubation in the operating or procedural room. The device cannot be used with patients whose mouth cannot be accessed or who have complete airway obstruction. Usage is also contraindicated: (1) if there is a need for high airway pressure to allow effective ventilation (i.e., decreased lung compliance); (2) in elective procedures where there is an increased risk of aspiration such as morbid obesity, later than the second trimester of pregnancy, nonfasting state, or upper gastrointestinal bleed; or (3) in an emergency when the patient is not profoundly unconscious or there is risk of aspiration due to conditions associated with delayed gastric emptying.

To insert an LMA, the cuff is first deflated. The cuff should form a smooth wedge shape without wrinkles. Lubrication is applied *only* to the posterior wall with a water-based lubricant. The patient is placed in sniffing position (head flexion, neck extension) and the position is maintained with the nondominant hand. The dominant hand inserts the LMA into the oral cavity. The mask is advanced into the pharynx using the index finger or the thumb to exert cephalad pressure while pushing the mask into position. Once resistance is found, the hand is removed while the LMA is held in place. The cuff is inflated and, if needed, a bite block placed.[52,53]

Improper insertion and inflation may result in mucosal or structural injury (including nerve palsy). There may also be mechanical obstruction of the airway from displacement of the epiglottis or penetration into the glottis, resulting in hypoventilation. There is risk of aspiration. Overall, it seems that the safety profile and incidence of perioperative complications is low.[54]

Currently Available Devices

LMAs are chosen based on the patient weight and/or approximate patient size (see **Table 5-8**). There are several manufacturers of LMAs (LMA, Inc.; Portex, Smiths-Medical; Sheridan, Teleflex Medical; King Systems; MEDLINE Industries, Inc.; Ambu, Inc.; and Vital Signs, Inc., among others). Specific characteristics for each device must be reviewed prior to operating that device. These characteristics also may change in the same device from year to year. Specifications of representative devices are shown in **Tables 5-9** and **5-10**.

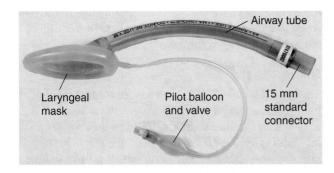

Airway tube

Laryngeal mask

Pilot balloon and valve

15 mm standard connector

FIGURE 5-4 Parts of the laryngeal mask airway.

TABLE 5-8
LMA Sizing Chart

Approximate Weight (kg), Patient Size	Size	Maximum Air in Cuff (mL)*
< 5, Neonates/infants	1	4
5–10, Infants	1.5	7
10–20, Infants/children	2	10
20–30, Children	2.5	14
30–50, Children/small adults	3	20
50–70, Adults	4	30
70–100, Large adults	5	40
> 100, Large adults	6	50

*The maximum air in the cuff and pressure generated by it may vary from model to model.[4] This information applies for the LMA Classic and Unique models. The optimal intra-cuff pressure is 60 cm H_2O.

Courtesy of Teleflex.

TABLE 5-9
LMA Tube Internal Diameter and Length

LMA Size	LMA Classic LMA Unique		LMA ProSeal		LMA Flexible		Single-Use LMA Flexible	
	ID	Length	ID	Length	ID	Length	ID	Length
1	5.3	115	NA	NA	NA	NA	NA	NA
1.5	6.1	135	6.4	135	NA	NA	NA	NA
2	7	155	6.4	135	5.1	215	5.1	215
2.5	8.4	175	8	160	6.1	230	6.1	230
3	10	220	9	170	7.6	255	7.6	255
4	10	220	9	170	7.6	255	7.6	255
5	11.5	235	10	170	8.7	285	8.7	285
6	11.5	235	NA	NA	8.7	285	NA	NA

ID: internal diameter in mm; Length: length in mm; NA: not applicable.

Reusable LMAs

The LMA Classic (LMA, Inc.) has aperture bars to prevent the epiglottis from obstructing the mask airway. The Ambu Aura 40 (Ambu, Inc.) does not have epiglottic bars. The LMA Classic Excel (LMA, Inc.) is reusable up to 60 times and has an epiglottic elevating bar to aid with intubation through the mask. Some devices have a removable and reusable airway connector to allow passing a larger ETT. The LMA Classic Excel allows intubation with tubes up to size 7.5 when the largest mask is used (size 5).

Disposable LMAs

The LMA Unique (LMA, Inc.) is identical to the Classic model with the exception that there is no size

6 available. The Portex Silicone is a single-use LMA available from size 2 to 5. The Portex Soft Seal uses a different mask material that is less permeable to nitrous oxide gas; it does not have epiglottic bars (it has different maximum cuff volumes).

Special Designs

The LMA Flexible (LMA, Inc.) has a wire-reinforced but flexible airway tube. The airway tube is also longer than the classic design. It is designed for ENT procedures because the reinforced tube is less prone to kinking with aberrant head positions. It is not used the in the emergency setting.

The LMA ProSeal (LMA, Inc.) has an additional channel for suctioning gastric contents. The channel

TABLE 5-10

Example LMA Maximum Size Bronchoscope and Endotracheal Tube

LMA Size	LMA Classic LMA Unique		LMA ProSeal		LMA Flexible		Single-Use LMA Flexible	
	ETT	FOB	ETT	FOB	ETT	FOB	ETT	FOB
1	3.5	2.7	NA	NA	NA	NA	NA	NA
1.5	4	3	4.5 UC	3.5	NA	NA	NA	NA
2	4.5	3.5	4.5 UC	3.5	NA	2.7	NA	2.7
2.5	5	4	4.5 UC	3.5	NA	3	NA	3
3	6 cuffed	5	5 UC	4	NA	3.5	NA	3.5
4	6 cuffed	5	5 UC	4	NA	3.5	NA	3.5
5	7 cuffed	5.5	6 cuffed	5	NA	4	NA	4
6	7 cuffed	5.5	NA	NA	NA	4	NA	NA

ETT: endotracheal tube; FOB: fiber-optic bronchoscope; UC: uncuffed; NA: not applicable. All sizes in mm.

opens in the tip of the LMA, which, when properly placed, should allow the passage of a gastric drain. It also allows ventilation with higher pressures (30 cm H_2O). It is designed for patients who require prolonged procedures or gastric access. The LMA Supreme, which is a newer design, is similar to the ProSeal and has a built-in bite block.

The LMA Fastrach (LMA, Inc.) is an intubating laryngeal mask airway (ILMA) designed to serve as a conduit for blind intubation. Although most LMA designs can serve to intubate, the LMA Fastrach has an insertion handle, a rigid shaft with anatomical curvature, and an epiglottic elevating bar designed to lift the epiglottis as the endotracheal tube passes. An important note: Standard endotracheal tubes are not recommended for use with the LMA Fastrach. The LMA Fastrach has its own specially designed endotracheal tubes that have a wire-reinforced wall and a high pressure–low volume cuff. If not using these types of ETT, then the operator must ensure that the endotracheal tube used be capable of passing through the LMA with the pilot balloon and valve. If the LMA is removed prior to extubation, a stabilizer rod is used to maintain the ETT in place while the LMA is removed. There are both reusable and disposable models. It is only available in sizes 3 to 5. Caution is suggested in patients with unstable cervical spine because it can cause cervical spine motion.

The Aura-i (Ambu, Inc.) does not have an insertion handle. The ETT tube size recommended for insertion is indicated in the airway connector.

Air-Q

The Air-Q (Cookgas) is also referred as an intubating laryngeal airway (ILA). (Note: This can easily be confused with the commonly used term intubating laryngeal mask airway, or ILMA.) It consists of an airway tube and a mask. It could be confused with an ILMA because it shares several features; however, the differences are that the mask has a series of ridges below the airway connector designed to improve the seal and it does not have an epiglottis bar. The Air-Q allows intubation with fiber-optic bronchoscope, stylet, or blindly. The Air-Q can be removed once the endotracheal tube is in place with a specially designed Air-Q removal stylet and a removable 15-mm adapter. There are several styles: disposable, reusable, the Air-Q SP (self-pressurized), and one with an esophageal blocker. It is color coded for each size 1.5 to 4.5. Recent studies compared the Air-Q to the ILMA in blind endotracheal intubation in the operating room; the Air-Q was successful 57–77% of the time, as compared to 95–99% for ILMA patients.[37,55]

Esophageal/Tracheal Tubes

Description

An **esophageal/tracheal tube** is a disposable double-lumen tube that has an esophageal (or tracheal) opening and a pharyngeal opening (**Figure 5-5**). It has an inflatable distal cuff and a much larger proximal cuff designed to occlude the oropharynx and nasopharynx. It is inserted blindly and usually enters the esophagus (95% of placements). Under these conditions, one port is used to ventilate and the other is used to pass a gastric tube. If the tip ends in the trachea, the tube is used as a regular endotracheal tube.[56]

Application

The esophageal/tracheal tube was designed for use during cardiac arrest, for which it continues to be recommended. The Advanced Cardiac Life Support guidelines give it a class IIa recommendation as an of studies of airways used in the prehospital setting demonstrated a pooled estimate for success of 85.4% (95% CI 77.3%–91.0%).[30]

Insertion of the esophageal/tracheal tube begins with testing both cuffs for leaks. Then the tube tip and pharyngeal balloon are lubricated with water-soluble jelly. A **laryngoscope** may be used to facilitate placement. The patient's head is placed in a neutral position and the nondominant hand performs a chin-lift maneuver. Then the dominant hand inserts the tube into the mouth, gently guiding the tip along the palate and posterior surface of the oropharynx. With a curving motion, the tube is guided inward and downward and caudally. The tube is advanced until the upper incisors or gums are between the two black guidelines. The proximal cuff is inflated and then the distal balloon. Ventilation is begun using the longer (blue) tube. The patient is observed for chest rise, bilateral breath sounds, and air gurgling over the epigastrium. If there is a chest rise and bilateral breath sounds, the tube is in the esophagus and ventilation is continued through the long (blue) port. Confirmatory testing such as end tidal capnography or capnometry is recommended. If no chest rise and no breath sounds are observed but epigastrium gurgling sounds are heard, the tube is likely in the trachea. Ventilation is begun through the shorter (white) tube and usual verification of placement is done. If neither connector can be ventilated, then the tube is most likely too deep. The tube should be withdrawn 2–3 cm at a time and placement reassessed.[56]

Improper insertion may result in mucosal or structural injury. There may also be mechanical obstruction of the airway from displacement of the epiglottis or penetration into the glottis, resulting in hypoventilation. There is a risk of aspiration.

Currently Available Devices
Combitube and Combitube SA

For the Combitube and Combitube SA (Covidien), the blue tube ends with eight ventilation holes in the pharyngeal area. The white tube ends in a single lumen at the distal tip. The airway cannot be accessed from the pharyngeal (blue) port by a bronchoscope or an endotracheal tube; thus, the trachea can't be suctioned with the Combitube. The proximal or oropharyngeal cuff contains latex. This tube comes with prefilled syringes for each cuff. Available sizes are shown in **Table 5-11**.

Rusch EasyTube

The Rusch EasyTube (Hudson RCI Teleflex Medical and Armstrong Medical Industries) is similar to the Combitube but is latex free. Another difference is that the design of the pharyngeal aperture allows insertion of a flexible bronchoscope, bougie, or suction catheter with a maximum external diameter of 3.9 mm into the trachea. Available sizes are small (28 Fr) and large (41 Fr).

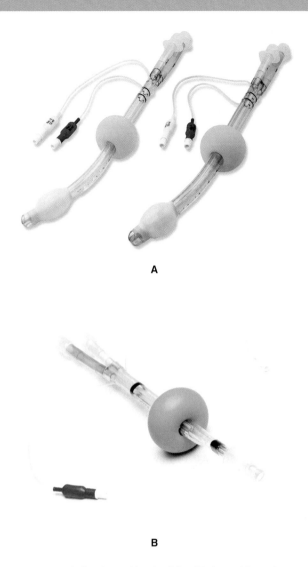

A

B

FIGURE 5-5 A. Esophageal/tracheal Combitube and Easytube. B. Parts of the Combitube.

Photo A reproduced with permission from Nellcor Puritan Bennett LLC, Boulder, Colorado, doing business as Covidien. Photo B courtesy of Teleflex.

alternative to bag-mask ventilation or endotracheal intubation for airway management. It is also used as a rescue airway when endotracheal intubation is difficult, hazardous, or unsuccessful.[30,49] It is used to establish an airway in the prehospital setting (where endotracheal intubation proficiency may be lower due to decreased experience). A major benefit of this device is that no neck movement or manipulation is needed for its placement, which makes it a viable alternative for trauma patients, intubations in limited space, or those in poor lighting conditions. A major benefit may be its use with patients with massive bleeding or regurgitation where views of the vocal cords may be limited. Use of this device is contraindicated when the patient's mouth cannot be opened or when there is complete airway obstruction. It should not be used in patients with esophageal disease (e.g., strictures, caustic ingestion, varices). A meta-analysis

TABLE 5-11
Combitube Sizing

	Size (Fr)	Patient Height (feet)	Proximal Oropharyngeal Cuff Volume (mL)	Distal Esophageal Cuff Volume (mL)
Combitube SA (small adult)	37	4–6	85	12
Combitube (adult)	41	> 5	100	15

Pharyngeal-Tracheal Lumen Tube

The pharyngeal tracheal lumen airway (PTL, Gettig Medical) is another two-lumen tube. The proximal cuff is large and seals the oropharynx proximally. A distal cuff occludes the esophagus distally, allowing for ventilation through the short tube. If the trachea is intubated by the long tube, ventilation can occur through the lumen, similar to an ETT.

Lower Airway Devices
Endotracheal Tubes

The first description of an endotracheal tube used for elective anesthesia was in 1878 by William Macewen; since then it has been widely adopted and multiple modifications to the technique and equipment have occurred.[57,58] Although the device has evolved in design, function, and specific application, the endotracheal tube remains essentially the same concept.[59] The basic requirements for proper design of the tube, cuff, and other accessories are described by the American Society of Testing and Materials (ISO 5361).[60]

Description

An endotracheal tube is a wide-bore conduit inserted into the trachea for establishing and maintaining a patent airway (**Figure 5-6**). The tube is most frequently inserted through the mouth (orotracheal) but also is placed through the nose (nasotracheal). The device is commonly made of PVC. The PVC's thermoplastic characteristic gives the endotracheal tube initial rigidity, which facilitates placement, yet it becomes softer at body temperature to improve comfort.[60] Polymeric silicone is also used, but it is more expensive and less thermoplastic than PVC. Some endotracheal tubes have a Magill curve; the radius of curvature is 12 to 16 cm, which refers to a curvature to conform to the anatomy of the airway. The endotracheal tube can be reinforced with a metal wire or be coated with silver (as an antimicrobial). The *tube* has proximal and distal markings. The proximal markings, usually in centimeters, refer to the depth of the tip; the distal markers either refer to the distance to the distal tip or

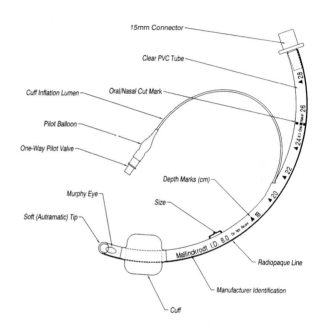

FIGURE 5-6 Endotracheal tube diagram.

are appropriate depth placement markers. (They should be aligned with the vocal cords.) A radio-opaque line to allow for visualization on radiographs lines the tube. The proximal end of the tube is fitted with a standard 15-mm adapter that allows connection to respiratory equipment. In the distal end of the endotracheal tube a *cuff or balloon* is commonly placed. (This is usually absent in pediatric and neonatal tubes.) The cuff holds the endotracheal tube in place, allows positive pressure ventilation, and attempts to isolate the airway from the oropharyngeal airway and esophagus. Some models use water for inflation or are filled with polyurethane foam (see later in this section). The cuff is inflated through an inflation tube, which is often embedded in the wall of the endotracheal tube. Near the proximal end, the inflation tube comes off the endotracheal tube as a single tube that ends in a *pilot balloon and valve*. The pilot balloon inflates in parallel to the cuff. It serves as a visual and manual marker of inflation. The valve allows inflation of the balloon with a syringe (Luer-Lok and slip tip). It is automatically closed by a spring once the syringe tip is removed. Finally, the *distal tip* is beveled (usually 38 ± 8 degrees with respect to the longitudinal axis of the tube); the opening faces left and is rounded to minimize trauma to the airways. There are three different designs for the distal tip (**Figure 5-7**).[61]

1. The Murphy tip has one or more oval openings, called "Murphy eyes," opposite to a beveled end. This allows ventilation in the event that the end of the tube either becomes occluded by secretions or rests against the tracheo-bronchial wall.
2. The Magill tip is also beveled but has no openings.
3. The Parker Flex-Tip (Parker Medical) has a soft, flexible, curved centered tip to help the tube advance over a fiber-optic scope or an endotracheal tube introducer.[59]

Application

An endotracheal tube is intended as an artificial airway. It serves as a bypass of the oral cavity and pharynx. Placement can be an elective or an emergent procedure.

The indications for endotracheal intubation can be divided into the following two categories:

1. *Procedural or diagnostic*, where the choice of tube and device are based on the procedure itself. For example, a patient undergoing general anesthesia will likely receive a standard endotracheal tube, for oral surgery a preformed RAE tube (see later in this chapter), or for lung isolation a double-lumen tube.
2. *Therapeutic*, where the endotracheal tube is placed to help maintain an airway (isolate the trachea from the pharynx), provide positive pressure ventilation, or remove airway secretions; for example, in acute respiratory failure or massive hemoptysis.

Granted, the endotracheal tube can have multiple indications in the same patient.

Although orotracheal intubation is the preferred route for placement of endotracheal tubes, there are

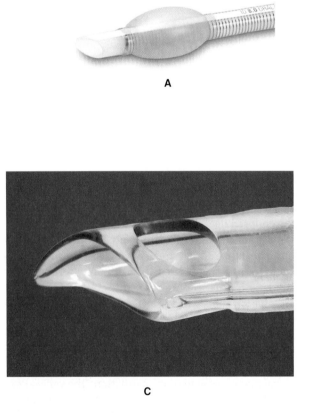

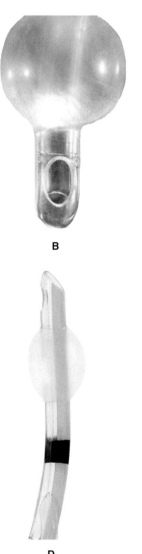

A

B

C

D

FIGURE 5-7 Endotracheal tube tips. A. Magill-tipped. B. Murphy-tipped with a Murphy eye. C. Parker tip. D. LMA Fastrach tip.

Photo A courtesy of Smiths Medical. Photo B courtesy of Dr. Dean Hess. Photo C courtesy of Parker Medical. Photo D courtesy of Teleflex.

circumstances in which nasotracheal intubation would be favored, such as awake intubation, surgery in the oral cavity or mandible, when the oral route access is difficult, poor visualization by direct laryngoscopy, or whenever mobilization of the neck is contraindicated. The nasal route should be avoided in patients with coagulopathy or basal skull fracture.

Hazards[59] of intubation include mucosal or structural injury, sympathetic response (tachycardia or bradycardia, hyper- or hypotension, bronchospams) during insertion, and laryngospasm. The endotracheal tube may become obstructed with secretions after a period of use, particularly if humidification of inspired gas is inadequate, eventually leading to hypoventilation. Prolonged intubation may result in mucosal or structural damage, which may manifest as tracheal stenosis or vocal cord damage. Nasotracheal intubation may result in trauma to the nasal and pharyngeal passage, leading to epistaxis. Nasotracheal intubation may have an increased risk of sinusitis.[62] The tube may kink in the oropharynx or nasopharynx, which will increase airway resistance and make ventilation or passage of suction catheters difficult. Overinflating the cuff can also cause pressure injury of the mucosa or cartilaginous structures, leading to mucosal necrosis, bleeding, stenosis, tracheobronchial rupture, or a tracheoesophageal fistula. In rare occasions, the cuff may inflate unevenly or herniate, covering the tube lumen or Murphy's eye leading to airway obstruction. Intraoperative nitrous oxide (N_2O) diffusion into the cuff may lead to overinflation.[63]

Sizing

When selecting the size of an ETT one must take into account the function for which the tube is placed. The two basic tube models are cuffed and uncuffed; however, there are multiple variations on each, all with different goals and specifications. The reader is cautioned that the following values are dependent on time (i.e., year manufactured) and manufacturer; thus, reviewing the latest specifications on each product is essential.

The size of an ETT is standardized and refers to the internal diameter. Sizes are presented in 0.5-mm increments and range from 2.5 to 10 mm. In general, the trachea of adult females will fit a 7.0- to 7.5-mm tube, and adult males 7.5 to 8.0 mm. The larger the tube, the less airflow resistance and the easier it is to suction or to pass a bronchoscope; however, larger sizes may also increase some of the hazards of endotracheal intubation. The reader is also cautioned that the inner diameter of the endotracheal tube will decrease with time due to secretions and deformation of the tube. This diameter reduction can be critical and present within 24 hours of intubation.[64] **Table 5-12** shows various ETT sizing methods.

Table 5-13 shows suggested ETT sizes for different sized patients. There are also multiple formulas for choosing the size of the ETT. Tube size may be estimated for 1- to 12-year-olds with the following formula:[65]

$$\text{Internal diameter ETT (mm)} = \frac{\text{Age} + 16}{4}$$

where age is in years.

To estimate the size of an endotracheal tube with a cuff for children older than 1 year of age and less than 8 years old, use the following:[66]

$$\text{Internal diameter ETT (mm)} = \frac{\text{Age}}{4} + 3.5$$

where age is in years and is rounded to the next number (e.g., if the age is 1 year and 1 month, it is rounded to 2 years old).

Formulas to predict the depth of insertion of the endotracheal tube for children are also available, using weight in kilograms and age in years; however, these have not been prospectively validated.[67]

For children younger than 1 year old:

$$\text{Nasotracheal insertion depth (cm)} = \frac{\text{Weight}}{2} + 9$$

$$\text{Orotracheal insertion depth (cm)} = \frac{\text{Weight}}{2} + 8$$

For children older than 1 year old:

$$\text{Orotracheal insertion depth (cm)} = \frac{\text{Age}}{2} + 13$$

$$\text{Nasotracheal insertion depth (cm)} = \frac{\text{Age}}{2} + 15$$

In 1979, Tochen described a simple calculation for determining the depth of ETT insertion for neonates.[68] The predicted depth of insertion was 1.17 multiplied by the infant's weight (in kg) plus 5.58. For example, an infant weighing 1 kg would be intubated to a depth of 7 cm, a 2-kg infant to a depth of 8 cm, and a 3-kg infant to a depth of 9 cm. This became known as the "7-8-9 Rule," and it continues to be endorsed by the Neonatal Resuscitation Program.[69] Simply expressed, it adds 6 cm to the infant's weight (e.g., 1 kg + 6 = 7 cm) to estimate the depth of ETT insertion.[70] Peterson et al. have shown that when the 7-8-9 Rule is applied to infants weighing less than 750 g, caution is warranted[71] because it may lead to an overestimated depth of insertion and may result in clinically significant consequences. They recommended placing the ETT in these patients at a depth at least 0.5 cm higher than the depth suggested by the 7-8-9 Rule (**Figure 5-8**).

TABLE 5-12
Approximate Equivalents of Various Endotracheal Tube Sizing Methods*

Diameter Sizing					Equivalent Connector Size (mm)
Internal (mm)	External (mm)	Magill Gauge	French Gauge	Equivalent Cuff (in.)	
2.5	4.0		12		3
3.0	4.5	00	12–14		
3.5	5.0	0–0	14–16	3/16	4
4.0	5.5	0–1	16–18	3/16	
4.5	6.0	1–2	18–20	1/4	5
5.0	6.5	1–2	20–22	1/4	
5.5	7.0	3–4	22	1/4	6
6.0	8.0	3–4	24	1/4	
6.5	8.5	4–5	26	1/4	7
7.0	9.0	5–6	28	5/16	
7.5	9.5	6–7	30	5/16	8
8.0	10.0	7–8	32	5/16	9
8.5	11.5	8	34	3/8	
9.0	12.0	9–10	36	3/8	10
9.5	12.5	9–10	38	3/8	11
10.0	13.0	10–11	40	7/16	12
10.5	13.5	10–11	42	7/16	
11.0	14.5	11–12	42–44	1/2	13
11.5	15.0	11–12	44–46	1/2	

*Because tube thickness varies from one manufacturer to another, data are intended as a guide only.

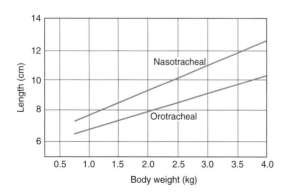

FIGURE 5-8 Graph for determining the appropriate length of insertion for infant endotracheal tubes. For infants weighing < 750 grams subtract 0.5 cm from predicted length.

Currently Available Devices

There are multiple manufacturers of endotracheal tubes. Most are PVC tubes that are differentiated by the cuff and/or specific designs for a given function.[72] Thus, we divided the available endotracheal tubes by type of cuff, uncuffed, and special designs.

Cuffed

Almost all adult endotracheal tubes are cuffed. Neonatal tubes are typically uncuffed because there is not enough room in small diameter tracheas to accommodate both the thickness of the tube wall and the extra thickness of the cuff. Pediatric tubes can be obtained both cuffed and uncuffed. The cuff on the endotracheal tube primarily serves three purposes: (1) to provide an adequate seal for positive pressure

TABLE 5-13
General Guide to Choice of Endotracheal Tube

Patient Size	French Size	Internal Diameter (mm)	Oral Length (cm)	Nasal Length (cm)	Suction Catheter (Fr)
< 1000 g	12	2.5	8	11	5
1000–2000 g	14	3.0	9	12	6
6 mo	16	3.5	10	14	8
1 yr	18–20	4.0–4.5	12	16	8
2 yr	22–24	5.0–5.5	14	17	8
2–4 yr	24–26	5.5–6.0	15	18	10
4–7 yr	26–28	6.0–6.5	16	19	10
7–10 yr	28–30	6.5–7.0	17	21	10
10–12 yr	30–32	7.0–7.5	20	23	10
12–16 yr	32–34	7.5–8.0	21	24	12
Adult (female)	34–36	8.0–8.5	22	25	12
Adult (male)	36–38	8.5–9.0	22	25	14

ventilation; (2) for airway protection, to prevent gastric and oral secretions from being aspirated into the lower airways; and (3) to provide optimal positioning of the endotracheal tube in the trachea to prevent the tip from injuring the mucosal lining.

The cuff, just like the ETT, has evolved over the years. The initial sealing procedure was provided by packing the oral cavity with gauze; later it evolved to a high pressure–low volume cuff, which generated a high incidence of tracheal injury.[73,74] Currently cuffs can be grouped essentially into two groups. *High pressure–low volume (HPLV) cuffs* are made of silicone and are reusable. When deflated, the cuff is small and has minimal residual volume. When inflated it requires high pressures to overcome the low compliance of the cuff. The trachea is deformed to a circular shape. This cuff minimizes aspiration and maximizes the visual field during intubation. Be aware that the pressure in the cuff does not reflect the pressure against the tracheal wall.[74] HPLV cuffs are rare, but one is present in LMA Fastrach endotracheal tubes (LMA, Inc.).[75] When using this tube the minimum occlusion volume cuff pressure should be used (see later in this chapter in the section Devices to Measure Cuff Pressure). *High volume–low pressure (HVLP) cuffs* are constructed of PVC or polyurethane and are disposable. The cuff has a larger diameter (1.5 to 2 times the size of the trachea) and high residual volume when deflated. The cuff is thin, has high compliance, and adapts to the shape of the trachea. The pressure in the cuff closely reflects the

TABLE 5-14
Recommended Endotracheal Tube Cuff Pressures for Adults

Pressure Level	cm H₂O	mm Hg
Ideal	20–30	15–22
High	> 40	> 30
Low	< 20	< 15

pressure against the wall of the trachea.[74] Besides air, the cuff may be inflated with lidocaine, methylene blue, saline, and sterile water. This is usually done for procedures where the cuff may be perforated (e.g., laser surgery) or the cuff may expand (e.g., use of nitrous oxide anesthesia).[76]

The American Society for Testing and Materials (ANS/ISO 5361) has defined the characteristics of the cuff. There is a standard distance from the cuff to tip, the cuff must not encroach on the Murphy eye, and it must inflate symmetrically.[59] There exists an opportunity of error from overinflating cuff due to the relationship among the volume inflated, the cuff compliance, and pressure exerted; that is, the design of the cuff will have implications on the amount of volume required to achieve the given pressure.[63] Regular monitoring of the cuff pressure may help decrease injurious pressures (**Table 5-14**).[77,78]

Types of Cuffs

Cuff construction and material change among endotracheal tubes. The material (PVC, latex, silicone, Lycra, or polyurethane) will determine the cuff compliance and apposition to the tracheal wall. The design of the cuff (conical, tapered, circular) may also decrease the penetration of secretions into the tracheal airway.[79-82] The interaction of the cuff with positive pressure should also be noted. As the pressure in the airway increases, the highly compliant cuffs are deformed. The pressure in the trachea generates retrograde compression and expansion of the cuff in the proximal area. This is called "self-sealing" because it improves the sealing capacity of the cuff.[81] In addition to cuff pressures, leakage across the cuff is inversely dependent on the positive end expiratory pressure and the peak inspiratory pressure.[83]

The following are some of the types of cuffs available:

- *Cylindrical cuff:* This is the most common shape of the cuff (Figure 5-9A). It inflates symmetrically, giving an even area of contact with the trachea wall. The cuff is an HVLP cuff, so when it is inflated, folds (more evident with PVC cuffs) remain that may serve as a conduit for supraglottic secretions[79] (Hi-Lo, Covidien; Bivona Mid-Range Aire-Cuf, Smiths-Medical).
- *Elongated cuff:* This type of HVLP cuff uses ultra-thin polyurethane to decrease microfolds and improve airway seal at lower cuff pressures[82] (Microcuff, Kimberly Clark).
- *Low profile cuff:* In order to improve visualization of the vocal cords, a cuff with a low profile when deflated is preferred (Figure 5-9B). The Lo-Pro/

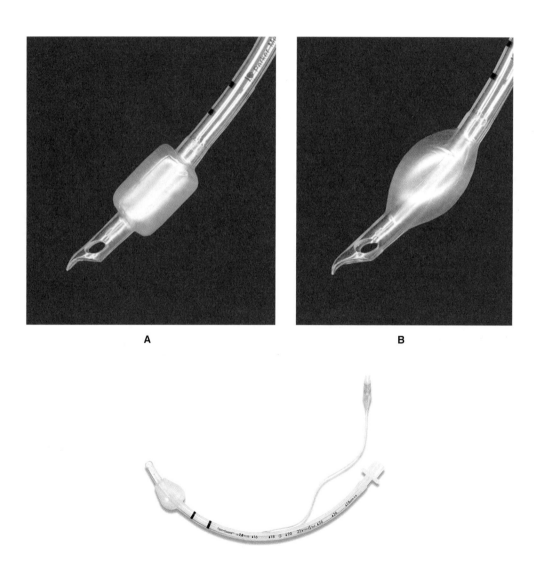

A   B   C

FIGURE 5-9 Endotracheal tube cuffs. A. Cylindrical cuff. B. Low profile cuff. C. Tapered cuff.

Lo-Contour (Covidien) does this with a low-volume, low-pressure balloon.

- *Tapered cuff:* In an attempt to decrease the micro-aspirations noted with conventional cuffs, the contour of this cuff is tapered (**Figure 5-9C**).[84] The aim is to avoid microfolds by better fitting the cuff to the trachea and improving the self-sealing phenomenon (TaperGard, Covidien; Soft Seal, Smiths-Medical; Teleflex ISIS HVT, Hudson RCI; Spiral-Flex Sheridan, Hudson RCI).
- *Foam cuff tube:* The foam-filled cuff (Bivona Adult Fome-cuf, Smiths-Medical) is an HVLP cuff that self-expands. During insertion, air is evacuated from the cuff, collapsing it over the tube. After intubation, the pilot balloon is opened to room air, allowing the foam to expand, thus filling the contours of the trachea. Because the foam is open to atmospheric pressure the theory is that no added pressure is applied, minimizing tracheal wall injury.[85] An adapter allows the pilot tube to be connected to the ventilator airway to increase intracuff pressure during mechanical ventilation breaths.
- *Water-filled cuff:* The Laser-Flex (Covidien) endotracheal tube is designed for laser surgery. It has two cuffs in case one of them is perforated by the laser during the procedure. Both are filled with sterile water, although some practitioners may fill the balloon with methylene blue in order to detect perforation during procedures.[86]

Integrated Automatic Monitoring of Cuff Pressure

Some endotracheal tubes are fitted with devices to maintain a target cuff pressure. These are different from devices that are designed to be used with *any* tube and monitor or maintain cuff pressure (see Devices to Measure Cuff Pressure).

The Lanz Pressure Regulating Valve (Covidien) has a balloon inside a protective cuff. The balloon is connected to a pressure-regulating valve that is connected to the endotracheal tube cuff. If the pressure in the cuff falls, the balloon contracts, transferring air and pressure to the cuff. If the pressure increases, the balloon expands. This design maintains intracuff pressures at approximately 30 cm H_2O, which is important in the presence of nitrous oxide.[87] There is a risk that this device might not form a seal when high ventilator pressures are used. It should not be used with laser surgery, and electrosurgical active electrodes should not be placed close to the device.

Uncuffed

Uncuffed endotracheal tubes come in the same standard sizes as the cuffed tubes, and are mostly used in the pediatric population. Traditionally, cuffed tubes are not used in children under 8 years of age. The reasons are that the narrowest portion of the airway is at the cricoid cartilage, which will achieve an appropriate seal; adding a cuff will reduce the size of the endotracheal tube being inserted (increasing airway resistance); and a cuff adds to the risk of mucosa and structural pressure injury.[88] A study in children undergoing general anesthesia demonstrated less need for fresh gas flow and anesthetic gas contamination when using a cuff.[88] Debate ensued. A recent randomized controlled trial comparing cuffed versus uncuffed tubes in children undergoing general anesthesia demonstrated a reduction in need for endotracheal tube exchanges as well as no increased risk in postextubation stridor.[89] It seems that consensus has shifted from prohibiting cuffed tubes to being safe for use if cuff pressures are maintained below 10–20 cm H_2O.[89–91]

In some tubes, the distal portion has reference depth marks (**Table 5-15**). The meaning of these varies according to brand, type of tube, and patient use (adult vs. pediatric vs. neonatal). In some, the depth markings are one or two reference lines at the distal end to aid in positioning below the vocal cords (2 cm). Some pediatric tubes show three reference lines (two in sizes 2.5–3.0), which are placed at 1-cm intervals; the distance from the distal tip to the first line varies with size. On some tubes, a dark line covers the tip of the tube; the vocal cords should be at the junction of the clear and black lines. Finally, some (RAE tubes) show a "center" mark that is intended to be placed in alignment with the lower incisors to indicate optimal depth.[92]

TABLE 5-15
Uncuffed Tubes' Reference Line Distance from Tip

ID Size (mm)	Distance from the Distal Tip to First Reference Line (mm)
2.0	20
2.5	22
3.0	24
3.5	26
4.0	28
4.5	30
5.0	32
5.5	34
6.0	36
6.5	39
7.0	41

Data adapted for Sheridan Ped-Soft Uncuffed endotracheal tubes from http://www.hudson.rci.com.

Specialty

Above the Cuff Suction ETT

Applying suction just above the cuff, also termed subglottic suctioning, has been integrated into the endotracheal tubes. This is based on the idea that aspiration of subglottic secretions leads to ventilator-associated pneumonia (VAP) and by suctioning them regularly the incidence of VAP should be reduced.[93] The tracheal tube has an integrated lumen that opens just above the cuff, in the dorsal aspect of the tube. The proximal end has a port designed to attach to a vacuum regulator. There is no consensus on the amount of vacuum pressure or the frequency with which it should be done.[94] Each brand of tube has differences in design (Teleflex ISIS HVT, Hudson RCI; SACETT, Smiths-Medical; Hi-Lo Evac, Covidien; Unomedical ETT suction, Convatec).

Spiralwire Reinforced

The spiralwire-reinforced tube has a flat spiral wire implanted in the wall of the tube, which gives it the characteristics of easy flexibility while being resistant to kinking and puncturing (**Figure 5-10**). The tube is used for neurosurgical, face, head, and neck surgeries where the position of the head may be extended or flexed, thereby increasing the chance of kinks in the tube. The tube has a larger outer diameter than a regular endotracheal tube (Mallinckrodt Reinforced cuffed and uncuffed, Covidien; Portex Reinforced Silicone Tubes (RST); UnoFlex, Unomedical).

Silver Coated

The silver-coated ETT (Agento I.C., Bard Medical) is lined with a hydrophilic silver coating, which has an antimicrobial effect.[95] In a large randomized multicenter trial, a silver-coated ETT was shown to

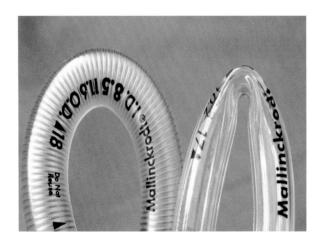

FIGURE 5-10 Reinforced endotracheal tubes. The figure shows the benefit of reinforced tubes to avoid kinking of the endotracheal tube.
Courtesy of howequipmentworks.com.

reduce the time to development and the incidence of ventilator-associated pneumonia.[96]

Laser Tracheal Tubes

Laser treatment is used frequently in the airway. The main risk is ignition of gas or the tube itself. Multiple case reports have evidenced this adverse effect.[97,98] There are special tubes designed for surgery of the larynx and other areas using a laser beam (CO_2, KTP, or Nd/YAG). The designs are different for each company, as is their performance. The goal is to avoid ignition of the tube as well as avoiding reflected beams from the tube that may cause accidental laser strikes to healthy tissue. Some devices have two distal cuffs with individual pilot balloons (to avoid having to change the tube if one perforates); others cover the cuff with material to avoid perforation or are filled with saline or methylene blue to prevent ignition. Finally, some practitioners wrap generic endotracheal tubes in foil tape (Mallinckrodt Laser-Flex, Covidien; Sheridan LASER-TRACH, Hudson RCI; Lasertubus Rusch, Teleflex Medical).

Directional Tip

This ETT has a controllable directional distal tip. A ring in the proximal end is attached to a thread, which travels through a channel embedded in the wall of the tube. When the ring is pulled, it curves the tip of the ETT anteriorly (toward the larynx). These tubes are designed for nasotracheal blind intubation and fiber-optic intubation (Endotrol, Covidien; Parker EasyCurve, Parker Medical).

Monitoring or Medication Lumen

A monitoring or medication delivery lumen integrated into the wall of the endotracheal tube opens at the distal tip. It can be used to monitor end tidal CO_2 or airway pressure (Sheridan ETCO2 Uncuffed, Hudson RCI, Teleflex Medical) or deliver medications (EMT Emergency medicine tube, Mallinckrodt, Covidien; Sheridan STAT-MED, Hudson RCI, Teleflex Medical). A tube with a port above the cuff to deliver topical anesthesia is also available (Sheridan LITA, Hudson RCI, Teleflex Medical).

RAE Preformed Tubes

RAE is an acronym for the names of the tube's inventors (Ring-Adair-Elwyn).[99] These ETTs are semi-rigid, preformed tubes developed to maintain a contour with the facial profile and facilitate positioning with the anesthesia circuit. The intention is also to decrease kinking and pressure injury. They are also termed "south facing" if the connector is directed caudally or "north facing" if directed coronally (Nasal or Oral RAE, Mallinckrodt, Covidien).

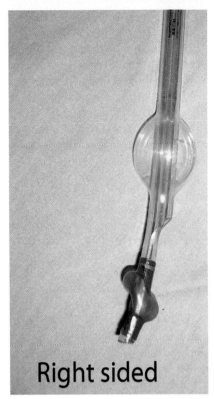
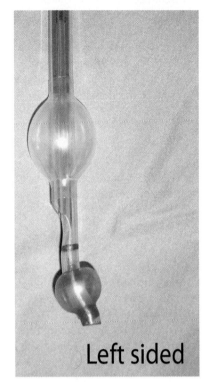

Right sided   **Left sided**

A

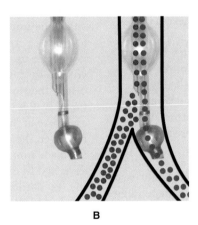

B

FIGURE 5-11 Double lumen tubes. A. Two types of double lumen tubes. Notice the right-sided cuff is irregular, to allow ventilation of the right upper lobe. B. A diagram demonstrating the ventilation of each lung through each lumen.

Photos courtesy of howequipmentworks.com.

Hi-Lo Jet Tube

The Hi-Lo jet endotracheal tube (Mallinckrodt Medical) was a triple-lumen uncuffed endotracheal tube. The main lumen allowed ventilation, the insufflation lumen delivered the jet ventilation, and the monitoring/irrigation lumen provided airway pressure measurement, medication administration, sample respiratory gases, and clearance of secretions during jet ventilation. With the development of the LifePort (Bunnell), a port that attaches to a conventional ETT, this type of tube is no longer needed. The device is no longer made, although it is still available in some places.

Double-Lumen Tubes

A double-lumen tube has the function of allowing each lumen to ventilate a specified lung. The tube is specifically designed for the right or the left main stem bronchus (**Figure 5-11**). The right-sided tube allows ventilation of the right upper lobe. The tracheal and bronchial lumens each have an independent cuff. The HVLP cuff (polyurethane or PVC), pilot balloons, and proximal lumens are color-coded to help identify bronchial and tracheal lumens. These tubes come in French sizes (size 28 to 41 Fr). The tubes have double connectors with ports that allow passage of suction catheters and bronchoscopes without disconnecting the ventilator circuit. An adapter allows ventilation of both lungs simultaneously (Bronchocath, Mallinckrodt, Covidien; Sheridan, Rusch and Portex). Some left-sided tubes come with a Carlens hook, or "carinal hook," for securing its correct position. These tubes require special knowledge for placement and monitoring of cuff pressures.[76,100]

Endotracheal Tube Adjuncts
Laryngoscope

A laryngoscope is a device for visualizing the larynx of a patient for diagnostic, therapeutic, and/or procedural intervention. The most common use is for visual guidance while inserting an endotracheal tube to provide a secure airway.

Description

The laryngoscope has three components: the handle, the blade, and the light source. Its construction is guided by the ASTM (F965) and ISO (7376:2009) standards. The *handle* is the structure used to hold the laryngoscope during insertion. It guides the blade and provides lift to view the vocal cords. Laryngoscopes are usually left-handed instruments, with the operator's dominant right hand used to pass the endotracheal tube. Right-handed handles are available. The handles are usually a standard size with different design blades being compatible with different manufacturers; this system is known as the *Green system* (**Figure 5-12A**). The handles also may serve as the power source for the light source (**Figure 5-12B**). They use alkaline or rechargeable batteries housed in the handle. The size of the device depends on the size of the battery, light source, and/or manufacturer's design. There are several types of handles routinely used in practice:

- *Standard handle (medium):* Most commonly used, 143–172 mm long by 27–38 mm wide (depending on battery size C or D).
- *Pen light or slender handle:* Thinner handle for improved balance with smaller blades (102–140 mm by 15–18 mm). Battery size AA.
- *Stubby handle:* Thicker and shorter handle for use in patients with a short neck or barrel-shaped chest; avoids chest or breast impingement (103 mm by 32 mm).
- *Pediatric handle:* For smaller blades.
- *Large handle:* Larger than the standard handle.
- *Adjustable handles:* The Penlon and Patil Syracuse design allow the blades to be positioned at varying angles, from 180 degrees to 135 degrees to 90 degrees or 45 degrees to ease use of the laryngoscope. The 180-degree position allows the blade to be introduced parallel to the handle when extension of the neck is contraindicated because of cervical spine instability. Visualization of the larynx is also facilitated in obese patients or those in halo traction.

The *blade* may be integrated into the handle or attached to it by a hook. The blade is the portion of the laryngoscope that is introduced into the oral cavity. Multiple styles (described later in this section) are available; however, in general the blade consists of the following components. The *tongue/spatula* is a horizontal shaft that passes over the dorsal surface of the tongue and compresses the soft tissues to obtain a view of the laryngeal inlet. It may be straight or curved in part or its entire length. The *flange* is the lateral projection arising from the spatula toward the roof of the mouth. The flange has two portions: (1) the web or vertical step, which is the upward vertical portion; and (2) the horizontal flange, which rests on top of the vertical step. The flange is used to displace the tongue and improve the visual field. The *tip/beak* of the spatula is thick and blunt to avoid soft tissue trauma. The tip may be mobile or disposable.

The traditional laryngoscope *light source* uses bulbs screwed or embedded into the blade. Others have the bulb in the handle, and the blades have fiber-optic fibers that transmit the light from the handle. Others, mainly disposable devices, are made of clear plastic that transmits light throughout the device. The bulbs are made with an incandescent filament (tungsten with halogen gas), xenon gas, or a light-emitting diode (LED). The bulb can have either a frosted or clear lens, and sometimes also includes a specialized reflector (common with bulb-on-handle designs). The *adapter* is a device used to improve the exposure of the larynx. These devices attach between the handle and the blade. The Howland adapter, ideally used with a traditional blade, allows a 45-degree angle, increasing the exposure of the larynx while minimizing jaw mobility. However, the angle also makes it difficult to introduce the blade into the mouth. The Jellicoe adapter is designed to increase the Macintosh blade angle from the standard 58 degrees to 90 degrees. The Dhara and Cheong adapters are multiple angle adapters (65, 90, 110, 130, 150, and 180 degrees). The Yentis adapter allows the blade to be inserted into the patient's mouth at a 90-degree angle with the handle to the right; after insertion, the handle is swung back to the normal position.[4]

Application

The technique for using each device may be different and the clinician must be trained and educated before using a device. Laryngoscopes must not be used by untrained practitioners and never on conscious patients without appropriate preparation (topical anesthesia, sedation, etc.). Indications for using a laryngoscope include diagnostic laryngoscopy, placement of an endotracheal tube, confirmation of endotracheal tube placement, and foreign body removal.

Hazards of using a laryngoscope include damage to the teeth during insertion or when leveraged backward

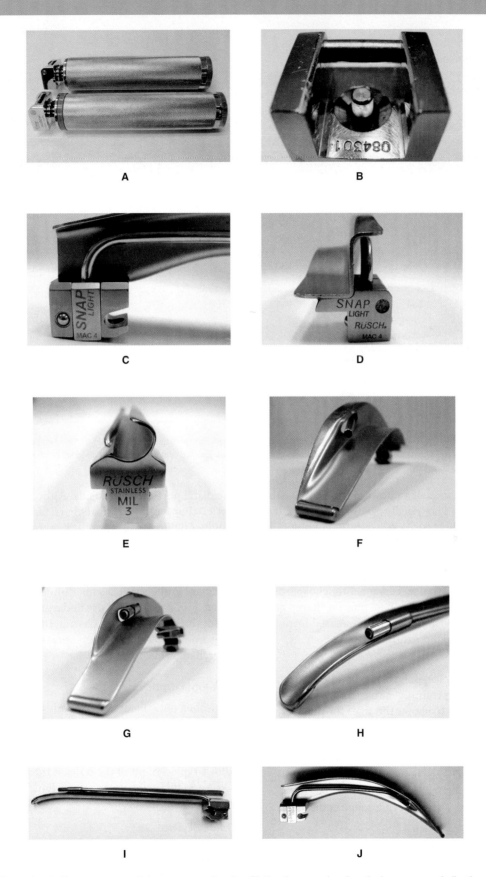

FIGURE 5-12 Deconstructed laryngoscopes. A. Laryngoscope handles. Notice the green band on the laryngoscope indicating it is Green system compatible. B. Securing bar and light source power contact. C. Hook used to secure blade. Notice the spring-loaded bearing to secure it in position. This model has a detachable light source. D. Rear view of a Macintosh blade. Notice the green dot indicating a fiber-optic light source. E. Rear view of a Miller blade. F. Frontolateral view of a fiber-optic Macintosh blade. G. Frontolateral view of a screw bulb Macintosh blade. H. Frontolateral view of a Miller blade. I. Lateral view of a Miller blade. J. Lateral view of a Macintosh blade.

TABLE 5-16
Sizes for Laryngoscopes

		Macintosh Blades						Miller Blades		
		American Profile		English Profile						
Size	Patient Selection	Length (mm)*	Length (mm)**	Length (mm)*	Length (mm)**	Size	Patient Selection	Length (mm)	Base to Tip Length (mm)
0	Newborn	80	NA	80	NA	00	Premature	65	36
1	Infant	87	63	92	70	0	Neonate	75	23
2	Child	108	82	100	90	1	Infant	102	79
3	Medium adult	128	101	130	110	1.5	Small child	125	NA
3.5***	Extra-medium adult	144	NA	144	NA	2	Child	155	132
4	Adult	159	135	155	130	3	Medium adult	195	172
5	Extra-large adult	176	NA	175	NA	4	Large adult	205	182

*Overall length, **Base to tip length, ***Profile IV Mac blade.

Data for Macintosh blades and Miller blades from http://www.welchallyn.com, http://www.sun-med.com, and HEINE laryngoscope brochure.

against the teeth instead of an upward lift. Damage to oral, pharyngeal, and laryngeal structures may occur during insertion. There is risk of aspiration of blood, teeth, or gastric contents. Adverse autonomic reactions to laryngoscopy include emesis, bradycardia, gagging, and diaphoresis. The patient may experience anxiety, pain, laryngospasm, laryngeal edema, bronchospasm, and aspiration. In some cases there may be altered gas exchange (e.g., hypoventilation) and increased intra-ocular and intracranial pressure.

Sizing
The practitioner's choice of the blade, handle, and adapters is made based on training, situation, patient, and availability. Table 5-16 shows the sizes for the most commonly used devices.

The ISO/ASTM standardized the size of the handle and blade connector; this is called the Green system, and it allows interchange between blades and handles from different manufacturers. Note, however, that there are still non-Green system laryngoscope equipment.

Currently Available Devices
Multiple manufacturers are available.

Blade Types
Fiber-Optic
The fiber-optic or bulb-on-handle systems have a light-conducting fiber. The fiber is made of glass or plastic that conveys the light from the top of the handle to the distal portion of the blade. Although called "fiber-optic," they have no optical fibers, per se. Glass fibers conduct light more efficiently, but are expensive. The disposable blades commonly use a light-conducting bundle made of plastic, whereas nondisposable blades use glass fiber bundles. In the United States, any blade or handle that uses fiber illumination has a green dot on the blade base and a green circle at the top of the handle. The blades and the handles of the fiber-optic and the non-fiber-optic systems are not interchangeable.

Non-Fiber-Optic
Non-fiber-optic blades or the bulb-on-blade designs (conventional blades) have a simple electrical connection between the blade and the handle. They may have a removable bulb or bulbs fused to the blade. The first allows replacement of the bulb, at the risk of becoming loose and flickering during operation. The latter makes the bulb nonreplaceable.

Blade Styles
Traditionally, two types of blades have been used, the straight and the curved blades. The straight blade laryngoscopes have a smaller displacement volume (defined by the dimensions of the spatula and flange) and are passed deeper with the goal of lifting the epiglottis directly. The curved blades have a larger displacement volume and are passed into the vallecula,

where the pressure pulls the hyoepiglottic ligament, lifting the epiglottis indirectly.

Miller

The Miller blade is a popular straight blade, introduced by Robert Miller in 1941.[101] The flange has a compressed *D*-shape (on longitudinal view) and a light placed at the distal tip on the right side of the spatula, opposite the flange and tilting toward midline to avoid being embedded in the tongue. There have been modifications to the initial design with changes in the flange height and changes to the bulb location (to the left flange edge, or recessed within the flange). Most Miller designs currently made for adults cannot accommodate an adult-sized tube down the barrel, unlike the older design. The narrow design of the modern blades necessitates careful paraglossal placement without sweeping the tongue from the extreme right corner of the mouth. The narrow blade limits the area for landmark identification down the barrel, which improves as the flange height and spatula size are increased, but increases the displacement volume making it harder to introduce the blade alongside the tongue and reach the larynx.

Macintosh

The Macintosh blade is the most common model of curved blade and was initially described in 1943 by Sir Robert Macintosh.[102] Though initially envisioned as a single-sized blade for an adult, the sizes were later expanded for broader use. There are now a variety of blade styles distinguishable by their flange height, flange shape, light position, and light type. Some blades are available as flangeless. The blade designs are labeled by their geographic origins (i.e., American or Standard, English or Classic, and German designs) (see Table 5-17). The German designs resemble the English except for the presence of a large fiber-optic glass bundle with the bulb in the handle. The common features are a gently curved spatula and a reverse Z-shaped flange.

The differences in size of flange with each design may hinder the use of a same-sized blade in an individual;

for example, due to its larger flange a size 4 Macintosh American blade might not be ideal for a small adult, whereas an English or German blade with their smaller flanges are easier to use. Because there are now a number of manufacturers, each of the blades is now available with fiber-optic illumination with a mix of design features.

Other Blades

There are many other types of blades, most named after their inventors. Their use is dependent on the type of patient, practitioner experience, and availability. There is scant head-to-head information for each of the devices, and when available it is not conclusive that a single blade is better than others.[103,104]

- Wisconsin blade: The Wisconsin blade has a straight spatula and flange that expands slightly toward the distal portion of the blade. This feature increases the visual field and supposedly reduces the possibility of trauma during intubation. The distal portion of the blade is wider and formed slightly to the right to better adapt it to lifting the epiglottis.
- Whitehead modification of the Wisconsin: This is a straight Wisconsin blade in which the flange has been reduced and widened. The goal is to increase visualization.
- Cranwall modification of the Miller blade: This blade has a smaller flange; other features are similar to the original Miller blade. It allows insertion through a restricted mouth opening.
- Wis-Hipple blade: This blade is a modification of the Wisconsin blade with a large circular flange. It is primarily designed for use in infants. The flange is straighter and runs parallel with the spatula and the tip is wider to lift the epiglottis.
- Phillips blade: A straight blade with a curved distal tip and an almost direct line approach to the trachea during intubation.
- Snow blade: This blade has a Miller spatula and the Wisconsin modification flange to reduce trauma during intubation. It curves back from the distal end and is designed for a better visual field.

TABLE 5-17
Differences Between the Macintosh American and English Blades

		American (Standard)	English (Classic)
Flange	Size	Large	Small
	Shape	Vertical, square-shaped	Curvilinear
	Location	Proximal does not extend to the tip	Proximal extends to the distal tip
Light source		Bulb-on-blade (traditionally), fiber-optic	Bulb-on-blade (traditionally), fiber-optic
		Longer light-to-tip distance	Shorter light-to-tip distance
		Frosted bulb or clear	Frosted bulb or clear

- Oxford blade: The Oxford blade was designed for premature infants, babies, and children up to the age of 4 years. There is sufficient overhang on the open side to prevent the lips from obscuring vision. The broad, flat lower surface is a help with small children with an extreme degree of cleft palate.
- Levering tip laryngoscope blade, Corazzelli-London-McCoy (CLM): This blade has the Macintosh design with a hinged distal tip that is activated by a lever in the handle. When it is activated, the tip elevates the tissue at the base of the tongue (improving epiglottis lift and laryngeal exposure). This allows improved visualization of the larynx without altering the axis of the handle, and eliminates contact with the upper teeth as it moves the fulcrum point to within the pharynx. The pediatric model, however, has a straight blade (HEINE FlexTip+).
- Polio blade: Originally designed for patients confined to the iron lung, the blade now may be used in patients with an increased antero-posterior chest diameter or restricted neck mobility. This blade is a modification of the Macintosh blade by mounting the blade at 135 degrees at the handle.
- Robertshaw blade: This blade is used in infants and children. It has a gentle curve over the distal third and is designed to lift the epiglottis indirectly in the manner of the Macintosh blade.
- Blechman blade: This is a modified Macintosh blade with the tip angled to further elevate the epiglottis in a patient of short spine, and sweep the tongue to the left with the ability to tip the blade upward with the handle between the teeth while viewing from the right side.
- E/C E-Mac English Channel blade: This is a modified "English" Macintosh laryngoscope blade with a channel created to add strength to the blade. The channel allows the passing of the ETT while visualizing the cords.
- Fiber-optic Sun-Flex blade (SunMed): A flexible tip blade with a replaceable fiber-optic bundle, an English Channel to help visualize the epiglottis, and a lever in the handle to control and elevate the epiglottis.
- Trueview EVO (Rusch, Teleflex Medical): The Trueview, which used to be called Viewmax, is a curved blade with a view tube lens system. There is only one size for adults and one for pediatrics. It has a port for continuous oxygen insufflation.
- Siker blade: This is a curved blade with a mirror located at the proximal tip at an angle of 135 degrees on the flange facing the spatula. The distal portion of the blade is 3 inches long. It is designed to minimize neck hyperextension. The mirror view of the larynx is inverted.
- Dorges blade: This is a low profile blade (height of 15 mm) with less mouth opening required compared to the Macintosh 3 or 4 size blade. It is considered a universal blade (it is graded according to patient weight) because the depth of insertion depends on the size of the patient.
- Oxiport blade: The Macintosh and Miller blades have a modified oxygen port allowing administration of oxygen or any gas mixture during intubation.

Insertion Techniques

The patient is preoxygenated, premedicated, and positioned. The standard position is one where there is alignment of the three axes (pharynx, larynx, and mouth), also called the sniffing position.[105] By convention, the handle is held with the left hand.

Miller

The straight Miller blade is inserted deep into the oropharynx, beyond the epiglottis. Sufficient lifting force is applied in parallel to the blade. The handle is raised up and away from the patient in a plane perpendicular to the patient's mandible. Care is provided to avoid posterior rotation. Under direct vision, the blade is slowly withdrawn until it slips over the anterior larynx and comes to a position that holds the epiglottis flat against the tongue and anterior pharynx, exposing the vocal cords.[106]

Macintosh

The curved Macintosh blade is inserted past the tongue or displaces it to the left and the tip is rested in the vallecula (at the base of the tongue). Sufficient lifting force is applied in parallel, with the handle being raised up and away from the patient in a plane that is perpendicular to the patient's mandible. Care is taken to avoid posterior rotation. Pressure is applied deep in the vallecula by the tip of the blade anterior to the epiglottis to expose the vocal cords.[106]

Video Laryngoscopes

These devices allow visualization of the glottis opening even when there is an inability to align the oral, pharyngeal, and laryngeal axes. Compared to a conventional laryngoscope, the rigid fiber-optic laryngoscopes permit minimal head manipulation. These devices are intended for use in routine intubation as well as in difficult airway algorithms, restricted oropharyngeal openings, in cases of blood or secretions in the airway, intubation of the morbidly obese patient, or for those with cervical spine immobilization.[107] Each device has its specific characteristics and subtleties (Figure 5-13). Understanding its performance and limitations, training, and regular use are needed for safe use.

Bullard Scope (Gyrus ACMI)

The Bullard laryngoscope is an indirect, rigid fiber-optic laryngoscope that allows visualization of the glottis opening even when there is an inability to align the oral, pharyngeal, and laryngeal axes. Compared to a conventional laryngoscope, the rigid fiber-optic laryngoscope permits minimal head manipulation. This laryngoscope permits both oral and nasal intubations. During nasal intubations, the Bullard laryngoscope is introduced into the mouth for visualization of the vocal cords but the ETT is not placed on the stylet. The Bullard can also be used for rapid sequence intubation, but requires an experienced user. The optical instrument needs to be defogged either by submersion in warm water or by using a defogging solution.

The major advantage of this device is its ability to be used in patients with a minimal mouth opening of as little as 6 mm. It also can be used with ease in patients with anterior larynx, unstable cervical spine, upper body burns, trauma, temporomandibular joint immobility, and micrognathia. The Bullard laryngoscope has been reported to be used successfully in awake and anesthetized patients and also with a double-lumen ET. This device should not be used in patients with preexisting uncontrolled oropharyngeal bleeding or orolaryngeal trauma. The choice between the adult or pediatric size laryngoscope is dependent on both the height of the patient (less than 5 feet pediatric, greater than 5 feet adult, greater than 6 feet adult with tip extender), and the minimal size of the ETT that can be fitted onto the adult stylet.

Glidescope (Verthon, Inc.)

The Glidescope is a video laryngoscope that transmits laryngeal images on an accompanying monitor. It can be used for intubating neonates. The blade is curved and angulated at approximately 290 degrees up from horizontal.[108] A rigid preformed stylet (GlideRite) helps direct the endotracheal tube into position. Sizing options are shown in **Table 5-18**.

Upsher Scope Ultra (Mercury Medical)

The Upsher Scope Ultra (Mercury Medical) is a rigid fiber-optic scope with a *J*-shaped blade that is narrow and rounded. In addition, on the posterior surface is

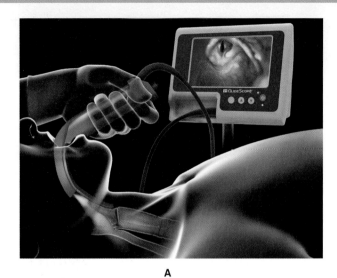

A

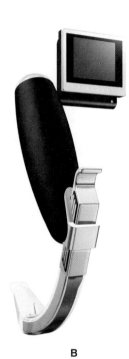

B

FIGURE 5-13 Examples of video laryngoscopes. A. Illustration of the GlideScope. B. McGrath video laryngoscope.

Illustration courtesy of Verthon, Inc. Photo courtesy of Teleflex Incorporated. Unauthorized use prohibited.

TABLE 5-18
Glidescope Sizes and Models

Device	Blade Sizes	Population	Reusable
Cobalt AVL and AVL Preterm/Neonate	0–4	Preterm (500 g) to adult	No
Ranger Single use	0–4	Preterm (500 g) to adult	No
GVL	2–5	Neonate (2 kg) to adult	Yes
Ranger	3–4	Child (10 kg) to adult	Yes

Data from Verathon, http://www.verathon.com.

an *L*-shaped tube guiding channel that accommodates ET tubes up to 7.5 mm interior diameter; however, the scope does not have a working channel.

AirVu and AirVu Plus (Mercury Medical)

A rigid fiber-optic scope, the AirVu has a curvature and an oxygenation port. Its eyepiece is prefocused. It uses a Green system laryngoscopy fiber-optic handle as a light source. The endotracheal tube is placed on the scope, so it works as a stylet.

Airtraq (Prodol Meditec)

The Airtraq is a disposable optical laryngoscope that uses a prism and a battery-powered light-emitting diode (LED) to visualize the larynx. It can be used with a wireless digital monitor. The Airtraq is not designed to be used with ETTs with an interior diameter less than 7 mm or greater than 8.5 mm. It cannot be used with active bleeding in the oropharyngeal area because suctioning is limited. Using the device requires active uplift, similar to the Macintosh or the Miller style, and the tip can be placed either in the vallecula or over the epiglottis, to visualize the vocal cords.

C-MAC (Storz)

The C-MAC integrates a fiber-optic bundle into the standard Macintosh blade (for adults) or a Miller blade (for pediatrics). The device has a camera lodged in the laryngoscope blade and a cable travels to an 8-inch monitor where images of the larynx can be seen.

McGrath Video Laryngoscope (LMA North America, Inc.)

This device has a digital camera in the base of the handle. A single-size adjustable-length curved blade is used for all patients, pediatric to adult. The blade is covered by a disposable sterile blade.

Ambu PENTAX Airway Scope (AWS) (Ambu, Inc.)

The AWS is a rigid portable laryngoscope. It has a fiber-optic channel that fits inside a disposable curved blade. The blade has one channel to guide the endotracheal tube and another for suction. The screen is part of the handle and is hinged. The screen has crosshairs to position the laryngeal opening between them, so they serve as a guide for where the endotracheal tube will go through.

Stylet

A stylet is a malleable, plastic-coated metal rod used to provide rigidity to the ETT. It is inserted into the ETT before intubation and can be molded to achieve an advantageous angle for passage into the trachea. A straight stylet that angles at the cuff to a 35-degree anterior bend (hockey stick) improves laryngeal views.[108] When inserting the stylet, it is important that its tip does not protrude from the end of the ETT; otherwise, tracheobronchial puncture or mucosal

TABLE 5-19
Stylet Sizes

Size	Outer diameter (OD) (mm)	Length (mm)
Pediatric	2.2	225
Adult	4.2–5	335–365
Extra Long	4–5	673–693

damage may result. Stylets come both with and without an adjustable 15-mm adapter. Table 5-19 shows some sizing options.

Currently Available Devices

Multiple simple stylets are available: Slick Disposable Endotracheal Stylet and Flexislip Stylet (Rusch, Teleflex Medical), and the Disposable Malleable Aluminum Stylet SHER-I-Slip (Sheridan, Hudson RCI, Covidien).

Parker Flex-It Directional Stylet

This is a disposable articulating stylet that is threaded into the ETT tube; depressing the proximal end gives an angle to the ETT. Its limitation is the fixed curvature, which might not be suitable for all oral anatomy.

Rigid

A few rigid stylets are available. These are designed to help enable the placement of the endotracheal tube with fiber-optic devices or video laryngoscopes (GlideRite Stylet, Verathon Inc.).

Frova Intubation Introducer (Cook Medical Inc.)

This is a combination of a tube exchanger and stylet. A removable stiffening cannula increases the rigidity of all except the distal 5 cm. There is an adapter that could allow ventilation or oxygenation if needed

Lighted Stylet

The lighted stylet is used for blind, awake, or laryngoscope-assisted intubation. It is also used as an esophageal confirmation device. (See the section Devices Used to Confirm Endotracheal Tube Placement.) The lighted stylet can be used in patients who failed laryngoscopy, who have poor cervical mobility or high Mallampati scores, who require remote site intubations with poor lighting conditions, or who are in suboptimal positions. The light wand needs to be lubricated before loading the endotracheal tube. The endotracheal tube (without the 15-mm adapter) is then loaded. The light wand is advanced to the bevel, but not protruding. The tip of the endotracheal tube is then angled anteriorly at a 120-degree angle. (For ease, set it up as if it were 11:15 on the face of a clock.)[109]

Gum Elastic Bougie

The bougie is a blunt-ended malleable rod about twice the length of an ETT used as a guide for intubation in difficult airways. The earliest versions of this thin endotracheal tube guide were made of gum elastic (latex) coated wire. Most bougies are now latex-free plastic. The bougie can be straight or bent at the tip (**Figure 5-14**) at a 35-degree angle, 2.5 cm from the distal end (coudé tip), which helps in passing it blindly in the midline upward beyond the base of the epiglottis.

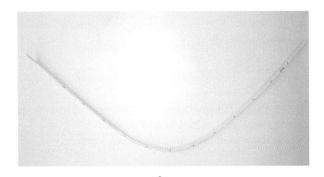

A

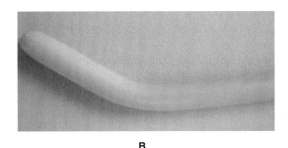

B

FIGURE 5-14 Bougie (A) and coudé (B) tips.

The bougie can be used in all routine intubations (operator dependent), when initial intubation attempts are unsuccessful, or when a difficult intubation is anticipated. It is contraindicated in patients less than 8 years old or when the ETT size is less than 6 mm. Excessive force, passage beyond the carina, or blind introduction may result in soft tissue damage or tracheal/bronchial rupture. Adult size is 15 Fr, 700 mm; pediatric size is 10 Fr, 600 mm.[110]

Endotracheal Tube Exchanger

ETT exchangers or airway exchange catheters are semirigid yet malleable hollow tubes with distal side holes that allow oxygenation using an included 15-mm or Luer Lok connector. They have graduation marks with depth markings that are designed to exchange an ETT without the need of a laryngoscope. These devices are used when there is damage to an ETT cuff or when there is a need to change the size of the tube. Tracheal or endobronchial rupture and pneumothorax can occur. The exchange catheter may come out from the Murphy's eye, which will make ETT removal harder and may lead to injury. Esophageal intubation may also occur. Specifications for common endotracheal tube exchangers are shown in **Table 5-20**.

Devices Used to Confirm Endotracheal Tube Placement

These devices are intended to confirm the placement of the endotracheal tube in the trachea. There are multiple devices available, and the common practice and multiple guidelines indicate to use more than one technique to confirm tracheal placement.[3,6,111,112] All patients who are intubated should have a physical

TABLE 5-20
Endotracheal Tube Exchangers

Brand	OD (mm)	ETT Range (ID, mm)	Length (cm)	Use
Sheridan TTX	2.0 3.3 4.8 5.8	2.5–4 4–6 6–8.5 7.5–10	56 81 81 81	Regular tube exchange
Sheridan ETX		35–41 Fr	100	Double lumen tubes
Sheridan JETTX		6.5–10	100	Provide jet ventilation or oxygen delivery
Cook Airway Exchanger Soft Tip and Extra Firm	11 Fr 14 Fr	≥ 4 ≥ 5	100 100	Provide jet ventilation or oxygen delivery; extra firm is for double lumen tubes
Cook Airway Exchange Catheter Regular	8 11 14 19	≥ 3 ≥ 4 ≥ 5 ≥ 7	45 83 83 83	
Aintree Intubation Catheter	19	≥ 7	56	

exam with auscultation of breath sounds on both sides of the chest and the absence of gurgling sounds in the abdomen. However, commonly seen features of endotracheal intubation (such as "breath" sounds, chest wall elevation and recoil with bag-valve ventilation, or tube fogging with exhalation) may be seen in esophageal intubation.[113,114]

There are several devices to confirm placement. They can be divided into two categories, mechanical and chemical. The most common mechanical device is one that generates suction and is connected to the ETT. Appropriate placement is concluded when, on repeated aspiration, there is no air return. Chemical devices rely on detection of carbon dioxide (CO_2), assuming that the atmosphere and esophagus have no significant amount of this gas. The device is connected to the ETT and will give either numerical, color change, or a graphic display of the end tidal CO_2 ($ETCO_2$). The $ETCO_2$ detectors can be disposable or reusable electronic devices. In simple terms, the presence of CO_2 in the exhaled breath, in consecutive breaths, indicates tracheal intubation.

Currently Available Devices
Capnography

There are two noninvasive methods to measure the exhaled carbon dioxide ($ETCO_2$) for detection of endotracheal intubation: the electronic capnometer and the colorimetric capnometer. We will focus on the latter. The American College of Emergency Physicians recommends using a secondary device, mainly an $ETCO_2$ device, to confirm placement.[115] The Adult Advanced Cardiac Life Support guidelines give a class I recommendation to waveform capnography for confirmation and monitoring of correct placement. A nonwaveform capnometer is considered a reasonable alternative if no other device is available (recommendation class IIa).[6] In patients with circulation, the sensitivity and specificity are high; however, in cardiac arrest the performance becomes less reliable.[116,117]

A colorimetric capnometer is a pH-sensitive chemical indicator that is connected between the endotracheal tube and the bag-valve or ventilator circuit (**Figure 5-15**). The pH-sensitive indicator changes color when exposed to CO_2.[118] The color varies between inspiration and exhalation; purple when there is no CO_2, changing to yellow when exposed to CO_2. The commonly cited pitfalls of this devices are the false negatives in the presence of cardiac arrest or lung hypoperfusion,[119] and false positives in the presence of carbonated drinks or vinegar ingestion.[120,121] These devices attach to the 15-mm standard adapter of the endotracheal tubes. Once the package is open, the device will be effective for up to 2 hours. In pediatric patients who weigh less than 10 kg, a pediatric model (Pedi-Cap Nellcor, Covidien; Mini StatCO$_2$, Mercury Medical) and a neonatal model

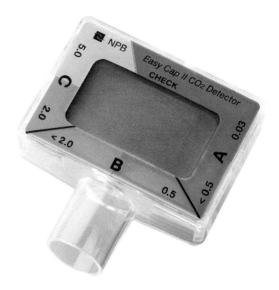

FIGURE 5-15 Capnometry. Colorimetric CO_2 sensor. It fits between the endotracheal tube and the bag valve device.

(Neo-StatCO$_2$, Mercury Medical) are available. For adults, models include the Easy Cap II Nellcor, Covidien; StatCO$_2$, Mercury Medical; and Portex CO_2 Clip, Smiths-Medical.

Esophageal (Intubation) Detection Device

This device applies suction to the 15-mm connector of the ETT. If the tube is in the trachea, the device will aspirate air easily (reexpanding immediately or in less than 3 seconds).[122] If it is in the esophagus, then the device will not aspirate air because the walls collapse around the ETT opening, obstructing the flow of air. The main caveat of these devices is that during resuscitation or intubation, aerophagia may occur and the test may be falsely positive (i.e., indicating tracheal intubation when the ETT is actually in the esophagus). On the other hand, it may be falsely negative (i.e., indicating esophageal intubation when the ETT is actually in the trachea). The latter may be more frequent in patients with morbid obesity, late pregnancy, status asthmaticus, or with aspiration or copious tracheal secretions.[123,124] These conditions cause the airway to collapse (low functional residual capacity) and decrease the expiratory flow or obstruct the ETT with suction. In a study of out-of-hospital cardiac arrest, the self-inflating bulb had a sensitivity of 72.3% and a specificity of 100% when an inflating time of less than 4 seconds was used.[123] In comparison, when used in the controlled setting (medical intensive care unit), the device sensitivity increased to 100% but the specificity was 91%.[114] The self-inflating bulb has a high rate of false negatives when used alone. The Adult Advanced Cardiac Life Support guidelines give the esophageal detector devices a class IIa recommendation for confirmation of endotracheal intubation.[6]

The following devices are available:

- Self-inflating bulb: This is a plastic bulb that is squeezed until it is collapsed and then it self-expands when compression is released. Examples are the Esophageal Intubation Detector (EID), Wolfe-Tory Medical Inc., and the AmbuTubeChek bulb style.
- Syringe: This is a large syringe that attaches to the ETT. The plunger is pulled to generate negative pressure. Examples are the Posi tube, PerSys Medical, and the Syrynge EID, Wolfe-Tory Medical, Inc.

Other Devices to Confirm Endotracheal Tube Placement
Lighted Stylet

This is a retractable or fixed stylet with a bright light at the end. It can be used during intubation or after intubation. When the endotracheal tube is correctly placed into the trachea, the light will transilluminate in the midline as an intense and circumscribed glow in the anterior neck, just below the thyroid prominence.[125] In contrast, when the esophagus is intubated, the transilluminated glow is diffuse and cannot be easily detected. A study evaluating the lighted stylet's performance by experienced providers in controlled medical intensive care unit settings found a sensitivity of 95% and specificity of 97%.[114] There are different devices such as Surch-Lite, Aaron Medical; Vital Signs, Inc.; and Trachlight by Rusch, Teleflex Medical.

SCOTI (Playa de los Vivos S.A., no distributor)

The SCOTI, an acronym for sonomatic confirmation of tracheal intubation, is a device that attaches to the proximal end of the endotracheal tube. It uses reflected sound to determine whether the ETT is in the trachea. The device monitors the acoustical impedance beyond the end of the tube and displays this with a number from 00 to 99. To assist the operator it also displays a red light indicating esophagus if the number is 15 or less and a green light indicating trachea if the number is 20 or greater. There is also an audible alarm that indicates the color of the light.[126] Its performance seems to be good in the hospital setting, with a sensitivity of 93% and specificity of 98%. The false positive cases were seen after prolonged bag-valve ventilation leading to gastric-esophageal distention[127] or when performing blind nasal intubation with PVC tubes with a Murphy eye.[128]

Tracheostomy Tubes

A tracheostomy is a surgical procedure in which an opening (stoma) is created in the trachea. This stoma is usually cannulated with a tube (**tracheostomy tube**) to maintain airway patency and allow function (e.g., breathing) and therapy (e.g., suction). There are multiple indications for a tracheostomy; the device used depends on the patient population, length of use, goals, and device available. The technique for placement can be divided into two categories: surgical and percutaneous. The surgical technique is the most common way to perform a tracheostomy. It is also termed an *open tracheostomy*. It can be performed in the operating room or in the room of a critically ill patient. The procedure is done under general anesthesia or local anesthesia with sedation. The patient's neck is moderately extended to expose the anterior neck and tracheal rings. A skin incision is made below the cricoid cartilage between the second and third tracheal rings. The muscles are retracted laterally. The thyroid gland isthmus is retracted or divided. A transverse or vertical incision is made between the second and third or third and fourth tracheal cartilages. The endotracheal tube is slowly withdrawn to just above the tracheotomy incision while a tracheostomy tube is inserted under direct vision.[129,130]

The percutaneous technique has become more common over the last 30 years. There are several variations in equipment and techniques.[130] It can be performed in the operating room; however, it gained popularity as a critical care in-room procedure. The procedure is done with local anesthesia and sedation. Bronchoscopic guidance and confirmation of placement are often used. The patient's neck is moderately extended to expose the anterior neck and tracheal rings. A small skin incision is made. A needle is introduced into the anterior wall of the trachea (between the first and second or second and third tracheal cartilages), through which a guidewire is advanced. From there on, the technique relies on progressive dilation of the tracheal aperture created by a needle using one or more dilators until it allows insertion of a tracheostomy tube.[72]

Description

A tracheostomy tube consists of a plastic (rubber, Teflon, silicone, polyethylene, or PVC) or metal (silver or stainless steel) hollow curved tube (**Figure 5-16**). There are several variations on the theme, but generally there are four basic parts. The *flange* is a ridge at the proximal end of the tube that sits at the skin opening. It prevents the tracheostomy from being displaced deeper or away from the tracheal stoma. It has slots where a securing device attaches from one end to the other around the neck. In some devices the flange position may be adjustable or be hinged to allow movement. The *outer cannula* is a curved or angled, stiff or flexible hollow tube that serves as the body of the tracheostomy. It connects the trachea with the environment. The proximal opening is where the flange is attached. The body of the outer cannula may be fenestrated or reinforced with metal wiring. If there is a cuff, it will be attached to the outer cannula. The distal opening should rest mid-trachea. The tip is blunted and does not have any Murphy's eye. The *inner cannula* is a hollow

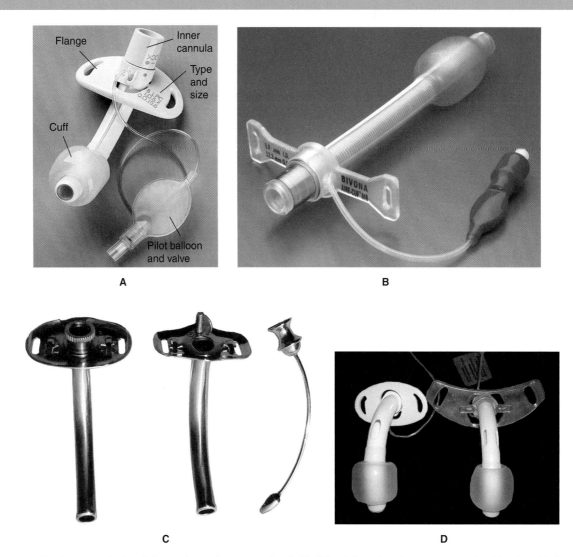

FIGURE 5-16 Tracheostomy design. A. Parts of a tracheostomy tube. B. Flexible reinforced tracheostomy cannula with adjustable flange. C. Metal tracheostomy tube, with inner cannula and obturator. D. Fenestrated tracheostomy tubes.

Photos A and D courtesy of Dr. Dean Hess. Photo B courtesy of Smiths Medical. Photo C courtesy of the Department of Otolaryngology - Head and Neck Surgery, Johns Hopkins Medicine.

tube that is smaller in diameter and tightly fits within the outer cannula. It usually has a 15-mm connector. It may be fenestrated as well. It may have an interlocking mechanism with the outer cannula to keep it in place. The distal portion of the outer cannula has a balloon or cuff. The cuff is inflated (some are self-inflating) to direct the flow of air through the tracheostomy rather than the larynx. The standard cuff is high volume and low pressure. A pilot balloon and inflation tube travel by the side or embedded in the outer cannula and hang outside the tracheostomy. The *obturator* is a device that fits inside the outer cannula. It occludes the distal lumen with a rounded tip to facilitate insertion. It is used *only* during insertion.

Application

A tracheostomy tube is used to bypass upper airway obstruction, stent the airway, aid in removal of secretions, and provide long-term mechanical ventilation

instead of an ETT (to avoid complications).[130] However, a tracheostomy tube is associated with many hazards itself.[72,129] These include tracheal injury, stenosis, granulation tissue, suction trauma, tracheomalacia, wound or stoma infection, subcutaneous emphysema, tube obstruction, stoma bleeding, and tracheo-innominate artery fistula bleeding (a potential cause of death).[130,131] Use of a tracheostomy may result in an inefficient cough due to bypassing the glottis whereby the cough mechanism can't be completed. The tube may become misplaced, causing esophageal perforation and a tracheoesophageal fistula. There may be scarring or a persistent stoma after decannulation. Bypassing the upper airway may lead to increased respiratory tract infection and problems with inadequate humidification of secretions. The tube may impede passage of food or adequate laryngeal mobility.[132]

The size, labeling, and performance of tracheostomy tubes are described by the American Society for Testing and Materials (ISO 5366-1 for adults, ISO 5366-3 for pediatrics).[60] In spite of regulations, there are variations in presenting information and even details as simple as measuring the tube length (**Figure 5-17**).

There are two ways to describe the size of a tracheostomy tube.[133,134] The Jackson System goes from 00 to 12 (**Table 5-21**) and refers to the outside diameter. For example, all Jackson size 4s have an outer diameter of approximately 8 mm (differences may exist between manufacturers). The Shiley dual cannula uses this system.

The second system is the International Organization for Standardization System and the American Society for Testing and Materials ISO 5366.[60] For single-cannula tracheostomy tubes the size is determined by the internal diameter (ID) of the outer cannula at its smallest dimension. For dual-cannula tubes, the ID of the tube is the functional ID (that is, the inner cannula ID). The outer diameter (OD) is the largest diameter of the outer cannula. **Tables 5-22** through **5-25** show various sizes.

Currently Available Devices

There are multiple manufacturers of tracheostomy tubes (see **Table 5-26**).

Specifications

Standard

A standard tracheostomy tube, as described earlier in this section, consists of a flange and an outer cannula. Additions to this basic model have been made to help with function, pathology, and/or therapy (e.g., fenestration to allow speech). The user must remember that the

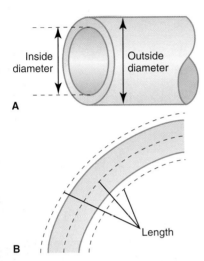

FIGURE 5-17 Tracheostomy tube measurements. A. Inner and outside measurements. B. Length measurements reported.

TABLE 5-21
Jackson Sizes for Tracheostomy Tubes

Jackson Size	Outside Diameter (mm)	Internal Diameter (mm)	Length (mm)
00	4.5	2.4	33
0	5	2.8	36–38
1	5.5	3.0	40–44
2	6	3.4	44–51
3	7	4.3	48–58
4	8	5.3	52–62
5	9	6.2	56–68
6	10	7.2	56–69
7	11	8.3	56–69
8	12	9.2	56–69
9	13	9.9	56–69
10	14	10.6	56–69
11	15.3	12.3	56–69
12	16.3	12.7	56–69

Data from Pilling tracheostomy manual. The size specifications may vary among manufacturers.

TABLE 5-22
Pediatric Cuffless Tracheostomy Without Inner Cannula

Shiley PED				Tracoe Mini 355-Pediatric				Bivona Uncuffed Pediatric			
Size	ID (mm)	OD (mm)	Length (mm)	Size	ID (mm)	OD (mm)	Length (mm)	Size	ID (mm)	OD (mm)	Length (mm)
				2.5	2.5	3.6	32	2.5	2.5	4	38
3	3	4.5	39	3	3	4.3	36	3	3	4.7	39
3.5	3.5	5.2	40	3.5	3.5	5	40	3.5	3.5	5.3	40
4	4	5.9	41	4	4	5.6	44	4	4	6	41
4.5	4.5	6.5	42	4.5	4.5	6.3	48	4.5	4.5	6.7	42
5	5	7.1	44	5	5	7	50	5	5	7.3	44
5.5	5.5	7.7	46	5.5	5.5	7.6	55	5.5	5.5	8	46
				6	6	8.4	62				

TABLE 5-23
Adult Cuffless Tracheostomy with Inner Cannula

Portex Blue Line					Shiley CFS				Tracoe 303				Bivona Uncuffed			
Size	ID (mm)	OD (mm)	Length (mm)	IC* ID (mm)	Size**	ID (mm)	OD (mm)	Length (mm)	Size	ID (mm)	OD (mm)	Length (mm)	Size	ID (mm)	OD (mm)	Length (mm)
									4	4	7.2	56				
					4	5	9.4	65	5	5	8.6	66	5	5	7.4	60
6	6	8.3	55		6	6.4	10.8	76	6	6	9.2	72	6	6	8.8	70
7	7	9.7	75	5					7	7	10.4	74	7	7	10	80
8	8	11	82	6	8	7.6	12.2	81	8	8	11.4	76	8	8	11	88
9	9	12.4	87	7	10	8.9	13.8	81	9	9	12.5	78	9	9	12.3	98
10	10	13.8	98						10	10	13.8	80				

*IC: inner cannula, **Shiley uses the Jackson sizing method

TABLE 5-24
Adult Cuffed Tracheostomy with Inner Cannula

Portex Blue Line					Shiley LPC				Tracoe Twist 302				Bivona Cuffed Aire Cuf			
Size	ID (mm)	OD (mm)	Length (mm)	IC* ID (mm)	Size**	ID (mm)	OD (mm)	Length (mm)	Size	ID (mm)	OD (mm)	Length (mm)	Size	ID (mm)	OD (mm)	Length (mm)
									4	4	7.2	56				
					4	5	9.4	65	5	5	8.6	66	5	5	7.4	60
6	6	8.3	55		6	6.4	10.8	76	6	6	9.2	72	6	6	8.8	70
7	7	9.7	75	5					7	7	10.4	74	7	7	10	80
8	8	11	82	6	8	7.6	12.2	81	8	8	11.4	76	8	8	11	88
9	9	12.4	87	7	10	8.9	13.8	81	9	9	12.5	78	9	9	12.3	98
10	10	13.8	98						10	10	13.8	80				

*IC: inner cannula, **Shiley uses the Jackson sizing method

TABLE 5-25
Nylon Cuffless Tracheostomy

AIR-LON				
Size	ID (mm)	OD (mm)	Inner Length (mm)	Outer Length (mm)
3	4	7	58	70
4	5	8	62	76
5	7	9	65	83
6	8	10	72	89
7	9	11	76	95
8	10	12	81	102

TABLE 5-26
Tracheostomy Tubes

Shiley Tracheostomy		
Product	Description	Sizes
DCT	Disposable cannula, low-pressure, cuffed tracheostomy tube	4–10
DFEN	Disposable cannula, fenestrated, low-pressure, cuffed tracheostomy tube	4–10
PERC	Disposable cannula, cuffed, percutaneous tracheostomy tube	4–10
SIC	Spare inner cannula	4–10
DIC	Disposable inner cannula	4–10
DCFS	Disposable cannula, cuffless tracheostomy tube	4–10
DCFEN	Disposable cannula, cuffless, fenestrated tracheostomy tube	4–10
Tracheosoft XLT	Disposable cannula, extended length in the proximal or distal cannula	5–8 ID
LPC	Low-pressure, cuffed tracheostomy tube	4–10
FEN	Fenestrated, low-pressure, cuffed tracheostomy tube	4–10
CFS	Cuffless tracheostomy tube	4–10
CFN	Cuffless fenestrated tracheostomy tube	4–10
LGT	Laryngectomy tube	6–10
NEO	Neonatal tracheostomy tube	3–4.5
PED	Pediatric tracheostomy tube	3–5.5
PDL	Long pediatric tracheostomy tube	5–6.5
PDC	Cuffed pediatric tracheostomy tube	4–5.5
PLC	Cuffed, long pediatric tracheostomy tube	5–6.5
SCT	Single-cannula, cuffed tracheostomy tube	5–10

(continues)

TABLE 5-26
Tracheostomy Tubes (*Continued*)

Tracoe	Product	Description	Sizes
Twist		Swivel neck plate, use inner cannula	
	301	Low-pressure, cuffed tube, nonfenestrated	4–10
	302	Low-pressure, cuffed tube, fenestrated	4–10
	303	Cuffless tube, nonfenestrated	4–10
	304	Cuffless tube, fenestrated	4–10
	305	Cuffless laryngectomy tube	5–10
	306	Low-pressure, cuffed tube with suction line, nonfenestrated	4–10
	307	Low-pressure, cuffed tube with oxygen supply line	4–10
	308	Cuffless tube with oxygen supply line, nonfenestrated	4–10
	309	Low-pressure, cuffed tube with air supply line for speaking, nonfenestrated	4–10
Vario		Adjustable flange, no inner cannula	
	450	Low-pressure, cuffed with spiral reinforcement	6–11
	455	Uncuffed with spiral reinforcement	6–11
	460	Low-pressure, cuffed	6–11
	465	Uncuffed	6–11
	Moore	Flexible, designed for tracheal stenosis	6 & 8
	Singer laryngectomy tube	To prevent stoma closure	24 sizes
Comfort		Clear plastic, flexible, low profile, long-term use	
	101	Standard length without inner cannula	3–14
	102	Standard length with inner cannula	3–14
	103	Standard length with silver speaking valve and inner cannula	3–14
	104	Standard length tube with swivel speaking valve	3–14
	105	Standard length tube with 15-mm inner cannula	3–14
	106	Laryngectomy tube with inner cannula	3–14
	201	Extra-long tube without inner cannula	3–14
	202	Extra-long tube with inner cannula	3–14
	203	Extra-long tube with silver speaking valve	3–14
	204	Extra-long tube with swivel speaking valve	3–14
	205	Extra-long tube with 15-mm inner cannula	3–14

TABLE 5-26
Tracheostomy Tubes (*Continued*)

Bivona			
Type	**Subtype**	**Description**	**Sizes**
Aire Cuff		No inner cannula	
	Mid-range, nonadjustable	Cuffed, nonfenestrated	6–9
	Mid-range, adjustable neck flange hyperflex	Cuffed, nonfenestrated, flexible wire reinforced, adjustable flange	6–9
	Mid-range with talk attachment	Cuffed, nonfenestrated, additional speaking device	5–9.5
	Neonatal		2.5–4
	Pediatric		2.5–5.5
Cuffless	Adult	Flexible, nonfenestrated, no inner cannula	5–9
	Pediatric		2.5–5.5
	Neonatal		2.5–4
	Cuffless laryngectomy	Flexible, nonfenestrated, no inner cannula	9.5–13
Fome-Cuff	Adult	Cuff is filled with foam that is collapsed when inserting	5–9.5
	Pediatric		2.5–5.5
	Neonatal		2.5–4
	with Talk attachment	Cuffed, nonfenestrated, additional speaking device	5–9.5
TTS		Cuff is tight to shaft	
	Adjustable neck flange, hyperflex	Cuffed, nonfenestrated, flexible wire reinforced, adjustable flange	5–9
	Adult	Cuffed, nonfenestrated	5–9
	Pediatric	Straight or V neck flange	2.5–4
	Neonatal	Straight or V neck flange	2.5–5.5
	Fixed neck flange, extra length, hyperflex	Cuffed, nonfenestrated, flexible wire reinforced	6–9
Flextend	Pediatric	Uncuffed, proximal flexible tube extension, different types of flanges (straight, V shape, extra length)	4–6
Blue line		No inner cannula	
	Extra horizontal length, cuffed, adjustable flange	No inner cannula	6–10
	Extra horizontal length, uncuffed, adjustable flange	No inner cannula	6–10
	Cuffed fenestrated	Low-pressure cuff, has inner cannula	7–9
	Extra vertical length with double cuff	Low-pressure cuffs, no inner cannula	7–10
	Ultra adult cuffed	105-degree angle	6–10

(*continues*)

TABLE 5-26
Tracheostomy Tubes (*Continued*)

Portex			
Type	**Subtype**	**Description**	**Sizes**
	Ultra fenestrated cuffed		6–10
	Adult cuffed		6–10
DIC		Disposable inner cannula, 15-mm adapter	
	Uncuffed		5–9
	Cuffed		6–10
	Cuffed fenestrated		6–10
	Uncuffed fenestrated		5–9
Flex DIC		Flexible, disposable inner cannula, 15-mm connector	
	Uncuffed		6–10
	Cuffed		6–10
Lo-profile		Minimally protruding inner cannula and flange	
	Uncuffed		6–10
	Uncuffed, fenestrated		6–10
	Cuffed		6–10
Trach-Talk		Inner cannula	7–9
Uni-Perc		Percutaneous insertion, adjustable flange, inner cannula	7–9
Neonatal		Uncuffed, 15-mm connector	2.5–3

use of an inner cannula will reduce the effective inner diameter, which results in an increase in airflow resistance and smaller access for devices.

Uncuffed

Uncuffed tracheostomy tubes maintain the stoma patent and may allow mechanical ventilation but do not protect against aspiration.[133] They are used most commonly for the following indications: (1) in children (0–6 years old) because the cricoid ring is narrower and the tracheal and laryngeal cartilages are softer, hence the cuff may cause more tracheal deformation with no increase in seal; (2) when there is no need for mechanical ventilation (e.g., laryngectomy, tumors, or severe sleep apnea); and (3) when patients are weaned off tracheostomy (i.e., progressive reduction in cannula size).

Cuffed

A cuff in the distal portion of the outer cannula, when inflated, has the following functions: (1) It directs the air from the trachea to the inner cannula; (2) it decreases the amount of oral/esophageal secretions that enter the airway; and (3) it facilitates the administration of positive pressure ventilation.[59] The cuff is filled with air (although some are filled with other substances, see the following section). The pressure in the cuff should be measured regularly to avoid injury. The cuff pressure should be maintained between 20 and 25 mm Hg (25–35 cm H_2O),[73] unless otherwise specified by the manufacturer.

Foam Cuff

The Bivona Fome-cuff uses a polyurethane foam that is inside a silicone cuff. The goal is to reduce the pressure induced by the tracheostomy cuff on the tracheal wall, thereby reducing tracheal wall injury (e.g., stenosis). The tracheostomy tube is inserted by evacuating the air from the silicone cuff surrounding the foam. This causes the collapse of the foam against the outer cannula. When the cannula is inserted, the pilot port is open to ambient (atmospheric) pressure and the foam expands.

It is important to recognize that the pressure against the tracheal wall depends on the appropriate sizing of the tracheostomy tube in relation to the trachea. If the tracheostomy tube is too small, there will not be appropriate apposition of the cuff against the tracheal wall, leading to leakage. If the tracheostomy tube is too large compared to the trachea, then the foam cuff may cause high pressure against the tracheal wall. Although the Fome-cuff was described in 1974,[135] there is very little literature on its use.

Tight-to-Shaft (TTS) Cuff

The TTS cuff is designed to allow mechanical ventilation and/or minimize aspiration, while maximizing the airflow in patients who need short-term cuff inflation. This is achieved by two features of its design. First, the cuff sits tightly against the outer cannula, hence decreasing the outer diameter and maximizing the ability of air to flow around the tracheostomy (e.g., allowing the patient to talk). Second, the cuff is a high pressure–low volume cuff that when inflated should minimize air leakage and aspiration. The cuff is inflated with sterile water (not saline, because it will crystallize) to avoid the problem of air leaking under high pressures.

Fenestrated

A fenestrated tracheostomy tube has one or more openings in the posterior wall of the outer cannula. These openings or fenestrations allow air to pass through the outer cannula. The reader is advised that there are variations among models (see the following section Talking Tracheostomy). Those described here are the most common. First, there may be a cuff, which is always placed below the fenestration. When the cuff is inflated the air will flow exclusively through the inner cannula and then through the fenestration, gaining access to the larynx. If the cuff is deflated, then the air may go around the tracheostomy and through the inner cannula and fenestration, thereby increasing the air reaching the larynx. This is not always true if there is an inner cannula. Second, there may be an inner cannula. The inner cannula comes in two models: fenestrated and not fenestrated. Be aware that if the inner cannula is *not* fenestrated, then the fenestration in the outer cannula is not patent to the airway. There are *two potentially dangerous* scenarios if a combination of events leads to capping the tracheostomy while leaving the cuff inflated. If a fenestrated inner cannula is in place, excessive airflow resistance may develop. If an unfenestrated inner cannula is in place, the patient will have a completely blocked airway!

Specialty Tubes

Custom
The anatomy of the patient may require a custom tracheostomy. Several companies offer this service and require measurements and ordering by an airway specialist.

Metal Tracheostomy Tubes
The metal tracheostomy tube is a remnant of the first tracheotomies. They are still available for use, however. Their main indications are the same as for a standard cuffless tracheostomy tube. The advantage is that they are reusable. The problems are that they are rigid, the flange angle is fixed, and most models lack a 15-mm connector. The metal tracheostomy tube can be fenestrated. A fenestrated metal tracheostomy tube may come with a Tucker valve (Pilling, Teleflex Medical). The valve is built into the inner tube and allows speech without covering the proximal opening of the tracheostomy. It consists of a valve that opens on inhalation, allowing air to go into the lungs, but closes on exhalation to direct the flow to the fenestration and the pharynx, thus allowing speech. The metal tracheostomy tubes can be also be custom made. There are several types of metal tracheostomy tubes, each with its own characteristics and all currently available: Jackson original, Jackson improved, Jackson extra-long, Mayo clinic tube, Holinger, Tucker, Martin, and Luer.

Nylon Tracheostomy Tubes
The Air-Lon trachea tube is a tracheostomy tube used to maintain the stoma patency. It is similar to the metal tracheostomy tube, but it is not fenestrated. Its low profile proximal opening and flange make it useful in the decannulation process or in the ambulatory setting.

Subglottic Suctioning or Above-the-Cuff Suction
This is a cuffed tracheostomy tube with an opening just above the cuff. The opening is attached to a suction line. The goal is that by intermittent use of supraglottic suctioning the aspiration of oral and esophageal/gastric content can be minimized. No study has been published in regard to this type of tracheostomy tube (Tracoe Twist Model 306, Boston Medical Products, Inc.).

Talking Tracheostomy
A talking tracheostomy tube is designed to allow patients to speak while the cuff is inflated. It is different from a fenestrated tracheostomy tube. The talking tracheostomy tube is designed for use by patients that still have vocal cord use, but need to have the cuff continuously inflated (i.e., need persistent mechanical ventilation). The device has one or several openings above the cuff that are connected to a gas source (air) at 4/6 L/min. The tubing has a port that, when occluded, directs the flow toward the larynx allowing speech (Tracoe Twist Model 309, Portex Trach-Talk, Bivona Aire-Cuff, and Fome-Cuf with talk attachment). A recent device, the Blom Tracheostomy and Speech Cannula (Pulmodyne)[136] allows phonation with the cuff inflated, while using an ingenious inner cannula and a fenestrated outer cannula. The inner cannula has a bubble valve that expands during inspiration (occluding the fenestration) and deflates during exhalation, and a flap valve that occludes the tip of the inner

cannula during exhalation. The effect is air being deviated during exhalation to the subglottic space.

Oxygen Supply Line

An oxygen supply line is built into the tracheostomy tube (Tracoe Twist Model 307 and 308, Boston Medical Products, Inc.). The oxygen port opens proximally to the outer cannula (near the proximal opening). The models available are both cuffed and uncuffed, and have inner cannulas that have a proximal fenestration.

Extended Length

The extended length tracheostomy tubes can be proximal or distal. The proximal extended length has a longer proximal segment that allows placement in patients with large necks (obese) or anatomical variations. The distal extended length has a longer distal tube that bypasses tracheal abnormalities. The distal extended length may have two cuffs (for sequential inflation to minimize injury). The proximal extended length is available with an adjustable flange to adjust the fit.

Montgomery T-Tubes

The Montgomery T-Tubes (Montgomery Safe-T-tubes, Boston Medical Products, Inc.) are flexible tracheostomy tubes that are different from the basic tracheostomy design. They were described in an article in 1965 for the management of tracheal stenosis.[137] The Montgomery tube is made of semirigid plastic with a *T* shape. It has a limb that comes through the tracheostoma; a lower limb goes to the trachea and the upper limb goes to the subglottic space. The main use is to provide support to a stenotic airway (tracheal stenosis, tracheomalacia, or reconstruction).[138] A standard 15-mm adapter is available for connection to respiratory equipment. It is available in six models (size given in millimeters): Pediatric (sizes 6–9); Standard (sizes 10–16); Thoracic, with an extra-long lower limb (sizes 10–16); Extra-long, designed to allow customization to measured lengths (sizes 10–16); Tapered, in which the upper limb is tapered to allow placement in glottic or subglottic stenosis (sizes 8/10 and 10/13); Hebeler, in which an internal balloon in the upper limb (subglottic) can be inflated to decrease the flow of air or gas to the subglottic area, allowing mechanical ventilation or anesthesia (sizes 12, 15–18); and finally the HMS System, which is used for surgical procedures and has an inner cannula that can be removed for cleaning without removing or disturbing the surgical site (sizes 7, 9, and 11 mm).

Tracheostomy Tube Adjuncts

Vocalization Devices

One of the main concerns of patients with a tracheostomy is speech.[139] Vocalization devices help patients with tracheostomies to speak. A speaking valve is different from a talking tracheostomy. A speaking valve is used with the cuff deflated. During inspiration, it allows the air to enter the airway, both from the upper airway and the tracheostomy. During exhalation, the valve closes or increases resistance to redirect air toward the larynx. In contrast, a talking tracheostomy maintains the tracheostomy cuff inflated and a gas source provides air to the subglottic space to allow speech. The talking tracheostomy is used when the patient requires continuous ventilation and cannot tolerate cuff deflation (e.g., need for positive end-expiratory pressure [PEEP]). A speaking valve seems to improve swallowing[140] and decrease secretions, and may decrease aspiration[141] and improve olfactory function.[142]

Description

The basic design of a vocalization device entails redirecting gas flow during exhalation from a path that goes through the tracheostomy tube to a path that goes through the larynx. Because gas flows to areas of least resistance, redirection of flow usually involves intermittent manual or mechanical obstruction of the tracheostomy tube. Some speaking valves can be used in conjunction with mechanical ventilation.[143] All are attached by friction fit to the tracheostomy and, if needed, to the ventilator circuit.

There are two types of valves: (1) diaphragm valves, which are either flapper (most) or disk valves, or (2) ball valves,[144] where a ball occludes the lumen during expiration. Speaking valves can also be classified in relation to the type of diaphragm construction: (1) bias-closed valve, in which the valve is closed at all times except on inspiration, when negative tracheal pressure opens the valve, or (2) bias-open valve, in which the valve is open at all times except on expiration. A bias-closed valve may require greater effort to achieve airflow, whereas a bias-open valve may have higher air loss during expiration, which may affect speech quality.[145,146] There are differences in the resistance to air flow and work of breathing between devices, and although this may not be clinically significant,[147] the construction and performance of the valve affects the speech quality.[148]

It is recommended that when a speaking valve is used, the tracheostomy tube should be not more than two thirds the size of the tracheal lumen, and if possible a cuffless tracheostomy tube should be used. Further, the use of tracheal manometry during passive exhalation to assess expiratory resistance may help identify patients who will tolerate its use. A value above 5 cm H_2O for adults[149] or 10 cm H_2O for children[150] should prompt the clinician to evaluate the airway for obstruction or consider a change of tracheostomy tube (cuffless or downsize). Vocalization devices are contraindicated in patients who are unconscious or have unstable respiratory status including large amounts of secretions or the need for high oxygen concentrations. Hazards include an increased work of breathing due to the increased resistance of the speaking valve.[147,151]

Currently Available Devices

Passy-Muir Speaking Valve (Passy-Muir, Inc.)

The Passy-Muir speaking valve uses a unidirectional diaphragm flapper valve, which allows inhalation but prevents exhalation through the tracheostomy tube. It is a bias-closed valve. There is an optional oxygen adapter (less than 6 L/min oxygen delivery) for selected models. Models are shown in **Table 5-27**.

Shikani-French Speaking Valve (Airway Company, Teleflex, Pilling)

The Shikani-French speaking valve uses a ball valve design.[144] Two models are available, one for use with plastic and another for metal tracheostomy tubes.

Montgomery Speaking Valve (Boston Medical Products, Inc.)

The Montgomery valve uses a unidirectional diaphragm flapper silicone valve, which allows inhalation but prevents exhalation through the tracheostomy. It has a "cough-release" mechanism whereby the excessive pressure from a cough is released to avoid device dislodgment. It can be connected to a standard tracheostomy tube, a Montgomery Long-Term cannula (see the section Stomal Maintenance Devices later in this chapter) or in-line with a ventilator (VENTRACH). It connects to a standard 15-mm connector. The outer diameter is 22 mm.

Shiley Phonate Speaking Valve (Covidien)

This is a diaphragm flapper silicone valve. It has a hinged cap to disable the speaking valve. A model with an oxygen port is available.

Tracoe Phon Assist I (Boston Medical Products, Inc.)

The Phon Assist I uses a unidirectional diaphragm valve. The device can be adjusted to allow speech or be switched to permit unrestricted breathing. It connects to a standard 15-mm connector. A model with an oxygen port is available.

Trachvox (Pulmodyne)

This device includes a heat and moisture exchanger (HME) and an oxygen port for supplemental oxygen. A valve allows suctioning and forceful breathing (bypassing the HME). The speech valve requires the patient to depress it with the finger; once released, a spring opens it to resume normal ventilation.

Hood Speaking Valve (Hood Laboratories)

This is a one-way valve designed for use with tracheal buttons, in particular the Hood Stoma stent (see the section Stomal Maintenance Devices later in this chapter). It is also available in a 15-mm model to adapt to a standard tracheostomy tube.

Medin Low Resistance Speaking Valve (Hood Laboratories)

This is a one-way valve that fits a standard 15-mm adapter.

Eliachar Speaking Valve (Hood Laboratories)

This is a one-way, silicone, low profile valve that only fits tracheal stomas (buttons) with an OD of 11 or 13 mm.

The Kistner and Olympic Trach Talk are no longer available.

Stomal Maintenance Devices

In patients in whom the tracheal stoma needs to remain patent, a series of devices are available. Some will just maintain the stoma patent; some allow access for suctioning. These are ideal for patients with preserved respiratory function because they preserve the tracheal stoma and minimally decrease the airway diameter.

TABLE 5-27
Passy-Muir Speaking Valve Models

Valve	Color	ID	OD	In-line Mechanical ventilation	Characteristics
PMV 005	White	15	23	Yes*	
PMV 007	Aqua	15	22	Yes	Designed to fit inside ventilator tubing, disposable and nondisposable
PMV 2000	Clear	15	23	Yes*	Low profile, may use oxygen adapter
PMV 2001	Purple	15	23	Yes*	Identical to PMV 2000
PMV 2020	Clear	15	23	No	Attaches to metal Jackson Improved tracheostomy with an adapter

* For use with short, wide mouth, flexible, nondisposable (rubber) ventilator tubing

Description

These devices are made of plastic, PVC, or silicone and consist of a straight, rigid, or flexible hollow cannula, which latches between the skin and the anterior wall of the trachea (Figure 5-18). Some have inner cannulas or caps that allow occlusion of the air channel. Most stomal maintenance devices are just inserted into the airway with no instrumentation. Each device has specific characteristics and techniques, of which the provider should be aware and train the patient. Another term for these devices is *tracheal buttons*.

Sizing

Appropriate sizing is essential for a snug fit, which leads to appropriate function and minimizes air and secretion leak. An ENT specialist will measure and fit the device.

Currently Available Devices

Tracoe Stoma Button (Boston Medical Products, Inc.)

This is a hollow structure made of silicone with two flanges on either end. One flange is flat and larger so as to fit against the skin. The other is smaller and fits against the anterior tracheal wall. One of the models (Tracoe Grid button) comes with a removable fine metallic mesh, to prevent aspiration into the airway, and lateral tabs to attach a neck strap. It fits stomas from 9 to 15 mm, and comes in three lengths: 16, 22, and 33 mm (Tracoe Larynx 601, 602, 603, 611, 612, 613). Optional accessories include a heat moisture exchanger, a stopper, and a speaking valve. (See Tracoe Phon Assist I [Boston Medical Products, Inc.] earlier in the chapter.)

Hood Stoma Stent (Hood Laboratories)

This is a hollow silicone structure. It has a curved tracheal portion and a flat skin flange to secure it in position. A stoma plug comes attached to the skin flange. There are straight and curved cannula models

that fit stomas from 8 to 15 mm and lengths from 11 to 50 mm. Optional accessories include the Hood Lab speaking valves (see earlier in the chapter) and a 15-mm standard connector.

Barton-Mayo Tracheostoma Button (InHealth Technologies)

This is a silicone tube; the tracheal portion is flanged and the skin portion has a cup-like device. It was designed for near-total laryngectomy and total laryngectomy patients. It comes in sizes 9 to 14, and lengths of 15, 22, and 30 mm. It can be used with a speaking valve (Blom-Singer Adjustable Tracheostoma Valve I, InHealth Technologies) or a heat moisture exchanger (Blom-Singer HumidiFilter, InHealth Technologies).

Olympic Trach-Button (Natus Medical, Inc.)

The trach-button is a hollow structure made of Teflon. On the trachea side there is a ring at the end that has been sliced open a little, creating ridges and petals. When the inner plug is inserted it extends the whole length of the cannula and snaps in place, forcing the ridges outward, thereby securing the device. The expansion lock completely occludes the stoma lumen. It fits stomas from 9 to 14 mm, comes in two lengths (27 or 44 mm), and has multiple spacers to adjust fit. Optional equipment are a standard 15-mm adapter in case ventilation is needed, a flange, and a retaining device to secure placement.

Montgomery Short- and Long-Term Cannulas (Boston Medical Products, Inc.)

This system is designed for patients who do not need a standard tracheostomy. The Montgomery Short-Term cannula is placed surgically while the tract matures. It consists of a hollow flexible silicone cannula. The tracheal end has flaps and is angled at a 27-degree

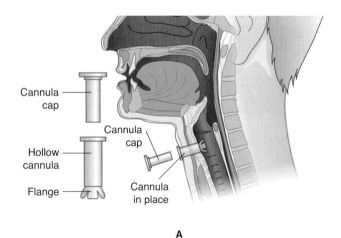

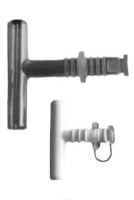

Cannula cap

Cannula cap

Hollow cannula

Flange

Cannula in place

A

B

FIGURE 5-18 A. Tracheostomy button. B. Montgomery Standard Safe-T-Tube.

Photo courtesy of Boston Medical Products, Inc.

angle. The flap is longer on the vertical orientation and shorter horizontally. This helps the cannula position properly in the stoma, and the flaps in the trachea keep it from rotating. The body of the cannula has ridges such that an adjustable flange can be anchored. The cannula length can be trimmed. Once the tract is mature, the device can be changed to the Long-Term cannula model.

The Montgomery Long-Term cannula also has the angled and flanged inner flaps; however, the body of the cannula is smooth until the proximal portion, where the ridges are present, to ensure the adjustable flange is secured. Sizes available are 4, 6, 8, and 10 mm and it has six length ranges (17 to 65 mm). It comes with a plug attached to a ring to occlude the airway. Optional equipment is a 15-mm standard adapter for ventilation.

Helsper Stoma Vent (Bentec Medical)

This is made of silicone. The skin flange has a conical shape, and the tracheal flange is either straight or can be slanted. It comes in sizes 5–12, and has a length from 14.5 to 20.3 mm. Special sizes are also available.

Moore Trachesotomy Button (Teleflex)

This is made of acrylic. The skin flange has a slight conical shape, and the tracheal flange is straight. It has an outer diameter size of 14 to 16 mm and a length of 10 to 15 mm.

Norris Tracheostomy Button (Teleflex)

This is made of white Teflon. The skin flange has a conical shape, and the tracheal flange is straight. It has an outer diameter size of 11 to 13 mm and a length of 19 mm.

Airway Care Equipment

Devices to Measure Cuff Pressure

There are four different methods to assess the inflation of a cuff in a tracheostomy or endotracheal tube.[152]

1. The minimal occlusive volume technique, where air is added to the cuff to create a seal and abolish air leak on inspiration (while on mechanical ventilation)[63]
2. The minimum leak technique, where just enough air is removed from the cuff to allow a small leak on inspiration
3. Manual, where the pilot balloon of the ETT is gently pressed to estimate the appropriate cuff pressure (subjective)
4. Pressure monitoring, in which a device is used to measure the pressure in the cuff

The tracheal capillary perfusion pressure is normally 25 to 35 mm Hg. (The reader is cautioned that measurements are also reported in cm H_2O.) The cuff used to seal the airway around any endotracheal device may cause high pressures against the mucosa. High cuff pressure will overcome the capillary perfusion pressure, leading to decreased perfusion and ischemia.[73] Conversely, low cuff pressures will allow supraglottic contents (oral, esophageal, or gastric) to enter the airway, leading to pneumonia.[153] Both situations may lead to complications. The recommendation is to keep the cuff pressure between 20 and 30 cm H_2O (15–22 mm Hg).[129,154] Devices that measure cuff pressure should be used to monitor the cuff pressure based on a standardized protocol.

Currently Available Devices

Aneroid Manometer
This is a reusable device that is rigged with a conventional manometer at the bedside. It involves connecting the cuff to the manometer with a hose and a three-way stopcock, so that pressure can be monitored while air is injected.[133]

Portex PressureEasy Cuff Pressure Monitor (Smiths-Medical)
This is a single-use device that uses a graded spring to show the cuff pressure. It has two connections: (1) to the pilot balloon, and (2) to an adapter to connect to the endotracheal tube. The cuff pressure is regulated manually and set in the "safe range" (20–30 cm H_2O). Because the device is connected to the airway pressure, when it increases, the pressure is transmitted to the cuff to increase the pressure and prevent leakage.

Posey Cufflator (Posey Co.)
This is a manometer that allows inflation and deflation of the cuff. The manometer is attached to an inflator bulb and has an integrated vent button. A green area is marked from 20 to 30 cm H_2O.

Rüsch Endotest (Teleflex Medical)
This is a manometer that allows inflation and deflation of the cuff. The manometer is attached to an inflator bulb and has an integrated vent button. A green area is marked from 15 to 25 cm H_2O.

Ambu Cuff Pressure Gauge (Ambu, Inc.)
This is a manometer that allows inflation and deflation of the cuff. The manometer is attached to an inflator bulb and has an integrated vent button. A green area is marked from 22 to 32 cm H_2O.

VBM Cuff Controller (VBM Medizintechnik GmbH)
This is a pressure controller connected to the pilot balloon. It automatically regulates the pressure in the cuff. It can be set in mm Hg or cm H_2O. This brand also has a cuff pressure gauge.

Tracoe Cuff Pressure Control (Tracoe Medical GmbH)
This is a pressure controller connected to the pilot balloon. It automatically controls the pressure in the cuff. It alarms with pressure changes that cannot be rapidly compensated (within 10 seconds).

Vacuum Regulators

Vacuum regulators are used to reduce the negative pressure produced by the hospital pneumatic system to a clinically safe level. A typical hospital head wall vacuum intake will produce between 550 and 760 mm Hg of suction. Vacuum regulators display pressures below atmospheric pressure (i.e., negative gauge pressure) but are labeled with positive numbers. The American Association for Respiratory Care (AARC) guidelines recommend that patients are never exposed to more suction than 150 mm Hg;[155] however, emergency situations may require higher amounts of suction. The use of a vacuum regulator gives clinicians the tools required to effectively control the level of suction.

There are two types, portable and wall mounted. The portable type uses a motor to drive a device to generate suction, whereas the wall-mounted unit uses the hospital main vacuum line. There are low suction pressures of up to 160 mm Hg, standard suction pressures of up to 200 mm Hg, and high suction pressures of up to 760 mm Hg. Because there are differences between regulatory agencies, the devices may be found in two standardized presentations:

1. *ISO/CE (International Organization for Standardization/Council of Europe):* The gauge moves counter-clockwise. For the high vacuum, the center of the regulator gauge display is yellow and the periphery black. For the standard (low) vacuum, the center is black and the periphery is yellow.

2. *ANSI (American National Standards Institute):* The gauge moves clockwise. The low pressure range is coded with green (0 to 80 mm Hg), medium range is yellow (80 to 120 mm Hg) and high range is orange (greater than 120 mm Hg). The low vacuum regulator gauge is color-coded green. The high vacuum regulator display and gauge needle are color-coded orange.

Application

The device is used to regulate the negative pressure used to suction fluids (oral care, airway secretions, nasogastric drainage, subglottic secretions, chest drainage, surgical). The devices have a range of vacuum pressures.

Currently Available Devices

Portable

All portable devices use a mechanical device to create negative pressure; most are electrically powered. A canister and a filter or valve separate the secretions from the vacuum source. **Table 5-28** summarizes currently available portable devices.

Stationary

Suction units can be found as mobile units (to wheel them around) and wall-mounted units. Information about the wall units can be found in the ANSI and ISO standards. The major manufacturers include Ohio Medical Corporation (now part of GE Healthcare), Amvex (a subsidiary of Ohio Medical), Boehringer Laboratories, Precision Medical, Allied Healthcare, and Taema Air Liquid, among others. In general, all manufacturers provide similar options:

- *Digital or analog:* A digital display is used instead of a gauge needle and dial.
- *Continuous/intermittent:* Suction is applied continuously versus intermittently. The timing between suctioning can be set in some models.
- *Two-mode (on and off) and three-mode (on, off, and max):* When the mode is set to on, it can be intermittent or continuous, and the vacuum pressure can be regulated.
- *High (up to 760 mm Hg):* Use is intended for surgery where large volumes of fluid may need to be removed rapidly.
- *Adult, pediatric, and/or neonatal:* As stated previously, the ranges of vacuum pressure and labeling will differ among models.
- *Surgical:* Intended for large volume, high flow suctioning. Usually equipped with larger canisters.
- *Mobile units:* Different models, with different use, from surgical to hospital and nursing home use.
- *Specialty*
  - MRI compatible
  - *Thoracic tube suction:* Dial is set in cm H_2O in increments of 1 cm H_2O. Some models have positive pressure relief valves.
  - *Subglottic suction:* For use with endotracheal and tracheostomy tubes with supraglottic suction, automatic intermittent, or continuous suctioning.
  - *Uterine suction:* Intended for gynecological and obstetric procedures.
  - *Gastric suction:* Intermittent suction of gastric or abdominal contents.

Suction Catheters

A suction catheter is a flexible or rigid hollow tube. It attaches on one end to a suction device. The other end has a hollow tip used to aspirate fluids or secretions. There are open and closed systems (to minimize contamination). Suction catheters are composed of several standard features. The proximal end of the catheter is designed to connect to the vacuum tubing. This is achieved by an increase in the catheter inner diameter such that the tubing or an adapter fits in, or it has a device to accept the vacuum tubing. Some catheters have a directional valve or a thumb port (finger-occluded opening) to help control suctioning in an on/off manner. When the port is not occluded, air flows through the port; when occluded, suctioning occurs through the distal tip. On some models there is a spring-operated valve

TABLE 5-28
Portable Suction Devices

Brand	Device	Vacuum (mm Hg)	Battery (min)	Flow rate (min)	Weight (lbs)
Gomco	OptiVac G180	25–550	60–180	30	11.4*
	405/4005	0–635	—	40	14.5*
	300/3001	0–559	—	29	23.5*
	309/3091	0–559	—	29	23*
	1180-1181	0–507	—	19	13*
	280-2801	0–559	—	12	18
DeVilbiss	VacuAide	50–550	60	27	3.37
	7305 Homecare	80–550	60	27	6.3
SSCOR	VX-2	50–525	?	30	10.5
	Quickdraw	120 or 500	30–180	12	1.18
	EVX	50–525	?	30	10.5
	TEN	125 or 525	?	30	10
	9	125 or 525	?	30	8
	III	125 or 525	?	30	7
	II	125 or 525	?	30	10
	New-Duet	50–525	?	30	10.5
	New-Sentinel	50–525	?	30	8.5
Rico	RS-5X/5	Manual	Manual	?	6
	RS-6	Manual	Manual	?	7
Laerdal	Laerdal Suction Unit	80, 120, 200, 350, 500	45–192	30	8.9
	Laerdal Compact Suction Unit 3 (300–800 mL)	0–550	45–60	27	3.3–3.7
	V-Vac Manual Suction	170–380	Manual	70	0.64
Impact	305/305GR	0–550	60–90	31	13
	305Vac-Pak	0–550	40	31	9
	308/308GR	0–550	29	31	13
	320/320GR	0–550	30	31	4.9–5.1
	321/321GR	0–550	30	31	5.1–5.4
	326	0–200 or 0–550	120	31	12
Ohio Medical Corporation	Car-e-vac 3	0–550	60	50	10.5
	Tote-l-vac	0–550	30	36	15.5

*Shipping weight

that when pressed allows the negative pressure to transmit to the catheter to allow suction. This is mostly present in the closed suction devices. The suction catheter itself may be rigid (e.g., Yankauer device commonly used for suctioning secretions from the mouth) or flexible, as in most suction catheters used for suctioning secretions from endotracheal tubes.

Catheters are made from silicone or PVC. Some tubes have graduation marks to gauge the depth of insertion. The distal tip of the suction catheter can have many different configurations: DeLee tip (rounded with side ports), whistle tip (round beveled tip with lateral holes), pig snout tip (tip edge is slightly raised with a central opening and several small side holes just below the "snout"), or coudé tip (French word for elbow or bent—the distal tip of the catheter is curved, which allows directing the catheter when intentionally suctioning a main stem bronchus).

Application

Suction devices are used to remove accumulated airway secretions (saliva, pulmonary secretions, blood, vomit, foreign material). They help maintain the patency and integrity of an artificial airway (e.g., endotracheal tube) and also provide a means to access liquid specimens (from the airway) for analysis.

When suctioning the airway (trachea) the AARC gives the following recommendations:[155]

- Sterile technique is encouraged.
- The diameter of the suction catheter should not occlude more than 50% of the endotracheal or tracheostomy tube in children and adults, and not more than 70% in neonates.
- Preoxygenate.
- Do not surpass a negative pressure of 100 mm Hg in neonates or more than 150 mm Hg in adults.
- Preferential use of shallow suctioning (described later in this section).
- Suction for less than 15 seconds.
- Establish a protocol for postsuctioning care.

Airway suctioning is contraindicated in patients with epiglottitis or croup, laryngospasm, myocardial infarct, or intracranial hypertension. Hazards include creation of atelectasis and resulting reduction of lung compliance and functional residual capacity and hypoxia. There may be trauma to the tissues of the upper or lower respiratory tract. Suctioning may induce bronchospasm and coughing, possibly leading to changes in cerebral blood flow and increased intracranial pressure, hypotension or hypertension, and cardiac dysrhythmias.[156] To avoid many of these side effects, sizing, vacuum settings, length of insertion, and timing have to be appropriate.

The goal is that the diameter of the catheter does not exceed one half[156-158] to two thirds (0.7)[156] of the ID of the artificial airway; that is, an endotracheal tube with an ID of 6 mm should have a catheter with an outer diameter no higher than 3–4 mm (9–12 Fr). Hence, the literature is filled with formulas[156] to estimate the appropriate size of the catheter (for suctioning endotracheal or tracheostomy tubes) in French using the catheter's ID in millimeters. Recall that to convert from mm to Fr you only need to multiply mm by 3. All of the following formulas[158,159] have been described and reach the same numbers in adults (for an 8 ID it is a size 14, which is approximately half of the radius).

$$\text{Suction catheter (Fr)} = \frac{\text{Tube ID} \times 3}{2}$$

For this formula you can use the next larger Fr size suction catheter.

$$\text{Suction catheter (Fr)} = \text{Tube ID} \times 2$$

For this formula use the next smallest size catheter.

$$\text{Suction catheter (Fr)} = (\text{Tube ID} - 1) \times 2$$

A proposed guideline for suction catheters in children and neonates based on a bench study[160] selection in pediatric patients is presented in **Table 5-29**.

Regarding depth of suctioning, there are two main techniques, deep and shallow. For deep suctioning, the catheter is inserted until resistance is met, followed by withdrawal of the catheter by 1 cm before suction is applied.[155] Shallow suctioning refers to insertion of the suction catheter to a predetermined depth, usually the length of the artificial airway plus the airway adapter.[155] When using endotracheal tubes, measure the length of the endotracheal tube adapter and add it to the length of the endotracheal tube. This will give the insertion distance. When using a tracheostomy tube, you may use the obturator as a measuring guide plus the length of any other adapters. Commercially available catheter lengths are shown in **Table 5-30**.

Currently Available Devices

There are multiple manufacturers of suction catheters. Differences between devices may exist, so consult the manufacturer's information for the specific product used.

Suction catheters are available with the following presentations:

- Open suctioning, alone, in sterile package
- Open suctioning kit with a sleeved catheter
- Sterile kits with the equipment required to do open suction
- Closed suction assembly to attach to endotracheal or tracheostomy tube
- Suction catheter attached to a Lukens trap

In a closed catheter system, the whole catheter is covered by a plastic sheath. The end where the suction

TABLE 5-29
Approximate Catheter Size Selection for Pediatric Suctioning

Age	Weight (kg)	ETT (mm, ID)	Mucus Consistency, Catheter Size in Fr		
			Liquid	Medium	Thick
Newborn	< 1	2	5	5	5
Newborn	1	2.5	5	5	6
Newborn	2	3	5	6	6
Newborn	3.5	3.5	5	6	7
3 months	6	3.5	5	6	7
1 year	10	4	6	7	7
2 years	12	4.5	6	7	8
3 years	14	4.5	6	7	8
4 years	16	5	7	8	8
6 years	20	5.5	7	8	8
8 years	24	6	8	10	10
10 years	30	6.5	8	10	12
12 years	> 30	7	8	10	12

Data from Morrow BM, Argent AC. *Pediatr Crit Care Med.* 2008;9:465-477.

TABLE 5-30
Available Suction Catheter Lengths

	Centimeters	Inches
Tracheostomy or pediatric	10–12	26–30
Regular or endotracheal tube	22–22	51–56

tubing is attached is not covered. The other end has a fitting to attach the catheter and sheath between the tracheostomy or endotracheal tube and patient circuit of a ventilator. When in use, the catheter is advanced through the fitting to the airway to the desired depth. Then suction is applied as the catheter is pulled back. The idea of this design is to minimize the risk of contamination during suctioning and to help maintain ventilating pressure. Closed suction systems can be used without changing for anywhere from 24 hours to every week, depending on the manufacturer's specifications.

A special type of closed system is the Lukens trap. This is a container that has a cap with two hose connections. The vacuum source is attached to one connection, and the suction device is attached to the other. As suction is applied the fluid/secretions fall into the container. These containers are usually sterile and used to collect samples for analysis.

References

1. Safar P, Escarraga LA, Chang F. Upper airway obstruction in the unconscious patient. *J Appl Physiol.* 1959;14:760-764.
2. Morrison JJ, Mellor A, Midwinter M, Mahoney PF, Clasper JC. Is pre-hospital thoracotomy necessary in the military environment? *Injury.* 2011;42:469-473.
3. American Heart Association. Part 7.1: Adjuncts for airway control and ventilation: 2005 American Heart Association guidelines for cardiopulmonary resuscitation and emergency cardiovascular care. *Circulation.* 2005;112(IV):51-57.
4. Hagberg CA, ed. *Benumof's airway management: Principles and practice.* Philadelphia: Mosby Elsevier; 2007:1320.
5. McIntyre JW. Oropharyngeal and nasopharyngeal airways: I (1880–1995). *Can J Anaesth.* 1996;43:629-635.
6. Neumar RW, Otto CW, Link MS, et al. Part 8: Adult advanced cardiovascular life support: 2010 American Heart Association

guidelines for cardiopulmonary resuscitation and emergency cardiovascular care. *Circulation.* 2010;122:S729-S767.

7. Marsh AM, Nunn JF, Taylor SJ, Charlesworth CH. Airway obstruction associated with the use of the Guedel airway. *Br J Anaesth.* 1991;67:517-523.

8. Bould MD, Thomas ML, Stylianou M. Variability of Guedel-type airways. *Anaesthesia.* 2006;61:1125-1126.

9. Dulak SB. Placing an oropharyngeal airway. *RN.* 2005;68: 20ac1-20ac3.

10. Berman JC. The Berman airway. *Anaesth Intensive Care.* 1998; 26:597.

11. Guedel AE. A nontraumatic pharyngeal airway. *JAMA.* 1933; 100:1862.

12. Berman RA. A method for blind oral intubation of the trachea or esophagus. *Anesth Analg.* 1977;56:866-867.

13. Greenland KB, Irwin MG. The Williams Airway intubator, the Ovassapian airway and the Berman airway as upper airway conduits for fibreoptic bronchoscopy in patients with difficult airways. *Curr Opin Anaesthesiol.* 2004;17:505-510.

14. Greenland KB, Lam MC, Irwin MG. Comparison of the Williams Airway intubator and Ovassapian fibreoptic intubating airway for fibreoptic orotracheal intubation. *Anaesthesia.* 2004;59:173-176.

15. Rogers SN, Benumof JL. New and easy techniques for fiberoptic endoscopy-aided tracheal intubation. *Anesthesiology.* 1983;59:569-572.

16. Roberts K, Whalley H, Bleetman A. The nasopharyngeal airway: Dispelling myths and establishing the facts. *Emerg Med J.* 2005;22:394-396.

17. Schade K, Borzotta A, Michaels A. Intracranial malposition of nasopharyngeal airway. *J Trauma.* 2000;49:967-968.

18. Stoneham MD. Nasopharyngeal airways and nasotracheal suction. *Anesthesiology.* 1994;80:480.

19. Stoneham MD. The nasopharyngeal airway. Assessment of position by fibreoptic laryngoscopy. *Anaesthesia.* 1993;48:575-580.

20. Luba K, Cutter TW. Supraglottic airway devices in the ambulatory setting. *Anesthesiol Clin.* 2010;28:295-314.

21. Cook TM, Hommers C. New airways for resuscitation? *Resuscitation.* 2006;69:371-387.

22. Woodall NM, Cook TM. National census of airway management techniques used for anaesthesia in the UK: First phase of the Fourth National Audit Project at the Royal College of Anaesthetists. *Br J Anaesth.* 2011;106:266-271.

23. Drolet P. Supraglottic airways and pulmonary aspiration: The role of the drain tube. *Can J Anaesth.* 2009;56:715-720.

24. Ruetzler K, Roessler B, Potura L, et al. Performance and skill retention of intubation by paramedics using seven different airway devices—a manikin study. *Resuscitation.* 2011;82:593-597.

25. Ruetzler K, Gruber C, Nabecker S, et al. Hands-off time during insertion of six airway devices during cardiopulmonary resuscitation: A randomised manikin trial. *Resuscitation.* 2011;82(8): 1060-1063.

26. Asai T, Shingu K. The laryngeal tube. *Br J Anaesth.* 2005;95: 729-736.

27. Hooshangi H, Wong DT. Brief review: The Cobra Perilaryngeal Airway (CobraPLA) and the Streamlined Liner of Pharyngeal Airway (SLIPA) supraglottic airways. *Can J Anaesth.* 2008;55: 177-185.

28. Park SH, Han SH, Do SH, Kim JW, Kim JH. The influence of head and neck position on the oropharyngeal leak pressure and cuff position of three supraglottic airway devices. *Anesth Analg.* 2009;108:112-117.

29. Sanuki T, Uda R, Sugioka S, et al. The influence of head and neck position on ventilation with the i-gel airway in paralysed, anaesthetised patients. *Eur J Anaesthesiol.* 2011;28:597-599.

30. Hubble MW, Wilfong DA, Brown LH, Hertelendy A, Benner RW. A meta-analysis of prehospital airway control techniques part II: Alternative airway devices and cricothyrotomy success rates. *Prehosp Emerg Care.* 2010;14:515-530.

31. Gaitini LA, Vaida SJ, Somri M, Yanovski B, Ben-David B, Hagberg CA. A randomized controlled trial comparing the ProSeal laryngeal mask airway with the laryngeal tube suction in mechanically ventilated patients. *Anesthesiology.* 2004;101:316-320.

32. Thee C, Serocki G, Doerges V, et al. Laryngeal tube S II, laryngeal tube S disposable, Fastrach laryngeal mask and Fastrach laryngeal mask disposable during elective surgery: A randomized controlled comparison between reusable and disposable supraglottic airway devices. *Eur J Anaesthesiol.* 2010;27:468-472.

33. Rumball CJ, MacDonald D. The PTL, Combitube, laryngeal mask, and oral airway: A randomized prehospital comparative study of ventilatory device effectiveness and cost-effectiveness in 470 cases of cardiorespiratory arrest. *Prehosp Emerg Care.* 1997;1:1-10.

34. Gaitini L, Yanovski B, Somri M, Vaida S, Riad T, Alfery D. A comparison between the PLA Cobra and the Laryngeal Mask Airway Unique during spontaneous ventilation: A randomized prospective study. *Anesth Analg.* 2006;102:631-636.

35. Galvin EM, van Doorn M, Blazquez J, et al. A randomized prospective study comparing the Cobra Perilaryngeal Airway and Laryngeal Mask Airway-Classic during controlled ventilation for gynecological laparoscopy. *Anesth Analg.* 2007;104:102-105.

36. Darlong V, Chandrashish C, Chandralekha, Mohan VK. Comparison of the performance of "Intubating LMA" and "Cobra PLA" as an aid to blind endotracheal tube insertion in patients scheduled for elective surgery under general anesthesia. *Acta AnaesthesiolTaiwan.* 2011;49:7-11.

37. Erlacher W, Tiefenbrunner H, Kastenbauer T, Schwarz S, Fitzgerald RD. CobraPLUS and Cookgas air-Q versus Fastrach for blind endotracheal intubation: A randomised controlled trial. *Eur J Anaesthesiol.* 2011;28:181-186.

38. Uppal V, Gangaiah S, Fletcher G, Kinsella J. Randomized crossover comparison between the i-gel and the LMA-Unique in anaesthetized, paralysed adults. *Br J Anaesth.* 2009;103:882-885.

39. Theiler LG, Kleine-Brueggeney M, Luepold B, et al. Performance of the pediatric-sized i-gel compared with the Ambu AuraOnce Laryngeal Mask in anesthetized and ventilated children. *Anesthesiology.* 2011;115:102-110.

40. Francksen H, Renner J, Hanss R, Scholz J, Doerges V, Bein B. A comparison of the i-gel with the LMA-Unique in non-paralysed anaesthetised adult patients. *Anaesthesia.* 2009;64:1118-1124.

41. Lange M, Smul T, Zimmermann P, Kohlenberger R, Roewer N, Kehl F. The effectiveness and patient comfort of the novel streamlined pharynx airway liner (SLIPA) compared with the conventional laryngeal mask airway in ophthalmic surgery. *Anesth Analg.* 2007;104:431-434.

42. Vaida SJ, Gaitini D, Ben-David B, Somri M, Hagberg CA, Gaitini LA. A new supraglottic airway, the Elisha Airway Device: A preliminary study. *Anesth Analg.* 2004;99:124-127.

43. Bledsoe BE, Slattery DE, Lauver R, Forred W, Johnson L, Rigo G. Can emergency medical services personnel effectively place and use the supraglottic airway laryngopharyngeal tube (SALT) airway? *Prehosp Emerg Care.* 2011;15:359-365.

44. Brain AI, McGhee TD, McAteer EJ, Thomas A, Abu-Saad MA, Bushman JA. The laryngeal mask airway. Development and preliminary trials of a new type of airway. *Anaesthesia.* 1985;40:356-361.

45. Voyagis GS, Photakis D, Kellari A, et al. The laryngeal mask airway: A survey of its usage in 1,096 patients. *Minerva Anestesiol.* 1996;62:277-280.

46. Porhomayon J, El-Solh AA, Nader ND. National survey to assess the content and availability of difficult-airway carts in critical-care units in the United States. *J Anesth.* 2010;24:811-814.

47. Ezri T, Szmuk P, Warters RD, Katz J, Hagberg CA. Difficult airway management practice patterns among anesthesiologists practicing in the United States: Have we made any progress? *J Clin Anesth.* 2003;15:418-422.

48. Wang HE, Mann NC, Mears G, Jacobson K, Yealy DM. Out-of-hospital airway management in the United States. *Resuscitation.* 2011;82:378-385.

49. Practice guidelines for management of the difficult airway: An updated report by the American Society of Anesthesiologists Task Force on Management of the Difficult Airway. *Anesthesiology.* 2003;98:1269-1277.

50. Brain AI. The development of the laryngeal mask—a brief history of the invention, early clinical studies and experimental work from which the laryngeal mask evolved. *Eur J Anaesthesiol Suppl.* 1991;4:5-17.

51. Agro FE, Cataldo R, Mattei A. New devices and techniques for airway management. *Minerva Anestesiol.* 2009;75:141-149.

52. Middleton P. Insertion techniques of the laryngeal mask airway: A literature review. *J Perioper Pract.* 2009;19:31-35.

53. Laryngeal Mask Company Limited. *Laryngeal mask airway instruction manual.* San Diego, CA: Laryngeal Mask Company Limited; 2011.

54. Yu SH, Beirne OR. Laryngeal mask airways have a lower risk of airway complications compared with endotracheal intubation: A systematic review. *J Oral Maxillofac Surg.* 2010;68:2359-2376.

55. Karim YM, Swanson DE. Comparison of blind tracheal intubation through the intubating laryngeal mask airway (LMA Fastrach) and the Air-Q. *Anaesthesia.* 2011;66:185-190.

56. Agro F, Frass M, Benumof JL, Krafft P. Current status of the Combitube: A review of the literature. *J Clin Anesth.* 2002;14:307-314.

57. Keys TE. Sir William Macewen (1848–1924). *Anesth Analg.* 1974;53:537.

58. Szmuk P, Ezri T, Evron S, Roth Y, Katz J. A brief history of tracheostomy and tracheal intubation, from the Bronze Age to the Space Age. *Intensive Care Med.* 2008;34:222-228.

59. Dunn PF, Goulet RL. Endotracheal tubes and airway appliances. *Int Anesthesiol Clin.* 2000;38:65-94.

60. St. John RE, Seckel MA. Airway management. In: Burns S, ed. *AACN protocols for practice. Care of mechanically ventilated patients.* Sudbury, MA: Jones and Bartlett; 2007:1-57.

61. Lee JH, Kim CH, Bahk JH, Park KS. The influence of endotracheal tube tip design on nasal trauma during nasotracheal intubation: Magill-tip versus Murphy-tip. *Anesth Analg.* 2005;101:1226-1229.

62. Holzapfel L, Chevret S, Madinier G, et al. Influence of long-term oro- or nasotracheal intubation on nosocomial maxillary sinusitis and pneumonia: Results of a prospective, randomized, clinical trial. *Crit Care Med.* 1993;21:1132-1138.

63. Bernhard WN, Yost L, Joynes D, Cothalis S, Turndorf H. Intracuff pressures in endotracheal and tracheostomy tubes. Related cuff physical characteristics. *Chest.* 1985;87:720-725.

64. Boque MC, Gualis B, Sandiumenge A, Rello J. Endotracheal tube intraluminal diameter narrowing after mechanical ventilation: Use of acoustic reflectometry. *Intensive Care Med.* 2004;30:2204-2209.

65. King BR, Baker MD, Braitman LE, Seidl-Friedman J, Schreiner MS. Endotracheal tube selection in children: A comparison of four methods. *Ann Emerg Med.* 1993;22:530-534.

66. Duracher C, Schmautz E, Martinon C, Faivre J, Carli P, Orliaguet G. Evaluation of cuffed tracheal tube size predicted using the Khine formula in children. *Paediatr Anaesth.* 2008;18:113-118.

67. Lau N, Playfor SD, Rashid A, Dhanarass M. New formulae for predicting tracheal tube length. *Paediatr Anaesth.* 2006;16:1238-1243.

68. Tochen ML. Orotracheal intubation in the newborn infant: A method for determining depth of tube insertion. *J Pediatr.* 1979;95:1050-1051.

69. Kattwinkel J, ed. *Textbook of neonatal resuscitation.* Dallas, TX: American Heart Association; 2006.

70. Niermeyer S, Kattwinkel J, Van Reempts P, et al. International guidelines for neonatal resuscitation: An excerpt from the Guidelines 2000 for Cardiopulmonary Resuscitation and Emergency Cardiovascular Care: International consensus on science. Contributors and reviewers for the Neonatal Resuscitation Guidelines. *Pediatrics.* 2000;106:E29.

71. Peterson J, Johnson N, Deakins K, Wilson-Costello D, Jelovsek JE, Chatburn R. Accuracy of the 7–8–9 rule for endotracheal tube placement in the neonate. *J Perinatol.* 2006;26:333-336.

72. Durbin CG, Jr. Tracheostomy: Why, when, and how? *Respir Care.* 2010;55:1056-1068.

73. Seegobin RD, van Hasselt GL. Endotracheal cuff pressure and tracheal mucosal blood flow: Endoscopic study of effects of four large volume cuffs. *Br Med J(Clin Res Ed).* 1984;288:965-968.

74. Leigh JM, Maynard JP. Pressure on the tracheal mucosa from cuffed tubes. *Br Med J.* 1979;1:1173-1174.

75. Riley E, DeGroot K, Hannallah M. The high-pressure characteristics of the cuff of the intubating laryngeal mask endotracheal tube. *Anesth Analg.* 1999;89:1588.

76. Jaeger JM. Special purpose endotracheal tubes. *Respir Care.* 1999;44:661-683.

77. Sole ML, Su X, Talbert S, et al. Evaluation of an intervention to maintain endotracheal tube cuff pressure within therapeutic range. *Am J Crit Care.* 2011;20:109-117; quiz 118.

78. Chadha NK, Gordin A, Luginbuehl I, et al. Automated cuff pressure modulation: A novel device to reduce endotracheal tube injury. *Arch Otolaryngol Head Neck Surg.* 2011;137:30-34.

79. Dullenkopf A, Gerber A, Weiss M. Fluid leakage past tracheal tube cuffs: Evaluation of the new Microcuff endotracheal tube. *Intensive Care Med.* 2003;29:1849-1853.

80. Kolobow T, Cressoni M, Epp M, Corti I, Cadringher P, Zanella A. Comparison of a novel Lycra tracheal tube cuff to standard PVC and polyurethane cuffs for fluid leak prevention. *Respir Care.* 2011 Aug;56(8):1095-1099.

81. Zanella A, Scaravilli V, Isgro S, et al. Fluid leakage across tracheal tube cuff, effect of different cuff material, shape, and positive expiratory pressure: A bench-top study. *Intensive Care Med.* 2011;37:343-347.

82. Dave MH, Frotzler A, Spielmann N, Madjdpour C, Weiss M. Effect of tracheal tube cuff shape on fluid leakage across the cuff: An in vitro study. *Br J Anaesth.* 2010;105:538-543.

83. Pitts R, Fisher D, Sulemanji D, Kratohvil J, Jiang Y, Kacmarek R. Variables affecting leakage past endotracheal tube cuffs: A bench study. *Intensive Care Med.* 2010;36:2066-2073.

84. Dave MH, Koepfer N, Madjdpour C, Frotzler A, Weiss M. Tracheal fluid leakage in benchtop trials: Comparison of static versus dynamic ventilation model with and without lubrication. *J Anesth.* 2010;24:247-252.

85. Lederman DS, Klein EF, Jr., Drury WD, et al. A comparison of foam and air-filled endotracheal-tube cuffs. *Anesth Analg.* 1974;53:521-526.

86. Sosis MB, Dillon FX. Saline-filled cuffs help prevent laser-induced polyvinylchloride endotracheal tube fires. *Anesth Analg.* 1991;72:187-189.

87. Beydon L, Gourgues M, Talec P. [Endotracheal tube cuff and nitrous oxide: Bench evaluation and assessment of clinical practice]. *Ann Fr Anesth Reanim.* 2011 Sep;30(9):679-684.

88. Khine HH, Corddry DH, Kettrick RG, et al. Comparison of cuffed and uncuffed endotracheal tubes in young children during general anesthesia. *Anesthesiology.* 1997;86:627-631; discussion 27A.

89. Weiss M, Dullenkopf A, Fischer JE, Keller C, Gerber AC. Prospective randomized controlled multi-centre trial of cuffed or uncuffed endotracheal tubes in small children. *Br J Anaesth.* 2009;103:867-873.

90. Taylor C, Subaiya L, Corsino D. Pediatric cuffed endotracheal tubes: An evolution of care. *Ochsner J.* 2011;11:52-56.

91. Lonnqvist PA. Cuffed or uncuffed tracheal tubes during anaesthesia in infants and small children: Time to put the eternal discussion to rest? *Br J Anaesth.* 2009;103:783-785.

92. Weiss M, Dullenkopf A, Bottcher S, et al. Clinical evaluation of cuff and tube tip position in a newly designed paediatric preformed oral cuffed tracheal tube. *Br J Anaesth.* 2006;97:695-700.

93. Dezfulian C, Shojania K, Collard HR, Kim HM, Matthay MA, Saint S. Subglottic secretion drainage for preventing ventilator-associated pneumonia: A meta-analysis. *Am J Med.* 2005;118:11-18.

94. Depew CL, McCarthy MS. Subglottic secretion drainage: A literature review. *AACN Adv Crit Care.* 2007;18:366-379.

95. Rello J, Afessa B, Anzueto A, et al. Activity of a silver-coated endotracheal tube in preclinical models of ventilator-associated pneumonia and a study after extubation. *Crit Care Med.* 2010;38:1135-1140.

96. Kollef MH, Afessa B, Anzueto A, et al. Silver-coated endotracheal tubes and incidence of ventilator-associated pneumonia: The NASCENT randomized trial. *JAMA.* 2008;300:805-813.

97. Sesterhenn AM, Dunne AA, Braulke D, Lippert BM, Folz BJ, Werner JA. Value of endotracheal tube safety in laryngeal laser surgery. *Lasers Surg Med.* 2003;32:384-390.

98. Lai HC, Juang SE, Liu TJ, Ho WM. Fires of endotracheal tubes of three different materials during carbon dioxide laser surgery. *Acta Anaesthesiol Sin.* 2002;40:47-51.

99. Ring WH, Adair JC, Elwyn RA. A new pediatric endotracheal tube. *Anesth Analg.* 1975;54:273-274.

100. Russell WJ. A logical approach to the selection and insertion of double-lumen tubes. *Curr Opin Anaesthesiol.* 2008;21:37-40.

101. Miller RA. A new laryngoscope for intubation of infants. *Anesthesiology.* 1946;7:205.

102. Scott J, Baker PA. How did the Macintosh laryngoscope become so popular? *Paediatr Anaesth.* 2009;19(Suppl 1):24-29.

103. Sethuraman D, Darshane S, Guha A, Charters P. A randomised, crossover study of the Dorges, McCoy and Macintosh laryngoscope blades in a simulated difficult intubation scenario. *Anaesthesia.* 2006;61:482-487.

104. Whittaker JD, Moulton C. Emergency intubation of infants: Does laryngoscope blade design make any difference? *J Accid Emerg Med.* 1998;15:308-311.

105. Greenland KB, Eley V, Edwards MJ, Allen P, Irwin MG. The origins of the sniffing position and the Three Axes Alignment Theory for direct laryngoscopy. *Anaesth Intensive Care.* 2008; 36(Suppl 1):23-27.

106. Levitan R, Ochroch EA. Airway management and direct laryngoscopy. A review and update. *Crit Care Clin.* 2000;16:373-388, v.

107. Niforopoulou P, Pantazopoulos I, Demestiha T, Koudouna E, Xanthos T. Video-laryngoscopes in the adult airway management: A topical review of the literature. *Acta Anaesthesiol Scand.* 2010;54:1050-1061.

108. Levitan RM, Heitz JW, Sweeney M, Cooper RM. The complexities of tracheal intubation with direct laryngoscopy and alternative intubation devices. *Ann Emerg Med.* 2010;57:240-247.

109. Davis L, Cook-Sather SD, Schreiner MS. Lighted stylet tracheal intubation: A review. *Anesth Analg.* 2000;90:745-756.

110. Sime J, Bailitz J, Moskoff J. The bougie: An inexpensive lifesaving airway device. *J Emerg Med.* 2011 Dec;43(6):e393-e395.

111. Kleinman ME, Chameides L, Schexnayder SM, et al. Part 14: Pediatric advanced life support: 2010 American Heart Association guidelines for cardiopulmonary resuscitation and emergency cardiovascular care. *Circulation.* 2010;122:S876-S908.

112. Kattwinkel J, Perlman JM, Aziz K, et al. Part 15: Neonatal resuscitation: 2010 American Heart Association guidelines for cardiopulmonary resuscitation and emergency cardiovascular care. *Circulation.* 2010;122:S909-S919.

113. Andersen KH, Hald A. Assessing the position of the tracheal tube. The reliability of different methods. *Anaesthesia.* 1989;44:984-985.

114. Knapp S, Kofler J, Stoiser B, et al. The assessment of four different methods to verify tracheal tube placement in the critical care setting. *Anesth Analg.* 1999;88:766-770.

115. Verification of endotracheal tube placement. *Ann Emerg Med.* 2009;54:141-142.

116. Grmec S. Comparison of three different methods to confirm tracheal tube placement in emergency intubation. *Intensive Care Med.* 2002;28:701-704.

117. Walsh BK, Crotwell DN, Restrepo RD. Capnography/capnometry during mechanical ventilation: 2011. *Respir Care.* 2011;56:503-509.

118. O'Flaherty D, Adams AP. The end-tidal carbon dioxide detector. Assessment of a new method to distinguish oesophageal from tracheal intubation. *Anaesthesia.* 1990;45:653-655.

119. MacLeod BA, Heller MB, Gerard J, Yealy DM, Menegazzi JJ. Verification of endotracheal tube placement with colorimetric end-tidal CO2 detection. *Ann Emerg Med.* 1991;20:267-270.

120. Leong MT, Ghebrial J, Sturmann K, Hsu CK. The effect of vinegar on colorimetric end-tidal carbon dioxide determination after esophageal intubation. *J Emerg Med.* 2005;28:5-11.

121. Li J. Capnography alone is imperfect for endotracheal tube placement confirmation during emergency intubation. *J Emerg Med.* 2001;20:223-229.

122. Salem MR, Wafai Y, Baraka A, Taimorrazy B, Joseph NJ, Nimmagadda U. Use of the self-inflating bulb for detecting esophageal intubation after "esophageal ventilation." *Anesth Analg.* 1993;77:1227-1231.

123. Tanigawa K, Takeda T, Goto E, Tanaka K. Accuracy and reliability of the self-inflating bulb to verify tracheal intubation in out-of-hospital cardiac arrest patients. *Anesthesiology.* 2000;93:1432-1436.

124. Baraka A, Khoury PJ, Siddik SS, Salem MR, Joseph NJ. Efficacy of the self-inflating bulb in differentiating esophageal from tracheal intubation in the parturient undergoing cesarean section. *Anesth Analg.* 1997;84:533-537.

125. Stewart RD, LaRosee A, Kaplan RM, Ilkhanipour K. Correct positioning of an endotracheal tube using a flexible lighted stylet. *Crit Care Med.* 1990;18:97-99.

126. Cardoso MM, Banner MJ, Melker RJ, Bjoraker DG. Portable devices used to detect endotracheal intubation during emergency situations: A review. *Crit Care Med.* 1998;26:957-964.

127. Li J. A prospective multicenter trial testing the SCOTI device for confirmation of endotracheal tube placement. *J Emerg Med.* 2001;20:231-239.

128. Trikha A, Singh C, Rewari V, Arora MK. Evaluation of the SCOTI device for confirming blind nasal intubation. *Anaesthesia.* 1999;54:347-349.

129. De Leyn P, Bedert L, Delcroix M, et al. Tracheotomy: Clinical review and guidelines. *Eur J Cardiothorac Surg.* 2007;32:412-421.

130. Mallick A, Bodenham AR. Tracheostomy in critically ill patients. *Eur J Anaesthesiol.* 2010;27:676-682.

131. Engels PT, Bagshaw SM, Meier M, Brindley PG. Tracheostomy: From insertion to decannulation. *Can J Surg.* 2009;52:427-433.

132. Romero CM, Marambio A, Larrondo J, et al. Swallowing dysfunction in nonneurologic critically ill patients who require percutaneous dilatational tracheostomy. *Chest.* 2010;137:1278-1282.

133. Hess DR. Tracheostomy tubes and related appliances. *Respir Care.* 2005;50:497-510.

134. Chatburn RL, Mireles-Cabodevila E. *Handbook of respiratory care.* Sudbury, MA: Jones & Bartlett Learning; 2011:274.

135. Kamen JM, Wilkinson CJ. A new low-pressure cuff for endotracheal tubes. *Anesthesiology.* 1971;34:482-485.

136. Kunduk M, Appel K, Tunc M, et al. Preliminary report of laryngeal phonation during mechanical ventilation via a new cuffed tracheostomy tube. *Respir Care.* 2010;55:1661-1670.

137. Montgomery WW. T-tube tracheal stent. *Arch Otolaryngol.* 1965;82:320-321.

138. Wahidi MM, Ernst A. The Montgomery T-Tube tracheal stent. *Clin Chest Med.* 2003;24:437-443.

139. Hess DR. Facilitating speech in the patient with a tracheostomy. *Respir Care.* 2005;50:519-525.

140. Suiter DM, McCullough GH, Powell PW. Effects of cuff deflation and one-way tracheostomy speaking valve placement on swallow physiology. *Dysphagia.* 2003;18:284-292.

141. Elpern EH, Borkgren Okonek M, Bacon M, Gerstung C, Skrzynski M. Effect of the Passy-Muir tracheostomy speaking valve on pulmonary aspiration in adults. *Heart Lung.* 2000;29:287-293.

142. Lichtman SW, Birnbaum IL, Sanfilippo MR, Pellicone JT, Damon WJ, King ML. Effect of a tracheostomy speaking valve on secretions, arterial oxygenation, and olfaction: A quantitative evaluation. *J Speech Hear Res.* 1995;38:549-555.

143. Prigent H, Garguilo M, Pascal S, et al. Speech effects of a speaking valve versus external PEEP in tracheostomized ventilator-dependent neuromuscular patients. *Intensive Care Med.* 2010;36:1681-1687.

144. Shikani AH, French J, Siebens AA. New unidirectional airflow ball tracheostomy speaking valve. *Otolaryngol Head Neck Surg.* 2000;123:103-107.

145. Fornataro-Clerici L, Zajac DJ. Aerodynamic characteristics of tracheostomy speaking valves. *J Speech Hear Res.* 1993;36:529-532.

146. Zajac DJ, Fornataro-Clerici L, Roop TA. Aerodynamic characteristics of tracheostomy speaking valves: An updated report. *J Speech Lang Hear Res.* 1999;42:92-100.

147. Prigent H, Orlikowski D, Blumen MB, et al. Characteristics of tracheostomy phonation valves. *Eur Respir J.* 2006;27:992-996.

148. Leder SB. Perceptual rankings of speech quality produced with one-way tracheostomy speaking valves. *J Speech Hear Res.* 1994;37:1308-1312.

149. Le HM, Aten JL, Chiang JT, Light RW. Comparison between conventional cap and one-way valve in the decannulation of patients with long-term tracheostomies. *Respir Care.* 1993;38:1161-1167.

150. Gereau SA, Navarro GC, Cluterio B, Mullan E, Bassila M, Ruben RJ. Selection of pediatric patients for use of the Passy-Muir valve for speech production. *Int J Pediatr Otorhinolaryngol.* 1996;35:11-17.

151. Brigger MT, Hartnick CJ. Drilling speaking valves: A modification to improve vocalization in tracheostomy dependent children. *Laryngoscope.* 2009;119:176-179.

152. Rose L, Redl L. Survey of cuff management practices in intensive care units in Australia and New Zealand. *Am J Crit Care.* 2008;17:428-435.

153. Rello J, Sonora R, Jubert P, Artigas A, Rue M, Valles J. Pneumonia in intubated patients: Role of respiratory airway care. *Am J Respir Crit Care Med.* 1996;154:111-115.

154. Lorente L, Blot S, Rello J. New issues and controversies in the prevention of ventilator-associated pneumonia. *Am J Respir Crit Care Med.* 2010;182:870-876.

155. American Association of Respiratory Care. Clinical practice guidelines. Endotracheal suctioning of mechanically ventilated patients with artificial airways 2010. *Respir Care.* 2010;55:758-764.

156. Morrow BM, Argent AC. A comprehensive review of pediatric endotracheal suctioning: Effects, indications, and clinical practice. *Pediatr Crit Care Med.* 2008;9:465-477.

157. Hess DR, Galvin WF, MacIntyre NR, Adams AB, Mishoe SC. *Respiratory care: Principles and practice.* Sudbury, MA: Jones & Bartlett Learning; 2012:1372.

158. Pedersen CM, Rosendahl-Nielsen M, Hjermind J, Egerod I. Endotracheal suctioning of the adult intubated patient—what is the evidence? *Intensive Crit Care Nurs.* 2009;25:21-30.

159. Wilkins RL, Stoller JK, Scanlan CL. *Egan's fundamentals of respiratory care.* St. Louis, MO: Mosby; 2003.

160. Morrow BM, Futter MJ, Argent AC. Endotracheal suctioning: From principles to practice. *Intensive Care Med.* 2004;30:1167-1174.

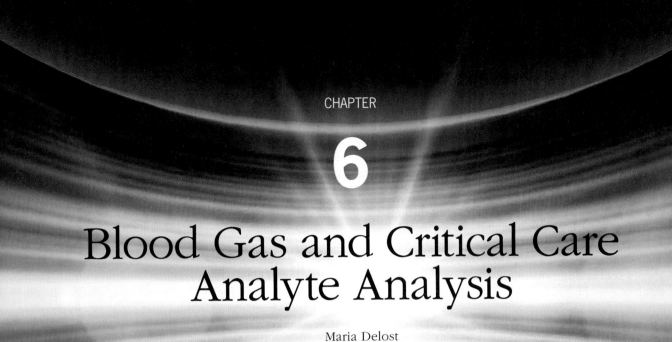

6

Blood Gas and Critical Care Analyte Analysis

Maria Delost

CHAPTER OBJECTIVES

1. List the types of samples that can be analyzed for blood gas and analyte concentrations.
2. Describe the three phases of analysis.
3. Explain the types of errors that can occur with blood gas analysis.
4. Calculate oxygen content.
5. Define Westgard rules.
6. Distinguish between shift and drift.
7. Describe the QC process for a point-of-care testing device.

KEY TERMS

Acid
Amperometry
Analyte
Anode
Base
Buffer
Cathode
CO oximetry

Electrochemical cell
Electrode
Oxidation
Partial pressure of oxygen
 (pO$_2$)
Potentiometric
Pulse oximetry
Reduction

Introduction

Blood gas analysis provides critical information to healthcare providers that assists in the diagnosis and treatment of a variety of metabolic and respiratory disorders. Historically, clinical laboratory testing was performed by medical laboratory scientists and medical laboratory technicians. Today, blood gas analysis is performed by trained personnel not only in the central or core laboratory, but by respiratory therapists[1] in satellite laboratories or with portable devices at the point of care (POC) in critical care areas such as the emergency department, neonatal and adult medical intensive care units, surgical intensive care units, and the operating room.[2]

The collection and analysis by portable or standard blood gas machines at or near the point of care minimizes the time needed to obtain and report laboratory values, which facilitates timely evaluation of results and prompt intervention.[3] Although the basic principles of operation for blood gas analyzers haven't changed significantly from earlier units, the components were notably adapted in 2005. At that time, self-contained cartridges were introduced into several analytical systems, paving the way for point-of-care testing and compact units. During this innovative period, additional **analytes** were incorporated into the testing menus. Today, healthcare facilities have the option of selecting analyzers to meet a variety of clinical needs and testing menus.[4]

Early blood gas analyzers were high maintenance and temperamental instruments that required operator-generated maintenance, calibration, and quality control. These units only measured the pH, partial pressure of oxygen (pO$_2$), and partial pressure of carbon dioxide (pCO$_2$) and provided calculated or derived values for other parameters. Today, auto-calibration and verification modes provide a more predictable testing atmosphere for the measurement of pH, pO$_2$, pCO$_2$, hemoglobin, electrolytes, and metabolites such as glucose, lactate, and creatinine.[5] Of course, calibration and quality control remain paramount in the accurate measurement and reporting of all values obtained from blood gas analyzers.

Percutaneous arterial puncture or arterial sampling from an indwelling catheter with measurement by a point of care or standard analyzer remains the "gold standard" for analysis. Fiber-optic catheters may be used for invasive in vivo analysis of pH, pCO_2, and pO_2. The indwelling catheters and analysis system allow for continuous blood gas monitoring with minimal blood loss.[6] Continuous monitoring of pCO_2, pO_2, and oxygen saturation can be accomplished through noninvasive methods by transcutaneous monitors and **pulse oximeters**, respectively. Noninvasive methods involve minimal risk to the patient and require no specimen; a continuous measurement is obtained by placing **electrodes** or probes on the body.

Common Nomenclature for Blood Gases and Analytes

Nomenclature and reference ranges for analytes and arterial blood gas parameters are summarized in Tables 6-1 and 6-2, respectively. Reference ranges may vary slightly and are based on the methodology, age of the patient, and reference values the particular healthcare facility adopts.[7] The reference ranges listed in this chapter are a guide. Blood gas instruments directly measure the pH, pO_2, and pCO_2; other parameters, such as the bicarbonate, oxygen saturation, and base excess, are derived or calculated values. Direct measurements are more accurate and reliable; the parameters automatically calculated by the analyzer may be subject to variables that are not accounted for, contributing to error.

Common Abbreviating Symbols and Acronyms

Symbols for electrolytes and analytes are summarized in Table 6-1. The testing of these analytes is described later in the chapter. Table 6-3 summarizes common symbols and acronyms used in blood gas testing.

Specimen Type and Origin Symbols

Blood gases can be analyzed on a variety of specimen types, including arterial, venous, and capillary samples. The collection site is based on the patient's diagnostic needs and clinical condition. In general, collection of an arterial specimen by percutaneous puncture or indwelling catheter is recommended. Heparin is the preferred anticoagulant used in the syringe for specimen collection.[8,9] Venous specimens may be suitable if pH, pCO_2, and bicarbonate values are needed. Results from venous specimens are affected by metabolism and peripheral circulation. Arterialized capillary samples can be collected from the earlobe, finger, toe, or heel. When collecting capillary blood from the heel, the site should first be massaged or carefully warmed. Heel collection is not suitable once an infant has reached 2 to 3 months of age. Capillary specimens are collected into heparinized micro-collection tubes.

TABLE 6-1
Analyte Nomenclature and Symbols

Analyte	Symbol	Reference Range	Comments
Potassium	K^+	3.5–5.1 mmol/L	Major intracellular cation
Sodium	Na^+	136–145 mmol/L	Major extracellular cation; important in maintaining osmotic pressure
Chloride	Cl^-	98–107 mmol/L	Major extracellular anion
Calcium	Ca^{2+}	8.8–10.2 mg/dL (total)	Occurs in three forms: bound to plasma proteins, complexed with ions such as bicarbonate, and ionized or free, which is the physiologically active form
Magnesium	Mg^{2+}	1.6–2.6 mg/dL	Role in many cellular enzymes for metabolism
Glucose		75–105 mg/dL	Increased in hyperglycemia and diabetes mellitus; decreased values termed hypoglycemia
Creatinine		0.5–1.5 mg/dL	Index of renal function and glomerular filtration
Blood urea nitrogen	BUN	6–20 mg/dL	Major nitrogen-containing end product of protein metabolism
Lactate		4.5–14.5 mg/dL (venous plasma) < 11.3 mg/dL (arterial blood in heparin)	Lactic acidosis may be hypoxic (shock, hypovolemia) or metabolic (diabetes mellitus, hepatic disease, neoplasms)

TABLE 6-2
Nomenclature and Symbols for Arterial Blood Gas Parameters

Parameter	Description	Reference Range	Comments
pH	Negative logarithm of the hydrogen ion concentration; measure of acid–base balance of blood.	7.35–7.45	Direct measure by pH (Sanz) electrode
pO_2	Partial pressure of oxygen in arterial blood. Also written as paO_2.	80–110 mm Hg	Direct measure by pO_2 (Clark) electrode
pCO_2	Partial pressure of carbon dioxide in arterial blood; mainly regulated by respiratory system. Also written as $paCO_2$.	35–55 mm Hg	Direct measure by pCO_2 (Stowe-Severinghaus) electrode
HCO_3	Bicarbonate; includes true bicarbonate, bicarbonate, and dissolved free CO_2.	21–28 mmol/L serum; 18–23 mmol/L arterial	Actual bicarbonate is a derived measurement calculated from the pH and pCO_2 of an aerobically drawn arterial specimen. Standard bicarbonate is derived from the Henderson-Hasselbalch equation and indicates the bicarbonate level in an oxygenated plasma specimen at 98.6°F (37°C) and pCO_2 of 40 mm Hg.
sO_2	Oxygen saturation of hemoglobin	95–100%	Derived value calculated using $sO_2\% = cO_2Hb/(cO_2Hb + cHHb) \times 100$. Calculated value does not account for other hemoglobins or actual pCO_2. Oxyhemoglobin is directly measured using oximetry.
P_{50}	pO_2 at which hemoglobin is 50% saturated with oxygen.		Calculated parameter
Buffer base	Total of all anionic buffers in the blood; includes hemoglobin, bicarbonate, inorganic phosphate, and proteins with a negative charge.	44–48 mmol/L	Calculated parameter; should not be affected by respiratory disorders.
Base excess	Number of millimoles of strong acid needed to titrate a blood sample to pH 7.4 at pCO_2 40 mm Hg.		Calculated parameter; should not be affected by respiratory disorders.

cHHb = content of deoxygenated hemoglobin; cO_2Hb = content of oxygenated hemoglobin

Introduction to General Measurement Concepts

Gas Tension

Gas tension is the partial pressure of a gas in blood. Partial pressure refers to the pressure exerted by a single gas in a mixture of gases or in a liquid. The pressure of the gas is related to the concentration of the gas to the total pressure of the mixture. For example, the concentration of oxygen in the atmosphere is 0.21. Atmospheric pressure is 760 mm Hg (at sea level). The **partial pressure of oxygen** in the atmosphere can be calculated by multiplying the concentration of this gas in the atmosphere (0.21) by atmospheric pressure (760 mm Hg).[10]

> Gas tension of oxygen in the atmosphere =
> 0.21×760 mm Hg = 160 mm Hg

pO_2 refers to the partial pressure or tension of oxygen; it may also be written as PO_2, PO_2, and pO_2. The reference range of pO_2 in arterial blood is 80–110 mmol/L. pCO_2 refers to the partial pressure or tension of carbon dioxide; it may also be written as PCO_2, PCO_2, or pCO_2. The reference range of pCO_2 for arterial blood is 35–45 mm Hg.

pH

The pH is a measure of the acidity or alkalinity of a solution and ranges from 1–14. Values less than 7.0 are acidic and greater than 7.0 are alkaline. An **acid** is a substance that produces or donates hydrogen ions [H^+] when dissolved in water, whereas a **base** or alkaline substance is one that produces or donates hydroxyl ions [OH^-] when dissolved in water. When there are equal numbers of [H^+] and [OH^-] ions, the

TABLE 6-3
Common Symbols and Acronyms Related to Blood Gas Testing

Symbol	Meaning
pO_2	Partial pressure of oxygen; also written as PO_2, pO_2, or PO_2
pCO_2	Partial pressure of carbon dioxide; also written as PCO_2, pCO_2, or PCO_2
$[H^+]$	Hydrogen ion concentration
$[OH^-]$	Hydroxyl ion concentration
Hb	Hemoglobin
COHb	Carboxyhemoglobin
HHb	Reduced or deoxygenated hemoglobin
O_2Hb	Oxygenated hemoglobin or oxyhemoglobin
THb	Total hemoglobin
sO_2	Oxygen saturation of hemoglobin
P_{50}	pO_2 at which 50% of hemoglobin is saturated
ctO_2	Oxygen content
QA	Quality assurance
QC	Quality control

solution is neutral and the pH is 7.0, as shown in the following equation:[10]

$$H^+ + OH^- \longleftrightarrow H_2O$$

Relationship Between pH and H+

The pH is the negative logarithm of the hydrogen ion concentration $[H^+]$ in moles/liter. For example, a pH of 6, a slightly acidic solution, would have an $[H^+]$ of 1.0×10^{-6}. Conversely, if a solution has an $[H^+]$ concentration of 1×10^{-12}, the pH of this solution would be 12, which is very alkaline.

The pH is measured in arterial blood to determine the degree of acidity or alkalinity. The acid–base balance of body fluids, including blood, is maintained through the hydrogen ion concentration. The reference range for the pH of arterial blood is 7.35–7.45.[10] **Buffers** are weak acids or bases that resist changes in pH when a strong acid or base is added. The body has several buffering mechanisms.

Sensors and Measurement Concepts

pH Electrode and Reference Electrode

Glass electrodes are commonly used to measure pH. The pH measurement system uses the Sanz electrode, which consists of two half cells connected by a potassium chloride (KCl) bridge. The measurement half

cell or electrode has a glass membrane with layers of hydrated and nonhydrated glass. It is permeable or sensitive to hydrogen $[H^+]$ ions. This measurement electrode consists of silver-silver chloride (Ag-AgCl), which is then placed into a phosphate buffer of pH 6.840, and thus has a known $[H^+]$ concentration. The reference half cell or electrode consists of mercury and mercurous chloride (Hg-HgCl) or calomel. This calomel electrode is placed into a solution of saturated KCl.[11]

The reference electrode provides steady voltage while the measuring electrode responds to the ions of interest in the sample. Thus, the reference electrode provides a baseline voltage against which the voltage measured by the measuring electrode is compared. A pH meter or voltmeter measures this potential difference, known as ΔE, between the two electrodes. This relationship is shown in the following equation:

$$\Delta E = \Delta E^0 + 0.05916/n \log a_1 \text{ at } 25°C$$

where:

ΔE = Potential difference
ΔE^0 = Standard potential of **electrochemical cell**
n = charge of analyte ion
a_1 = activity of ion

There is a change of + 59.16 millivolts (mV) at 25°C for a 10-fold increase in $[H^+]$ activity and a decrease in pH units. At 37°C, the change in one pH unit causes a 61.5 mV change in the electrical potential.[12]

Functional Requirements and Characteristics of the pH System

It is postulated that sodium ions in the hydrated glass drift out and are replaced by the smaller hydrogen ions that are present in the sample. This results in a net increase in the external membrane potential, which travels through the thin, dry membrane to the inner hydrated glass surface. Chloride ions in the buffer solution migrate to the internal glass layer, creating a potential difference at the pH electrode that, in turn, signals the external reference electrode. The difference in voltage is converted and displayed as the pH.

pCO_2 Electrode System

Functional Requirements and Characteristics of the pCO_2 Electrode

The pCO_2 electrode is a modified pH electrode that was first described by Stowe and later by Severinghaus;[13] today it is known as a Stowe-Severinghaus electrode. The electrode has an outer semipermeable membrane consisting of Teflon or silicon elastic (Silastic). CO_2 diffuses into an electrolyte layer; a bicarbonate buffer covers the electrode glass. When CO_2 reacts with the buffer, carbonic acid forms, which then dissociates into a bicarbonate ion [HCO_3^-] and hydrogen ions [H^+].[14]

$$CO_2 + H_2O \rightarrow H_2CO_3 \rightarrow H^+ + HCO_3^-$$

The hydrogen ions diffuse across the glass electrode and the change in [H^+] activity is measured using the same principle as for the pH electrode. The pCO_2 is determined from the pH value using the Henderson-Hasselbalch equation:

$$pH = pk + \log [HCO_3^-]/pCO_2$$

pO_2 Electrode System

Functional Requirements and Characteristics of the pO_2 Electrode

The partial pressure of oxygen (pO_2) is measured using the Clark electrode, which is a complete electrical cell. The Clark electrode consists of a small platinum **cathode** and a silver-silver chloride (Ag-$AgCl_2$) **anode** immersed in a phosphate buffer that contains additional potassium chloride. The platinum electrode is covered with a small layer of electrolyte and a thin gas-permeable membrane made of a material such as polypropylene. The membrane separates the test specimen from the electrode and is selectively permeable to oxygen, which diffuses into the electrolyte to contact the cathode. The cathode potential is adjusted to a constant voltage potential of -0.65 volts (V). When there is no oxygen present in the solution, the cathode is polarized and the current is approximately equal to 0 volts. When oxygen is present in the test specimen, a current is produced and oxygen

diffuses from the sample solution and then through the membrane, where it is reduced.[15] Electrons are drawn from the anode surface to the cathode to reduce the oxygen. The current is proportional to the pO_2 of the test solution.

The sensitivity of the pO_2 electrode is related to the thickness of the membrane and the size of the cathode area. A micro-ampmeter measures movement of electrons between the anode and cathode, which forms the electrical current. There are four electrons drawn for each mole of O_2 that is reduced. The reaction at the cathode is summarized as follows:

$$O_2 + 4e^- \rightarrow 2\,O^-$$

$$2\,O^- + 2\,H_2O \rightarrow 4\,OH^-$$

Next, elemental silver present at the anode is oxidized and then ionized, forming four electrons before combining with chloride to form silver chloride. The reaction at the anode is summarized as follows:

$$4\,Ag \rightarrow 4\,Ag^+ + 4\,e^-$$

$$4\,Ag^+ + Cl^- \rightarrow 4\,AgCl$$

Other gases may pass through the membrane, but the degree of the polarizing voltage does not permit them to be reduced at the cathode. The membrane prevents proteins and other oxidizing agents from reaching the cathode surface. Protein build-up on the membrane is an important source of measurement error; proteins may alter the diffusion of the gases and hinder the electrode response. The sensitivity of the electrode is related to the thickness of the membrane and the size of the cathode area.

Calculated Values

Hemoglobin/Oxygen Saturation

Oxygen saturation of hemoglobin is the percentage of oxygenated hemoglobin divided by total hemoglobin present capable of binding with oxygen. Oxygen saturation (sO_2) is calculated using the following equation:

$$sO_2\% = cO_2Hb/(cO_2Hb + cHHb) \times 100$$

where cO_2Hb is the concentration of oxyhemoglobin and $cHHb$ is the concentration of reduced or deoxyhemoglobin; the sum of oxy- and deoxyhemoglobin represents the total functional hemoglobin. Oxygen saturation is a derived value for most blood gas analyzers. It is only measured by analyzers that have hemoximetry capabilities. A hemoximeter directly measures the amount of hemoglobin present and capable of binding with oxygen.[16] Therefore, the microprocessors of analyzers that calculate sO_2 assume normal O_2 affinity of the hemoglobin. It is important for the clinician to recognize this calculation may be approximate and should be interpreted with caution.

Oxygen saturation may also be calculated using the following formula:

$$sO_2\% = cO_2Hb/ctHb \times 100\%$$

where $ctHB$ includes the carboxyhemoglobin, methemoglobin, and sulfhemoglobin fractions. Using this equation, the $sO_2\%$ will never reach 100% if any of these nonfunctional hemoglobin fractions are present. This calculation should not be used because the dishemoglobins, mentioned above, are present in the blood and the findings may be misleading. For example, if a patient had 10% carboxyhemoglobin, the sO_2 could not be any higher than 90%, even in fully saturated blood, which might indicate an increase in oxygen shunting to the lungs, which would not be accurate.[10]

Total Hemoglobin Measurement: Oxyhemoglobin and Dishemoglobinemias

Total hemoglobin ($ctHb$ or tHb) must be measured because the value is needed to calculate several other blood gas values. Total hemoglobin is a measure of all of the hemoglobin fractions detected by the spectrophotometer of the analyzer. The hemoglobin molecule that is bound to oxygen is known as oxyhemoglobin, whereas deoxyhemoglobin or reduced refers to a hemoglobin molecule that does not contain oxygen. Carboxyhemoglobin contains bound carbon monoxide instead of oxygen, and methemoglobin is a hemoglobin fraction that contains iron in the ferric (Fe^{3+}) form. These fractions are summarized in **Table 6-4**.

Blood gas analyzers measure total hemoglobin spectrophotometrically.[17] Once in the analyzer, the hemolyzer unit hemolyzes or ruptures the red blood cells in an aliquot of the specimen. A portion of the hemolyzed sample is transferred to a measuring chamber, also known as a cuvette. A tungsten halogen lamp or other light source provides polychromatic light, which is directed toward the sample in the cuvette. Depending on the concentration of hemoglobin in the sample, light is transmitted through the hemolyzed sample and toward the spectrophotometer. The specific wavelengths that transmit the color of each hemoglobin fraction are selected through a monochromater. Transmitted light contacts photodetectors that produce a voltage that corresponds to the amount of light transmitted and photons of light produced. The microprocessor converts the voltage through calculations into the hemoglobin

TABLE 6-4
Hemoglobin Fractions

Hemoglobin Fraction	Abbreviation	Description	Comments
Total hemoglobin	ctHb or tHb	Concentration of total hemoglobin or all fractions measured by spectrophotometer	
Oxyhemoglobin or fraction of oxyhemoglobin	O_2Hb or FO_2Hb	Concentration of hemoglobin that is oxygenated	Normal adult hemoglobin includes 1.5–3.5% HbA_2, less than 2% HbF, and ~95% HbA, which is the major adult hemoglobin
Deoxyhemoglobin or fraction of deoxyhemoglobin	HHb or FHHb	Concentration of hemoglobin that is deoxygenated and is not bound to oxygen	
Carboxyhemoglobin or fraction of carboxyhemoglobin	COHb or FCOHb	Concentration of hemoglobin that is combined with carbon monoxide	Hb affinity for CO is 200 times higher than for O_2; increased in city dwellers and smokers; extreme elevation and anoxia in carbon monoxide poisoning
Methemoglobin or fraction of methemoglobin	MetHb or FMetHb	Concentration of hemoglobin that contains iron in its ferric (Fe^{3+}) state	MetHb cannot bind oxygen; normally less than 1.5% of total Hb; increased in cyanosis and hypoxia; causes include exposure to nitrates and/or benzocaine products
Fetal hemoglobin or fraction of fetal hemoglobin	HbF or FHbF	Concentration of hemoglobin F or fetal hemoglobin; HbF can bind oxygen very tightly	Makes up 50–80% of total hemoglobin at birth and less than 2% in adults; the concentration of HbF is increased in some hemoglobinopathies and in some cases of hypoplastic anemia, pernicious anemia, and leukemia
Sulfhemoglobin or fraction of sulfhemoglobin	SulfHb or FSulfHb	Sulfur molecule attaches to hemoglobin and oxygen cannot be transported; may combine with CO to form carboxysulfhemoglobin	Normally less than 2.0%; cyanosis when increased; occupational exposure to sulfur compounds and pollutants

concentrations or fractions. Most blood gas analyzers detect oxyhemoglobin, as well as deoxyhemoglobin, carboxyhemoglobin, and methemoglobin fractions.

The hemoglobin unit must be calibrated using a known total hemoglobin standard. A calibration curve is electronically developed based on the voltage produced and is sent to the microprocessor. Sample results cannot be reported if the analyzer fails to calibrate successfully. Also, quality control using two different levels of a hemoglobin control must be performed with acceptable results before reporting patient values.[18]

Hematocrit Measurement

The hematocrit formerly was known as the packed cell volume (PCV). When a whole blood specimen is centrifuged, the red blood cells sediment to the bottom, the white blood cells and platelets form a middle layer, and plasma forms the upper layer. The percentage of red blood cells in the whole blood specimen is known as the hematocrit.

Bicarbonate Content

Bicarbonate constitutes a large fraction of the ions in plasma. Bicarbonate includes true bicarbonate, carbonate, and CO_2 bound in plasma carbamino compounds. True bicarbonates are the largest contributor to bicarbonate content.

Oxygen Content

Oxygen content can be measured directly or calculated by the oxygen content equation.

$$ctO_2 = (Hb \times 1.36 \times sO_2) + (0.003 \times pO_2)$$

where

ctO_2 is the oxygen content
Hb is the hemoglobin in g/dL
sO_2 is the oxygen saturation in %
pO_2 is the partial pressure of oxygen in mm Hg

However, the tO_2 can be determined with results obtained from an arterial blood sample using the **CO-oximetry** test panel, which includes fractional concentration of oxyhemoglobin, reduced hemoglobin, carboxyhemoglobin, and methemoglobin. The sum total of these hemoglobin derivatives yields the total hemoglobin concentration. Many current blood gas analyzers either measure or calculate all variables needed to calculate the ctO_2.

Base Excess

Base excess can be defined as the concentration of titratable base when a fluid is titrated to a pH of 7.40 at a pCO_2 of 40 mm Hg. However, in practical terms, the base excess is calculated using a nomogram or with the Van Slyke equation.[19] The base excess is useful in evaluating the patient's acid–base balance in metabolic disorders. A positive base excess occurs when there is a surplus of HCO_3^- and a negative base excess when there is a deficit of HCO_3^-. The calculation of base excess requires the hemoglobin value, pCO_2, and HCO_3^-; the base excess at pH of 7.40, pCO_2 of 40 mm Hg, and Hb of 15 g/dL at a temperature of 37°C is zero.

$$\text{Base excess} = (1.0 - 0.0143\ Hb)(HCO_3^-) - (9.5 + 1.63\ Hb)(7.4\ pH) - 24$$

Today, this value is automatically calculated by the microprocessor in the blood gas analyzer.[20] The reference range for base excess in adults is from − 2 to + 3.

Biosensors and Methods Used in the Measurement of Analytes

Whole blood can be analyzed for many analytes, including the electrolytes potassium (K^+), sodium (Na^+), and calcium (Ca^{2+}) and metabolites such as glucose, lactate, blood urea nitrogen (BUN), and creatinine. The sensors used for these measurements are ion-specific or ion-selective electrodes (ISE). These sensors are membrane-based electrochemical transducers that respond to a specific ion. Biosensors are used in analyzers in the traditional clinical laboratory, but also in point-of-care (POC) testing devices. Biosensors use biologically sensitive material that contacts the appropriate transducer responsible for converting the biochemical signal into an electrical signal (**Figure 6-1**).

Electrolytes are determined by **potentiometric** measurements, a form of electrochemical analysis.[21] In potentiometry, the potential or voltage is measured between two electrodes in a solution. These potentials can also be produced when a metal and ions of that metal are present in a solution. By using a membrane that is semipermeable to the ion, different concentrations of the ion can be separated. These systems use a reference and a measuring electrode. A constant voltage is applied to the reference electrode; the difference in voltage between the reference and measuring electrode is used to calculate the concentration of the ion in solution.

Ion-selective electrodes are based on a modification of the principal of potentiometry.[21] The potential difference or electron flow is created by selectively transferring the ion to be measured from the sample solution to the membrane phase. The ISE measures the free ion concentration of the desired analyte on a selectively produced membrane. Membranes have a complex composition and contain organic solvents, inert polymers, plasticizers, and ionophors. Ionophors are molecules that increase the membrane's permeability to the specific ion.

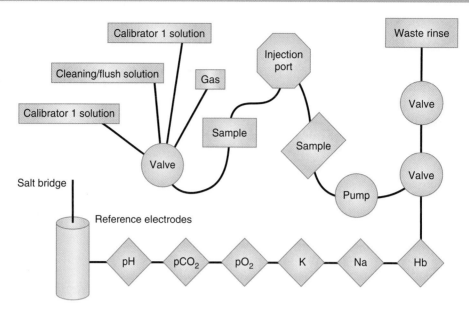

FIGURE 6-1 Schematic of a typical analyzer used to measure blood gas and electrolytes.

Because ISEs produce a direct measurement, there is no need for reagents or the production of a standard curve. Results are precise, accurate, sensitive, and specific for the analyte that is being tested. Ion-selective electrodes are also cost effective, have a rapid analysis time, and are easily maintained and adapted toward automation.

The corresponding membrane component is unique for a specific ISE membrane. For example, the sodium ISE membrane contains silicate in glass; the potassium ISE membrane contains valinomycin; the chloride ISE membrane contains solvent polymeric membranes. ISEs are also available for chloride (Cl^-), calcium (Ca^{2+}), magnesium (Mg^{2+}), and lithium (Li^+).

Amperometric methods measure the current flow produced from **oxidation-reduction** reactions. Types of **amperometry** include enzyme electrodes, such as the glucose oxidase method and the Clark pO_2 electrode, previously discussed. These types of designs are known as biosensors and are adaptable for testing in the clinical laboratory as well as for point-of-care (POC) testing.

Enzyme-based biosensor technology was first developed to measure blood glucose. A solution of glucose oxidase is placed between the gas-permeable membrane of the pO_2 electrode and an outer membrane that is semipermeable.[22] Glucose in the blood diffuses through the semipermeable membrane and reacts with the glucose oxidase. Glucose is converted by glucose oxidase to hydrogen peroxide and gluconic acid. A polarizing voltage is applied to the electrode, which oxidizes the hydrogen peroxide and contributes to the loss of electrons. Oxygen is consumed near the surface of the pO_2 electrode and its rate of consumption is measured. The loss of electrons and rate of decrease in pO_2 is directly proportional to the glucose concentration in the sample. Enzyme-based biosensors are also used to measure cholesterol, creatinine, and pyruvate.

There are also enzyme-based biosensors with potentiometric and conductimetric detection methods.[23] Conductimetric methods utilize chemical reactions that produce or consume ionic substances and alter the electrical conductivity of a solution. In this technology, polymembrane ion-selective electrodes are used. Blood urea nitrogen (BUN), glucose, and creatinine may be measured using this technology. The BUN biosensor immobilizes the enzyme urease at the surface of an ammonium ISE; the urease catalyzes the breakdown of urea to ammonia (NH_3) and CO_2. Subsequently the ammonia forms ammonium, which is detected by the ISE. The signal produced by the ISE is related to the concentration of blood urea nitrogen in the sample.

Biosensor systems can also use optical detection to measure glucose, bilirubin, and other analytes. The sensors include immobilized enzymes and indicator dyes and may be detected using spectrophotometer, fluorescence, reflectance, or luminescence.[24]

Phases of Analysis

Within the test setting, control of variables that may affect the three phases of analysis must be evaluated. Preanalytical test variables that may alter patient results include correct patient identification, turnaround time, transcription errors, patient preparation, specimen collection, and specimen transport. There are many individuals involved in the preanalytical testing phase; therefore, a coordinated effort among the healthcare providers involved in the process is essential. Following specimen collection and transport, the sample must be correctly processed or maintained prior to analysis.

The analytical stage includes the actual testing of the specimen. A specific testing protocol with standard operating procedures (SOPs) for each analyzer is needed. This includes criteria to accept or reject specimens. All specimens must be analyzed consistently by the testing personnel, who must follow the specific procedure directions outlined in the procedure manual. The process that occurs during sample analysis is provided in **Figure 6-2**. Quality control (QC) is a very significant component to assess the quality of the analytical testing phase. Quality control is used to monitor and assess the accuracy of specimen analysis. QC uses samples with known values of each analyte with a range of acceptable values given. In the postanalytical phase, the results are evaluated for error and proximity to normal limits.

Of course, technical competence is a requirement for all testing phases. Proper training of personnel who perform the analysis is essential and should include education standards, learning objectives, an evaluation of technical competence, in-services, and continuing education. Work quality must be evaluated and corrective actions suggested if needed.

Preanalysis Phase: Specimen Handling and Special Considerations

Arterial blood collection begins by confirming the identification and location of the patient. The test order, or requisition, and patient identification must agree. Any identification discrepancies must be resolved and corrected before proceeding to collect the specimen. Correct specimen collection and transport are essential to ensure accurate results for the patient. Failure to properly collect or transport the sample can lead to erroneous results that may affect the diagnosis, treatment regimen, and clinical outcome.[25] Arterial blood gas specimens are most often collected using a single percutaneous needle puncture from the radial artery, although specimens may also be collected from brachial, femoral, or pedis arteries. The temporal artery may also be used for collection in newborns. Capillary blood gas collections from the heel or earlobe of infants are also acceptable for analysis; however, reference

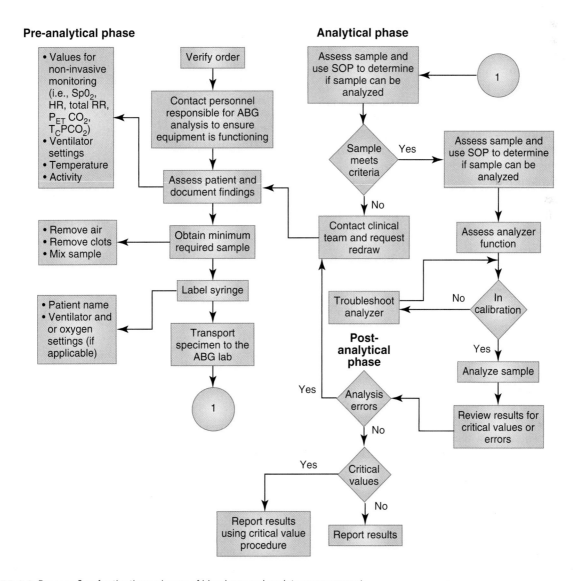

FIGURE 6-2 Process flow for the three phases of blood gas and analyte measurement.

ranges and results differ from arterial samples. Venous specimens are commonly used for venous pH, pCO_2, and bicarbonate testing. Attempts should be made to keep sample sizes as small as is technically feasible to limit blood loss, particularly in neonates.[2] Once collected, the specimen must be accurately labeled with the patient's name, identification number, location, F_IO_2, and temperature as well as the collector's initials, date, and time of collection.[2] Specimen labeling must occur even in cases where the individual collecting the specimen also performs the analysis.[26]

Following collection of percutaneous samples, all air bubbles must be immediately removed by gently tapping the side of the syringe. The syringe should not be agitated. Significant error may occur when even a small amount of air bubbles is found in the sample.[27]

When collecting specimens from indwelling arterial catheters, first remove 1–2 mL of blood from adults and 0.2–0.5 mL from infants. Flush the cannula with sterile, physiologic saline to prevent clotting in the cannula. Saline and heparin in catheter lines can dilute the sample and falsely decrease the pCO_2 and hemoglobin.[28,29]

Temperature Correction for Blood Gas Values

Patient temperature affects blood gas values. Blood gas analyzers assume the patient's temperature is 98.6°F (37°C). In cases of hypothermia due to surgery or prolonged exposure to cold, where the body temperature may be significantly lower than 98.6°F (37°C), or hyperthermia due to fever, the patient's actual body temperature may be manually entered into the analyzer so that temperature-corrected pH, pCO_2, and pO_2 values can be calculated.[30] The algorithms used for these calculations are generally found in the instrument operator's manual. The use of the temperature correction is not standardized, and there is a lack of agreement in the literature regarding its use. Some report corrected values provide a more correct indication of the acid–base balance and oxygenation state of the patient. For example, pO_2 changes approximately 7% for each 1°C deviation from 37°C. Thus, it is advisable to perform temperature corrections for measured pO_2 even for a 1°C deviation. Both the pO_2 value measured under the standard temperature of 98.6°F (37°C) and the temperature-corrected value should be reported.[31] It is generally accepted that it is not necessary to correct the pH and pCO_2 for hyperthermia and they are generally reported only when requested by the physician.[32] A temperature correction does not affect the calculated HCO_3^-.

Key Points for Specimen Collection/Preparation for Analysis

Blood gas specimens must not be exposed to room air during collection, transport, or measurement. Room air has a pO_2 of approximately 150 mm Hg, which can affect the value of oxygen in the sample. Specimens must be transported for analysis within 10 minutes of collection when held at room temperature. Specimens that cannot be analyzed immediately must be placed within an ice slurry and maintained at a temperature of 32–39.2°F (0–4°C) for no longer than 30 minutes. Specimens should not be held in ice alone because the sample may freeze and red cells may hemolyze. Oxygen may be metabolized by white blood cells after specimen collection, especially if the patient has an elevated white blood cell count. Delays in transport may also increase diffusion of gases through the plastic syringe and increase the likelihood of potassium diffusion from the red cells. Preanalytical error may lead to measurement error and improper medical diagnosis.

Prior to analysis, gently mix the specimen to obtain a homogeneous sample; this can be accomplished by gently inverting the sample or by rolling the syringe in the palms of the hands. Never shake the specimen because this may hemolyze the red cells, releasing potassium and altering the results.

Preanalysis Phase: Calibration Principles

High and low calibration is required for all measured and reported laboratory analytes in order to verify the analyzer is operating correctly. Today, most blood gas analyzers are self-calibrating, controlled through the microprocessor and monitored constantly. The frequency and type of calibration that is programmed into the instrument varies and is based on the manufacturer, accreditation standards, and the facility's operation schedule.

A one-point calibration uses only one calibration standard; the electrical output is adjusted to a single standard. A one-point calibration of pO_2 and pCO_2 is generally automatically performed every 30 minutes. One-point calibrations should be manually performed prior to sample analysis. In a two-point calibration, the response of the electrode is measured against known values for both a high and low standard. The values are plotted and a linear calibration curve is derived; all subsequent measurements are compared against the calibration line. Most blood gas analyzers automatically perform a two-point calibration every 8 hours.

Functional Requirements of Calibration

The pH system is calibrated against primary calibration buffers that are phosphate solutions and that must meet the standards of the National Institute of Standards and Technology (NIST). These calibrators are prepared from standard reference materials—potassium dihydrogen phosphate and disodium monohydrogen phosphate—according to a specific protocol to produce two buffer solutions. The first has a pH of 6.841 at 98.6°F (37°C) and the second has a pH of 7.383 at 98.6°F (37°C). The buffers must meet NIST specifications; they are commercially available and manufactured to a size and shape to fit into the reservoirs of the analyzer. The tolerance for calibrators should be ± 0.003 in order to achieve standard deviations of ± 0.005 to ± 0.01.

The calibration of the gas system requires known concentrations of O_2 and CO_2 gases to be introduced into the measurement chamber. Pure O_2, CO_2, and N_2 can be purchased as compressed gases with a certificate of analysis provided by the manufacturer and then mixed into the required composition, or they can be purchased commercially in the appropriate calibration mixture. The low gas mixture calibrator and high gas mixture calibrator compositions are shown in Table 6-5. Calibration using these mixtures will provide a calibration range of 0–152 mm Hg for O_2 and 38–80 mm Hg for CO_2. The pO_2 electrode can be calibrated using "no atmosphere" air as the low calibrator and "room air" as the other calibrator. Today, gas calibrators are included in the testing cartridges for most blood gas analyzers.

During calibration of the gas system, gas released from the tanks is pumped into the calibration buffers. The solutions are mixed, warmed to 98.6°F (37°C), and a small aliquot moved to make contact with the surface of the pO_2 and pCO_2 electrodes. A voltage measurement is taken, which is corrected for the barometric pressure; the microprocessor analyzes the values and derives a calibration curve for pH, pO_2, and pCO_2. Some analyzers have an internal barometer or transducer so that the

barometric pressure value is known to the microprocessor, which then calculates the pO_2 and pCO_2 based on Dalton's law. Other models require that the operator manually enter the barometric pressure.

Analysis Phase: Laboratory Blood Gas Analyzers

Principles of Operation

The basic principles of operation for laboratory blood gas analyzers are the previously described electrodes for pH, pCO_2, and pO_2; spectrophotometric analysis of hemoglobin; and ion-specific electrodes for the measurement of electrolytes. The principle of operation is shown in Figure 6-3. Approximately 50–120 µL of a well-mixed arterial blood sample are injected through the inlet and sample probe into the measuring chamber. The specimen contacts the surface of each electrode for several seconds.

Calibration

Calibrator gases and buffers enter through the valve to the chamber area maintained in a fluid and metal bath at a constant temperature of 98.6°F (37°C) ± 0.1°C. The measuring and reference electrodes are located in this chamber. The high pH and low pH calibrators enter in alternating mode into the chamber, generating electrical responses for the upper and lower pH limits

TABLE 6-5
Gas Calibration Mixtures

	pO$_2$ (%)	O$_2$ (mm Hg)	pCO$_2$ (%)	CO$_2$ (mm Hg)	N$_2$ (%)
Low gas mixture	0	0	5	59	95
High gas mixture	20	150 mm Hg	10	80 mm Hg	70

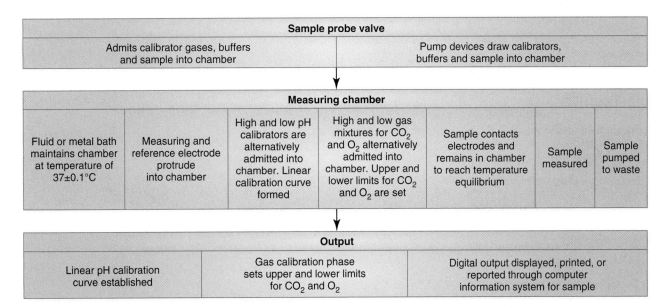

FIGURE 6-3 Process that occurs during the analysis of whole blood for gas and analyte measurement.

and producing a linear pH curve. The high and low gas calibrators for pO_2 alternatively enter the chamber, the electrical responses are measured, and a standardized linear curve is generated. The same process also occurs for pCO_2 with the high and low calibrator gases entering the measuring chamber, generating voltages, and producing a linear calibration curve. After an acceptable calibration, the blood sample is introduced and analyzed. The electrodes have a threaded neck with a leak-proof fit and the sample contacts the tip of each electrode. The pH electrode has glass that is sensitive to $[H^+]$ ions.

An electrical output is generated for each parameter of the sample and then sent to the microprocessor; the results are sent to the computer screen or printer. A report is generated, which can be sent through the laboratory information system to the patient's location or healthcare provider. Patient demographics, sample type, F_IO_2, and temperature are entered by the operator prior to sample analysis.

Analysis Phase: Sources of Measurement Error

Most errors in blood gas analysis occur in the preanalytical phase, including specimen collection and handling. Insufficient sample and/or inadequate mixing of the blood specimen prior to analysis may lead to a nonhomogeneous distribution of red blood cells across the electrode junction. Analytical errors such as problems with maintaining the temperature control can lead to

measurement error if the sample does not reach 98.6°F (37°C) ± 0.1°C. The analysis process is outlined in Figure 6-3. Temperature control errors may result from pinched or clogged tubing within the analyzer or from clogs or spaces in the sample stream. Point-of-care testing devices may be more vulnerable to analytical errors and have a higher rate of error when compared to analyzers in a core or satellite laboratory.[33] Sources of error associated with blood gas analysis are summarized in Table 6-6.

Postanalysis Phase: Quality Control and Reporting Principles

Assessment of Analyzer Performance

Total quality management (TQM) is a management process designed to improve quality of care, maintain patient safety, and control the cost of care. In terms of laboratory analysis, TQM includes quality assurance (QA) and quality control (QC). Quality assurance deals with the wider measures of laboratory performance, such as turnaround time, specimen and patient identification, and appropriate test utilization. Through QA processes, problems are identified and solutions provided to mitigate the problem.

Analyzers must be maintained to ensure proper performance; careful maintenance of the analyzer and specimen quality are important in providing accurate and timely results. The microprocessor of the analyzer displays the diagnostic maintenance routine required

TABLE 6-6
Sources of Error Associated with Blood Gas Analysis

Preanalytical Errors	Analytical Errors	Postanalytical Errors
Wrong patient drawn	Insufficient sample	Reporting incorrect result to clinician
Poor drawing technique	Calibration set points not accurate	Transcription errors
Failure to follow protocol for specimen collection	Quality control not run or out of control	Failure to recognize and interpret flags and instrument errors
Failure to mix heparin sufficiently with sample	Maintenance not performed	
Air introduced into syringe	Failure to run calibration	
Specimen exposed to air	Temperature control errors	
Delay in transportation for testing		
Sample not kept cold during transport		
Failure to mix sample adequately before analysis		
All air bubbles are not removed from the sample		
Presence of fibrin clots in the sample		
Analysis of a clotted specimen		

by the manufacturer and also displays warnings or indicators of problems that must be addressed and corrected. Regular maintenance in accordance with the manufacturer's recommendations is required for all blood gas analyzers; the schedule should be adjusted to the needs of the particular facility. This includes routine maintenance, which is performed on a daily, weekly, or monthly basis.

Corrective maintenance is required if there are problems with quality control or performance concerns with the analyzer. The instrument manual provides specific guidelines for routine, preventative, and corrective maintenance requirements for each analyzer. In general, frequency of maintenance is directly related to the number of blood gas analyses performed on the instrument.

It is important to maintain a clean sample chamber and path. Although automatic flushing to clean the sample chamber and pathway is an element of most blood gas analyzers, it may still be necessary to manually clean these areas with implements or solutions recommended by the manufacturer. Fibrin strands or small clots may be present in samples or may develop in the sample as it is warmed in the temperature chamber. Fibrin and clots will alter calibrations and measurements by affecting the contact of blood, gases, or buffers with electrode membranes.

Quality control is a required component of laboratory analysis. It is not only necessary to ensure that the analyzer is operating correctly and producing accurate results, but also required for accreditation by agencies, including the College of American Pathologists, and to comply with the Clinical Laboratory Improvement Act of 1988.[1]

Proficiency testing is an external quality assessment process in which simulated patient specimens are produced from a common pool and analyzed by participating laboratories. The purpose is to evaluate each laboratory's performance on specific analytes. Target values are established for each tested parameter as well as for the method of analysis. Typically, proficiency testing occurs in three cycles per year; there are five specimens required for each specific analyte. For laboratories to be graded "successful" in most clinical laboratory areas, including chemistry, correct results must be produced for that analyte on four out of the five specimens. A minimal score of 80% must be achieved in three consecutive cycles. All unacceptable performances must be assessed and an explanation provided for the measurement error. Of course, the problem causing the error must be identified and corrected. As a component of the laboratory accreditation process, proficiency testing is mandatory.[1]

Quality control materials should be analyzed after a successful calibration, following completion of routine maintenance procedures, and after completing any corrective maintenance or troubleshooting of the analyzer.

State and federal accreditation agencies require that three levels (low, normal, and elevated) of each analyte must be tested in each 24-hour period. Most facilities analyze all three levels in each 8-hour shift.

Postanalytical variables, the third stage of analysis, include the accurate recording and reporting of results. Results must be correctly reported to the appropriate healthcare provider in a timely manner. Patient results not within the reference range, and in particular critical values, must be reported to and documented with the healthcare provider.

Reporting Values

Reference ranges for some common parameters are summarized in **Table 6-7**. Results must be reported through the information system, electronic medical record, or instrument interface in a timely manner.

Importance of/Rationale for Critical Values for Blood Gases and Analytes

Critical values, also known as panic values, are those testing results that present a life-threatening situation for the patient.[34] Timely and accurate reporting of critical values to licensed medical professionals is required by laboratory accrediting bodies and is recognized as an important patient safety initiative.[35] Critical limits may vary with the laboratory and the medical facility. **Table 6-8** shows the upper and lower limits for pertinent clinical chemistry laboratory tests.[36]

Assessment of Analyzer Performance: Quality Control

It is essential to only report patient results that are accurate and precise so that the healthcare provider can make a reliable diagnosis and treatment regimen. Error refers to deviations from the true value. Testing errors are categorized as either random/wild or systematic. All test systems attempt to identify and minimize measurement errors. Systematic error occurs in some predictable manner. The measurement value is either overestimated or underestimated, but not both. It is controlled through proper calibration and quality control of the testing system. Systematic error is explainable and has a correctable cause. Systematic error may be caused by an inaccurate calibrator or standard, improper handling of samples or reagents, or instrument malfunction. It can generally be identified and corrected through quality control by identifying shifts, trends, and violations of the Westgard Rules (see more on these rules later in this section).[37] By contrast, random error is unpredictable and results from uncontrollable factors. It is introduced by chance and can be minimized, but never eliminated. Random errors may appear on both the high and low sides of the true value.

TABLE 6-7
Reference Values

Test	Specimen Type	Reference Range
Blood Gases		
pH	Arterial	7.35–7.45
pH (newborn)	Arterial	7.25–7.45
pCO_2	Arterial	35–45 mm Hg
pCO_2 (newborn)	Arterial	27–40 mm Hg
pO_2*	Arterial	83–108 mm Hg
pO_2 (newborn)	Arterial	55–90 mm Hg
HCO_3	Arterial	21–28 mmol/L
HCO_3 (newborn)	Arterial	17–24 mmol/L
$T CO_2$	Venous	22–29 mmol/L
$T CO_2$ (newborn)	Venous	13–22 mmol/L
sO_2	Arterial	95–98%
sO_2 (newborn)	Arterial	40–90%
Base excess	Arterial	–2 to +3
Base excess (infant)	Arterial	–10 to –2
Chemistry		
Glucose (adult: fasting)	Whole blood, serum, or plasma	60–95 mg/dL
Glucose (infant and child)	Whole blood, serum, or plasma	70–100 mg/dL
Glucose (newborn)	Whole blood, serum, or plasma	50–80 mg/dL
Potassium	Whole blood, serum, or plasma	3.5–5.1 mmol/L
Potassium (newborn)	Whole blood, serum, or plasma	3.0–5.8 mmol/L
Sodium	Whole blood, serum, or plasma	136–145 mmol/L
Sodium (infant)	Whole blood, serum, or plasma	139–146 mmol/L
Chloride	Whole blood, serum, or plasma	98–107 mmol/L
Chloride (newborn)	Whole blood, serum, or plasma	98–113 mmol/L
Hematology		
Hemoglobin (male)	Whole blood	13.5–17.5 g/dL
Hemoglobin (female)	Whole blood	12.0–16.0 g/dL
Hemoglobin (newborn)	Whole blood	10.0–17.0 g/dL
Hematocrit (male)	Whole blood	37–48%
Hematocrit (female)	Whole blood	35–45%

* pO_2 decreases with age and high altitude.

TABLE 6-8
Critical Values for Some Common Laboratory Analytes

Test	Specimen Type	Lower Limit	Upper Limit
Blood Gases			
pH	Arterial and capillary	7.20	7.60
pCO_2	Arterial and capillary	20 mm Hg	70 mm Hg
pO_2	Arterial	40 mm Hg	
HCO_3	Arterial and capillary	10 mmol/L	40 mmol/L
Chemistry			
Glucose (adult)	Whole blood, serum, or plasma	40 mg/dL	450 mg/dL
Glucose (infant < 1 year)	Whole blood, serum, or plasma	40 mg/dL	400 mg/dL
Glucose (newborn)	Whole blood, serum, or plasma	30 mg/dL	200 mg/dL
Potassium	Whole blood, serum, or plasma	2.8 mmol/L	6.2 mmol/L
Potassium (newborn)	Whole blood, serum, or plasma	2.8 mmol/L	6.5 mmol/L
Sodium	Whole blood, serum, or plasma	120 mmol/L	160 mmol/L
Sodium (infant)	Whole blood, serum, or plasma	125 mmol/L	150 mmol/L
Hematology			
Hemoglobin (adult)	Whole blood	6 g/dL	20 g/dL
Hemoglobin (newborn)	Whole blood	10 g/dL	20 g/dL

Their effect can be reduced by producing repeated measures of the same quality. Random error exhibits a Gaussian or normal data distribution, which enables us to make probability statements about measurement accuracy. An outlier is a value that is found outside of the normally distributed data.

Quality control (QC) should be performed at least once per shift. Electronic QC, which is a feature of many analyzers, uses an analyzer signal that mimics a sample. It is economical, easy to run, and reliable; however, it does not evaluate the operator or all systems within the analyzer. Thus, it is essential when appropriate to also analyze commercially available QC materials. The frequency of QC analysis depends on the instrument, its stability, and the manufacturer's specification, as well as government regulations and the policy of the healthcare system. Daily instrument setup involves calibration and running QC. Normal and abnormal QC with known results are analyzed and compared to known ranges. The result rarely perfectly matches the mean value every time. Limits of variation are established. If QC results are within the limits, we can assume that patient results are also acceptable and reportable.

Repeated measures of a given analyte on a given instrument will cluster around the mean. Plotting the frequency of each result against the concentration or amount of the analyte should produce a normal, Gaussian distribution. Based on the analysis of the QC material, parameters are established for results that are plus or minus 1 standard deviation ($\pm$ 1 SD), plus or minus 2 standard deviations ($\pm$ 2 SD), and plus or minus 3 standard deviations ($\pm$ 3 SD) from the mean. Laboratory limits are generally set to $\pm$ 2 SD, which means that based on the Gaussian distribution, 95.0% of the QC results will be within 2 SDs of the mean. Thus, 5% or 1 out of 20 QC results will fall outside of the limits as a result of random error.

Levey-Jennings plots are used to track QC performance over a period of time. This process assists in identification of shifts and trends that alert the operator to possible problems in the testing system. A shift shows that the results are biased and "shifted" in one direction. The values are all shifting either above or below the mean. Shifts are sudden and show an abrupt change in consecutive results. Shifts are most often attributable to instrument malfunction or errors in operator technique. A Levey-Jennings plot showing a shift is provided in **Figure 6-4**.

By contrast, a trend is a gradual change in consecutive control results with all results going upward or downward. A trend results from systematic drift due to

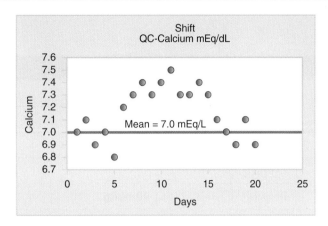

FIGURE 6-4 Shift.

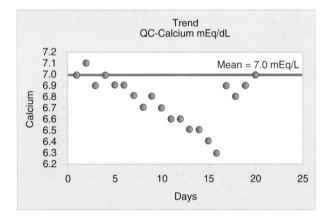

FIGURE 6-5 Trend.

deterioration of a reagent or control material. Trends may also be caused by failure of a component within the analyzer. An example of a trend is shown in the Levey-Jennings plot in **Figure 6-5**.

A high level of precision indicates reproducible measurements; precise results are reproducible, reliable, and consistent. They are most affected by random error. The greater the random error, the less precise is the measurement. Precision is enhanced by the use of standardized measurement methods, which include training and certification of the operator.[38] Poor precision results from poor technique. Precision is also enhanced by refining instruments through automation and by repeating the measure to reproduce the results.

Accuracy is the degree to which the test system measures the analyte of interest. Accuracy refers to agreement with the true value. It is most affected by systematic error; the greater the systematic error, the less accurate is the result. Accuracy is assessed by comparing the results to the "gold standard" of testing, or the reference technique considered to be the most accurate for a laboratory parameter. Accuracy is affected by both specificity and sensitivity. Tests with high specificity detect and measure only the characteristic of interest whereas tests with low specificity

will detect the characteristic when it is not present. Thus, test systems with low specificity will have a high percentage of false positive results. Sensitivity is the ability to detect small amounts of the characteristic of interest; highly sensitive tests will detect small amounts of the analyte and will also differentiate between small amounts of different amounts of the analyte. Tests with poor sensitivity will produce a high percentage of false negatives; the phenomenon is not detected when it is indeed present. In a perfect test setting, all methods would achieve 100% sensitivity and 100% specificity; because the parameters are inversely related, this of course is not possible. Thus, test systems that are at least 90% sensitive and 90% specific are recommended. Screening tests generally promote a higher level of sensitivity and a lower level of specificity, so as to not miss a characteristic or condition. This generally prompts follow-up testing that is more specific, but perhaps less sensitive. Calibration that fails or quality control values that are not within control limits must be investigated and corrective action taken. All corrective measures must be documented.

In summary, internal quality control requires that controls are a part of internal QC and it should be run as often as specified by the instrument manufacturer. It should also be run whenever there is concern about results or the quality of the testing system. Of course, QC should be rerun if previous controls were not in control. It is important to emphasize that the operator cannot report patient results if QC results are not within control.

The Westgard Rules are six rules used to examine quality control charts to determine possible problems.[39] The type of error, random or systematic, can be identified. At least two levels of control must be run. If any of the six rules are broken, patient results cannot be reported. Once the problem is identified and corrective action taken and documented, it may be necessary to reanalyze patient samples from previous testing, especially if a systematic error is identified. Laboratories may choose to use all or some of the Westgard rules; however, they must use at least one for random and one for systematic error detection.

The 1_{2s} rule is a warning rule that describes random error; it states that there is a problem if one QC value falls more than 2 SD above or below the mean. Random error is also associated with violations of the 1_{3s} and R_{4s} rules; violation of either of these rules requires that the run be rejected. The 1_{3s} rule violation occurs when one result falls outside of the 3 SD limit; the R_{4s} rule violation occurs if the difference between the highest and lowest results exceeds a total range of 4 SD. Systematic error is associated with violations of the 2_{2s}, 4_{1s}, and 10_x; in each case the run should be rejected. The 2_{2s} violation occurs when two consecutive controls exceed either the +2 SD or −2 SD limits; the 4_{1s} violation occurs when four consecutive controls exceed either the +1 SD

TABLE 6-9
Westgard Rules

Rule	Description	Type of Error
1_{2s}	At least one QC value falls more than 2 SD above or below the mean. Warning.	Random
1_{3s}	Result falls outside of 3 SD limit. Reject Run.	Random
2_{2s}	Two consecutive controls exceed the +2 SD or −2 SD limit. Reject Run.	Systematic
R_{4s}	Difference between highest and lowest result of a run exceeds 4 SD. Reject Run.	Random
4_{1s}	Four consecutive controls exceed the +1 SD or −1 SD limit. Reject Run.	Systematic
10_{x}	Ten consecutive controls fall on the same side of the mean. Reject Run.	Systematic

or −1 SD limits. When 10 consecutive controls fall on the same side of the mean, the 10_x rule is violated. The Westgard rules are summarized in **Table 6-9**.

Emerging Technology: Point-of-Care Analyzers

Point-of-care testing is a rapidly growing part of healthcare and takes place in critical care units, surgery, the emergency department, cardiac care units, and neonatal and pediatric units. Other uses for POC testing include interfacility transport and physician office testing. Benefits of POC include rapid turnaround time and enhanced patient management. The goal of POC testing is to offer a test whose result provides a more rapid, yet still accurate result to the healthcare provider that leads to a more timely medical decision and the initiation of appropriate care.

POC technologies are built on principles similar to those of clinical laboratory analyzers. Electrochemistry has been developed for the POC analysis of glucose, pH, blood gases, electrolytes, BUN, and creatinine. Lateral flow-immunoassay is used to identify infectious agents such as group A streptococcus (*Streptococcus pyogenes*), viruses such as influenza, human chorionic gonadotropin (hCG) for pregnancy, and certain cardiac markers. These methods were first developed for qualitative testing, or to identify the presence of an analyte or compound, but now have quantitative capabilities when combined with a detection system. The test system consists of layers of a porous material that contains reagents specific to react with the analyte to be tested. The top layer contains a semipermeable membrane that will trap red blood cells and other larger molecules that may interfere with the test. As the sample diffuses through the membrane, if present, the analyte will react with the reagents and form a chromogen, or colored compound. The color intensity is proportional to the amount of analyte present. This can be quantitated using principles of light scattering, reflectometry, electrochemistry, or turbimetric methods.

Biological sensors or immunosensors have been developed to measure troponin, infectious agents, and antibodies to identify an immunologic response to infectious agents. In this type of flow-through technology, a gold-labeled antibody is bound to a porous surface matrix. If the sample contains the analyte to be tested for, the analyte binds to the antibody. Next, a second antibody is added that is labeled with biotin or another measureable compound, forming a sandwich containing the first antibody, the analyte, and then the second antibody. This complex is trapped on the membrane, but can travel laterally along the membrane until it reaches the "capture area," where the compound streptavidin is bound to a solid, nonmovable phase. Biotin in the antibody binds to the streptavidin, which immobilizes the complex. It is visualized as a colored band, which is measured and then quantitated using the reflectometer.

Other technologies adapted to POC testing include light scattering, used in coagulation testing; spectrophotometry for bilirubin, hemoglobin, and chemistry analytes; electrical impedance for hematology blood cell counts, and fluorescence for C-reactive protein (CRP), cardiac markers, and drugs.

POC blood gas analyzers permit in vitro analysis at the patient's bedside, in the emergency room, or in the intensive care unit. These units use solid state sensors with fluorescence or thin-film electrodes. The microchips, reagents, calibrators, and a sampling device are all contained within a disposable cartridge system for single analysis. Healthcare facilities can select cartridges with additional test options, including potassium, glucose, BUN, and lactate. These are usually battery operated, but some also offer the advantage of operating using an electrical output. Manufacturers provide a range of flexibility as to the number of tests per cartridge (single or multiple) and test menu based on the needs of the facility.

The standard components of most POC units include an operator interface, a bar code device to easily identify the type of test being performed, a sample delivery method, a reaction cell, sensors, quality control, data management, storage, and a retrieval system.

Advantages of POC devices include their ease of use and rapid results—most results can be available in minutes. Because whole blood can be tested, minimal specimen processing is needed; the sample does not have to centrifuged and the plasma separated from the red blood cells prior to testing. There are minimal operating steps and the units are small and portable. The reagent cartridges eliminate the need to prepare reagents and there are flexible test menus that can be aligned with the needs of the unit. Calibration and quality control are integrated into the unit, which eliminates the need for separate calibrators and QC material. The calibration and QC, however, cannot be overridden, so the operator cannot report a patient result if the calibration fails or if the QC is out of control.

There are, however, potential concerns with POC testing. With diverse testing personnel from a variety of education, or lack of education, backgrounds, testing may not be performed correctly. Preanalytical errors involving sample identification, collection, and input are also possible concerns. Those who are not educated on the importance of sample collection and testing protocol may perform tests incorrectly and report invalid results. These results may negatively impact patient care. Therefore, problems with training and competency of operators remain a large concern. Quality control and a proficiency testing protocol with corrective actions and documentation need to be provided for any instrument malfunctions or out of control situations. Although some testing devices provide auto-verification and prevent reporting of patient results when calibration or quality control fails, other analyzers permit the operator to override and report the results. There may be problems with the accurate and timely recording of data, including QC, calibration, and patient results. Because some operators are not trained sufficiently to learn the importance of laboratory testing, significant errors may occur in each phase of testing. The desire to turn out a result, any result—accurate or not—may be the overriding goal because the operator has other responsibilities to their patient. Some POC devices are not electronically interfaced into the patient's medical record and may not be compatible with the laboratory's information management system. In these cases, results need to be manually entered into the medical record or laboratory information management system, increasing the propensity for transcription error. Transcription errors can compromise patient care, especially if the error goes unrecognized and the patient is treated on erroneous results.

There may also be duplication in testing, which is costly and not efficient. Patients may have specimens collected and tested in the core laboratory while having the same or similar tests performed via POC. POC testing, although convenient, uses many consumable cartridges and supplies, which can add cost to the facility and to the patient. Duplicate testing systems for the same analyte add cost to the facility and to the laboratory when considering the cost to purchase or rent the analyzer as well as costs for supplies, reagents, and maintenance. Finally, POC testing does not always completely correlate with values obtained on traditional laboratory analyzers, due to specimen type and methodology. Thus, the healthcare provider must be cognizant of the type of analysis performed before altering a diagnosis or treatment regimen. Even with broader menu flexibility, POC testing does not offer the comprehensive testing menu of the core clinical laboratory. Yet POC testing fulfills important and critical healthcare needs of patients and providers, and is indeed here to stay. Future developments in the area of POC testing will most likely continue.

Current Blood Gas Technology

Prior to 2005, blood gas analyzers directly measured pH, pO_2, and pCO_2 and provided calculated parameters for HCO_3^-, percent oxygen saturation, and base excess. These were large analyzers with gas tanks and manual quality control. Sampling was more cumbersome and specimens could be easily exposed to air during collection and sample analysis. Today's analyzers provide a variety of test menus, which may include electrolytes and other measured analytes and self-contained reagent cartridge systems. Quality control is electronically generated and there are features for auto-calibration and auto-verification. Manufacturers offer a complete testing approach that includes a corresponding sample collection device, methods of analysis, and reporting of results, which often can be directly entered into the patient's electronic medical record. Rear-venting syringes with lyophilized heparin improve the sample collection by reducing exposure to oxygen and minimizing the fibrin clot formation.

Matching Analyzer Type to Clinical Setting

Today's blood analyzers used in POC settings with low- to medium-volume testing use self-contained reagent cartridges. Single-use cartridges contain the calibration solution and miniaturized electrochemical sensors that are needed for analysis. These single-use systems are portable and easy to transport. They are recommended for settings with a test volume of less than 10 samples per day. Sensor electrodes in single-use cartridge systems are self-calibrating and can flag calibration errors. The analyzer and electrodes require little, if any, maintenance and a calibration is performed before any measurement is released. In the event of a calibration error, the calibration is flagged and the results are suppressed. Problems due to blockage from fibrin clots are confined to the cassette in use. The cartridge containing the waste, blood, and calibration fluid is removed from the analyzer and disposed of in a biohazard container.

In settings with medium- to high-volume sample testing, a multiuse cartridge system is used. These cartridges can be customized to the specific analyte menu and to the volume of testing. The number of samples measured on a cartridge may vary from 25 to 750. Once loaded onto the analyzer, the cartridge has an in-use life of between 14 and 30 days. For cost effectiveness, the appropriate size cartridge is selected to meet the unit's workload volume.

There are also larger analyzers that provide sensor electrodes and reagents, such as calibrators, wash solutions, and quality control materials in either a modular format or as individual reagent containers. These systems include a closed waste system and feature reduced downtime compared with earlier models. These larger analyzers may require more maintenance to replace or to remembrane sensor electrodes, replace tubing or peristaltic pumps, or replace a gas cartridge when compared to the smaller volume analyzers. Thus, the larger analyzers may require additional technical support and expertise.

As discussed previously in this chapter, modern analyzers utilize a variety of technologies to measure and report results. These include potentiometry, amperometry, and fluorescence. Ion-selective electrodes are used to measure the electrolytes, Na^+, K^+, Ca^{2+}, Cl^-, and Mg^{2+}. The hematocrit is measured using conductivity, and hemoglobin is measured using spectrophotometry. CO-oximetry measurement is based on optical measurements of analytes at a number of wavelengths of light.

Laboratory Processes: Calibration and Quality Control

Calibration allows the analyzer responses to be set and adjusted to a known standard reference. Newer analyzers use aqueous tonometered solutions for calibration. These are available in sealed units. A one-point calibration adjusts the electrode to one level, either high or low. It is frequently performed and is automatically conducted by some analyzers before each measurement is released. A two-point calibration adjusts the electrode at two levels, high and low, and is set by the operator at intervals ranging from every 2 to every 24 hours. Calibrations can be preset at scheduled intervals.

Internal quality control is designed to detect and monitor errors in the testing procedure, but will not detect errors in sample collection and handling. Internal QC assures the operator that the reagents and analyzer are operating correctly; it will identify many analytical errors. The frequency of QC depends on the level of testing done and the specifications of the manufacturer and standards of the accrediting agencies. Internal QC

may also be conducted manually using individual gas ampules that contain aqueous control solutions that are equilibrated with gas mixtures. Today, most analyzers utilize automatic on-board quality control materials that simplify the process and reduce operator workload, while producing a more consistent quality control program. Electronic QC requires no user input and automatically detects, corrects, and monitors the status of the analyzer's internal electronics.

Because QC can be automatically scheduled into the analyzer, it doesn't get delayed if the healthcare provider is attending to patient care issues. The automatic QC can be scheduled to run three levels at three times a day; the operator must still verify the results. Further, operators cannot attempt to analyze expired QC or incorrect QC materials, another concern with older testing systems. In the past, operators may have had to rerun a calibration or QC to obtain values that are accepted or are in range. This practice delayed patient care and perhaps compromised patient results, and also added to the cost of the test.

Currently Available Analyzers and Units Used for Blood Gas Analysis

In the early days of blood gas analysis, there were four major equipment manufacturers: Corning (now Siemens), Instrument Laboratories (IL), Nova Biomedical, and Radiometer. These four manufacturers still exist, and there are several other vendors worldwide, including Roche.

Each manufacturer has product lines that meet the needs of the testing facility, based on the volume of testing, test menu, and speed of analysis. There is also flexibility when choosing the degree of operator-initiated and internal quality control, calibration, and verification. Whereas surgery requires a POC analyzer that produces fast and accurate results, the needs of the neonatal ICU are directed more toward trending, and what the patient's results are from day to day. For example, smaller critical care units may opt for a bench top unit, such as Siemen's 405, which offers tests for blood gases, glucose, hemoglobin, hematocrit, calcium, electrolytes, and a full co-oximeter panel. The QC is automatically run by the analyzer, but does require operator verification. Larger volume critical care units may choose larger analyzers that can accommodate a higher test volume, such as the Siemens 1265. Adult medical and surgical critical care units may rely primarily on specific parameters, such as the blood gases, whereas pediatric testing in neonatal units often requires a broader test menu. There is also flexibility in the cartridge size; for example, Siemens offers a 450-specimen and a 700-specimen cartridge for the 405 series analyzers. Again, a facility can choose the more cost-effective and appropriate cartridge for its testing setting.

Larger volume analyzers generally require increased maintenance, which includes checking the electrodes, calibrating the barometer, and deproteinizing the electrodes. Linearity studies, calibration verification, and other surveys required by the College of American Pathology (CAP) are also required throughout the year. However, even large-volume modern blood gas analyzers require significantly less manual maintenance than did their predecessors. Whereas older analyzers required pathways to identify the problem, today's analyzers offer more self-maintenance. The testing cartridge contains the reagents and components, in place of reagent bottles and ampules that would have to be replaced. Cartridge-based systems provide flexibility in the test menu and can be selected based on the testing volume. Because cartridges last 2 to 4 weeks, the menu and type of cartridge can be adjusted to meet the needs of the facility. The electrode module is similar to that of earlier units, and therefore requires appropriate maintenance.

By choosing the same manufacturer, units can be selected that meet the needs of the core laboratory, critical care units, surgery, neonatal care units, and emergency room. Consolidation to a single vendor as compared to using different analyzers and vendors for different departments is both cost effective and beneficial for inventory management. There are less items to inventory and to order and less products to be knowledgeable about. Further, there is consistency in the results from the POC units to the larger units that may be used in the respiratory department or laboratory. The ability to communicate with one vendor and to become familiar with its products minimizes issues with testing. Further, there is a greater agreement with patient values when the same product line or methodology is used.

The Siemens products also interface into the laboratory's information system, so that the operator can review historical data, tracking, test ordering and canceling, and quality audits.

The Instrument Laboratory (IL) also offers products with POC and traditional central core laboratory capabilities. The GEM 3000 series provides self-contained plug-in cartridges, eliminating the need to prepare reagents and to pump in the gas mixtures. There are also important quality control features, including IL's proprietary Intelligent Quality Management (IQM) System. Quality control between the central laboratory and POC is more consistent and standardized through the IQM system. Auto-validation is another feature of the IL analyzers; the system runs a fully automated QC sequence immediately after the aspiration of each patient sample and before test results are released. In the past, it was necessary to aspirate blood gases two times in a row to determine precision. Other features of the IL system include enhanced clot detection, low sample warning flags, and detection of biosensor

malfunctions. However, because of these technology checks, the analysis time is extended from 1 minute to approximately 4 minutes from aspiration to result. The IL analyzers run over 100 QC each day on average, which further assists with compliance and consistency of results.

Other advantages of modern analyzers include the concept that the instrument is continuously up and running. Clogged aspiration probes, electrode drift, or replacing electrode membranes used to be labor-intensive procedures requiring a skilled professional. Upon completion of such tasks, a calibration and full QC were required, which often led to instrument down time and delays for patient results.

Less staff time is needed to test daily QC and to install and recalibrate gas cylinders, and there is a more efficient mechanism to document errors. For IL analyzers, new electrodes are included in each GEM cartridge, so there is no need to remembrane or replace failed electrodes. Other advantages include integrated sample collection devices. For example, the GEM systems use a flexible heparin tube for pediatric patients whose volume is sufficient to perform blood gases, and also electrolytes and other analytes.

The GEM system also offers an add-on module for CO-oximetry analysis (GEM-OPL), which is interfaced into the main testing unit. The GEM-OPL uses six wavelengths of light, but does not require hemolysis of the sample. It uses thin-slide translucency technology that requires only 50 μL of blood and a disposable cuvette. The full CO-oximetry panel is reported within 10 seconds.

Roche's line of analyzers includes the cobas b 221, which is also a multiparameter analyzer for blood gases, CO-oximetry, electrolytes, and metabolites. It is designed to be a high-volume analyzer, and is not considered to be a portable unit. These units also use reagents to generate the gases, eliminating metal tanks for O_2 and CO_2. Roche's cobas b 123 is a POC system that features a mobile blood gas analyzer with a selection of 15 parameters. The system uses a patented thick-film sensor technology and a broad test menu with results within 2 minutes. Another feature of the cobas b 123 is its four-level clot protection system as well as automatic linearity testing and calibration. Roche's Electronic Quality Assurance Program (eQAP) assists with QC, regulatory compliance, and the ability to participate in peer review and benchmarking of quality control.

Radiometer, manufacturer of the ABL line of analyzers, patented its "First Automatic" technology, designed to improve workflow by improving sample collection, processing, analysis, and reporting. Its goal is to provide a system with fewer preanalytical errors; better identification of patient, sample, and results; and less paperwork. Radiometer's ABL 800 Flex analyzer offers a comprehensive test menu of 18 analytes and rapid

TABLE 6-10
Currently Available Analyzers

| Manufacturer | Model | Category | Blood Gas | Electrolytes | Measured Analytes | | Volume | Features |
					Metabolites and Other Tests	CO-Oximetry		
Siemens	RAPIDLab 1200 Systems	POC	pH, pCO_2, pO_2	Sodium (Na^+), Potassium (K^+), Calcuim (Ca^{2+}), Chloride (Cl^-)	Glucose, lactate, neonatal total bilirubin	Total hemoglobin (tHb), deoxyhemoglobin (HHb), oxyhemoglobin (O_2Hb), Oxygen saturation (sO_2), Carboxyhemoglobin (COHb), Methhemoglobin (MetHb)	Medium to high	Clot detection and clearance sampling system, automatic QC, comprehensive menu
	RAPIDPoint 350	POC	pH, pCO_2, pO_2	Na^+, K^+, Ca^{2+}, Cl^-	Hematocrit		Low to medium	Single reagent cartridge; dialysate mode; 75–120 µL sample
	RAPIDPoint 340	POC	pH, pCO_2, pO_2				Low to medium	Single reagent cartridge; dialysate mode; 75–120 µL sample
	RAPIDLab 248	Critical care	pH, pCO_2, pO_2				Critical care testing	Small sample size, 50–95 µL; analysis in 45 seconds
	RAPIDLab 348	Critical care	pH, pCO_2, pO_2	Na^+, K^+, Ca^{2+}, Cl^-	Hematocrit		Critical care testing	Small sample size, 50–95 µL; analysis in 50 seconds
	RAPIDLab 348	POC	pH, pCO_2, pO_2	Na^+, K^+, Ca^{2+}, Cl^-	Hematocrit			Dialysate mode; low volume; enhanced operator features
	RAPIDPoint 500	POC	pH, pCO_2, pO_2	Na^+, K^+, Ca^{2+}, Cl^-	Glucose, lactate	tHb, HHb, O_2Hb, sO_2, COHb, MetHb, neonatal total bilirubin		Data management system
Instrument Laboratory (IL)	GEM Premier 4000	POC	pH, pCO_2, pO_2	Na^+, K^+, Ca^{2+}, Cl^-	Glucose, lactate, neonatal total bilirubin, hematocrit	tHb, HHb, O_2Hb, sO_2, COHb, MetHb		Self-contained, multiuse cartridges, Intelligent Quality Management (IQM) System

(continues)

TABLE 6-10
Currently Available Analyzers (Continued)

Manufacturer	Model	Category	Blood Gas	Electrolytes	Measured Analytes		Volume	Features
					Metabolites and Other Tests	CO-Oximetry		
Instrument Laboratory (IL)	GEM Premier 3500	POC	pH, pCO_2, pO_2	Na^+, K^+, Ca^{2+}, Cl^-	Glucose, lactate, hematocrit			Self-contained, multiuse cartridges, IQM
	GEM Premier 3000	POC and centralized testing	pH, pCO_2, pO_2	Na^+, K^+, Ca^{2+}, Cl^-	Glucose, lactate, hematocrit, prothrombin time (PT), activated partial thromboplastin time (APTT), activated clotting time (ACT), activated clotting time—low range (ACT-LR)	tHb, HHb, O_2Hb, sO_2, COHb, MetHb	Large volume	Comprehensive test menu; customizable cartridges; car add coagulation and CO-oximetry units
Roche	cobas b 123 POC	Critical care	pH, pCO_2, pO_2	Na^+, K^+, Ca^{2+}, Cl^-	Glucose, lactate, hematocrit	tHb, HHb, O_2Hb, sO_2, COHb, MetHb	Medium to small volume	Results within 2 minutes; thick-film sensor technology
	cobas b 121	Critical care	pH, pCO_2, pO_2					Small sample size
	cobas b 221 system	Critical care	pH, pCO_2, pO_2	Na^+, K^+, Ca^{2+}, Cl^-	Glucose, lactate, hematocrit, BUN, bilirubin	tHb, HHb, O_2Hb, sO_2, COHb, MetHb	Medium to high	
Radiometer	ABL 800 FLEX	POC and centralized testing	pH, pCO_2, pO_2	Na^+, K^+, Ca^{2+}, Cl^-	Glucose, lactate, creatinine, bilirubin	tHb, HHb, O_2Hb, sO_2, COHb, MetHb	Medium to high volume	First automatic and FlexQ features
	ABL 90 FLEX	Acute care	pH, pCO_2, pO_2	Na^+, K^+, Ca^{2+}	Glucose, lactate, bilirubin	tHb, HHb, O_2Hb, sO_2, COHb, MetHb	Medium volume	Comprehensive acute care panel, 35-second turnaround time
	ABL 80 FLEX		pH, pCO_2, pO_2	Na^+, K^+, Ca^{2+}, Cl^-	Glucose, hematocrit	tHb, HHb, O_2Hb, sO_2, COHb, MetHb	Medium to low volume	

Note: Table is not comprehensive and includes only measured, not derived, parameters.

analysis. Its FLEXQ module automatically identifies, mixes, and measures up to three samples in succession.

Although some blood gas systems permit the integration of POC results into the electronic medical record, other systems have this capability only for the centralized laboratory or respiratory care unit. Concerns continue with the ability of some analyzers to handle fibrin clots, which relates to the expertise of the individual drawing the arterial blood sample. Cleaning the arterial line to avoid diluted samples and avoiding clots within the specimen are dependent upon each person's training. Although the newer analyzers can detect clots and bubbles, a clot will still cause problems with the system until it is removed.

Today many hospitals use POC instruments in conjunction with stand-alone instruments to verify results obtained on POC analyzers. Both POC and stand-alone analyzers are subject to Clinical Laboratory Improvement Amendments of 1988 (CLIA) regulations. Some of the currently available analyzers are summarized in **Table 6-10**.

The accuracy and precision of results are related to the degree of technology, but equally important is the expertise of the testing personnel. Testing in the central laboratory is conducted by appropriately educated laboratory professionals who maintain regulatory compliance. Nonlaboratory personnel who use POC systems may not be fully cognizant of the influence of physiologic and analytical factors on the final result, which could lead to improper treatment decisions. Up to 68% of errors in blood gas measurements in point-of-care are related to sample collection, handling, and preparation that invalidate the results regardless of the technology of the analyzer.

References

1. Department of Health and Human Services, Health Care Financing Administration, Public Health Service. Clinical laboratory improvement amendments of 1988; final rule. *Federal Register.* 1992 February 28. Available at: https://www.federalregister.gov/clinical-laboratory-improvement-program. Accessed June 14, 2014.
2. National Committee for Clinical Laboratory Standards (NCCLS). Procedures for the collection of arterial blood specimens, 1999. Available at: http://www.ncbi.nlm.nih.gov/pmc/articles/PMC87384. Accessed June 26, 2014.
3. Browning JA, Kaiser DL, Durbin CG Jr. The effect of guidelines on the appropriate use of arterial blood gas analysis in the intensive care unit. *Respir Care.* 1989;34(4):269-276.
4. Jordan A. Blood gas: A brief anecdotal history by one who has been there. MLO-online. 2012. Available at http://www.mlo-online.com/articles/201209/blood-gas-a-brief-anecdotal-history-by-one-who-has-been-there.php. Accessed July 10, 2014.
5. Paxton A. Blood gas analyzers—the old and the new. CAP Today. August 2007. Available at: http://www.cap.org/apps/portlets/contentViewer. Accessed June 25, 2014.
6. Shapiro BA, Mahutte CK, Cane RD, Gilmour IJ. Clinical performance of a blood gas monitor: A prospective, multicenter trial. *Crit Care Med.* 1993;21(4):487-494.
7. Klæstrup E, Trydal T, Pedersen JF, Larsen JM, Lundbye-Christensen S, Kristensen SR. Reference intervals and age and gender dependency for arterial blood gases and electrolytes in adults. *Clin Chem Lab Med.* 2011;49(9):1495-1500.
8. Crockett AJ, McIntyre E, Ruffin R, Alpers JH. Evaluation of lyophilized heparin syringes for the collection of arterial blood for acid base analysis. *Anaesth Intensive Care.*1981;9(1):40-42.
9. Thomson JM. Blood collection and preparation techniques: Pre-analytical variation. In: Jespersen J, Bertina RM, Haverkate F, eds. *ECAT Assay Procedures: A Manual of Laboratory Techniques.* Dordrecht, Netherlands: Kluwer Academic; 1992:13-20.
10. Pruden EL, Siggaard-Andeson L, Tietz NW. Blood bases and pH. In: Burtis CA, Ashwood ER, eds. *Tietz Fundamentals of Clinical Chemistry.* Philadelphia: WB Saunders; 1996:211-223.
11. Adams AP, Morgan-Hughes JO, Sykes MK. pH and blood-gas analysis. Methods of measurement and sources of error using electrode systems. *Anaesthesia.* 1967;22(4):575-597.
12. Beetham R. A review of blood pH and blood-gas analysis. *Ann Clin Biochem.* 1982;19(Pt 4):198-213.
13. Severinghaus JW, Astrup PB. History of blood gas analysis. I. The development of electrochemistry. *J Clin Monit.* 1985; 1(3):180-192.
14. Severinghaus JW, Astrup PB. History of blood gas analysis. III. Carbon dioxide tension. *J Clin Monit.* 1986;2(1):60-73.
15. Reynafarje B, Costa LE, Lehninger AL. O_2 solubility in aqueous media determined by a kinetic method. *Anal Biochem.* 1985;145(2):406-418.
16. Gehring H, Duembgen L, Peterlein M, Hagelberg S, Dibbelt L. Hemoximetry as the "gold standard"? Error assessment based on differences among identical blood gas analyzer devices of five manufacturers. *Anesth Analg.* 2007;105(6 Suppl):S24-S30.
17. Toobiak S, Sher EA, Shaklai M, Shaklai N. Precise quantification of haemoglobin in erythroid precursors and plasma. *Int J Lab Hematol.* 2011;33(6):645-650.
18. Kazmierczak SC. Laboratory quality control: Using patient data to assess analytical performance. *Clin Chem Lab Med.* 2003; 41(5):617-627.
19. Siggaard-Andersen O. The van Slyke equation. *Scand J Clin Lab Invest Suppl.* 1977;146:15-20.
20. Lang W, Zander R. The accuracy of calculated base excess in blood. *Clin Chem Lab Med.* 2002;40(4):404-410.
21. Albert V, Subramanian A, Rangarajan K, Pandey RM. Agreement of two different laboratory methods used to measure electrolytes. *J Lab Physicians.*2011;3(2):104-109.
22. Ronkainen NJ, Halsall HB, Heineman WR. Electrochemical biosensors. *Chem Soc Rev.* 2010;39(5):1747-1763.
23. D'Orazio P. Biosensors in clinical chemistry. *Clin Chim Acta.* 2003;334(1–2):41-69.
24. Borisov SM, Wolfbeis OS. Optical biosensors. *Chem Rev.* 2008; 108(2):423-461.
25. Carraro P, Plebani M. Errors in a stat laboratory: Types and frequencies 10 years later. *Clin Chem.* 2007;53(7):1338-1342.
26. Bonini P, Plebani M, Ceriotti F, Rubboli F. Errors in laboratory medicine. *Clin Chem.* 2002;48(5):691-698.
27. Biswas CK, Ramos JM, Agroyannis B, Kerr DN. Blood gas analysis: Effect of air bubbles in syringe and delay in estimation. *Br Med J (Clin Res Ed).* 1982;284(6320):923-927.
28. Davies MW, Mehr S, Morley CJ. The effect of draw-up volume on the accuracy of electrolyte measurements from neonatal arterial lines. *J Paediatr Child Health.*2000;36(2):122-124.
29. Weibley RE, Riggs CD. Evaluation of an improved sampling method for blood gas analysis from indwelling arterial catheters. *Crit Care Med.* 1989;17(8):803-805.
30. National Committee for Clinical Laboratory Standards (NCCLS). C46-P Blood gas and pH analysis and related measurements. 2000. Available at: http://www.ncbi.nlm.nih.gov/pmc/articles/PMC87384. Accessed June 26, 2014.

31. Bisson J, Younker J. Correcting arterial blood gases for temperature: (When) is it clinically significant? *Nurs Crit Care.* 2006;11(5):232-238.

32. Westgard JO, Klee GG. Quality management. In: Burtis CA, Ashwood ER, eds. *Tietz fundamentals of clinical chemistry,* Philadelphia: WB Saunders; 1996:211-223.

33. O'Kane MJ, McManus P, McGowan N, Lynch PL. Quality error rates in point-of-care testing. *Clin Chem.* 2011;57(9):1267-1271.

34. Piva E, Plebani M. Interpretative reports and critical values. *Clin Chim Acta.* 2009;404(1):52-58.

35. Rensburg MA, Nutt L, Zemlin AE, Erasmus RT. An audit on the reporting of critical results in a tertiary institute. *Ann Clin Biochem.* 2009;46(Pt 2):162-164.

36. Kost CJ. Critical limits for urgent clinical notification of US medical centers. *JAMA.* 1990;263(5):704-707.

37. Schoenmakers CH, Naus AJ, Vermeer HJ, van Loon D, Steen G. Practical application of Sigma Metrics QC procedures in clinical chemistry. *Clin Chem Lab Med.* 2011;49(11):1837-1843.

38. Harel O, Schisterman EF, Vexler A, Ruopp MD. Monitoring quality control: Can we get better data? *Epidemiology.* 2008;19(4):621-627.

39. Westgard JO. Internal quality control: Planning and implementation strategies. *Ann Clin Biochem.* 2003;40(Pt 6):593-611.

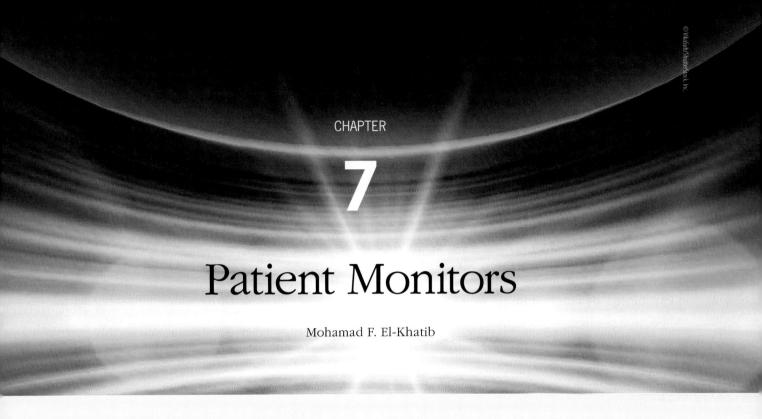

7

Patient Monitors

Mohamad F. El-Khatib

CHAPTER OBJECTIVES

1. Understand the basic principles of operation of noninvasive patient monitors commonly used by respiratory therapists.
2. Be familiar with most of the currently available noninvasive patient monitors used in clinical practice and compare their technical specifications.
3. Know the preutilization requirements in terms of calibration to assure accurate performance of these devices.
4. Identify the potential sources of error that can influence the performance of these devices.

KEY TERMS

Carbon dioxide
Esophageal pressure
Exhaled nitric oxide
Indirect calorimetry
Inhaled helium
Inhaled oxygen

Neonatal apnea monitors
Pulse oximeter
Transcutaneous carbon
  dioxide
Transcutaneous oxygen

Introduction

Monitoring patients who are suffering from cardio-pulmonary diseases and are receiving medical gas therapy and/or other forms of ventilatory support is a critical and paramount responsibility of respiratory therapists. The disease process, respiratory care interventions, and the patients' responses to such interventions largely affect the patient outcomes. These factors are dynamic processes that need to be continuously assessed and evaluated so that appropriate adjustments to the patients' care plan can be made. It is only with appropriate and accurate monitoring of respiratory care interventions and of the patients' responses to those therapeutic modalities that the effectiveness of any applied treatment can be judged.

In the practice of respiratory care, several patient monitors are at the disposal of respiratory therapists. Basic knowledge of the principles of monitoring and correct interpretation of data by respiratory therapists is imperative; failure to obtain this information can result in misdirected therapy and unfavorable patient outcomes. This chapter will review the operational principles of monitors used in the delivery of inhaled medical gases such as oxygen and helium and in the monitoring of exhaled gases such as carbon dioxide and nitric oxide. It also will cover monitors used in the assessment of gas exchange and adequacy of ventilation, such as pulse oximeters and transcutaneous oxygen and carbon dioxide monitors. Finally, this chapter will discuss specialized patient monitors such as indirect calorimetry, esophageal pressure, and neonatal apnea monitors.

Inhaled Gases

Oxygen

Oxygen is an essential gas for almost all forms of life. In medical practice, supplementation of oxygen gas at concentrations greater than what is available in room air (i.e., greater than 21%) can be lifesaving. However, **inhaled oxygen** gas should be treated like any other medical drug, and patients should never receive more oxygen than is needed because inhaled oxygen can potentially be toxic.[1,2] Several effects of oxygen toxicity are well known and include mucociliary depression and poor bronchial hygiene, nitrogen washout and absorption atelectasis, carbon dioxide narcosis and cessation of breathing in patients with chronic carbon dioxide retention, bronchopulmonary dysplasia and lung tissue damage, and retrolental fibroplasia and retinopathy of prematurity in neonates.[1,2] The respiratory therapist can play an important role in administering, monitoring, and adjusting the fraction of inspired oxygen (F_IO_2) diligently and correlating it with patient history and symptoms in order to determine and recommend an appropriate "dose" of inhaled oxygen. The goal is to preserve adequate oxygen delivery and tissue oxygenation while preventing oxygen toxicity. Oxygen analyzers, also known as oxygen monitors, are commonly used by respiratory care practitioners to measure the concentrations of inhaled oxygen administered to patients.

Principles of Operation

In clinical practice, oxygen monitors most commonly use galvanic or polarographic cells (both electrochemical) to measure the oxygen concentration in a gas mixture. A galvanic cell is a self-energizing, oxygen-powered battery in which the electrical voltage changes with the concentration of oxygen in the gas mixture. The cell's sensor consists of an anode and a cathode surrounded by an electrolyte, and it has a semipermeable membrane that permits oxygen to enter but prevents electrolytes from escaping (**Figure 7-1**). The oxygen diffuses into the cell through the membrane and electrolyte to the cathode, where it reacts to form hydroxide ions. These ions diffuse to the anode, where they give up electrons and generate voltage. The rate at which oxygen diffuses into the cell and generates voltage is directly proportional to the oxygen concentration of the gas outside the membrane.[3] An electrical cable connects the sensor to the analyzer, which displays the percentage of oxygen in the gas mixture.

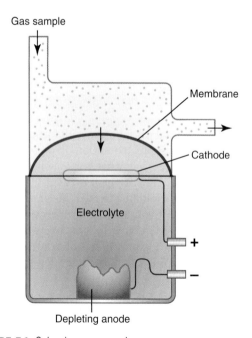

FIGURE 7-1 Galvanic oxygen analyzer.

A polarographic cell operates on the same principle, except that it conducts current from an external electrical source (usually a battery) in varying amounts, depending on the oxygen concentration. The polarographic oxygen analyzer incorporates an electrochemical sensor that responds to changes in the partial pressure of the oxygen in a gas mixture (**Figure 7-2**). The sensor cell consists of a sensing electrode (cathode), a reference electrode (anode), and an electrolyte. The cathode is separated from the sample gas by a permeable membrane that permits the diffusion of oxygen from the sample gas into the measurement cell. A predetermined voltage selected to make the sensor specific for oxygen is applied between the two electrodes. When the sensor is exposed to a sample gas, the oxygen in the sample diffuses through the membrane to the sensing surface of the cathode, where it is electrochemically reduced and a linear output current that is proportional to the partial-pressure changes of the oxygen in the sample is produced.[3] The output current is displayed as percent oxygen by the oxygen monitor.

Calibration and Troubleshooting

Because of several factors that can influence the performance of inhaled oxygen monitors (e.g., humidity, temperature, altitude and pressure, consumption of sensor's cell, etc.), calibration of inhaled oxygen monitors prior to use is essential. A two-point calibration should be done with known concentrations of oxygen. Room air (21% oxygen) and pure oxygen (100% oxygen) are two gas samples that can be easily used for the calibration process.

The galvanic oxygen sensor is rugged and insensitive to shock and vibration. The sensor can be packaged as a relatively small, self-contained, disposable cell. Some sensors can be refurbished rather than replaced by replacing the sensor anode. Galvanic sensors have several major disadvantages.[4] Because they operate on a battery principle, their life expectancy is a function of usage. Furthermore, as these sensors age, they have a tendency to read erroneously low due to a loss in sensitivity. As a result, analyzers that use battery-type sensors must be recalibrated on a frequent basis, sometimes as often as once per day. Another major drawback of battery-type sensors, particularly when used for trace oxygen measurements, is their susceptibility to "oxygen shock." If exposed to a large concentration of oxygen, these sensors can take several hours to recover.

The polarographic electrochemical oxygen sensor is insensitive to shock and vibration. The rate at which the sample gas flows over the sensor is not critical because sampling is diffusion-controlled through the membrane. The sensor can be stored for long periods of time; the anode is not consumed until power is applied to the sensor. Some disadvantages are also inherent in polarographic analyzers.[5,6] They generally have a slow response time during operation because the oxygen has

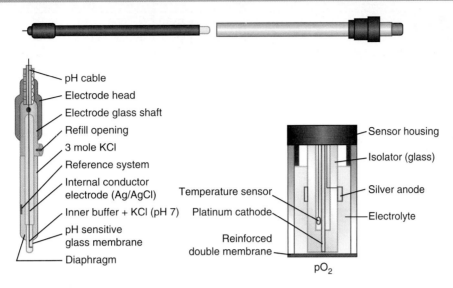

FIGURE 7-2 Polarographic oxygen analyzer.

to diffuse through the membrane. These analyzers also tend to be quite pressure- and temperature-sensitive. Regular use results in gradual degradation of the anode material and electrolyte solution, causing drift and erroneous low readings and requiring frequent calibrations. Because the sensor anode and electrolyte solutions are consumed in making oxygen measurements, the sensor requires replacement or refurbishing at intervals of 6 to 12 months, depending on usage. Polarographic analyzers are affected by temperature and humidity and their accuracy is affected if they are calibrated with a dry gas and then used with a humidified gas sample. For this reason, the analyzer should be placed before the humidification or aerosol-generating device.

Various factors affect the output and lifetime of the oxygen cells. The temperature of the oxygen gas affects its diffusion through the membrane (higher temperatures increase diffusion) and therefore the output of the cell. Oxygen diffusion and migration through the membrane and electrolyte are also slowed by accumulated electrolyte residues on the membrane and by oxidation of the electrode. As a result, the cell does not produce enough current to permit calibration, and its response becomes sluggish. At this point, galvanic cells must be replaced. Polarographic cells can be either replaced or renovated by adding more electrolyte gel and replacing the membrane. Because the operation of most oxygen monitors depends on sensing cells and batteries that have a limited life span, daily checks are essential to ensure proper accuracy and response. Some units are equipped with circuits that automatically activate visual signals when batteries or cells need to be replaced.

Currently Available Devices

There are many commercially available devices to monitor oxygen concentrations in inhaled gases. The types and specifications of such devices and monitors are presented in **Table 7-1**.

Helium

Helium (He) is a rare, naturally occurring gas that is nonflammable, colorless, odorless, tasteless, nontoxic, inert, and monatomic.[7] Helium has an extremely low density (0.1786 kg/m^3) that is about seven times lighter than air. In medical practice, helium is used for both diagnostic applications and therapeutic interventions. During pulmonary function testing, helium is used in the determination of lung volumes, in the assessment of airway obstruction, and in the carbon monoxide diffusing capacity (DL$_{CO}$) test. However, when mixed with oxygen in the form of heliox (*heli*um + *ox*ygen), helium is commonly used to treat patients with various forms of obstructive airway diseases including acute upper airway obstruction,[8] acute asthma,[9] and acute exacerbation of chronic obstructive pulmonary disease (COPD).[10]

Whereas heliox is available in prefilled cylinders with known concentrations of helium and oxygen (e.g., He:O$_2$ mixture of 80:20, 70:30, or 60:40), helium needs to be accurately measured during diagnostic procedures for pulmonary function testing. Several helium analyzers are available for accurate and continuous monitoring of helium gas concentrations. These analyzers are mainly of two types: handheld or incorporated into a pulmonary function testing system.

Principles of Operation

Helium analyzers measure the helium content based on the distinctively high thermal conductivity of helium gas. The analyzers consist of two main components: one is a sensor block and the other is an electronic circuit.[11,12] The unknown gas mixture flows through the sensing chamber and is sealed inside for measurement. Once the gas mixture is sealed inside the sensing chamber, the electronic circuit then measures the difference between the thermal conductivity of the gas

TABLE 7-1
Types and Specifications of Inhaled Oxygen Monitors

SPECIFICATIONS	ENMET ISA-60m/MRI-5175	ENMET MedAire 2200	ENMET RECON, O2	ENMET SDS-1100-97D	HUDSON 5800 SERIES	HUDSON 5810	MAXTEC OM-25ME & MEL	SIERRA MONITOR 4501-03	SIERRA MONITOR 5100-03-IY	TELEDYNE 3350	TELEDYNE AX300	TELEDYNE MX300	VASCULAR TECHNOLOGY VTI OXYGEN ANALYZER/MONITOR
Monitor													
Measurement Range	0–30%	0–30%	0–30%	0–30%	16–100%	0–100%	0–100%	0–25% Vol	0–25%	0–25%	0–100%	0–100%	0–100% oxygen
Resolution	0.10%	Not specified	Not specified	Not specified	0.10%	1%	0.10%	0.2% Vol	0.10%	0.50%	Not specified	Not specified	Not specified
Accuracy	± 0.1%	± 0.1%	± 0.1%	± 0.1%	± 1%	± 2%	± 1%	Not specified	± 0.1%	± 2%	± 2%	± 2%	± 2%
Linearity	Not specified	Not specified	Not specified	Not specified	± 1%	± 2%	± 1%	± 0.2%	± 0.2%	± 1%	± 1%	Not specified	Not specified
Sensor													
Sensor Type	Electrochemical	Electrochemical	Electrochemical	Electrochemical	Galvanic	Galvanic	Galvanic fuel cell	Fuel cell	Electrochemichal	Micro-fuel cell	Galvanic	Galvanic	Class R17MED
Warm-up Time	NA	NA	NA	NA	None	None	None required		1.0 minute	Not specified	Not specified	Not specified	Not specified
Expected Sensor Life	4–5 years	1–2 years		1.5–2 years	1 year plus	1 year plus	36 months	20 months	24 months		36 months in air (10 months in 100% O2)	36 months in air (10 months in 100% O2)	36 months in air at 25°C
Response Time	90% of final value in < 10 sec	90% of final value in < 15 sec	90% of final value in < 10 sec	90% of final value in < 10 sec	97% of final value in < 10 sec	97% of final value in < 10 sec	90% of final value in < 15 sec	90% of final value in < 10 sec	90% of final value in < 10 sec	90% of final value in < 20 sec	90% of step change in < 8 sec	90% of step change in < 8 sec	90% in < 6 seconds
Operating Conditions													
Operating Temperature	32°F to 104°F (0°C to 40°C)	32°F to 77°F (0°C to 25°C)	-4°F to 122°F (-20°C to 50°C)	-4°F to 104°F (-20°C to 40°C)	32°F to 104°F (0°C to 40°C)	32°F to 104°F (0°C to 40°C)	59°F to 104°F (15°C to 40°C)	-4°F to 122°F (-20°C to 50°C)	32°F to 122°F (0°C to 50°C)	Not specified	50°F to 104°F (10°C to 40°C)	50°F to 104°F (10°C to 40°C)	32°F to 104°F (0°C to 40°C)

MODEL

SPECIFICATIONS	ENMET	ENMET	ENMET	ENMET	HUDSON	HUDSON	MAXTEC	SIERRA MONITOR	SIERRA MONITOR	TELEDYNE	TELEDYNE	TELEDYNE	VASCULAR TECHNOLOGY
	ISA-60m/ MRI-5175	MedAire 2200	RECON, O2	SDS-1100-97D	5800 SERIES	5810	OM-25ME & MEL	4501-03	5100-03-IY	3350	AX300	MX300	VTI OXYGEN ANALYZER/ MONITOR
Humidity	10–99% RH	0–99% RH	5–95% RH	NA	0–100% RH	0–100% RH	0–95% RH	15–90% RH	15–90% RH	0–95% RH	0–50% RH	0–50% RH	0–50% RH
Interfering Gases	Not specified	Not specified	Not specified	Not specified	Not specified	Not specified	None specified	Not specified	None	None specified	None	None	Not specified
Alarms													
Low Alarm Range	Yes	Yes	0–30%	Yes	15–99%	NA	15–99%	Not specified	Yes		Yes	Yes	18–100%
High Alarm Range	Yes	Yes	Yes	Yes	16–100%	NA	18–99%	Not specified	Not specified		No	Yes	19–100%
Display Type	LCD	LCD	LCD	LCD	LCD	LCD	LCD	LCD	LED	LED	LCD	LCD	LCD
Power Requirements	100–240 VAC and/or 12 VDC, 15 watts	100–240 VAC	3.6 VDC, lithium battery, rechargeable	24 VDC	2 AA 1.5-volt alkaline batteries	9-volt alkaline battery	2 AA alkaline batteries (2 × 1.5 volts)	24 VDC nominal: 14–30 VDC	14 VDC and 30 VDC	AC 100–240, 12V DC lead acid battery	3 AA alkaline batteries	AC 100 to 240 Vac @ 50/60 Hz, 0.3A Max; battery backup: 12 VDC lead acid battery	3 AA alkaline batteries
Dimensions W × H × D, cm (in)	2 × 2 × 1.6 (5 × 5 × 4)	4.3 × 3.5 × 2.4 (11 × 9 × 6)	60 × 10 × 3.3 (2.4 × 3.9 × 1.3)	6.6 × 12 × 4.7 (2.6 × 4.79 × 1.9)	5.6 × 3.6 × 1.5 (5.6 × 3.6 × 1.5)	11.72 × 6.4 × 3.6 (4.6 × 2.5 × 1.4)	8.9 × 14 × 3.8 (3.5 × 5.5 × 1.5)	17.8 × 9.1 × 11.2 (7.0 × 3.6 × 4.0)	21.6 × 10.2 × 10.2 (8.5 × 4 × 4)	20.3 × 25.4 × 15.2 (8 × 10 × 6)	14 × 8.84 × 7.62 (5.5 × 3.5 × 3)	14 × 8.84 × 7.62 (5.5 × 3.5 × 3)	6.6 × 11.5 × 3.3 (2.5 × 4.5 × 1.25)
Weight, g (lb)	3,624 (8)	3,624 (8)	140 (0.3)	454 (1)	215 (0.48)	200 (0.45)	317 (0.70)	1,000 (2.2)	1,000 (2.21)	Not specified	454 (1)	454 (1)	Not specified
Green Features	Not specified	Not specified	Not specified	Not specified	Not specified	None specified	None specified	None specified	None specified	None specified	None specified	None specified	None specified
FDA Clearance	Not specified	Not specified	Not specified	Not specified	Yes	Yes	Yes	Not specified	No	No	Yes	Yes	No
CE Mark	Not specified	Not specified	Not specified	Not specified	Yes	Yes	Yes	Not specified	Yes	Yes	Yes	Yes	Yes

mixture and that of the reference gas. The helium content is then calculated by the circuit and displayed.

Calibration and Troubleshooting

Usually helium analyzers are supplied fully calibrated from the factory but will require calibration checks and recalibration every 30 days or less to maintain the best accuracy. Factors such as humidity, temperature, and pressure can affect the performance of **inhaled helium** monitors.[11,12] A two-point calibration should be done at two known concentrations of helium. Zeroing the sensor is done with room air. During zero calibration, there must be no residual gases other than air in the sample line of the instrument. This can be done with an air flow for at least 2 minutes, after which the sensor should read or be adjusted to 0.1%. The span calibration of a helium sensor is performed with a source of 100% helium. After 2 minutes at a flushing flow rate of 2 L/min, the sensor should read or be adjusted to 100%. Verification of calibration might be needed with known concentrations of helium gas other than zero or 100%.

Inhaled helium monitors require very little maintenance, other than calibration and checking and changing the helium sensor. Routine maintenance consists of periodic cleaning and leak checking the gas lines. Should any part of the instrument malfunction or fail to perform, the sensor should be removed from service and returned to the manufacturer for repair and calibration. Helium sensors are vibration-sensitive devices, and mechanical shock should be avoided. Dropping the unit on a hard floor may result in damage to the sensor.

The reading of helium concentrations can be taken 1 minute after turning on the power switch. When the unit/sensor is not used, the sensor should be exposed to ambient air.

Many recent helium analyzers do not require calibration in the hospital or clinic. Once calibrated at the manufacturing point, the helium sensor should not need recalibration. If, however, a known source gas shows erratic readings, the unit should be returned to the manufacturer for recalibration or replacement of the sensor.

Currently Available Devices

Several inhaled helium monitors are commercially available. Some of them incorporate oxygen gas sensors as well. **Table 7-2** is a comparison chart for technical specifications of commercially available helium monitors.

Exhaled Gases

Since the early days of the profession, respiratory care applications of medical gas therapy involved the delivery and monitoring of inhaled medical gases and mainly inhaled oxygen. This was a major function to the extent that respiratory care practitioners used to be called "inhalation therapists." However, the recent scientific evidence suggest that monitoring of exhaled gases, such as exhaled carbon dioxide and exhaled nitric oxide, is a valuable tool for assessment of patients and can accurately reflect the status and progression of diseases of the respiratory system.

Carbon Dioxide

End Tidal CO_2

Carbon dioxide (CO_2) is a by-product of cellular metabolism in humans as well as many other living species. It is eliminated to the atmosphere as an exhaled gas through the circulatory and respiratory systems. Exhaled-gas CO_2 monitors measure the partial pressure of CO_2 (pCO_2) in an exhaled breath (**Figure 7-3**). Usually, the CO_2 concentration reaches its maximum level at the end of exhalation of the tidal volume, at which point it is referred to as end-tidal carbon dioxide ($ETCO_2$) (**Figure 7-4**).

The $ETCO_2$ reflects changes in metabolic rate and, under conditions of normal pulmonary function, the status of the circulatory and pulmonary systems. Increased $ETCO_2$ can indicate hypoventilation, increased dead space ventilation, and hypermetabolic conditions such as sepsis and malignant hyperthermia.[13,14] Decreased $ETCO_2$ can be caused by hyperventilation, lowered cardiac output, cardiac arrest, pulmonary embolism, or hypothermia.[13,14]

$ETCO_2$ monitors are used in the operating rooms, intensive care units, and other locations in the hospital to monitor patients during anesthesia and mechanical ventilation, and to assess respiration (ventilation and perfusion) in various clinical applications. CO_2 monitors are valuable in alerting clinicians to inadequate ventilation, patient-circuit disconnections, and airway leaks. CO_2 monitoring can also detect ventilator failure and the inadvertent placement of the endotracheal tube in the esophagus, and can assess the adequacy of perfusion during cardiopulmonary resuscitation. In addition, CO_2 monitors can be used in pulmonary function and exercise laboratories and for metabolic studies.

There are two basic types of CO_2 monitors: the capnometer and the capnograph. Capnometers continuously measure CO_2 and display discrete numeric values, usually the partial pressure of $ETCO_2$ ($pETCO_2$) in mm Hg and respiration rate in breaths/minute (**Figure 7-5**). Capnographs measure CO_2 during each inspiratory/expiratory cycle and display both a CO_2 waveform, known as a capnogram, and numeric data for $pETCO_2$ in mm Hg and respiration in breaths/min (**Figure 7-4**). A capnometer connected to a patient monitor and/or recorder becomes a capnograph if a

TABLE 7-2
Types and Specifications of Inhaled Helium Monitors

SPECIFICATIONS	MODEL					
	ANALOX	CEA INSTRUMENTS INC.	C-SQUARED INC	NUVAIR	OXYCHEQ	TELEDYNE
	ANALOX 8000	K6050	HELIUM ANALYZER	HE ANALYZER	EXPEDITION ANALYZER	MIXCHEK HELIUM/ OXYGEN ANALYZER
Sensor						
Type	Thermal conductivity sensor	Not specified	Thermal conductivity	Electrochemical	Not specified	Micro-fuel cell and thermal conductivity cell
Life	Up to 10 years	Not specified	60 months	36 months	10 years plus	35 months
Measurement						
Range	0.1–100%	0–100%	0–100%	0.1–100%	0.1–100%	0–100%
Accuracy	± 0.5%	± 1%	± 1%	± 1%	± 1%	± 1%
Response time	15 seconds to T90	Not specified	< 1 minute to T90	< 6 seconds to T90	< 1 minute to T90	< 1 minute to T90
Warm-up Time	< 15 seconds	Not specified	Not specified	Not specified	Not specified	Not specified
Gas Flow Rate	20 L/hr	100–300 mL/min	Not specified	Not specified	Not specified	Not specified
Display	4-digit high-brightness red LED	Dot-matrix LCD	Not specified	LCD	Not specified	LCD
Environmental						
Operating temperature	32°F to 122°F (0°C to 50°C)	23°F to 104°F (–5°C to +40°C)	32°F to 122°F (0°C to 50°C)	32°F to 104°F (0°C to 40°C)	32°F to 104°F (0°C to 40°C)	32°F to 104°F (0°C to 40°C)
Relative humidity	95% at 40°C (noncondensing)	Not specified	0–95%	0–99% RH (noncondensing)	Not specified	Not specified
Operating pressure	Atmospheric pressure ± 350 mbar (± 5 psi)	Not specified	Not specified	Sensitive to partial pressure	Not specified	NA
Alarms	Optional	Not specified	Not specified	Not specified	Not specified	None
Outputs	0–1 volt	0–1 volt analog	Not specified	Not specified	Not specified	None
Power Supply	85 to 264 VAC, 47 to 63 Hz, 12 to 32 VDC	240 VAC, rechargeable battery 12 VDC	Rechargeable battery	9-volt alkaline battery	Portable, rechargeable batteries	120 VAC (6 VDC adapter) or 4 AA batteries
Dimensions W × H × D, in (cm)	9.45 × 5.24 × 9.25 (24 × 13.3 × 23.5)	13.3 × 6.38 × 11.61 (33.8 × 16.2 × 29.5)	Not specified	Not specified	Not specified	7.5 × 3.8 × 8.8 (19.05 × 9.65 × 22.35)
Weight, g (lb)	25,000 (55.1)	5,200 (11.46)	181 (0.4)	Not specified	12.47 (0.44)	84.48 (2.98)
Green Features	None specified	None specified	None specified	None specified	None specified	None specified
FDA Clearance	Not specified	Not specified	Not specified	Not specified	Not specified	NA
CE Mark	Not specified	Not specified	Not specified	Not specified	Not specified	NA

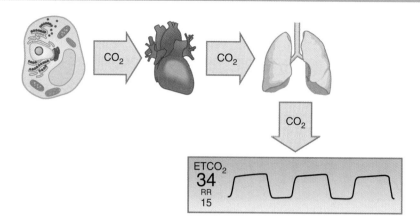

FIGURE 7-3 Carbon dioxide production, transport, and elimination.
Reproduced with permission from CareFusion.

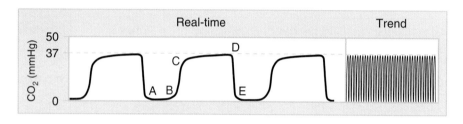

FIGURE 7-4 ETCO$_2$ tracing. A–B: Baseline (inspiratory phase); B–C: Expiratory upstroke; C–D: Expiratory plateau; D: End-tidal CO$_2$; D–E: Inspiration begins.
Reproduced with permission from CareFusion.

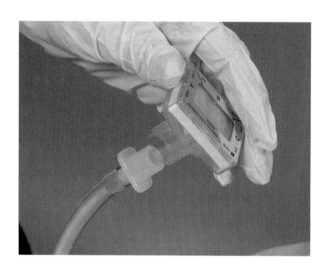

FIGURE 7-5 A capnometer.
© Jones & Bartlett Learning. Courtesy of MIEMSS.

CO$_2$ waveform is available and the recorder can print graphics.

Principles of Operation

CO$_2$ monitors use infrared (IR) absorption spectroscopy to measure partial pressure of carbon dioxide (pCO$_2$) in an exhaled breath.[14,15] CO$_2$ molecules absorb infrared light energy of a specific wavelength (4.26 μm). Because the amount of IR light absorbed is proportional to the absorbing CO$_2$ concentration, the sample's CO$_2$ concentration can be determined by comparing its absorbance to that of a standard of known concentration.

The monitor's CO$_2$ sensor typically consists of an IR source, optical filter, sample chamber, reference chamber, and detector (**Figure 7-6**). Light from the IR source (e.g., a lightbulb or light-emitting diode) strikes the optical filter, which excludes all wavelengths of light except those corresponding to the absorption peak of CO$_2$. This narrow-bandwidth light is passed through the sample and reference chambers. In the sample chamber, CO$_2$ absorbs the narrow-bandwidth light; because there is no CO$_2$ in the reference chamber, no absorption takes place as the light passes through it. At the end of the chambers, opposite the IR source, a solid-state detector converts light intensity to voltage. Once the monitor is calibrated with known CO$_2$ concentrations, it automatically converts the voltage to concentration of CO$_2$.

Carbon dioxide monitors measure gas concentration either directly, by using a sensor located in the patient breathing circuit (mainstream) (**Figure 7-7**), or remotely, by sampling from the patient's airway (sidestream) (**Figure 7-8**). With mainstream monitors, the sensor is connected to the breathing circuit with an airway adapter between the patient's ET tube and the "Y" of the breathing circuit. Sidestream carbon dioxide monitors contain a small suction pump that aspirates the exhaled gas from the patient's airway through a

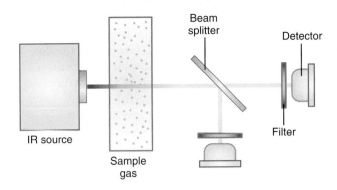

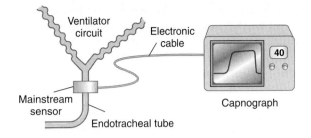

FIGURE 7-7 Mainstream CO_2 monitor; sensor is placed in the patient circuit.

FIGURE 7-6 CO_2 sensor.

Reproduced with permission from CareFusion.

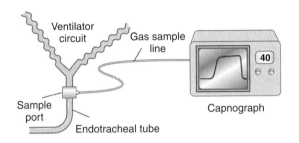

FIGURE 7-8 Sidestream CO_2 monitor; sensor is inside the monitor rather than in the patient circuit.

fine-bore tubing to the sensor. The tubing is connected to a T-piece placed on the tracheal tube or anesthesia-mask connector or is inserted into the patient's nostril to the pharynx (**Figure 7-9**). The mainstream system has a faster response time and less damping effect than the sidestream system, but it imposes a mechanical dead space that can affect total minute ventilation, particularly when using small tidal volumes.

Calibration and Troubleshooting
To provide accurate measurements, end-tidal CO_2 monitors must be calibrated at regular intervals. It is advisable to calibrate capnometers prior to each patient use. The two-point calibration involves the use of two reference carbon dioxide concentrations. A zero-point calibration can be done with room air and another calibration is usually performed with a 5% CO_2 gas mixture. The accuracy should be within ± 10%.

Several important factors such as water vapor, atmospheric pressure, anesthetic vapors, and nitrous oxide (N_2O) can affect the use and accuracy of capnometry. In sidestream systems, the condensed water and patient secretions that enter the mainstream sensor or the sampling tube are probably the most significant problem encountered that can lead to instrument failure. To prevent such incidents, some manufacturers use special sampling tubing that allows water vapor to diffuse through the tubing's wall (e.g., Nafion Tubing). Other manufacturers include water traps and/or

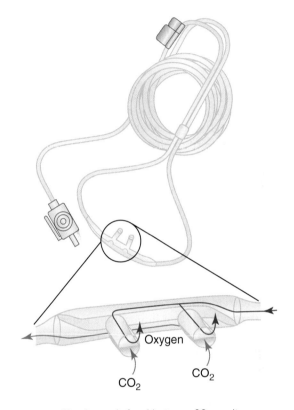

FIGURE 7-9 Nasal cannula for sidestream CO_2 monitor.

moisture-absorbent filters to protect against any water condensate effect on the performance of the monitor. In mainstream CO_2 monitors, water vapor can condense on the windows of the sensor cell and cause falsely high CO_2 readings; water vapor condensation needs to be prevented by heating the sensor to above body temperature.

Most CO_2 monitors automatically compensate for changes in barometric pressure or provide a chart for manual correction. In normal ventilation outside the operating room, anesthetic gases are not used; however, induction of anesthesia frequently involves high concentrations of inhaled anesthetic agents and nitrous oxide, resulting in falsely high CO_2 readings. The presence of inhaled anesthetic agents and nitrous oxide will produce a "collision broadening effect" that will affect the absorption band for CO_2 and subsequently cause falsely high CO_2 measurements. Correction factors to adjust for such effects are known and can be used to correct for the presence of gases and vapors other than carbon dioxide in the mixture of gas being analyzed. Some units automatically correct for this gas interference or have a user-actuated electronic offset.

Currently Available Devices

$ETCO_2$ monitors are available as stand-alone monitors or as modules incorporated into comprehensive patient vital sign monitors. Stand-alone units are usually portable and can be battery operated to facilitate use during in-hospital and out-of-hospital transport. A detailed list and specifications of currently available end-tidal CO_2 monitors are presented in **Table 7-3**.

Volumetric CO_2

Volumetric capnography is the combination of mainstream CO_2 and airway flow measurements.[16] It provides a quantitative assessment of the net quantity of CO_2 exhaled (VCO_2) on a breath-by-breath basis (**Figure 7-10**). Monitoring VCO_2 provides a valuable marker for describing the patient's current cardiorespiratory status and, more importantly, assessing changes in the status of a ventilated patient over time. Also, observing changes in the volumetric capnogram while making ventilator changes provides direct feedback of the patient's gas exchange on a breath-by-breath basis in response to ventilator settings. Volumetric capnography may prove to be a valuable tool when attempting to wean a patient off mechanical ventilation.[17] Another important application of VCO_2 monitoring in the intensive care unit (ICU) is the determination of physiological dead space ratio (Vd/Vt).[18] Optimization of positive end-expiratory pressure (PEEP) can be effectively achieved by monitoring VCO_2 and the slopes of the different phases of the volumetric capnogram.[19] Monitoring of VCO_2 can also be used in the detection of pulmonary embolism.[20] More recently, monitoring VCO_2 has also been shown to be useful in the assessment of pulmonary perfusion and noninvasive determination of cardiac output.[21]

Principles of Operation

Volumetric capnography is a technique that analyzes the pattern of CO_2 elimination as a function of expired tidal volume. The capnogram represents the total amount of CO_2 eliminated by the lungs during each breath. Expired gas receives CO_2 from three sequential compartments, forming three recognizable phases on the expired capnogram (**Figure 7-10**). Phase I contains gas from apparatus dead space and proximal conducting airways. Phase II represents the transitional region characterized by increasing CO_2 concentration, which results from progressive CO_2 emptying from more proximal alveoli to central airways. Phase III represents essentially alveolar gas and is known as the alveolar

plateau.[16] Volumetric CO_2 monitors are basically capnometers incorporating a pneumotachometer for measuring the exhaled flow and integrating the flow signal to determine the exhaled volume and subsequently display the partial pressure of CO_2 as a function of the exhaled volume.

Calibration and Troubleshooting

Calibration and troubleshooting of volumetric CO_2 monitors is identical to those tasks for end-tidal CO_2 monitors with the additional task of calibrating and troubleshooting the pneumotachometer (i.e., flow measuring device) used for the measurement of exhaled flow and determination of exhaled volume by electronic integration of the flow signal. Usually, volumetric CO_2 monitors have a combined CO_2 airway adapter and flow sensor (CO_2/flow sensor). Generally, flow sensor calibration is not necessary due to the consistency from one flow sensor to another. Modern volumetric CO_2 monitors will automatically zero the flow sensor periodically by internal valves. However, when needed, calibration should be done with gas of a viscosity similar to the gas that is to be measured. Because temperature affects viscosity, the temperature of the calibrating gas should also be similar to that being measured.

The flow sensor's principle of measurement is valid for measuring laminar flow, and thus turbulence should be minimized during calibration and use. Using a cone-shaped-diameter resistance element is a common strategy to minimize turbulence. Electronic linearizers that reduce the gain from the pressure transducer at high flow rates are also used to compensate for the presence of turbulence.

Similar to end-tidal CO_2 monitors, the combined CO_2/flow sensor should be protected by preventing "rain-out," moisture, and the patient's secretion from draining into and blocking the airway adapter and flow sensor tubing. It is always recommended not to place the airway adapter and flow sensor in a gravity-dependent position. Also, the flow sensor and tubing should be periodically checked for excessive moisture or secretion buildup.

Currently Available Devices

Volumetric CO_2 monitors are available as stand-alone monitors or as modules incorporated into comprehensive monitoring systems. Stand-alone units are usually portable and can be battery operated to facilitate use during in-hospital and out-of-hospital transport. A detailed list and specifications of currently available volumetric CO_2 monitors are presented in **Table 7-3**.

Nitric Oxide

Nitric oxide (NO) is a gas that is ubiquitously produced in the human body. It serves as a signaling molecule with numerous regulatory effects on multiple human organ systems such as blood vessels, the lungs, the heart, the nervous system, and the immune system.[22] NO is also produced by airway epithelial cells, airway and circulatory endothelial cells, and trafficking inflammatory cells in both large and peripheral airways and alveoli.[23] The fraction of exhaled NO (FeNO) can be measured easily and is well established in research, with more than 2,000 peer-reviewed publications on FeNO and its increasing adoption into clinical practice. It is now possible to estimate the predominant site of increased FeNO and its potential pathologic and physiologic role in various pulmonary diseases. In asthma, where exhaled NO promises to be very useful, it has been proposed to use this as a marker for diagnosis,[24] to monitor the response to anti-inflammatory medications,[25] to verify adherence to therapy,[26] and to predict upcoming asthma exacerbations.[27] In COPD, large/central airway maximal NO flux and peripheral/small airway/alveolar NO concentration may be normal and the role of FeNO monitoring is less clear and therefore less established than in asthma.[28] Furthermore, concurrent smoking reduces FeNO. Monitoring FeNO in pulmonary hypertension and cystic fibrosis has opened up a window to the role NO may play in their pathogenesis and possible clinical benefits in the management of these diseases.

In Europe, clinical testing of FeNO was commenced in the late 1990s, and the U.S. Food and Drug Administration approved the first NO analyzer (Aerocrine AB) for clinical monitoring of anti-inflammatory therapy in asthma in 2003. Online measurement of FeNO refers to FeNO testing with a real-time display of NO breath profiles, whereas offline testing refers to collection of exhalate into suitable receptacles for delayed analysis.[29] FeNO is expressed in parts per billion (ppb), which is equivalent to nanoliters per liter. The exhalation flow rate used for a particular test can be expressed as a subscript of the flow rate in liters/second (e.g., $FeNO_{0.05}$ is equivalent to exhaled NO concentration at a flow of 0.05 liters/second).

The use of FeNO measurement as a clinical tool requires the adoption of a standardized measurement technique followed by collection of reference data in all age groups. To date, several authors have published exhaled NO values in healthy subjects, but variable measurement techniques and methods reduce the utility of the data.[30,31]

Principles of Operation

It was first demonstrated in 1991 that NO could be detected in the exhaled gas of animals and humans in the range of 3 to 20 parts per billion (ppb) by using chemiluminescence analysis.[32] Chemiluminescence analysis allows the determination of NO concentration in the gas phase by reacting NO in the sample with ozone to produce nitrogen dioxide in an excited state. As nitrogen dioxide moves to a relaxed state, light is emitted in a stoichiometric relationship with the amount of NO

present in the gas sample. However, NO measurement based on alternative technologies, including luminol-/H_2O_2-based chemiluminescence, tunable diode laser absorption spectrometry, and laser magnetic resonance spectroscopy, is currently available or in development. New technologies offer potential advantages regarding increased portability, reduced cost, and auto-calibration. Performing the **exhaled nitric oxide** test is simple and straightforward, and most school-aged children are able to perform the test.[33]

The reference range of FeNO is sometimes referred to as the normal range, although this may be misleading because healthy individuals sometimes fall outside the range and individuals with a certain condition occasionally fall within the range.[34] However, the reference range varies considerably according to the sex, atopy status, and smoking status of the individual, suggesting that different reference ranges should exist for individuals with different combinations of these characteristics (**Table 7-4**).

Calibration and Troubleshooting

A reliable NO-free calibration gas is essential for the zeroing of exhaled NO analyzers and the provision of accurate measurements of FeNO. Zero gas or NO-free gas can be generated by exposing ambient air to NO scavengers (e.g., $KMnO_4$ and/or charcoal) or to an ozone generator, which converts NO to NO_2. The use of medical-grade air as an NO-free gas is not recommended because of the reported presence of highly variable NO concentrations in medical-grade air, up to many parts per billion, depending on the source and purification system.

For each exhaled NO analyzer, an initial linear validation should be performed using at least three-point calibration (zero and two higher NO concentrations). Specially prepared NO calibration gases with

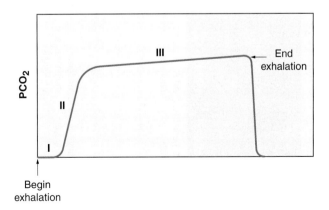

FIGURE 7-10 Volumetric exhaled carbon doxide. Phase I: Gas from apparatus dead space and proximal conducting airways. Phase II: Transitional region of progressive CO_2 emptying from more proximal alveoli to central airways. Phase III: Alveolar gas.

TABLE 7-3
Types and Specifications of End-Tidal CO_2 Monitors

SPECIFICATIONS	COMDEK MD-660P	CRITICARE EVISION	CRITICARE NCOMPASS MODEL 8100 H	CRITICARE NGENUITY MODEL 8100E1	DRAEGER MEDICAL INFINITY ETCO₂ MICROSTREAM SMARTPOD	DRAEGER MEDICAL INFINITY ETCO₂ MODULE	DRAEGER MEDICAL INFINITY ETCO₂ SMARTPOD	GE HEALTHCARE CAPNOSTAT MAINSTREAM CO₂ MODULE	GE HEALTHCARE COMBINATION CO₂ MODULE	GE HEALTHCARE SIDESTREAM CO₂ (LO FLOW) MODULE
Patient Population	Adult, pediatric, neonate	Adult, pediatric, neonate	Adult, pediatric, neonate	Adult, pediatric, neonate	Adult, pediatric, neonate	Adult, pediatric, neonate (mainstream configuration only)	Adult, pediatric, neonate (mainstream configuration only)	Adult, neonate	Adult, neonate	Not specified
Configuration										
Unit	Modular capnograph	Modular multiparameter vital signs monitor	Multiparameter vital signs monitor	Multiparameter vital signs monitor	Modular capnograph	Modular capnograph	Modular capnograph	Modular capnograph	Modular capnograph	Modular capnograph
Sensor	Sidestream	Sidestream	Sidestream	Sidestream	Sidestream	Mainstream, sidestream	Mainstream, sidestream	Mainstream	Mainstream, sidestream	Sidestream, low flow
CO₂ Measurement										
Range, mm Hg	0–100	0–99	0–99	0–99	0–99	0–99	0–99	0–100	0–100	0–100
Interference compensation										
Atmospheric pressure	Automatic	Automatic	Automatic	Automatic	Automatic	Automatic or user selectable	Automatic or user selectable	User adjustable	User adjustable	User adjustable
Calibration method	Daily zero recommended	Automatic	Automatic	Automatic	Every 12 months or 4,000 operating hours	Daily zero recommended	Daily zero recommended	None required (occasionally zero only)	None required (occasionally zero only)	None required (occasionally zero only)
Response time, msec	Depends on flow rate	170	170	170	60	60	60	< 150	< 150	< 200
Sampling Flow, mL/min	50, 70, 150, 250, selectable	200	200	200	50 ± 15	Mainstream, sidestream	Mainstream, sidestream	NA	180 ± 10	50 ± 10
Purging Mode	Yes	High suction occlusion clearing	High suction occlusion clearing	High suction occlusion clearing	NA	NA	NA	NA	No	No
Liquid Trap/ Filter	Filter	Yes/yes (22 mL capacity)	Yes/yes (22 mL capacity)	Yes/yes (22 mL capacity)	NA	NA	NA	NA	Yes/yes	Yes/yes

TABLE 7-3
Types and Specifications of End-Tidal CO_2 Monitors (Continued)

SPECIFICATIONS	COMDEK MD-660P	CRITICARE EVISION	CRITICARE NCOMPASS MODEL 8100 H	CRITICARE NGENUITY MODEL 8100E1	DRAEGER MEDICAL INFINITY ETCO2 MICROSTREAM SMARTPOD	DRAEGER MEDICAL INFINITY ETCO2 MODULE	DRAEGER MEDICAL INFINITY ETCO2 SMARTPOD	GE HEALTHCARE CAPNOSTAT MAINSTREAM CO2 MODULE	GE HEALTHCARE COMBINATION CO2 MODULE	GE HEALTHCARE SIDESTREAM CO2 (LO FLOW) MODULE
Alarms	On mounting system	Yes	Yes	Yes	On monitoring system	On monitoring system	On monitoring system	Yes	Yes	Yes
Visual/audible	Yes/yes	Yes/yes	Yes/yes	Yes/yes	Yes/yes	Yes/yes	Yes/yes	Not specified	Not specified	Not specified
High inspired CO_2	NA	Yes	Yes	Yes	User selectable	User selectable	User selectable	Adjustable	Adjustable	Adjustable
Low inspired CO_2	NA	No	No	No	No	No	No	No	No	No
Respiration rate	User selectable	Yes	Yes	Yes	User selectable	User selectable	User selectable	Adjustable	Adjustable	Adjustable
Apnea	No	Adjustable	Adjustable	Adjustable	Yes	Yes	Yes	Adjustable	Adjustable	Adjustable
Occlusion	No	Yes	Yes	Yes	NA	NA	NA	Yes	Yes	Yes
Display										
CO_2 concentration	On monitoring system	ETCO2, INCO2	ETCO2, INCO2	ETCO2, INCO2	On monitoring system	On monitoring system	On monitoring system	End-tidal and inspired	End-tidal and inspired	End-tidal and inspired
Respiration rate	On monitoring system	Yes	Yes	Yes	On monitoring system	On monitoring system	On monitoring system	Yes	Yes	Yes
Continuous CO_2	On monitoring system	Adjustable waveforms	Adjustable waveforms	Adjustable waveforms	On monitoring system	On monitoring system	On monitoring system	Waveform on display	Waveform on display	Waveform on CRT
Analog Output	Available through monitor as USB transmission	Yes	Yes	Yes	Available through monitor	Available through monitor	Available through monitor	Yes	Yes	Yes
Power										
Line voltage, VAC	110–230	100–240, 50/60 Hz	100–240, 50/60 Hz	100–240, 50/60 Hz	Powered by monitor	Powered by monitor	NA (powered by monitor)	Not specified	Not specified	Not specified
Battery	Yes	Yes	Yes	Yes	Powered by monitor	Powered by monitor	Powered by monitor	Not specified	Not specified	Not specified
Low battery indicator	Yes	Yes	Yes	Yes	NA	NA	NA	Not specified	Not specified	Not specified

(continues)

TABLE 7-3
Types and Specifications of End-Tidal CO_2 Monitors (Continued)

SPECIFICATIONS	COMDEK MD-660P	CRITICARE EVISION	CRITICARE NCOMPASS MODEL 8100 H	CRITICARE NGENUITY MODEL 8100E1	DRAEGER MEDICAL INFINITY $ETCO_2$ MICROSTREAM SMARTPOD	DRAEGER MEDICAL INFINITY $ETCO_2$ MODULE	DRAEGER MEDICAL INFINITY $ETCO_2$ SMARTPOD	GE HEALTHCARE CAPNOSTAT MAINSTREAM CO_2 MODULE	GE HEALTHCARE COMBINATION CO_2 MODULE	GE HEALTHCARE SIDESTREAM CO_2 (LO FLOW) MODULE
H × W × D, cm (in)	17 × 8.8 × 4.4 (6.7 × 3.5 × 1.7)	32.4 × 38.1 × 17.5 (12.8 × 15 × 6.9)	30.5 × 36.8 × 29.2 (12 × 14.5 × 11.5)	28 × 33 × 26.2 (11 × 13 × 10.3)	14 × 14 × 5.1 (5.5 × 5.5 × 2)	15 × 9.3 × 6.5 (5.9 × 3.6 × 2.6)	14 × 14 × 5.1 (5.5 × 5.5 × 2)	4.1 × 11.4 × 28.6 (1.6 × 4.5 × 11.25)	4.1 × 11.4 × 28.6 (1.6 × 4.5 × 11.25)	8 × 10.2 × 6.5 (3.1 × 4 × 2.6)
Weight, kg (lb)	0.34 (0.75) without batteries	7.3 (16)	6.4 (14)	6.4 (14)	0.48 (1.05)	0.5 (1.1)	0.5 (1.1)	0.5 (1.1)	0.5 (1.1)	< 0.45 (< 1)
Green Features	Recyclable materials, low power consumption	Recyclable and reusable packaging	Recyclable and reusable packaging	Recyclable and reusable packaging	None specified	None specified	None specified	None specified	None specified	None specified
FDA Clearance	Submitted	Yes	Yes	Yes	Yes	Yes	Yes	Yes	Yes	Yes
CE Mark	Yes	Pending	Yes	Yes	Yes	Yes	Yes	Yes	Yes	Yes

SPECIFICATIONS	IVY BIOMEDICAL VITAL-GUARD 450C MAIN	IVY BIOMEDICAL VITAL-GUARD 450C MICRO	MAQUET CRITICAL CARE CO_2 ANALYZER MODULE SERVO-I	NELLCOR OXIMAX N-85	NIHON KOHDEN OLG-2800	ORIDION CAPNOSTREAM 20	ORIDION MICROCAP PLUS	ORIDION MICROCAP	PHASEIN EMMA	PHILIPS M3014A
Patient Population	Not specified	Not specified	Adult, pediatric, neonate	Not specified	Adult, pediatric	Adult, pediatric, neonate	Adult, pediatric, neonate	Adult, pediatric, neonate	Adult, pediatric, neonate	Adult, pediatric, neonate
Configuration										
Unit	Configured	Configured	Modular capnometer	Handheld capnograph/oximeter	Portable, battery-operated	Stand-alone and/or linked to a central monitor system	Stand-alone and/or linked to a central monitor system	Stand-alone and/or linked to a central monitor system	Modular capnograph	Extension
Sensor	Mainstream	Mainstream: microstream	Mainstream	Sidestream	Mainstream for intubated and nonintubated patients	Microstream	Microstream	Microstream	Mainstream	Mainstream or sidestream
CO_2 Measurement										
Range, mm Hg	0–99	0–99	0–100	0–99	0–100	0–99	0–99	0–99	0–99	0–150

TABLE 7-3
Types and Specifications of End-Tidal CO$_2$ Monitors (Continued)

SPECIFICATIONS	IVY BIOMEDICAL — VITAL-GUARD 450C MAIN	IVY BIOMEDICAL — VITAL-GUARD 450C MICRO	MAQUET CRITICAL CARE — CO$_2$ ANALYZER MODULE SERVO-I	NELLCOR — OXIMAX N-85	NIHON KOHDEN — OLG-2800	ORIDION — CAPNOSTREAM 20	ORIDION — MICROCAP PLUS	ORIDION — MICROCAP	PHASEIN — EMMA	PHILIPS — M3014A
Interference compensation										
Atmospheric pressure	Manual	Automatic	Automatic	Automatic	Yes	BTPS	BTPS	BTPS	Automatic	Yes (based on entered altitude)
Calibration method	None required; optional zero	Once per year or 4,000 operating hr with 5% CO$_2$; auto zero	Verification or cell zero	Certify gas mixture annually	Automatic	Initially after 1,200 operating hr, then 1/yr or after 4,000 operating hr: 5% CO$_2$ gas annually	Initially after 1,200 operating hr, then 1/yr after 4,000 operating hr: 5% CO$_2$ gas annually	Initially after 1,200 operating hr, then 1/yr or after 4,000 operating hr: 5% CO$_2$ gas annually	No calibration required; gas span check recommended once every year	Zeroing before use; annual
Response time, msec	< 50	2.9 sec	< 25	2.5	120–200	177	190–240	190–240	< 0.5	60 (mainstream); 240 (sidestream)
Sampling Flow, mL/min	50	50	50	50	NA	50	50	50	NA	50 sidestream
Purging Mode	NA	Yes	Yes	Not specified	NA	Yes	Yes	Yes	NA	No
Liquid Trap/Filter	NA	No	NA	No/yes	NA	Incorporated into filtered line	Incorporated into filtered line	Incorporated into filtered line	NA	NA
Alarms	Yes	Yes	Yes	Yes	Yes	Yes	Yes	Yes	On monitoring system	Yes
Visual/audible	Not specified	Not specified	Not specified	Yes	Yes/yes	Not specified	Not specified	Not specified	Yes/yes	Yes/yes
High inspired CO$_2$	Yes	Yes	Yes	Adjustable	Yes	Yes	Yes	Yes	Yes	Yes
Low inspired CO$_2$	No	No	NA	No	No	Yes	Yes	Yes	NA	No
Respiration rate	Yes	Yes	NA	Yes	Yes	Yes	Yes	Yes	Yes	Yes
Apnea	Apnea off, 5, 10, 15, 20 sec	Apnea off, 5, 10, 15, 20 sec	Yes	10–60 sec adjust, no breath detection	Yes	Yes	Yes	Yes	Yes	Yes
Occlusion	Yes	Yes	Yes	Yes	NA	Yes	Yes	Yes	NA	NA

(continues)

TABLE 7-3
Types and Specifications of End-Tidal CO_2 Monitors (Continued)

SPECIFICATIONS	IVY BIOMEDICAL VITAL-GUARD 450C MAIN	IVY BIOMEDICAL VITAL-GUARD 450C MICRO	MAQUET CRITICAL CARE CO_2 ANALYZER MODULE SERVO-I	NELLCOR OXIMAX N-85	NIHON KOHDEN OLG-2800	ORIDION CAPNOSTREAM 20	ORIDION MICROCAP PLUS	ORIDION MICROCAP	PHASEIN EMMA	PHILIPS M3014A
Display										
CO_2 concentration	Yes	Yes	Yes	Yes	Yes	Yes	Yes	Yes	Yes	Yes
Respiration rate	Yes	Yes	Yes	Yes	Yes	Yes	Yes	Yes	Yes	Yes
Continuous CO_2	Yes	Yes	Yes	Waveform	Yes	Waveform, trend	Waveform, trend	Waveform, trend	Yes	Waveform
Analog Output	Yes	Yes	No	No	Yes	Yes	Yes	Yes	NA	No
Power										
Line voltage, VAC	Not specified	Not specified	Not specified	Not specified	100–127, 220–240	100–240	100–240	100–240	NA	Not specified
Battery	Not specified	Not specified	Integrated with ventilator	Not specified	Yes	Yes	Yes	Yes	Yes	NA
Low battery indicator	Not specified	Not specified	Not specified	Not specified	Yes	Yes	Yes	Yes	Yes	NA
H × W × D, cm (in)	25.9 × 27.7 × 21.1 (10.1 × 10.9 × 8.3)	25.9 × 27.7 × 21.1 (10.1 × 10.9 × 8.3)	43 × 90 × 154 (16.9 × 35.4 × 60.6) module	20.6 × 8.8 × 5.3 (8.1 × 3.5 × 2.1)	6.2 × 21 × 16.4 (2.4 × 8.3 × 6.5)	16.7 × 22 × 19.2 (6.6 × 8.7 × 7.6)	20.6 × 8.9 × 5.3 (8.1 × 3.5 × 2.1)	20.6 × 8.9 × 5.3 (8.1 × 3.5 × 2.1)	5.2 × 3.9 × 3.9 (2.1 × 1.5 × 1.5)	4 × 9.8 × 19 (1.6 × 4 × 7.5)
Weight, kg (lb)	8.6 (19)	8.6 (19)	0.45 (1) module	0.85 (1.87)	1.3 (2.9)	3.5 (7.7)	0.8 (1.8)	0.8 (1.8)	0.06 (0.?) with batteries	0.45 (0.99)
Green Features	None specified	None specified	None specified	None specified	None specified	None specified	None specified	None specified	Recyclable material, low power consumption	None specified
FDA Clearance	Yes	Yes	Yes	Yes	Yes	Yes	Yes	Yes	Yes	Yes
CE Mark	Yes	Yes	Yes	Yes	Submitted	Yes	Yes	Yes	Yes	Yes

TABLE 7-3
Types and Specifications of End-Tidal CO$_2$ Monitors (Continued)

SPECIFICATIONS	PHILIPS M3015A	SMITHS MEDICAL PM CAPNOCHECK	SMITHS MEDICAL PM CAPNOCHECK II	SMITHS MEDICAL PM CAPNOCHECK PLUS	SPACELABS HEALTHCARE 91517 MS/SS CAPNOGRAPH	WELCH ALLYN 1500 PATIENT MONITOR	WELCH ALLYN ATLAS	WELCH ALLYN PROPAQ CS	WELCH ALLYN PROPAQ ENCORE
Patient Population	Adult, pediatric, neonate	Adult, pediatric	Not specified	Not specified	Adult, pediatric, neonate	Adult, pediatric, neonate	Adult, pediatric	Adult, pediatric, neonate	Adult, pediatric, neonate
Configuration									
Unit	Extension	Quantitative capnometer	Handheld capnograph/oximeter	Stand-alone capnograph	Modular capnograph	Optional parameter within a multiparameter system	Optional parameter within a multiparameter system	Optional parameter within a multiparameter system	Optional parameter within a multiparameter system
Sensor	Sidestream	Mainstream	Sidestream	Sidestream	Mainstream, sidestream	Sidestream	Sidestream	Mainstream and/or sidestream	Mainstream and/or sidestream
CO$_2$ Measurement									
Range, mm HG	0–150	0–99	0–100	0–100	0–99 (0–13%)	0–99	0–98	0–99	0–99
Interference compensation									
Atmospheric pressure	Automatic	Not specified	Yes	Yes	Automatic, 0–10,000 feet	Automatic	Automatic	Automatic	Automatic
Calibration method	Automatic zeroing, annual (use reference gas)	Not specified	Manual two-point	Two-point from air and cylinder (45 sec), automatic room air	Two-point, zero and REF cells on the mainstream sensor cable	Automatic	Monthly CO$_2$ reset	Automatic	Automatic
Response time, msec	190 (neonate); 240 (adult/pediatric)	< 0.5 sec	2.46 sec	375	< 550 (mainstream)	Not specified	180	30–60 (mainstream), 180 (sidestream)	30–60 (mainstream), 180 (sidestream)
Sampling Flow, mL/min	50	Not specified	120	140	50	50	175 nominal	90 or 175, user selectable	90 or 175, user selectable
Purging Mode	Yes	Not specified	NA	NA	NA	NA	NA	NA	NA
Liquid Trap/Filter	Nafion tubing	Not specified	No/yes	Yes/yes	NA (mainstream), filter built into sampling line (sidestream)	Not needed	Yes	Not needed	Not needed
Alarms	Yes	Yes	Yes	Yes	Yes	Yes	Yes	Yes	Yes
Visual/audible	Yes/yes	Yes/yes	Not specified	Not specified	Yes/yes	Not specified	None specified	Not specified	Not specified
High inspired CO$_2$	Yes	Not specified	Adjustable	Adjustable	Adjustable, 1–40 mm Hg (0.1–9.9%)	Adjustable, 5 mm Hg default	NA	Adjustable, 5 mm Hg default	Adjustable, 5 mm Hg default
Low inspired CO$_2$	No	Not specified	Adjustable	Adjustable	NA	NA	NA	NA	NA

(continues)

TABLE 7-3
Types and Specifications of End-Tidal CO_2 Monitors (Continued)

					MODEL				
	PHILIPS	**SMITHS MEDICAL PM**	**SMITHS MEDICAL PM**	**SMITHS MEDICAL PM**	**SPACELABS HEALTHCARE**	**WELCH ALLYN**	**WELCH ALLYN**	**WELCH ALLYN**	**WELCH ALLYN**
SPECIFICATIONS	M3015A	CAPNOCHECK	CAPNOCHECK II	CAPNOCHECK PLUS	91517 MS/SS CAPNOGRAPH	1500 PATIENT MONITOR	ATLAS	PROPAQ CS	PROPAQ ENCORE
Respiration rate	Yes	Not specified	NA	No	Adjustable, 15–150/0–145	Adjustable, defaults depend on patient settings	Adjustable	Adjustable, defaults depend on patient settings	Adjustable, defaults depend on patient settings
Apnea	Yes	Not specified	NA	No	Adjustable timeout, 20–45	Yes	No	Yes	Yes
Occlusion	NA	Not specified	NA	Yes	Mainstream	Yes	Yes	Yes	Yes
Display									
CO_2 concentration	Yes	Not specified	Yes	Yes	Yes	Yes	Yes	Yes	Yes
Respiration rate	Yes	Not specified	Yes	Yes	Yes	Yes	Yes	Yes	Yes
Continuous CO_2	Waveform	Not specified	Waveform	Waveform	Yes	Waveform and numerics	Waveform and numerics	Waveform and numerics	Waveform and numerics
Analog Output	No	Not specified	No	3 channels	No	No	No	No	No
Power									
Line voltage, VAC	NA	Not specified	Not specified	Not specified	Supported by displays and monitor	100, 240	120, 240	120, 240	120, 240
Battery	NA	Yes	Yes	Yes	Supported by displays and monitor	Yes	Yes	Yes	Yes
Low battery indicator	NA	Yes	Not specified	Not specified	NA	Yes	Yes	Yes	Yes
H × W × D, cm (in)	3.8 × 9.7 × 18.8 (1.5 × 3.8 × 7.4)	5.2 × 3.9 × 2.9 (2.1 × 1.5 × 1.1)	12.7 × 11.1 × 7.4 (5 × 4.4 × 2.9)	8.9 × 25.4 × 14 (3.5 × 10 × 5.5)	11.2 × 5.6 × 20.3 (4.4 × 2.2 × 8)	39.6 × 28.4 × 8.1 (15 × 11 × 3)	35 × 23 × 25 (13.8 × 9 × 9.8)	28.8 × 24.4 × 19.7 (11.3 × 9.6 × 7.8)	24.4 × 21 × 19 (9.6 × 8.3 × 7.5)
Weight, kg (lb)	0.55 (1.2)	0.06 (0.13)	0.63 (1.4)	2.27 (5)	0.8 (1.8)	4.6 (10.1)	4.3–5.5 (9.5–12.1)	3.4–6.5 (7.6–14.4)	2.8–6.1 (6.3–13.5)
Green Features	None specified	None specified	None specified	None specified	None specified	None specified	None specified	None specified	None specified
FDA Clearance	Yes	Yes	Yes	Yes	Yes	Yes	Yes	Yes	Yes
CE Mark	Yes	Not specified	Yes	Yes	Yes	Yes	Yes	Yes	Yes

known and stable concentrations of NO are required. Commonly available concentrations currently range from 200 ppb to 500 ppm. An analyzer accuracy of ± 2% or better is recommended to optimize accuracy and reproducibility of exhaled and nasal gas sample NO analysis. It is highly desirable that exhaled NO analyzers be calibrated in the expected range of sample values (e.g., 10 to 100 ppb for exhaled samples and 0.4 to 50 ppm for nasal samples).

Daily calibration using the zero gas and one other standard NO concentration is recommended, but not absolutely essential; each analyzer manufacturer should recommend a desirable frequency of calibration. However, confirmation of stable ambient conditions (e.g., temperature, barometric pressure, humidity) is highly recommended for the calibration process. In the presence of unstable ambient conditions, frequent recalibration should be considered; at the very least, the zero point should be rechecked before each sample.

The chemiluminescence signal is very sensitive to changes in reaction chamber pressure, of which the major determinant is analyzer inlet gas sample flow. Thus, it is recommended that NO analyzer calibration and sample analysis always be performed at a constant inlet sample flow. Moreover, this inlet sample flow rate should be checked at regular intervals, depending on the stability of ambient laboratory conditions. Ozone chemiluminescence analyzers are sensitive to ambient conditions, including temperature, humidity, and exposure to sunlight.[35]

Exhaled and nasal gas samples are presumed to be fully saturated with water vapor; however, the drying of samples by passing through various drying agents (e.g., Drierite) is not recommended because of possible absorption of NO. An acceptable approach is the equilibration of sample humidity with ambient humidity (e.g., use Nafion tubing as the sample line). In all measurement systems, calibration gases (ambient temperature and pressure, dry [ATPD]) and clinical gas samples (body temperature [98.6°F/37°C] and pressure, saturated [BTPS]) should be measured under uniform humidity and temperature conditions. It is recommended that the quantitative effect of humidity on NO measurement should be measured and reported by the manufacturer of each NO analyzer. Quenching by water vapor should be less than 1% of measured NO signal per 1% volume H_2O.[35]

Major interferences with measurements of exhaled NO (eNO) include volatile anesthetic gases, which may be hazardous to the measurement system regarding chemical reactions; oxidation of analyzer and tubing materials; and risk of spontaneous combustion (e.g., O_3, electrical sparks in NO analyzers). Quenching by CO_2 should be less than 1% NO per 1% CO_2.[35] Also, alcohol-containing disinfectants can affect the analyzer performance and thus interfere with NO analysis.[36]

TABLE 7-4
Factors That Will Cause Increases or Decreases in Concentration of Exhaled Nitric Oxide

Increased Exhaled NO	Decreased Exhaled NO
Air pollution exposure	Alcohol ingestion
Chemical exposure	Caffeine
Chlorine dioxide	Chemical exposure
Fluoride	100% oxygen
Formaldehyde	Carbon dioxide
Latex	Heptane
Ozone	Nitrous oxide
Drugs	Water vapor
Enalapril	Drugs
L-arginine	Oxymetazoline
Papaverin	NO synthase inhibitors
Sodium nitroprusside	Exercise
Ingestion of arginine or nitrite-/nitrate-rich foods	Hypothermia
Upper respiratory tract infections	Menses
	Moderate altitude
	Repeated spirometry
	Smoking
	Sputum induction

Furthermore, expiratory flow, contamination by nasal NO, and dead space volume can all affect measurement of eNO.[37] A number of other factors that can influence eNO results are listed in Table 7-4.[38]

Currently Available Devices

As newer NO analyzers based on different measurement technologies become available, different specifications and specific guidelines may be required. Moreover, future equipment specifications will depend critically on clinical requirements. For example, analysis of FeNO during tidal breathing and in mechanically ventilated patients will require equipment with faster response times. Thus, the specifications in Table 7-5 are limited to the proposed application of measurement of FeNO and nasal NO in spontaneously breathing subjects using ozone-/NO_2-chemiluminescence–based analyzers.

TABLE 7-5
Types and Specifications of Exhaled Nitric Oxide Monitors

SPECIFICATIONS	MODEL			
	AEROCRINE NioxFlex	AEROCRINE NIOX MINO	ECO MEDICS CLD 88 sp	GE HEALTHCARE NOA 280i
Patient Population	Children: 4–17 years, adults	Children: 7–17 years, adults	Infants/children/adults	Infants/children/adults
Sensor				
Type	Chemiluminescence gas analyzer	Chemiluminescence gas analyzer	Not specified	Not specified
Life	Not specified	Not specified	Not specified	Not specified
Measurement				
Range	2–200 ppb	5–300 ppb	0.1–5,000 ppb	< 1–500,000 ppb
Accuracy	± 2.5 ppb of measured value < 50 ppb ± 5% of measured value > 50 ppb	± 5 ppb or max 10%	± 2%	± 5%
Detection level	2 ppb	5 ppb	0.06 ppb	Not specified
Linearity	< 2.5 ppb integral linearity	± 3 ppb	± 1% full scale	Not specified
Precision	< 2.5 ppb of measured value < 50 ppb < 5% of measured value > 50 ppb	< 3 ppb of measured value < 30 ppb < 10% of measured value ≥ 30 ppb	Not specified	1 ppb
Offset	± 3 ppb/14 days	Not specified	< 0.5 ppb per 6 hr	Not specified
Interference	< 10% of measurement value at 5% volume H_2O and 5% volume CO_2	Not specified	0.03 ppb	Not specified
Environmental				
Operating temperature	59°F to 85°F (15°C–30°C)	60°F to 85°F (16°C to 30°C)	50°F to 104°F (10°C–40°C)	32°F to 86°F (0°C to 30°C)
Relative humidity	30–75% (noncondensing)	20–60% RH (noncondensing)	5–95% RH (noncondensing)	0–90%
Operating pressure	860–1,060 hPa	10–15 psi (700–1,060 hPa)	Not specified	Not specified
Sampling				
Frequency	20 Hz	Not specified	Not specified	Not specified
Flow	Not specified	Not specified	Selectable type 1 or 3 (110 or 330 mL)	10–300 mL/min
Lag time	< 0.8 sec	Not specified	< 0.5 sec, software compensated	1 sec
Response time	< 1.5 sec	< 2 min	Not specified	67 milliseconds to 90% full scale
Rise time	10–90% in < 0.7 sec	Not specified	< 100 milliseconds	Not specified
Fall time	90%–100% in < 1 sec	Not specified	Not specified	Not specified
Calibration Interval	Recommended every 14 days, or whenever system is restarted or moved.	Not specified	Not specified	Not specified
Display	Not specified	PC screen	Not specified	Back-lit LCD screen ppb/ppm

(continued)

TABLE 7-5
Types and Specifications of Exhaled Nitric Oxide Monitors (*Continued*)

	MODEL			
	AEROCRINE	AEROCRINE	ECO MEDICS	GE HEALTHCARE
SPECIFICATIONS	NioxFlex	NIOX MINO	CLD 88 sp	NOA 280i
Outputs	USB ports	USB cable to PC	Printer	Analog: 0–1 V, 0–10 V, RS232, printer
Power Supply	100–240 VAC, 50–60 Hz	100–240 VAC, 50–60 Hz, 6 VDC (external power supply)	100–240 VAC, 50–60 Hz	120 V, 60 Hz (6A); 100 V, 50 or 60 Hz (7A); 230 V, 50 Hz (3A)
Dimensions W × H × D, in (cm)	11.81 × 19.68 × 15.75 (30 × 50 × 40)	5 × 9.1 × 3.8 (12.8 × 23 × 9.6)	5.25 × 19 × 17 (50 × 13.5 × 54)	6.2 × 16 × 20 (16 × 41 × 51)
Weight, g (lb)	4,000 (0.09)	800 (1.8)	2,400 (5.29)	1,600 (35)
Green Features	None specified	None specified	None specified	None specified
FDA Clearance	Yes	Yes	Not specified	Not specified
CE Mark	Yes	Yes	Yes	Not specified

Pulse Oximeters

Since their introduction into clinical practice, **pulse oximeters** have assumed a commanding position among noninvasive monitors in the clinical management of patients in a wide variety of situations, from anesthesia to critical care to home care.[39] Pulse oximeters provide noninvasive and continuous monitoring of hemoglobin oxygen saturation (SpO_2), generally expressed as a percentage (**Figure 7-11**). Pulse oximeters are of two types: stand-alone or modular units. Because they are based on light-absorbance changes resulting from arterial blood flow pulsations, pulse oximeters also provide a noninvasive, continuous, and instantaneous monitoring of pulse rate.[39] Pulse oximeters can provide early detection of hypoxia before other signs such as cyanosis are observed, and they may reduce the frequency of arterial puncture and invasive blood gas analysis when assessing the patient's oxygenation status.[40] Also, pulse oximeters can provide immediate detection of sudden changes in pulse rate (e.g., bradycardia and tachycardia). Most pulse oximeters also offer other display features, including alarm limits on oxygen saturation and pulse rate, plethysmograms, perfusion index, bar graphs indicating pulse amplitude, trending capabilities, and various system-status and error messages. For modular units, these displays are part of the patient's main vital signs monitor to which the unit is connected. A few manufacturers have developed pulse oximeters that can be safely used during magnetic resonance imaging (MRI) studies. MRI-compatible units typically use nonconductive fiber-optic cables

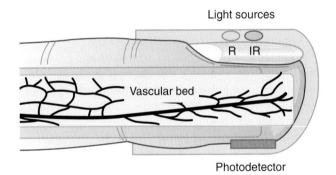

Light sources

R IR

Vascular bed

Photodetector

FIGURE 7-11 Pulse oximetry.

that will not cause radio-frequency (RF) burns and can reduce the occurrence of artifacts in magnetic resonance (MR) images. Several manufacturers have also introduced portable, battery-powered, handheld pulse oximeters for spot checks, short-term bedside monitoring, outpatient assessment, or emergency transport of patients.

Pulse oximetry is a standard of care throughout inpatient (anesthesia and critical care) and outpatient clinical settings. It is beneficial during sedation, while weaning from mechanical ventilation and/or supplemental oxygen, and in evaluating patient response to therapy and activity.[39,41] Pulse oximeters are also used during in-hospital transport, in diagnostic areas such as sleep laboratories and cardiac catheterization laboratories, and in outpatient centers and home care for spot checks and short-term monitoring.[39,41]

Principles of Operation

Pulse oximetry combines the principles of optical plethysmography and spectrophotometry to determine arterial hemoglobin oxygen saturation.[42] Optical plethysmography uses light absorption technology to reproduce waveforms produced by pulsatile blood. The changes that occur in the absorption of light due to vascular bed changes are reproduced by the pulse oximeter as plethysmographic waveforms. Spectrophotometry is the scientific technology that uses various wavelengths of light to perform quantitative measurement of light absorption through given substances.

Pulse oximeters' sensors are applied to an area of the body, such as a finger, a toe, an ear, or a forehead. Two wavelengths of red light at approximately 660 nm and infrared light at 930 nm are transmitted through the skin into the tissue by the sensor's light-emitting diodes (LEDs). These wavelengths are differentially absorbed by the blood's oxyhemoglobin (HbO_2), which is red and absorbs infrared light, and deoxyhemoglobin, which is blue and absorbs red light. The sensor's photodetector, which is on the opposite side of the LED, converts the transmitted light into electrical signals proportional to the absorbance; these are processed by the unit's microprocessor and saturation is displayed as a percent value.

When light is transmitted through a tissue, some of that light is absorbed by each constituent of the tissue; however, the only variable absorption is due to arterial pulsations. Each pulse of arterial blood causes cyclic variations in the path length of the transmitted light through the sensor site, varying the amount of light absorbed by the arterial blood. This varying absorption is translated into a plethysmographic waveform at both the red and infrared wavelengths.[42] A portion of the light passing through the sensor site is absorbed by venous blood, tissue, or bone components; however, this absorption is relatively constant over short periods of time and the microprocessor can isolate this constant when performing calculations. Most current units will have advanced signal-processing techniques that can read through motion artifact and/or conditions of low perfusion.[43] Also, to reduce small variations in displayed oxygen saturation values and to counter any false values from artifactual waveforms, pulse oximeters use algorithms to average data over few seconds.

Audible alarms on pulse oximeters sound when SpO_2 or pulse-rate alarm limits are violated. Most audible alarms can be manually temporarily silenced. Visual alarms can include all audible alarm conditions as well as low perfusion, low signal strength, low battery, probe status, silenced audible alarm, and system status.

Both disposable and reusable sensors are available for many oximeters.[44] Reusable sensors include finger probes, toe probes, ear probes, nasal probes, and foot probes. Disposable sensors, for single-patient use, are usually adhesive-style sensors that can be applied to a measurement site (e.g., finger, toe, foot). The probes are available in adult, pediatric, and neonatal sizes. To obtain valid data, the manufacturer's instructions must be followed regarding proper placement of the probe. Also, it is important to use the sensor type designed for the patient and site being monitored (Figure 7-12). Sensors used on the finger, toe, foot, nose, and ear are transmittance sensors; however, it is possible to use flat reflectance sensors, which measure the intensity of light reflected (backscattered) from the skin (e.g., forehead sensors). Depending on the application, one sensor type may be preferred (e.g., reflectance forehead sensors may be advantageous in the operating room for trauma patients who have damaged or poorly perfused transmittance sensor sites). Reflectance sensors may respond more quickly to desaturation than transmittance sensors do, especially in patients having poor peripheral perfusion.[45]

Calibration and Troubleshooting

Pulse oximeters are unique among noninvasive monitors in that they cannot be calibrated, nor is it common for calibration to be verified or accuracy assured by an external device when measurements are questioned. Each brand of pulse oximeter has its own empirically derived calibration algorithm to relate light transmission to oxygen saturation.

Several attempts have been made to verify the accuracy of pulse oximeters.[46] Volsko et al. used the Nonin Finger Phantom (Nonin Medical) to simulate SpO_2 values of 80%, 90%, and 97% as well as pulse rates of 120, 84, and 60 beats per minute to evaluate the function of several commercially available oximeters and probes used in the clinical setting.[47] They concluded that spot checks consisting of single measurements with the Nonin Finger Phantom device are probably adequate for evaluating the performance of pulse oximeters.[47] This device is commercially available, marketed as the BC Biomedical FingerSim.

Several factors can affect the performance and accuracy of pulse oximeters.[48,49] Interference from the surrounding environment can limit the use of pulse oximeters. Ambient light sources such as surgical lighting, bilirubin lights, and infrared sources (e.g., radiant warmers) can interfere with pulse oximeter sensors. Carefully covering or wrapping the sensor site with gauze or a towel can eliminate ambient light interference. Reusable clip-style sensors are generally less susceptible to ambient light interference than are disposable sensors. Reusable sensors have a design that is more rugged and more impermeable to light.

In low perfusion states caused by poor peripheral blood flow (e.g., hypotension, hypovolemia, hypothermia, and the administration of vasoactive agents), pulse oximeters may not be able to adequately differentiate between arterial pulsations and background noise.[49] As a result, the pulse oximeter may display readings that are

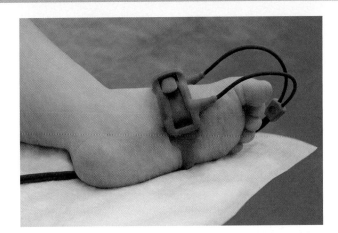
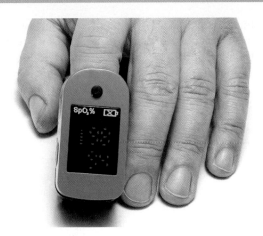
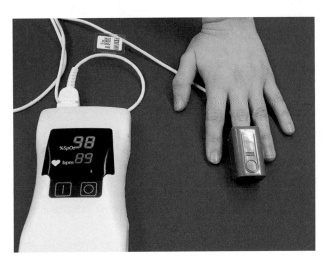

FIGURE 7-12 Different types of pulse oximeter sensors.

Top left photo © beerkoff/ShutterStock, Inc. Top right photo © RobByron/ShutterStock, Inc.

intermittent or absent. Reduction in pulse signal may also render the pulse oximeter more susceptible to interferences from other factors (e.g., motion artifact, ambient light). If the pulse amplitude is poor, the clinician may elect to choose an alternate site or sensor. Digital signal processing techniques offered by several suppliers allow assessment of perfusion (i.e., perfusion index) and for pulse oximeters to accurately read through low-perfusion conditions; an alarm will sound should a low-perfusion or no-pulse condition be detected.[50]

Pulse oximeters are also subject to motion artifact, which is a frequent cause of erratic measurement and spurious alarm conditions.[51] Motion artifacts are very common during transport and during frequent movement of the extremity being sampled, shivering, and seizures. Motion artifacts are usually reflected by an erratic pulse rate and/or an absent or distorted plethysmographic signal on the oximeter. Motion artifact can be reduced by selecting a less active sampling site for placement of sensor, by using snugly fitting sensors, by digital signal processing and adjusting the oximeter for a longer averaging time, and by electrocardiographic synchronization.

Because most pulse oximeters use two-wavelength spectrography, dysfunctional hemoglobins (e.g., carboxyhemoglobin, methemoglobin) may result in an inaccurately measured SpO_2 in most commercially available pulse oximeters. In the presence of carboxyhemoglobin, the pulse oximeters overestimate the true oxygen saturation by an amount roughly equal to the carboxyhemoglobin level.[52] In the presence of methemoglobin, the pulse oximeters read inaccurately low oxygen saturation when the oxygen saturation is high and inaccurately high when the oxygen saturation is low.[53] Pulse oximeters are accurate in the presence of fetal hemoglobin.[54]

A number of other factors can affect pulse oximetry measurements.[48,49] The accuracy of pulse oximeters may be affected by venous pulsation. To avoid spectral interference, nail polish should be removed if the pulse oximeter sensor is placed on the finger or toe. Dark skin pigmentation can decrease the accuracy and reliability of pulse oximeters. Extreme forms of anemia (i.e., hemoglobin levels less than 5 mg/dL) can prevent sufficient light from penetrating through to the photodetectors to obtain accurate results. Generally, bilirubin does not interfere significantly with pulse oximetry and may be insignificant even with bilirubin concentrations greater than 10 mg/dL. Other factors that may rule out pulse oximetry are the use of tourniquets, blood pressure cuffs, or intravenous infusion (which can cause vaso-constriction) in the same extremity as the oximeter.

Currently Available Devices

Pulse oximetry has become one of the most important clinical diagnostic tools and is a standard of care for almost every clinical situation. Because of its wide acceptance and use, several manufacturers are constantly releasing new, improved, and updated pulse oximeters that can be used as both stand-alone units and modular units with the capability of interfacing with anesthesia units or physiologic monitoring systems. Detailed descriptions of features and specifications of currently available pulse oximeters are presented in Appendix 7-A.

Transcutaneous Oxygen and Carbon Dioxide Monitors

Transcutaneous oxygen and **transcutaneous carbon dioxide** monitors use a combination electrode placed directly on the skin to measure skin PO_2 ($tcPO_2$) (**Figure 7-13**) and PCO_2 ($tcPCO_2$) (**Figure 7-14**). Measurement of transcutaneous PO_2 and PCO_2 is dependent on diffusion of oxygen and carbon dioxide from the circulation through the skin to the transcutaneous electrode that rests on the skin.[55] These measurements are not always equal to the arterial partial pressure of oxygen (pO_2) and carbon dioxide (pCO_2), but can be useful indicators of those values. In general, $tcPO_2$ is often similar to arterial pO_2 (particularly in neonates) whereas $tcPCO_2$ is higher than arterial pCO_2; some manufacturers incorporate a correction factor to account for this effect.

Continuous and noninvasive transcutaneous pO_2 and pCO_2 measurements can be used as alternatives for frequent invasive drawing and analyzing arterial blood samples. A number of factors affect the relationship between arterial blood gas levels and the transcutaneous blood levels of oxygen and carbon dioxide.[56,57] First, there is consumption of oxygen by the skin between the vascular bed and the transcutaneous electrode, which tends to decrease the $tcPO_2$ and increase the $tcPCO_2$. Second, the electrode heats the underlying skin, which tends to increase the $tcPO_2$ and $tcPCO_2$. Instrument response to acute changes in $tcPO_2$ and $tcPCO_2$ should be quick enough to show all clinically significant changes. The response time can be influenced by the material and size of the cathode, the pH of the electrolyte used in the sensor, and the membrane material.[55]

Transcutaneous monitors are available either as stand-alone units or as modules that can be integrated into physiologic monitoring systems. Some

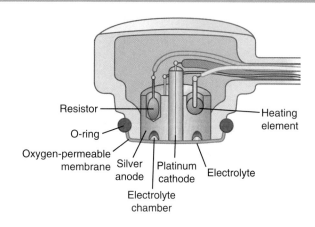

FIGURE 7-13 Schematic of the $tcPO_2$ electrode.

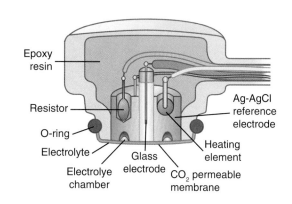

FIGURE 7-14 Schematic of the $tcPCO_2$ electrode.

stand-alone models incorporate microprocessors for storing transcutaneous blood gas trends, real-time blood gas readings, histograms, heating power trends, and thermistor's temperature and alarms for high and low $tcPO_2$ and $tcPCO_2$ limits. Additional alarms monitor system malfunctions such as disconnected sensors, unbalanced or inoperative thermistors, and deviations from preset temperatures. Transcutaneous O_2 and CO_2 monitors that are modular components of physiologic monitoring systems can be integrated with other monitors, such as those for electrocardiography, respiration, pressure, temperature, and pulse oximetry.

Researchers continue to look for the most stable and practical sensor materials, especially those that minimize skin irritation and those that require lower temperatures. In addition, researchers continue to add to the range of transcutaneous monitoring applications, including use in neonatal intensive care units and shock trauma units.

Principles of Operation

Measurement of tcPO₂

Transcutaneous PO_2 is measured with a miniaturized polarograhic Clark electrode. The electrode consists of a silver anode surrounding a platinum or gold cathode, an electrolyte, a semipermeable membrane, and a heating element (Figure 7-13). A principle unique to transcutaneous PO_2 measurement is that the electrode is heated to some temperature greater than body temperature (usually to 109.4°F–113°F [43°C–45°C]), depending on the patient's age and skin thickness).[55] This significantly increases the arterial blood supply to the dermal capillary bed by capillary vasodilation. Higher skin temperatures also enhance blood gas diffusion by increasing the rate at which O_2 dissociates from hemoglobin in the red blood cells, by elevating the rate at which the vital cells of the skin consume O_2 and generate CO_2, and by melting the lipid component of the stratum corneum to facilitate O_2 diffusion across the skin surface. The sensor uses a thermistor to monitor and maintain the desired temperature of the heating ring. After permeating the skin surface, O_2 diffuses through the sensor's membrane, usually made of either Teflon, polyethylene, or polypropylene, to the cathode where reduction of the oxygen generates an electrical current that is directly proportional to the concentration of oxygen against the outer membrane surface. The electrical current is measured and converted to millimeters of mercury (mm Hg) for display on the monitor.[58]

Measurement of $tcPCO_2$

Transcutaneous PCO_2 is measured with a miniaturized Severinghaus electrode. The electrode consists of a pH electrode, a reference electrode, an electrolyte solution, a Teflon membrane, and a heating element (Figure 7-14).[57] Similar to the $tcPO_2$ sensor, the $tcPCO_2$ sensor contains a heating element to warm the skin to a temperature of 107.6°F–113°F (42°C–45°C). The CO_2 diffuses through the stratum corneum by the warming of the skin and across the sensor membrane to react with the electrolyte to form hydrogen and bicarbonate ions. The hydrogen ions produced are linearly related to the amount of CO_2 diffusing across the membrane, as described in the Henderson-Hasselbalch equation. The hydrogen ions generate a voltage change between the two cells that is measured and converted to a $tcPCO_2$ reading in mm Hg.[57] This value is then shown on a digital display.

Some transcutaneous oxygen and carbon dioxide monitors measure both $tcPCO_2$ and $tcPO_2$ by using either two separate sensors or one sensor that has the ability to detect both parameters. The $tcPCO_2/tcPO_2$ sensor is a composite of separate $tcPCO_2$ and $tcPO_2$ sensors, consisting of a pH electrode, an O_2 cathode and heated reference electrode, a Teflon membrane, and bicarbonate ethylene glycol electrolyte, enclosed in a shielded cup with the sensor's electronics. Operation of the combination sensor is the same as that described for each type of transcutaneous sensor.

Measurement of SpO_2

Some transcutaneous oxygen and dioxide monitors also measure SpO_2 with a single sensor, typically attached to the earlobe. This measurement is based on the same principal as for the regular pulse oximeters previously described.

Calibration and Troubleshooting

There are several nonphysiologic factors that can affect measurements of $tcPO_2$ and $tcPCO_2$.[56,59] These factors include ambient-air temperature, humidity, barometric pressure, membrane thickness, rate of O_2 and CO_2 diffusion across the electrolyte, and the polarization voltage of the electrode. All transcutaneous oxygen and carbon dioxide monitors developed in recent years adjust automatically for these variables, but because some of these factors are dynamic and can fluctuate widely, the sensors must be periodically calibrated.

Calibration of the $tcPO_2$ Sensor

The $tcPO_2$ monitor is zeroed either by the addition of a drop of zero solution (i.e., solution with no free O_2) to the sensor membrane or by an electronic method that specifically adjusts the monitor's sensing circuitry to a zero current level. After zeroing, the unit's sensor is exposed to ambient air having an oxygen concentration of 20.9% for several minutes to set the high point. Some units can preset the values for barometric pressure, temperature, and/or relative humidity and automatically calibrate the PO_2; other units require manual adjustment using a chart supplied by the manufacturer that lists PO_2 values in relation to barometric pressure.

Calibration of the $tcPCO_2$ Sensor

One-point and two-point calibrations are generally required to ensure reliable $tcPCO_2$ electrode response. One-point calibration consists of exposing the electrode surface to 5% CO_2 gas for several minutes, then comparing the displayed value to the calculated calibration value. A variance of approximately ± 2 mm Hg is within acceptable drift limits. This one-point calibration is usually performed every 4 hours during continuous use and after any discontinuance of use. A two-point calibration consists of performing the procedure with both 5% and 10% CO_2 gas. A two-point calibration is usually performed at least once during a 24-hour period of continuous use, after membrane and electrolyte change, and whenever the clinical reliability of the values is in doubt. Calibration readings that vary more than 4 mm Hg from the calculated values indicate problems that must be identified and corrected.

With continuous use, a weekly cleaning of dried electrolyte from the electrode surface and applying a new membrane are recommended. Transcutaneous O_2 and CO_2 monitors not in use for more than 24 hours should be turned off to minimize evaporation of the electrolyte by the heating element. If the electrode has a newly applied electrolyte and membrane, it can be stored in this way for up to 1 week and be used at any time after a one-point calibration for the $tcPO_2$ electrode or a two-point calibration for the $tcPCO_2$ electrode.

The results from transcutaneous O_2 and CO_2 monitors should be compared regularly with arterial blood gas levels. Because of differences in skin permeability, cellular metabolic effects, unusual capillary configurations, and differences in temperature between capillary and arterial blood, readings of $tcPO_2$ and $tcPCO_2$ are not always a direct reflection of PaO_2 and $PaCO_2$.[55] Also, impaired peripheral circulation, as in cases of shock or peripheral vascular disease or very low core body temperature, can prevent the transcutaneous O_2 and CO_2 sensor from adequately tracking arterial blood gas levels.[60,61]

The sensor's elevated temperature and long duration of use in the same location can lead to varying degrees of burns. Therefore, frequent sensor relocation can help prevent burns; however, this means frequent recalibrations and interruption of measurements. In addition, adhesive-fastened sensors can fall off the skin, requiring recalibration and stabilization. Other factors may interfere with transcutaneous oxygen and carbon dioxide measurements. When a sensor is taped to a patient, mechanical pressure may compress underlying blood vessels and reduce the $tcPO_2$ value. During surgery, electrosurgical unit activation can cause the transcutaneous monitor to display inaccurate values. The performance and safety characteristics of $tcPO_2$ monitors during defibrillation are also not well known; users should remove the $tcPO_2$ sensor before defibrillating patients.

Failure to remove zero solution from the sensor's membrane as soon as possible following calibration can result in electrolyte contamination because of zero-solution diffusion through the membrane, necessitating membrane replacement. Failure to periodically check the sensor using a zero solution or calibration gas can result in inaccurate gas readings. The user must determine and set the appropriate high and low alarm limits for each patient, and differences among patients and their therapies must be considered when setting these limits.

Currently Available Devices

Transcutaneous oxygen and carbon dioxide monitors continue to be a stable technology, largely unchanged in the last few decades. Manufacturers have made improvements to instrument ease of use, reliability, and automated features such as calibration. Greater interfacing capabilities allow users to quickly and easily transfer patient data or incorporate additional patient monitoring devices. Technical features and specifications of currently available monitors are shown in Appendix 7-B.

Indirect Calorimetry

Indirect calorimetry is the method by which energy expenditure and the type and rate of substrate utilization are estimated in vivo. It is the calculation of energy expenditure and estimation of carbohydrates, fats, and proteins consumption. This technique is noninvasive and can be advantageously combined with other clinical methods to evaluate numerous aspects of nutrient assimilation,[62] mechanical ventilation and weaning invasive ventilatory support,[63] thermogenesis, the energetics of physical exercise, and the pathogenesis of metabolic diseases.[64] Until the late 1970s, the technology to measure energy expenditure in mechanically ventilated patients was not available. Recent technical progresses and research findings have led to the availability of indirect calorimetry as a valuable clinical tool in intensive care units, during anesthesia, as well as on general patients' wards. Although many systems have been devised, all indirect calorimetry works by one of two methods: the open-circuit method or the closed-circuit method.

Principles of Operation

Indirect calorimetry is based on the theory that all of a person's energy is derived from the oxidation of carbohydrates, fats, and proteins, and that the ratio of carbon dioxide produced to oxygen consumed (i.e., the respiratory quotient) is characteristic of the fuel being burned.[65]

Open-Circuit Method

The open-circuit method can be used to measure energy expenditure in spontaneously and mechanically ventilated patients. With the open-circuit method, the concentrations and volumes of inspired and expired gases are measured to determine oxygen consumption ($\dot{V}O_2$) and carbon dioxide production ($\dot{V}CO_2$). These measurements are converted to energy using the Weir equation:[66]

$$\text{Energy} = [\dot{V}O_2 \times 3.941) + (\dot{V}CO_2 \times 1.11)] \times 1,440$$

where energy is in cal/day, and $\dot{V}O_2$ and $\dot{V}CO_2$ are in mL/min.

Open-circuit calorimeters use oxygen and carbon dioxide analyzers, a volume measuring device, and a mixing chamber. Expired gases are directed into a collecting chamber containing baffles to ensure adequate mixing of gases. A vacuum pump withdraws a small sample of the mixed expired gas over the analyzers for determination of oxygen and carbon dioxide concentrations. At preselected intervals, the inspired oxygen and carbon dioxide concentrations are measured for determination of the inspired to expired oxygen and carbon dioxide concentration differences.

The entire volume of gas then exits through a volume transducer for measurement of minute ventilation. A pressure transducer ensures pressure-compensated gas measurements and a thermistor is used for correction of volumes to body temperature pressure saturated. A microprocessor controls all the indirect calorimeter functions, performs all the necessary calculations, stores the data, and provides a printed copy of all the measurements and calculations.

Closed-Circuit Method

The closed-circuit method differs from the open-circuit technique only in the measurement of oxygen consumption. The key components of a closed-circuit calorimeter are a volumetric spirometer, mixing chamber, carbon dioxide analyzer, and carbon dioxide absorber. The measurement of oxygen consumption is made by filling the spirometer with a known volume of oxygen and connecting it to the patient by either mask, mouthpiece, endotracheal tube, or tracheostomy. As the patient breathes from the spirometer, oxygen is consumed and carbon dioxide is produced. The decrease in volume over time will be equal to the oxygen consumption.

Calibration and Troubleshooting

Calibration of indirect calorimeters involves the calibration of gas analyzers, pressure transducer, and flow sensor. Most indirect calorimeters offer an automatic gas calibration through internal valves and tubings from a gas cylinder (95% oxygen and 5% carbon dioxide) connected to or inside the monitors. Manual calibration through a sampling line from external gas cylinders is also possible. Manual calibration should never be done with gases containing nitrous oxide. Usually, the pressure calibration should be made every 6 months for accurate measurement of barometric pressure, unless there are major fluctuations in barometric pressure. The flow sensors are usually calibrated using the alcohol burning test once every 2 to 6 months depending on the stability of the flow sensor.

It is recommended that metabolic monitors should be calibrated once every day for gas analyzers, preferably immediately before each measurement to ensure optimum accuracy. Most manufacturers provide an easy-to-follow, step-by-step algorithm to calibrate and troubleshoot indirect calorimeters.

Open-Circuit Method

For accurate measurements of energy expenditure with the open-circuit technique, the fraction of inspired oxygen (F_IO_2) must be stable (± 0.005%). This can be achieved with the use of an air–oxygen blender that will provide a stable fraction of mixed air–oxygen concentration. Also, the whole system must be leak free because loss of gas from the system does not allow for complete gas collection, and addition of gas from the atmosphere causes dilution of gas concentrations. In the event of significant drifts in the measurements of gas concentrations, the operator must check and ensure that all connections are tight and the system is leak free. For spontaneously breathing patients, leaks around the face mask are common. However, in mechanically ventilated patients with either a tracheostomy or endotracheal tube, leaky cuffs are the main reason for inaccurate measurements.[67] Also, it is difficult to ensure accurate measurements in patients with bronchopleural leaks. Finally, in mechanical ventilators using continuous-flow systems, the inspired and expired gases must be completely separated to be able to perform accurate measurements of energy expenditure with the open-circuit technique.

Closed-Circuit Method

As with the open-circuit technique, prevention of leaks is essential for the accurate measurement of oxygen consumption and carbon dioxide production. Also, as the volume of the spirometer decreases to a critical point, the measurement must be interrupted until the spirometer is refilled with oxygen. Furthermore, when closed-system calorimetry is used with mechanically ventilated patients, there is an increase in compressible volume, and sensitivity for triggering assisted breaths is decreased. Depending on peak airway pressure, the ventilator volume may have to be increased by 50% to 75% to ensure adequate minute ventilation of the patient. Generally, the closed-circuit system should not be used with low-rate intermittent mandatory ventilation or continuous-flow systems.

Currently Available Devices

Recent advances in microprocessor technology have made it relatively easy for clinicians to accurately measure energy needs and substrate utilization patterns in hospitalized patients, whether they are spontaneously breathing or receiving invasive mechanical ventilation. Several devices have been developed as either stand-alone or modular units to be part of the patient monitoring/management armamentarium. The features and specifications of such devices are provided in Appendix 7-C.

Esophageal Pressure

The measurement of **esophageal pressure** with balloon-tipped catheters has been used with great success over the past half century to delineate the physiology of the mechanical respiratory system. Pleural pressure values estimated from esophageal pressure measurements allow differentiation between and analysis of lung and chest wall compliances.[68] With this technique, a balloon-tipped catheter (**Figure 7-15**) attached to a pressure transducer is introduced into the lower esophagus, adjacent to the pleura, and used to measure

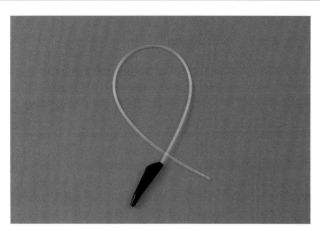

FIGURE 7-15 Esophageal balloon catheter.

esophageal pressure as an indirect measurement of pleural pressure. This allows the most accurate measurement of the transpulmonary pressure (i.e., the distending pressure of the alveoli), which is defined as the difference between the pressure applied at the airway and the pleural pressure.[68] Not only will esophageal manometry allow measurement of chest wall mechanics, but it also may be useful in determination of auto-PEEP, work of breathing, adjustment of PEEP during mechanical ventilation of acute respiratory distress syndrome (ARDS) patients, and weaning patients from mechanical ventilation.[69-71]

Principles of Operation

Esophageal manometry is not an automated procedure. It is measured from an air-filled balloon placed in the lower third of the esophagus. The proximal end is connected to a standard pressure transducer for continuous measurement and display of the pleural pressure. Some of these transducers are built into modern mechanical ventilators (e.g., Avea, Carefusion) whereas others are stand-alone respiratory monitoring systems (Bicore and Ventrak, both no longer commercially available). Experience is needed to ensure accurate balloon placement and to interpret results. Initially, the catheter is inserted into the stomach where positive pressure is observed during inspiration. Then the catheter is slowly withdrawn until negative pressure is observed during inspiration. The balloon is initially inflated with 6 to 10 mL of air to expand it completely, after which all of the air except 0.5 to 1.5 mL is removed. Gastric tubes are commercially available with a built-in esophageal balloon, which allows esophageal pressure monitoring during enteral feeding.

There has been debate as to whether esophageal balloons accurately represent pleural pressure, particularly in the mechanically ventilated patient.[72] A number of assumptions must be made, including that the transmural esophageal pressure is negligible and that there is no compression of the esophagus by other intrathoracic structures (heart and mediastinum). These measurements are most easily made in awake, cooperative patients who can perform maneuvers to help confirm optimal balloon placement. Unfortunately, direct measurement is invasive, so comparison with a gold standard is difficult. Some of these concerns have been addressed. For example, Washko and colleagues[73] evaluated esophageal pressures in healthy subjects in both the sitting and supine position. There was a small change, partly explained by changes in relaxation volume (functional residual capacity [FRC]) in the two positions, and partly by the change in position. The magnitude of change was less than 3 cm H_2O. Baydur and colleagues[74] also evaluated esophageal manometry at a variety of lung volumes and balloon positions within the esophagus; there were only small changes. However, it may not be valid to extrapolate data from normal subjects to those of critically ill mechanically ventilated patients.

Calibration and Troubleshooting

Calibration of the esophageal balloon involves mainly the calibration of the pressure transducer after making sure that all connections are made appropriately and the balloon is placed in the appropriate position. Whether it is part of a stand-alone monitor or incorporated into a mechanical ventilator, calibration is an automatic procedure with step-by-step instructions for any operator's intervention. Usually the operator will select the calibration option/menu and follow the step-by-step instructions. Generally the first step in the calibration process is to perform the leak/fill test by maximal inflation of the balloon, then deflation, and finally partial reinflation.

Esophageal pressure monitoring is not commonly used, owing to its semi-invasive nature and technical difficulties with proper placement of the esophageal balloon. The use of an esophageal catheter is contraindicated in patients with esophageal disease including esophageal varices, tumors, ulcerations, or diverticulitis. In all cases, insertion of the esophageal catheter must be done with extreme care to avoid trauma to the catheter balloon and the esophageal mucosa and/or epistaxis. If resistance is felt or epistaxis occurs during a nasal insertion, the catheter should be withdrawn and insertion through the other nare should be attempted. Although nasal insertion is preferred, the esophageal catheter may also be placed orally. If vomiting occurs during insertion, the esophageal catheter should be removed to allow the patient to stabilize and another attempt should be made as tolerated.

In patients already having endotracheal tubes in place, caution should be taken to not insert the esophageal catheter into the trachea. The position of the esophageal catheter should be checked after insertion and on a daily basis thereafter following the proper procedure or by using x-rays. To ensure optimal functioning of the esophageal

TABLE 7-6
Mechanical Ventilators with Esophageal Pressure Monitoring

SPECIFICATIONS	MODEL	
	CAREFUSION	HAMILTON MEDICAL
	AVEA	GALILEO
Esophageal Port	Yes	Yes
Esophageal Catheter	Yes	No (alternative vendor)
Calibration/Balloon Filling	Automatic	Manual

catheter, most manufacturers recommend replacing the esophageal catheter after 29 days of use. These catheters are intended for single patient use. Prior to removing the esophageal catheter, the balloon should be completely deflated. Disconnection and displacement of the catheter are possible causes of failure of the esophageal monitor. After confirmation of proper placement of the balloon, a good fixation of the gastric tube incorporating the esophageal balloon will prevent such failures.

Currently Available Devices

Although measurement of esophageal pressure during spontaneous breathing and during mechanical ventilation is theoretically appealing, no clinical trial has yet shown an outcome benefit of routine esophageal manometry in patients with acute respiratory failure. As a result, the balloon-tipped catheters and associated monitoring equipment are not commonly available for clinical use (**Table 7-6**). The subject requires more studies and findings on the utility of esophageal pressure monitoring as a valuable monitoring tool at the bedside.

Neonatal Apnea Monitors

An apnea monitor is a complete monitoring system intended to detect and to alarm primarily upon the cessation of breathing timed from the last detected breath. The apnea monitor also includes indirect methods of apnea detection such as monitoring of heart rate and other physiological parameters linked to the presence or absence of adequate respiration, such as heart rate and/or oxygen saturation. Apneas in neonates can result in a fast drop in oxygen concentration levels in the blood and tissues, which can lead to irreversible brain damage and, if prolonged and undetected, death.[75] Premature and low-birth-weight infants are particularly likely to exhibit apneic breathing patterns (i.e., apneic spells) for some time after birth and until full maturity of their respiratory control system.[75,76] Because the onset of apnea is unpredictable and its effects can be devastating,

apnea monitors are necessary to provide constant monitoring of those patients at risk.

Principles of Operation

Neonatal apnea monitors are designed to sense breathing activity in neonates and to trigger visual or audible alarms when a certain length of time elapses without the detection of a breath (**Figure 7-16**). Current detection methods include impedance pneumography, thermistors, infrared CO_2 sensors, mattress pressure pads, and pneumatic abdominal sensors.[77-79]

Impedance pneumography is most often used in home apnea monitoring units. The monitor detects small changes in electrical impedance as lung volumes change from air entering and leaving the lungs during respiration. These monitors pass a safe, low-amplitude, high-frequency (20 to 120 kHz) current through the chest by means of two electrodes placed on the right and left sides of the chest. Impedance variations in the thorax result in voltage variations in the monitor's detector circuit; these variations are interpreted as breaths. The same electrodes are also used to monitor the electrical activity of the heart and determine heart rate.

Thermistors, proximal airway pressure sensors, and carbon dioxide sensors are more direct methods

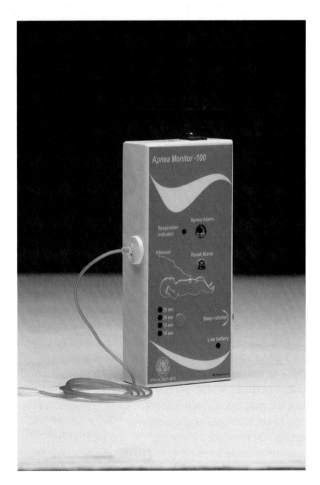

FIGURE 7-16 Neonatal apnea monitor.
Courtesy of Phoenix Medical Systems.

for monitoring of respiration by detecting airflow into and out of the lung. A thermistor is a temperature-sensitive device typically placed in front of the mouth and/or under the nose. As the patient breathes, the cool inhaled gas entering the lungs and the warm exhaled gas from the lungs change the thermistor temperature and affect its electrical resistance. These changes are registered as breaths. Infrared (IR) CO_2 sensors measure the partial pressure of CO_2 in the patient's exhaled gases. A cannula is placed in front of the nose and connected with tubing to a pump that continuously draws gas from in front of the nose that contains CO_2 whenever the patient is breathing. The changes in the CO_2 concentration are interpreted as breaths.

Mattress-type motion sensors monitor changes in the capacitance or resistance of a mattress transducer, and the changes in pressure caused by respiratory motion are interpreted as breaths by the monitor.

Pneumatic abdominal sensors use a pressure-sensitive capsule that is placed on the abdomen. Where pressure changes caused by the expansion and contraction of the abdomen occur during respiration, these are interpreted as breaths.

Even though various methods are used to sense respiration, all units use a similar approach to detect apnea. Apnea is detected and alarms are activated when the time elapsed since the last detected breath exceeds a limit preset by the operator. This time span can range from 0 to 60 seconds. Several apnea monitors have respiration and/or electrocardiogram (ECG) sensitivity settings, which are adjusted based on the size of the signal that is to be interpreted as a breath or heartbeat. Instrument sensitivity can be set manually or automatically and is usually set low enough to detect weak respiratory signals yet high enough to disregard extraneous signals (e.g., artifact).

In addition to detecting apnea, many apnea monitors incorporate a heart rate monitor. Even if respiration-detection circuitry fails to indicate a prolonged apneic episode, the heart rate monitor will detect bradycardia, which can be associated with hypoxia, and an alarm will sound. Similarly, some models include tachycardia (fast heart rate) alarms and display numerical heart rate data. Options for monitoring blood pressure and hemoglobin oxygen saturation by pulse oximetry (SpO_2) are available with some apnea monitors.

Some apnea monitors have the ability to record two or more channels of patient event data ranging from several hours to several months, depending on the amount and format of data and the parameters stored. Recorded data fall into two categories: patient (e.g., respiratory rate, heart rate) and equipment (e.g., power on/off, low battery). These data can be used to ensure that the monitor is being used properly, to distinguish true from false alarms, and to troubleshoot equipment problems. The data stored in the memory can be managed one of three ways. Some units overwrite the old data with more recent events; others keep the data that satisfies specific criteria based on the duration of the events; and some stop storing data when the memory is filled.

Calibration and Troubleshooting

Neonatal apnea monitors do not need frequent or extensive calibration, but they need to run a functional self-test to check that all the features of the unit are functioning properly. These functional self-tests are usually performed at least once a week or whenever a lead wire or the patient's cable is changed.

Some apnea monitors may fail to alarm during an apneic episode because they sense artifact as respiration.[80] Typical artifacts include vibrations from nearby instruments, heart activity, and patient movement. Electromagnetic emissions from electronic devices (e.g., home appliances) can also cause interference, possibly leading to false breath and heartbeat detection. Misinterpreting impedance changes because of heartbeats perceived as breaths is especially likely when instrument sensitivity is improperly adjusted to be too sensitive. Some monitors attempt to reduce the incidence of such signal misinterpretation by using artifact detection and rejection algorithms. In such cases, the respiration signal will not be counted when the measured respiratory rate coincides with the measured heart rate. Apnea monitoring by means of impedance pneumography or motion detection may also misinterpret diaphragmatic activity (e.g., gasping during upper-airway obstruction) as a breath.

Loose leads are a common problem encountered with neonatal apnea monitors. Also, it is possible that connections between electrodes, lead wires, and patient cable are not properly made, or lead wires, patient cable, and electrodes become defective. Clinicians should verify that the baby's skin underneath the electrodes is clean, that the electrodes are clean, and that the lead wires are fully inserted into the electrodes and patient cable. Lead wires, patient cable, and electrodes should be evaluated for possible replacement.

Currently Available Devices

Apnea monitoring has been used in hospitals and in patients' homes since the early 1970s. As monitor designs progressed, features such as heart rate detection, noise suppression, automatic sensitivity adjustment, and signal-processing algorithms were added for improved performance. Most current designs include the ability to record, display, and print patient and equipment data. As the technology advances, these monitors will be able to record more channels of information for longer periods of time. The description and technical specifications of currently available neonatal apnea monitors are shown in **Table 7-7**.

Neonatal Apnea Monitors   205

TABLE 7-7
Description and Technical Specifications of Neonatal Apnea Monitors

	MODEL							
	BERTOCCHI	BERTOCCHI	GETEMED	HISENSE	PHILIPS CHILDREN'S MEDICAL VENTURES	PHILIPS CHILDREN'S MEDICAL VENTURES	PHILIPS CHILDREN'S MEDICAL VENTURES	PHOENIX
SPECIFICATIONS	GB 62	GB 62AC	VITAGUARD VG 2100	BABYSENSE CU-100/2	SMARTMONITOR 2 4002: SMARTMONITOR 2 4003	SMARTMONITOR 2 PROFESSIONAL SERIES	SMARTMONITOR 2 PROFESSIONAL SERIES LIGHT	100 AM
Patient Population	Infant	Infant	Adult, pediatric, infant	Infant	Infant	Adult, pediatric, infant	Adult, pediatric, infant	Infant
Application	Home, hospital	Home, hospital	Ambulatory and clinical	Home, hospital, nursery	Home, hospita	Home, hospital	Home, hospital	Home, hospital
Configuration	Stand-alone	Stand-alone	Stand-alone	Stand-alone	Stand-alone	Stand-alone	Stand-alone	Stand-alone
Detection Method	Pneumatic sensor	Pneumatic sensor	Impedance	Piezoelectric pad	Impedance	Impedance	Impedance	Pressure sensor
Breath Detector								
Max sensitivity, Ω	NA	NA	0.2	NA	0.2	0.2	0.2	NA
Sensitivity adjust	Automatic	Automatic	Automatic	Automatic	Fixed	Fixed	Fixed	Automatic
Breath indicator	Audible and visual	Audible and visual	LED/LCD	Audible and visual	Visual	Visual	Visual	Audible
Apnea delay, sec	10, 20	10, 20	8–34, user-selectable	20	10, 15, 20, 25, 30, 40	10, 15, 20, 25, 30, 40	10, 15, 20, 25, 30, 40	10, 10, 15, 20
Alarm disable	No	No	No	No	No	≤ 60 sec in hospital mode only	≤ 60 sec in hospital mode only	No
Disable indicator	NA	NA	NA	NA	NA	NA	NA	NA
Apnea alarm silence	Automatic	Automatic	30–120	No	Automatic	Automatic	Automatic	Manual
Visual alarm memory	No	No	Yes	No	Yes	Yes	Yes	No
Breath rate meter	No	No	Yes	No	Yes	Yes	Yes	No
Type	NA	NA	Not specified	NA	Not specified	Not specified	Not specified	NA
Range, breaths/min	NA	NA	4–120	NA	0–120	0–120	0–120	NA

(continued)

TABLE 7-7
Description and Technical Specifications of Neonatal Apnea Monitors *(Continued)*

					MODEL			
	BERTOCCHI	BERTOCCHI	GETEMED	HISENSE	PHILIPS CHILDREN'S MEDICAL VENTURES	PHILIPS CHILDREN'S MEDICAL VENTURES	PHILIPS CHILDREN'S MEDICAL VENTURES	PHOENIX
SPECIFICATIONS	GB 62	GB 62AC	VITAGUARD VG 2100	BABYSENSE CU-100/2	SMARTMONITOR 2 4002: SMARTMONITOR 2 4003	SMARTMONITOR 2 PROFESSIONAL SERIES	SMARTMONITOR 2 PROFESSIONAL SERIES LIGHT	100 AM
Low/high alarm, breaths/min	NA	NA	No (central apnea only)	NA	4 (low)	4 (low)	4 (low)	NA
ECG Functions	No	No	Yes	No	Yes	Yes	Yes	No
QRS sensitivity, mV	NA	NA	0.2	NA	0.2	0.2	0.2	NA
Ratemeter	NA	NA	Yes	NA	Yes	Yes	Yes	NA
Heart rate alarm	NA	NA	Yes	NA	Yes	Yes	Yes	NA
Low/high, bpm	NA	NA	20–300	NA	40–100/90–270	40–100/90–270	40–100/90–270	NA
Lead Fault Alarm	Audible and visual	Audible and visual	Yes	Audible and visual	Audible and visual	Audible and visual	Audible and visual	Audible and visual
Memory	No	No	Yes	No	2 MB	4 MB	4 MB	No
Configuration	NA	NA	Event, FD, trend compliance	NA	Internal	Internal	Internal	NA
Data types	NA	NA	Respiration, ECG, HR, basal impedance, status, analog imputs	NA	Waveform	Waveform	Waveform	NA
Computer required	NA	NA	Yes	NA	For data	For data	For data	NA
Mode	NA	NA	Download via USB	NA	Event, event log, continuous	Event, event log, continuous	Event, event Icg, continuous	NA
Documented parameters	NA	NA	Respiration, ECG, HR, alarm types	NA	Bradycardia, tachycardia, apnea; can also trigger from external devices such as pulse oximeters	Bradycardia, tachycardia, apnea, SpO$_2$; can also trigger from external devices	Bradycardia, tachycardia, apnea; can also trigger from external devices	NA

TABLE 7-7
Description and Technical Specifications of Neonatal Apnea Monitors (*Continued*)

	MODEL							
	BERTOCCHI	BERTOCCHI	GETEMED	HISENSE	PHILIPS CHILDREN'S MEDICAL VENTURES	PHILIPS CHILDREN'S MEDICAL VENTURES	PHILIPS CHILDREN'S MEDICAL VENTURES	PHOENIX
SPECIFICATIONS	GB 62	GB 62AC	VITAGUARD VG 2100	BABYSENSE CU-100/2	SMARTMONITOR 2 4002: SMARTMONITOR 2 4003	SMARTMONITOR 2 PROFESSIONAL SERIES	SMARTMONITOR 2 PROFESSIONAL SERIES LIGHT	100 AM
Max no. events logged	NA	NA	200	NA	1,000	1,000 patient, 1,000 equipment	1,000 patient, 1,000 equipment	1
Max no. waveforms logged	NA	NA	All, 2 min before and 1 min after event	~180	~180	≥ 300 including QRS	≥ 300 including QRS	NA
Battery backup	NA	NA	Yes	Battery operated	Yes	Yes	Yes	Yes
External inputs	NA	NA	2 analog	NA	4 auxiliary channels	4 auxiliary channels, 2 external trigger channels	4 auxiliary channels, 2 external trigger channels	Yes
Other features	NA	NA	Online data output, nurse call, external alarm unit	Analysis of breathing	None specified	None specified	None specified	Low-battery indicator
Display	No	No	Yes	No	No	Yes	Yes	No
Channels	NA	NA	2 (respiration and ECG)	NA	NA	Heart rate, respiration rate, SpO$_2$	Heart rate, respiration rate, SpO$_2$	NA
Sweep speed, mm/sec	NA	NA	12.5	NA	NA	NA	NA	NA
Trending	NA	NA	7 days	NA	NA	NA	NA	NA
Recorder	No	No	No	No	Event, event log, continuous	Event, event log, continuous	Event, event log, continuous	No
Channels	NA	NA	NA	NA	ECG, respiration, heart rate, respiratory rate	ECG, respiration, heart rate, respiratory rate, SpO$_2$, plethysmograph, pulse rate	ECG, respiration, heart rate, respiratory rate	NA

(continued)

TABLE 7-7
Description and Technical Specifications of Neonatal Apnea Monitors (Continued)

SPECIFICATIONS	BERTOCCHI GB 62	BERTOCCHI GB 62AC	GETEMED VITAGUARD VG 2100	HISENSE BABYSENSE CU-100/2	PHILIPS CHILDREN'S MEDICAL VENTURES SMARTMONITOR 2 4002: SMARTMONITOR 2 4003	PHILIPS CHILDREN'S MEDICAL VENTURES SMARTMONITOR 2 PROFESSIONAL SERIES	PHILIPS CHILDREN'S MEDICAL VENTURES SMARTMONITOR 2 PROFESSIONAL SERIES LIGHT	PHOENIX 100 AM
Paper speed, mm/sec	NA	NA	NA	NA	NA	NA	NA	NA
Power								
Line voltage, VAC	Standard	NA	120/240	NA	100/134 or 220/240	100/134 or 220/240	100/134 or 220/240	230
Battery type	9 V or lithium	9 V or lithium; GF22 for stimulator	Ni-MH power pack or four 1.5 V alkaline LR6	Four AA alkaline	Ni-MH	Lithium ion, alkaline backup	Lithium ion, alkaline backup	Ni-Cd
Operating time, hr	~1 month	~1 month	24	4,000 (6 months)	20	20	20	24
H × W × D, cm (in)	3.4 × 8.2 × 15.5 (1.3 × 3.2 × 6.1)	3.4 × 8.2 × 15.5 (1.3 × 3.2 × 6.1)	45 × 20.3 × 13.5 (1.8 × 8 × 5.3)	16 × 12 × 3 (6.3 × 4.8 × 1.2)	5.8 × 18.8 × 22.4 (2.3 × 7.4 × 8.8)	5.8 × 18.8 × 22.4 (2.3 × 7.4 × 8.8)	5.8 × 18.8 × 22.4 (2.3 × 7.4 × 8.8)	19.5 × 8.8 × 3.5 (7.7 × 3.5 × 1.4)
Weight, kg (lb)	0.2 (0.44)	0.27 (0.6)	0.66 (1.5)	0.25 (0.55)	1.18 (2.6)	1.3 (2.9)	1.3 (2.9)	0.4 (0.9)
Green Features	None specified	None specified	None specified	None specified	None specified	None specified	None specified	None specified
FDA Clearance	Not specified	Not specified	No	No	Yes	Yes	Yes	No
CE Mark	Yes	Yes	Yes	Yes	No	Yes	Yes	No

References

1. Buonocore G, Perrone S, Tataranno ML. Oxygen toxicity: Chemistry and biology of reactive oxygen species. *Semin Fetal Neonatal Med.* 2010;15(4):186-190.

2. Auten RL, Davis JM. Oxygen toxicity and reactive oxygen species: The devil is in the details. *Pediatr Res.* 2009;66(2): 121-127.

3. Bageant RA. Oxygen analyzers. *Respir Care.* 1976;21(5):410-416.

4. Meyer RM. Oxygen analyzers: Failure rates and life spans of galvanic cells. *J Clin Monit.* 1990;6(3):196-202.

5. Abraham E, Gallagher TJ, Fink S. Clinical evaluation of a multi-parameter intra-arterial blood-gas sensor. *Intensive Care Med.* 1996;22(5):507-513.

6. Erdmann K, Jantzen JP, Etz C, Dick WF. Evaluation of two oxygen analyzers by computerized data acquisition and processing. *J Clin Monit.* 1986;2(2):105-113.

7. Harris PD, Barnes R. The uses of helium and xenon in current clinical practice. *Anaesthesia.* 2008;63(3):284-293.

8. Smith SW, Biros M. Relief of imminent respiratory failure from upper airway obstruction by use of helium-oxygen: A case series and brief review. *Acad Emerg Med.* 1999;6(9):953-956.

9. Valli G, Paoletti P, Savi D, Martolini D, Palange P. Clinical use of heliox in asthma and COPD. *Monaldi Arch Chest Dis.* 2007; 67(3):159-164.

10. Kumar D, Saksena RK. Use of heliox in the management of acute exacerbation of COPD. *Emerg Med J.* 2007;24(1):45-48.

11. Harris PD, Barnes R. The uses of helium and xenon in current clinical practice. *Anaesthesia.* 2008;63(3):284-293.

12. Gillespie DJ. Use of an acoustic helium analyzer and microprocessor for rapid measurement of absolute lung volume during mechanical ventilation. *Crit Care Med.* 1985;13(2):118-121.

13. St. John RE. End-tidal carbon dioxide monitoring. *Crit Care Nurse.* 2003;23(4):83-88.

14. Eipe N, Doherty DR. A review of pediatric capnography. *J Clin Monit Comput.* 2010;24(4):261-268.

15. Anderson CT, Breen PH. Carbon dioxide kinetics and capnography during critical care. *Crit Care.* 2000;4(4):207-215.

16. Blanch L, Romero PV, Lucangelo U. Volumetric capnography in the mechanically ventilated patient. *Minerva Anestesiol.* 2006;72(6):577-585.

17. Romero PV, Lucangelo U, Lopez Aguilar J, Fernandez R, Blanch L. Physiologically based indices of volumetric capnography in patients receiving mechanical ventilation. *Eur Respir J.* 1997; 10(6):1309-1315.

18. Tusman G, Sipmann FS, Borges JB, Hedenstierna G, Bohm SH. Validation of Bohr dead space measured by volumetric capnography. *Intensive Care Med.* 2011;37(5):870-874.

19. Böhm SH, Maisch S, von Sandersleben A, et al. The effects of lung recruitment on the Phase III slope of volumetric capnography in morbidly obese patients. *Anesth Analg.* 2009;109(1):151-159.

20. Moreira MM, Terzi RG, Cortellazzi L, et al. Volumetric capnography: In the diagnostic work-up of chronic thromboembolic disease. *Vasc Health Risk Manag.* 2010;6:317-319.

21. Rocco M, Spadetta G, Morelli A, et al. A comparative evaluation of thermodilution and partial CO_2 rebreathing techniques for cardiac output assessment in critically ill patients during assisted ventilation. *Intensive Care Med.* 2004;30(1):82-87.

22. Blitzer ML, Loh E, Roddy MA, Stamler JS, Creager MA. Endothelium-derived nitric oxide regulates systemic and pulmonary vascular resistance during acute hypoxia in humans. *J Am Coll Cardiol.* 1996;28(3):591.

23. Barnes PJ, Liew FY. Nitric oxide and asthmatic inflammation. *Immunol Today.* 1995;16(3):128.

24. Smith AD, Cowan JO, Filsell S, et al. Diagnosing asthma: Comparisons between exhaled nitric oxide measurements and conventional tests. *Am J Respir Crit Care Med.* 2004;169:473-478.

25. Yates DH, Kharitonov SA, Robbins RA, Thomas PS, Barnes PJ. Effect of a nitric oxide synthase inhibitor and a glucocorticosteroid on exhaled nitric oxide. *Am J Respir Crit Care Med.* 1995;152:892-896.

26. Beck-Ripp J, Griese M, Arenz S, Koring C, Pasqualoni B, Bufler P. Changes of exhaled nitric oxide during steroid treatment of childhood asthma. *Eur Respir J.* 2002;19:1015-1019.

27. Harkins MS, Fiato KL, Iwamoto GK. Exhaled nitric oxide predicts asthma exacerbation. *J Asthma.* 2004;41:471-476.

28. Hogman M, Holmkvist T, Wegener T, et al. Extended NO analysis applied to patients with COPD, allergic asthma and allergic rhinitis. *Respir Med.* 2002;96:24-30.

29. Deykin A, Massaro AF, Drazen JM, Israel E. Exhaled nitric oxide as a diagnostic test for asthma: Online versus offline techniques and effect of flow rate. *Am J Respir Crit Care Med.* 2002;165:1597-1601

30. Tsang KW, Ip SK, Leung R, et al. Exhaled nitric oxide: The effects of age, gender and body size. *Lung.* 2001;179:83-91.

31. Baraldi E, Azzolin NM, Cracco A, Zacchello F. Reference values of exhaled nitric oxide for healthy children 6–15 years old. *Pediatr Pulmonol.* 1999;27:54-58.

32. Gustafsson LE, Leone AM, Persson MG, Wiklund NP, Moncada S. Endogenous nitric oxide is present in the exhaled air of rabbits, guinea pigs and humans. *Biochem Biophys Res Commun.* 1991;181(2):852.

33. Buchvald F, Baraldi E, Carraro S, et al. Measurements of exhaled nitric oxide in healthy subjects age 4 to 17 years. *J Allergy Clin Immunol.* 2005;115(6):1130.

34. Smith AD, Cowan JO, Taylor DR. Exhaled nitric oxide levels in asthma: Personal best versus reference values. *J Allergy Clin Immunol.* 2009;124(4):714.

35. van der Mark TW, Kort E, Meijer RJ, Postma DS, Koeter GH. Water vapour and carbon dioxide decrease nitric oxide readings. *Eur Respir J.* 1997;10:2120-2123.

36. Meijer RJ, Kerstjens HA, Postma DS, Koeter GH, van der Mark TW. Exhaled nitric oxide concentration is influenced by alcohol containing disinfectants. *Eur Respir J.* 1996;9:1111.

37. Kharitonov SA, Barnes PJ. Exhaled markers of pulmonary disease. *Am J Respir Crit Care Med.* 2001;163(7):1693.

38. American Thoracic Society, European Respiratory Society. ATS/ERS recommendations for standardized procedures for the online and offline measurement of exhaled lower respiratory nitric oxide and nasal nitric oxide, 2005. *Am J Respir Crit Care Med.* 2005;171(8):912.

39. Valdez-Lowe C, Ghareeb SA, Artinian NT. Pulse oximetry in adults. *Am J Nurs.* 2009;109(6):52-59.

40. Walters TP. Pulse oximetry knowledge and its effects on clinical practice. *Br J Nurs.* 2007;16(21):1332-1340.

41. Rajkumar A, Karmarkar A, Knott J. Pulse oximetry: An overview. *J Perioper Pract.* 2006;16(10):502-504.

42. Sinex JE. Pulse oximetry: Principles and limitations. *Am J Emerg Med.* 1999;17(1):59-67.

43. Lima AP, Beelen P, Bakker J. Use of a peripheral perfusion index derived from the pulse oximetry signal as a noninvasive indicator of perfusion. *Crit Care Med.* 2002;30(6):1210-1213.

44. Pulse oximetry: Choosing the right sensor and applying it correctly. *Health Devices.* 2007;36(3):98-99.

45. Hodgson CL, Tuxen DV, Holland AE, Keating JL. Comparison of forehead Max-Fast pulse oximetry sensor with finger sensor at high positive end-expiratory pressure in adult patients with acute respiratory distress syndrome. *Anaesth Intensive Care.* 2009;37(6):953-960.

46. Webb RK, Ralston AC, Runciman WB. Potential errors in pulse oximetry. II. Effects of changes in saturation and signal quality. *Anaesthesia.* 1991;46(3):207-212.

47. Volsko T, Chatburn R, Kallstrom T. Evaluation of a commercial standard for checking pulse oximeter performance. *Respir Care.* 1996;41(2):100-104.

48. Ralston AC, Webb RK, Runciman WB. Potential errors in pulse oximetry. I. Pulse oximeter evaluation. *Anaesthesia*. 1991; 46(3):202-206.

49. Ralston AC, Webb RK, Runciman WB. Potential errors in pulse oximetry. III: Effects of interferences, dyes, dyshaemoglobins and other pigments. *Anaesthesia*. 1991;46(4):291-295.

50. Hummler HD, Engelmann A, Pohlandt F, Högel J, Franz AR. Decreased accuracy of pulse oximetry measurements during low perfusion caused by sepsis: Is the perfusion index of any value? *Intensive Care Med*. 2006;32(9):1428-1431.

51. Grace RF. Pulse oximetry. Gold standard or false sense of security? *Med J Aust*. 1994;160(10):638.

52. Hampson NB. Pulse oximetry in severe carbon monoxide poisoning. *Chest*. 1998;114(4):1036.

53. Barker SJ, Tremper KK, Hyatt J. Effects of methemoglobinemia on pulse oximetry and mixed venous oximetry. *Anesthesiology*. 1989;70(1):112.

54. Vardon D, Hors Y, Grossetti E, Creveuil C, Herlicoviez M, Dreyfus M. Fetal pulse oximetry: Clinical practice. *J Gynecol Obstet Biol Reprod (Paris)*. 2008;37(7):697-704.

55. Weaver LK. Transcutaneous oxygen and carbon dioxide tensions compared to arterial blood gases in normals. *Respir Care*. 2007;52(11):1490-1496.

56. Got I. Transcutaneous oxygen pressure (TcPO2): Advantages and limitations. *Diabetes Metab*. 1998;24(4):379-384.

57. Eberhard P. The design, use, and results of transcutaneous carbon dioxide analysis: Current and future directions. *Anesth Analg*. 2007;105(6 Suppl):S48-S52.

58. Capovilla J, VanCouwenberghe C, Miller WA, et al. Noninvasive blood gas monitoring. *Crit Care Nurs Q*. 2000;23(2):79-86.

59. Cuvelier A, Grigoriu B, Molano LC, Muir JF. Limitations of transcutaneous carbon dioxide measurements for assessing long-term mechanical ventilation. *Chest*. 2005;127(5):1744-1748.

60. Ueno H, Fukumoto S, Koyama H, et al. Regions of arterial stenosis and clinical factors determining transcutaneous oxygen tension in patients with peripheral arterial disease. *J Atheroscler Thromb*. 2010;17(8):858-869.

61. Herrejón A, Inchaurraga I, Palop J, Ponce S, Peris R, Terrádez M, Blanquer R. Usefulness of transcutaneous carbon dioxide pressure monitoring to measure blood gases in adults hospitalized for respiratory disease. *Arch Bronconeumol*. 2006;42(5):225-229.

62. Headley JM. Indirect calorimetry: A trend toward continuous metabolic assessment. *AACN Clin Issues*. 2003;14(2):155-167.

63. McClave SA. Indirect calorimetry: Relevance to patient outcome. *Respir Care Clin N Am*. 2006;12(4):635-650.

64. Perseghin G. Pathogenesis of obesity and diabetes mellitus: Insights provided by indirect calorimetry in humans. *Acta Diabetol*. 2001;38(1):7-21.

65. da Rocha EE, Alves VG, da Fonseca RB. Indirect calorimetry: Methodology, instruments and clinical application. *Curr Opin Clin Nutr Metab Care*. 2006;9(3):247-256.

66. Weir J. New method for calculating metabolic rate with special reference to protein metabolism. *J Physiol*. 1949;109:1-9.

67. Lev S, Cohen J, Singer P. Indirect calorimetry measurements in the ventilated critically ill patient: Facts and controversies—the heat is on. *Crit Care Clin*. 2010;26(4):e1-e9.

68. Sarge T, Talmor D. Transpulmonary pressure: Its role in preventing ventilator-induced lung injury. *Minerva Anestesiol*. 2008;74(6):335-339.

69. Talmor D, Sarge T, Malhotra A, et al. Mechanical ventilation guided by esophageal pressure in acute lung injury. *N Engl J Med*. 2008;359(20):2095-2104.

70. Brochard L. Intrinsic (or auto-) PEEP during controlled mechanical ventilation. *Intensive Care Med*. 2002;28(10):1376-1378.

71. MacIntyre NR. Respiratory mechanics in the patient who is weaning from the ventilator. *Respir Care*. 2005;50(2):275-286; discussion 284-286.

72. Talmor DS, Fessler HE. Are esophageal pressure measurements important in clinical decision-making in mechanically ventilated patients? *Respir Care*. 2010;55(2):162-172.

73. Washko GR, O'Donnell CR, Loring SH. Volume-related and volume-independent effects of posture on esophageal and transpulmonary pressures in healthy subjects. *J Appl Physiol*. 2006;100(3):753-758.

74. Baydur A, Sassoon CS, Carlson M. Measurement of lung mechanics at different lung volumes and esophageal levels in normal subjects: Effect of posture change. *Lung*. 1996;174(3):139-151.

75. Abu-Shaweesh JM, Martin RJ. Neonatal apnea: What's new? *Pediatr Pulmonol*. 2008;43(10):937-944.

76. Martin RJ, Abu-Shaweesh JM. Control of breathing and neonatal apnea. *Biol Neonate*. 2005;87(4):288-295.

77. Perfect Sychowski S, Dodd E, Thomas P, Peabody J, Clark R. Home apnea monitor use in preterm infants discharged from newborn intensive care units. *J Pediatr*. 2001;139(2):245-248.

78. Grögaard JB. Apnea monitors. *Acta Paediatr*. 1993;82(Suppl 389):111-113.

79. Nobel JJ. Apnea monitors. *Pediatr Emerg Care*. 1991;7(5):307-309.

80. Abendroth D, Moser DK, Dracup K, Doering LV. Do apnea monitors decrease emotional distress in parents of infants at high risk for cardiopulmonary arrest? *J Pediatr Health Care*. 1999;13(2):50-57.

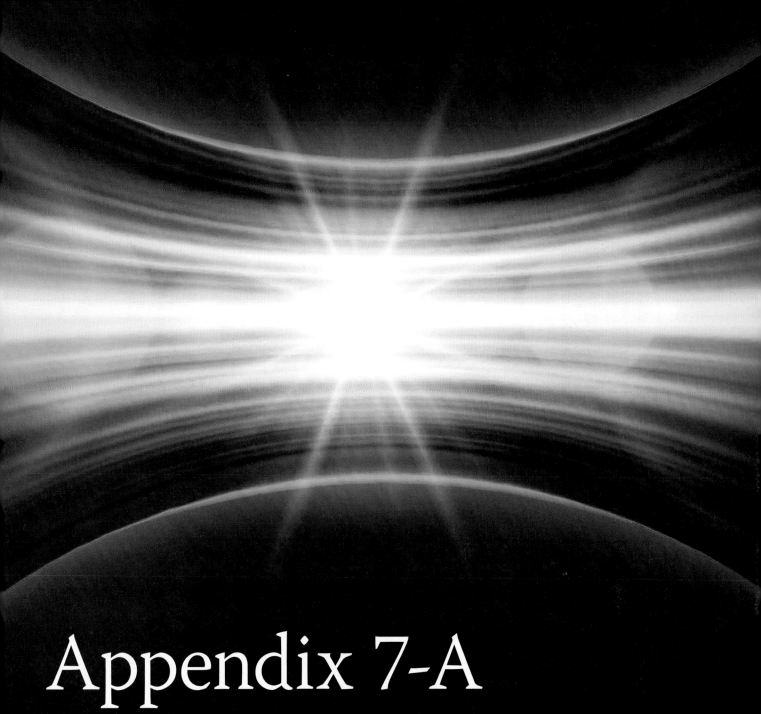

Appendix 7-A

APPENDIX 7-A
Descriptions of Features and Specifications of Pulse Oximeters

SPECIFICATIONS	ARMSTRONG AD-1500 SPECTRO2 10	ARMSTRONG AD-2500 SPECTRO2 30	COMDEK MD-600P	COMDEK MD-610P	COMDEK MD-620P	COMDEK MD-630P	COMDEK MD-650P	COMDEK MD-670P	COMDEK MD-680P
Modular/ Stand-alone	Stand-alone	Stand-alone	Not specified	Not specified	Not specified	Not specified	Not specified	Not specified	Not specified
MRI compatible	No	No	No	No	No	No	No	No	No
SpO$_2$ range, %	0–99	0–99	0–100	0–100	0–100	0–100	0–100	0–100	0–100
Accuracy, %	Adult/pediatric: ± 2 (70–99)	Adult/pediatric: ± 2 (70–99), neonate: ± 3 (70–99)	± 2 (80–100)	± 1 (90–100), ± 2 (80–89), ± 3 (65–79)	80–100 ± 2, 65–79 ± 3	± 1 (90–100), ± 2 (80–89), ± 3 (65–79)	± 2 (80–100), ± 3 (65–79), unspecified (0–65)	± 2 (80–100), ± 3 (65–79)	± 1 (90–100), ± 2 (80–89), ± 3 (65–79)
Pulse rate, bpm	30–254	20–300	30–250	30–250	30–250	30–250	30–250	30–250	30–250
Accuracy	Not specified	Not specified	1%	1%	1%	1%	1%	1%	1%
Probe Types									
Disposable	Yes	Yes	Finger, ear, toe	Finger, ear, toe	Finger, ear, toe	Finger, ear, toe	Not specified	Finger, ear, toe	Not specified
Reusable	Yes	Yes	Finger, ear, toe	Finger, ear, toe	Finger, ear, toe	Finger, ear, toe	Built-in finger	Finger, ear, toe	Built-in finger
Patient range	Adult, pediatric, infant, neonate	Adult, pediatric, infant, neonate	Adult, pediatric, infant, neonate	Adult, pediatric, infant, neonate	Adult, pediatric, infant, neonate	Adult, pediatric, infant, neonate	Adult, pediatric	Adult, pediatric, infant, neonate	Adult, pediatric
Perfusion Index and/or Signal Strength Indicator	Not specified	Not specified	Not specified	Not specified	Not specified	Not specified	Not specified	Not specifiec	Not specified
Response Time, sec	NA	NA	6	6	6	6	6–8	6	6–8
Start-Up Time, sec or pulses	Not specified	Not specified	4–6 sec	4–6 sec	4–6 sec	4–6 sec	4–6 sec	4–6 sec	4–6 sec
Averaging Time, sec	8	8 or 16	Not specified	Not specified	Not specified	Not specified	Not specified	Not specified	Not specified
Data Management									
Data stored	SpO$_2$, pulse rate, pulse amplitude index	SpO$_2$, pulse rate, pulse amplitude index	Not specified	Not specified	Yes	Yes	Not specified	Not specified	Not specified
Data storage, hr	144	72	Not specified	Not specified	48	0.5	Not specified	72	Not specified
External output	Not specified	USB, dock connection	None	None	USB	No	No	USB	No

APPENDIX 7-A
Descriptions of Features and Specifications of Pulse Oximeters (Continued)

SPECIFICATIONS	ARMSTRONG AD-1500 SPECTRO2 10	ARMSTRONG AD-2500 SPECTRO2 30	COMDEK MD-600P	COMDEK MD-610P	COMDEK MD-620P	COMDEK MD-630P	COMDEK MD-650P	COMDEK MD-670P	COMDEK MD-680P
Displays	SpO_2, pulse rate, quantitative pulse strength	SpO_2, pulse rate, quantitative pulse strength	SpO_2, pulse rate, pulse search indicator, low battery alarm	SpO_2, pulse rate	SpO_2, pulse rate, pulse search indicator, low battery alarm	SpO_2, pulse rate	SpO_2, pulse rate, pulse search indicator, low battery alarm	SpO_2, pulse rate, SpO_2 waveform	SpO_2, pulse rate, pulse search indicator, low battery alarm
Printer-Recorder	Optional	Optional	None	None	Optional IR printer	Built-in thermal printer	No	Yes	No
Alarms									
Audiovisual	No	Pulse rate, SpO_2	High/low SpO_2 and pulse rate, sensor off, sensor disconnected, low battery	Sensor off, sensor disconnected, low battery	High/low SpO_2 and pulse rate, sensor off, sensor disconnected, low battery	High/low SpO_2 and pulse rate, sensor off, sensor disconnected, low battery	Sensor off, sensor disconnected, low battery	High/low SpO_2 and pulse rate, sensor off, sensor disconnected, low battery, clock and symbol function, SpO_2 waveform display	Sensor off, sensor disconnected, low battery
Visual	Low battery	Low battery	High/low SpO_2 and pulse rate, low battery	Low battery	High/low SpO_2 and pulse rate, low battery	High/low SpO_2 and pulse rate, low battery	Low battery	High/low SpO_2 and pulse rate, low battery	Low battery
Alarm override	No	No	Yes	Not specified	Yes	Yes	Not specified	Yes	Not specified
Reactivation method	NA	Yes	Manual	Not specified	Manual	Manual	Not specified	Manual	Not specified
Volume control	NA	Yes	Yes	Not specified	Yes	Yes	Not specified	Yes	Not specified
Power									
VAC	Yes	Yes	110/120/220/240	110/120/220/240	110/120/220/240	110/120/220/240	Battery only	110/120/220/240	Battery only
Batteries	AA (4)	AA (4)	AA	AA	AAA alkaline	AAA alkaline	AAA alkaline	AA alkaline	AAA alkaline
Life, hr	32	17	24	24	Not specified	Not specified	~16	Not specified	Not specified
Rechargeable	Optional	Optional	Yes	Yes	Not specified	Not specified	Not specified	Not specified	Not specified
Low battery notice	Yes	Yes	Yes	Yes	Yes	Yes	Yes	Yes	Yes
H × W × D, cm (in)	8.4 × 15.5 × 4.3 (3.3 × 6.1 × 1.7)	8.4 × 15.5 × 4.3 (3.3 × 6.1 × 1.7)	17.2 × 9 × 3.6 (6.8 × 3.5 × 1.4)	17.2 × 9 × 3.6 (6.8 × 3.5 × 1.4)	11.5 × 6.5 × 4.3 (4.5 × 2.6 × 1.7)	16.8 × 8.8 × 5 (6.6 × 3.5 × 2)	7.3 × 4.5 × 3.9 (2.9 × 1.8 × 1.5)	17 × 8.8 × 4.4 (6.7 × 3.5 × 1.7)	9 × 6.6 × 2.2 (3.5 × 2.6 × 0.9)

(continues)

APPENDIX 7-A
Descriptions of Features and Specifications of Pulse Oximeters (*Continued*)

| | ARMSTRONG | ARMSTRONG | COMDEK | COMDEK | COMDEK | COMDEK | COMDEK | COMDEK | COMDEK |
| | AD-1500 SPECTRO2 10 | AD-2500 SPECTRO2 30 | MD-600P | MD-610P | MD-620P | MD-630P | MD-650P | MD-670P | MD-680P |
SPECIFICATIONS					**MODEL**				
Weight, kg (lb)	0.3 (0.8)	0.3 (0.8)	0.24 (0.53)	0.24 (0.53)	0.16 (0.35) including batteries	0.33 (0.73)	0.06 (0.1) without batteries	0.25 (0.6) without batteries	0.09 (0.02)
Green Features	None specified	None specified	None specified	None specified	None specified	Low power consumption	None specified	None specified	Low power consumption, auto power off
FDA Clearance	Yes	Yes	Submitted	Submitted	Submitted	Submitted	Submitted	Submitted	Submitted
CE Mark	Yes	Yes	Yes	Yes	Yes	Yes	Yes	Yes	Yes

| | COMDEK | CRITICARE | CRITICARE | DIGICARE | DIMA ITALIA | EMCO | GE HEALTHCARE | GE HEALTHCARE | GE HEALTHCARE |
SPECIFICATIONS	MD-700	503DX MiniSpO2T	504DX SERIES	DIGIOXI PO 930	O2 FLOW REGULATOR MODEL 106	2060	TruSat	TruSat WITH TREND DOWNLOAD	TuffSat HANDHELD (SPOT CHECK MODEL)
Modular/Stand-alone	Stand-alone	Stand-alone	Stand-alone	Stand-alone	Stand-alone	Stand-alone	Stand-alone	Stand-alone	Stand-alone
MRI compatible	Not specified	No	No	No	No	No	No	No	No
SpO₂ range, %	0–100	0–99	0–99	0–100	30–100	0–100	1–100	1–100	1–100
Accuracy, %	± 2 (80–100)	± 2 (70–99), ± 3 (40–69), unspecified < 40	± 2 (70–99), ± 3 (40–69), unspecified < 40	± 2 (70–100), ± 3 (50–69)	± 3 (70–100), not specified < 70	± 2 (70–99)	70–100 (± 2 digits without motion, ± 3 digits during clinical motion, ± 2 digits during clinical low perfusion), below 70% unspecified	70–100 (± 2 digits without motion, ± 3 digits during clinical motion, ± 2 digits during clinical low perfusion), below 70% unspecified	± 2 (70–100), unspecified below 70%
Pulse rate, bpm	30–250	20–300	20–300	0–250	30–250	18–300	30–250	30–250	40–255

APPENDIX 7-A
Descriptions of Features and Specifications of Pulse Oximeters (Continued)

SPECIFICATIONS	COMDEK MD-700	CRITICARE 503DX MiniSpO2T	CRITICARE 504DX SERIES	DIGICARE DIGIOXI PO 930	DIMA ITALIA O2 FLOW REGULATOR MODEL 106	EMCO 2060	GE HEALTHCARE TruSat	GE HEALTHCARE TruSat WITH TREND DOWNLOAD	GE HEALTHCARE TuffSat HANDHELD (SPOT CHECK MODEL)
Accuracy	1%	1% or 1 bpm	1% or 1 bpm	± 2	3 digits	3 ± 1 digit	30–250 bpm (± 2 digits or ± 2% without motion, ± 5 digits during clinical motion, ± 3 digits during clinical low perfusion)	30–250 bpm (± 2 digits or ± 2% without motion, ± 5 digits during clinical motion, ± 3 digits durirg clinical low perfusion)	40–100: ± 2 bpm, 100–255: ± 2%
Probe Types									
Disposable	Finger, ear, toe	Adhesive disposables (foam or fabric type)	Adhesive disposables (foam or fabric type)	Finger, universal wrap	Finger, clip, wrap, foot, flex	Finger, ear, neonatal	OxyTip+, TruSignal adhesive	OxyTip+, TruSignal adhesive	OxyTip+, TruSignal adhesive
Reusable	Finger, ear, toe	Finger clip (adult, pediatric), soft (adult, pediatric), Y-sensor, ear	Finger clip (adult, pediatric), soft (adult, pediatric), Y-sensor, ear	Wrap, ear	Finger, clip, wrap, foot, flex	Finger, pediatric, universal Y	Finger, FingerTip, ear, wrap/SE sensor	Finger, FingerTip, ear, wrap/SE sensor	Finger, FingerTip, ear, wrap/SE sensor
Patient range	Adult, pediatric, infant, neonate	Adult, pediatric, neonate	Adult, pediatric, neonate	Adult, pediatric, infant, neonate	Adult, pediatric, infant, neonate	Adult, pediatric, infant, neonate	Adult, pediatric, infant, neonate	Adult, pediatric, infant, neonate	Adult, pediatric, infant, neonate
Perfusion Index and/or Signal Strength Indicator	Not specified	None specified	None specified	Not specified	Plethysmographic amplitude and strength-bar indicator	3-color perfusion LED	Yes	Yes	Yes
Response Time, sec	6–8	6–12, pulse to pulse	4–16, pulse to pulse	9	Any pulse	5	1 (display update interval)	1 (display update interval)	1 (display update interval)
Start-Up Time, sec or pulses	4–6 sec	6–12 sec	10–16 sec	9 sec	5 sec	8 sec	< 10 sec	< 10 sec	≤ 12 sec

(continues)

APPENDIX 7-A
Descriptions of Features and Specifications of Pulse Oximeters (Continued)

SPECIFICATIONS	COMDEK MD-700	CRITICARE 503DX MiniSpO2T	CRITICARE 504DX SERIES	DIGICARE DIGIOXI PO 930	DIMA ITALIA O2 FLOW REGULATER MODEL 106	EMCO 2060	GE HEALTHCARE TruSat	GE HEALTHCARE TruSat WITH TREND DOWNLOAD	GE HEALTHCARE TuffSat HANDHELD (SPOT CHECK MODEL)
Averaging Time, sec	Not specified	12	User selectable: 3, 6, 9, 12, 15, 18, 21	Not specified	Not specified	4, 8, 16 (auto averaging)	12	12	12
Data Management	Yes	Not specified	Yes	Not specified	Yes	Yes	No	Yes	No
Data stored	Not specified	Not specified	All displayed parameters	Not specified	Not specified	SpO$_2$, pulse rate	NA	Trend memory with SpO$_2$, pulse rate, alarm conditions	NA
Data storage, hr	72	Not specified	24	Not specified	12	144	NA	48	NA
External output	USB	No	Analog, digital, RS232 compatible	RS232, optional	Serial	Parallel port	NA	Digital RS232 serial	NA
Displays	SpO$_2$, pulse rate	SpO$_2$, pulse rate, pulse amplitude	SpO$_2$, pulse rate, pulse amplitude, alarm messages	SpO$_2$, pulse rate, alarm limits, plethysmogram, pulse strength sensor, and system status	SpO$_2$, pulse rate, alarms, time, date	SpO$_2$, pulse rate, plethysmogram	SpO$_2$, pulse rate, plethysmogram, perfusion index, international icon, battery, volumes, alarm limits	SpO$_2$, pulse rate, plethysmogram, perfusion index, international icon, battery, volumes, alarm limits	SpO$_2$, perfusion index, pulse rate, plethysmography
Printer-Recorder	No	No	Optional thermal printer	Optional	No	Optional	NA	NA	NA
Alarms									
Audiovisual	Sensor off, sensor disconnected, low battery	No	Full alarms (user selectable), high/low SpO$_2$ and pulse rate	High/low SpO$_2$ and pulse rate, sensor off, no sensor connected, low battery	High/low SpO$_2$, pulse rate, loose connection, low battery, memory full	Sensor/patient disconnect, alarm-limit violation, low battery	SpO$_2$, pulse rate, system probe errors, low battery	SpO$_2$, pulse rate, system probe errors, low battery	No audio

APPENDIX 7-A
Descriptions of Features and Specifications of Pulse Oximeters (Continued)

MODEL

SPECIFICATIONS	COMDEK MD-700	CRITICARE 503DX MiniSpO2T	CRITICARE 504DX SERIES	DIGICARE DIGIOXI PO 930	DIMA ITALIA O2 FLOW REGULATER MODEL 106	EMCO 2060	GE HEALTHCARE TruSat	GE HEALTHCARE TruSat WITH TREND DOWNLOAD	GE HEALTHCARE TuffSat HANDHELD (SPOT CHECK MODEL)
Visual	Low battery	Sensor, low battery	Sensor, low battery, alarm silence, neonate mode, external power	Weak pulse/check site, alarm silenced	Flashing LCD	Sensor/patent disconnect, alarm-limit violation, low battery	Audio off, low battery, AC power connected	Audio off, low battery, AC power connected	Low battery, system failure, probe failure
Alarm override	Not specified	No	Yes	Yes	Yes	2 min silence	2 min and permanent	2 min and permanent	No
Reactivation method	Not specified	NA	Automatic after 2 min or manual	Automatic after 2 min or manual	Automatic, manual	Alarm silence switch	Automatic after 2 min	Automatic after 2 min	NA
Volume control	Not specified	NA	Yes	Beep and alarm	No	Yes	Yes	Yes	NA
Power									
VAC	100/200, 50/60 Hz	Battery only	110/120, 220/240	110/120, 220/240, selectable	100/200, 50/60 Hz	220/240	100–240, 50/60 Hz	100–240, 50/60 Hz	
Batteries	AA alkaline	AA alkaline	Sealed lead-acid	Sealed lead-acid	1.2 V Ni-MH	Sealed lead-acid 6 V, 1.2 mAh	Rechargeable Ni-MH	Rechargeable Ni-MH	1.5 V AA
Life, hr	~4	24	6	7	16	6	35	24	17–20
Rechargeable	No	Not included	Yes	Yes	Yes	Yes	Yes	Yes	No
Low battery notice	Yes	Yes	Yes	Yes	Visual and audible	LED indicator	Yes	Yes	Yes
H × W × D, cm (in)	6.7 × 14.8 × 19 (2.6 × 5.8 × 7.5)	14.6 × 9.1 × 3.3 (5.7 × 3.6 × 1.3)	14.4 × 17.8 × 12.2 (5.6 × 7 × 4.8)	7.8 × 24 × 21 (3.1 × 9.4 × 8.3)	15 × 10 × 5.5 (5.9 × 3.9 × 2.2)	8 × 23.4 × 16.5 (3.2 × 9.2 × 6.5)	21.8 × 11.5 × 10.3 (8.5 × 4.5 × 4)	21.8 × 11.5 × 10.3 (8.5 × 4.5 × 4)	15 × 7 × 3 (6 × 2.8 × 1.2)
Weight, kg (lb)	0.5 (1)	0.28 (0.62)	1.52 (3.4)	3.5 (7.7)	0.45 (1)	2 (4.4)	1.3 (2.8)	1.5 (3.3)	0.26 (0.6) with batteries
Green Features	None specified	None specified	None specified	None specified	None specified	None specified	None specified	None specified	None specified
FDA Clearance	Yes	Yes	Yes	No	No	Submitted	Yes	Yes	Yes
CE Mark	Yes	Yes	Yes	Yes	Yes	Yes	Yes	Yes	Yes

(continues)

APPENDIX 7-A
Descriptions of Features and Specifications of Pulse Oximeters (Continued)

SPECIFICATIONS	GETEMED VitaGuard VG 310	INVIVO 4500-MRI	MASIMO RAINBOW SET 2011 RADICAL-7	MASIMO RAINBOW SET PRONTO	MASIMO RAINBOW SET PRONTO-7	MASIMO RAINBOW SET RAD-57	MASIMO RAINBOW SET RAD-87	MASIMO RAINBOW SET RADICAL-7	MASIMO SET RAD-5
Modular/Stand-alone	Stand-alone	Stand alone or in conjunction with Invivo 1400 MRI NIBP monitor	Stand-alone	Stand-alone	Stand-alone	Handheld	Stand-alone	Stand-alone	Handheld
MRI compatible	No	Yes	No	No	No	No	No	No	No
SpO$_2$ range, %	1–100	50–100	1–100	1–100	1–100	1–100	1–100	1–100	1–100
Accuracy, %	± 3 > 70%	2–2.5 (70–100)	± 2 (70–100), ± 3 (60–80)	± 2 (70–100), ± 3 (60–80)	± 2 (70–100)	± 2 (70–100), ± 3 (60–80)	± 2 (70–100), ± 3 (60–80)	± 2 (70–100), ± 3 (60–80)	± 2 (70–100), ± 3 (60–80)
Pulse rate, bpm	25–240	20–250	25–240	25–240	30–250	25–240	25–240	25–240	25–240
Accuracy	± 3 without motion, ± 5 during motion	Not specified	± 3 (no motion), ± 5 digits (motion)	± 3 (no motion), ± 5 digits (motion)	± 3	± 3 (no motion), ± 5 digits (motion)	± 3 (no motion), ± 5 digits (motion)	± 3 (no motion), ± 5 digits (motion)	± 3 (no motion), ± 5 digits (motion)
Probe Types									
Disposable	Masimo LNOP and LNCS types	Grip sensor	Digit, hand, foot, toe	Digit	Digit	Digit, hand, foot, toe	Digit, hand, foot, toe	Digit, hand, foot, toe	Digit, hand, foot, toe
Reusable	Masimo LNOP and LNCS types	Grip sensor and finger clip sensor	Digit, hand, foot, ear, forehead	Digit	Digit	Digit, hand, foot, ear, forehead	Digit, hand, foot, ear, forehead	Digit, hand, foot, ear, forehead	Digit, hand, foot, ear, forehead
Patient range	All	Adult, pediatric, infant, neonate	Adult, pediatric, infant, neonate	Adult, pediatric	Adult, pediatric	Adult, pediatric, infant, neonate	Adult, pediatric, infant, neonate	Adult, pediatric, infant, neonate	Adult, pediatric, infant, neonate
Perfusion Index and/or Signal Strength Indicator	0.02–20%	Pulse strength light bar	Yes	Yes	Yes	Yes	Yes	Yes	Yes
Response Time, sec	< 10	3, 6, 12 selectable	Every second	NA	NA	Every second	Every second	Every second	Every second

APPENDIX 7-A
Descriptions of Features and Specifications of Pulse Oximeters (Continued)

			MODEL						
	GETEMED	INVIVO	MASIMO RAINBOW SET	MASIMO RAINBOW SET	MASIMO RAINBOW SET	MASIMO RAINBOW SET	MASIMO RAINBOW SET	MASIMO RAINBOW SET	MASIMO SET
SPECIFICATIONS	VitaGuard VG 310	4500-MRI	2011 RADICAL-7	PRONTO	PRONTO-7	RAD-57	RAD-87	RADICAL-7	RAD-5
Start-Up Time, sec or pulses	10 sec	3, 6, 12 sec	15 sec	15 sec	15 sec	15 sec	15 sec	15 sec	10 sec
Averaging Time, sec	4, 6, 8, 10, 12, 14, 16	Not specified	2, 4, 6, 8, 10, 12, 14, or 16	NA	NA	2, 4, 6, 8, 10, 12, 14, or 16	2, 4, 6, 8, 10, 12, 14, or 16	2, 4, 6, 8, 10, 12, 14, or 16	2, 4, 6, 8, 10, 12, 14, or 16
Data Management	Yes	Not specified	Yes	Yes	Yes	Yes	Yes	Yes	Yes
Data stored	Event, trends, and full disclosure	Not specified	Yes	Yes	Yes	Yes	Yes	Yes	Yes
Data storage, hr	≥ 72, trends; ≥ 8; full disclosure; ≥ 200, events	Not specified	72 at 2-sec resolution, 18 days at 10-sec resolution	Spot check storage (> 10,000) checks	Spot check storage (> 10,000) checks	72 at 2-sec resolution	72 at 2-sec resolution	72 at 2-sec resolution, 18 days at 10-sec resolution	72
External output	Online data (SpO$_2$, pulse, plethysmogram, signal IQ)	Analog, digital, RS232	USB A/B, Ethernet, Wireless 802.11, DVI (video), analog, serial, ASCII 1, ASCII 2, binary	Serial, ASCII 1	Mini USB, Wireless 802.11	Serial, ASCII 1	Serial, Patient SafetyNet, nurse call, Philips VueLink, ASCII 1, ASCII 2	Analog, serial, ASCII 2, binary	Serial, ASCII 1
Displays	SpO$_2$, pulse, plethysmogram, signal IQ, perfusion index	Alarms, SpO$_2$, pulse rate, pulse bar	SpO$_2$, SpHb, SpMet, SpCO, SpOC, RRa, pulse rate, perfusion index, PVI, Signal IQ, plethysmogram, trends, sensitivity, status message, Fast Sat, AC power, battery life, alarm status	SpO$_2$, SpHb, pulse rate, perfusion index, Signal IQ, battery life	SpO$_2$, SpHb, pulse rate, perfusion index, battery life	SpO$_2$, SpHb, SpMet, SpCO, pulse rate, perfusion index, Signal IQ, status message, Fast Sat, battery life, alarm status	SpO$_2$, SpHb, SpMet, SpCO, SpOC, RRa, pulse rate, perfusion index, PVI, Signal IQ, plethysmogram, trends, sensitivity, status message, Fast Sat, AC power, battery life, alarm status	SpO$_2$, SpHb, SpMet, SpCO, SpOC, RRa, pulse rate, perfusion index, PVI, Signal IQ, plethysmogram, trends, sensitivity, status message, Fast Sat, AC power, battery life, alarm status	SpO$_2$, pulse rate, perfusion index, Signal IQ, sensitivity, status message, Fast Sat, battery life, alarm status

(continues)

APPENDIX 7-A
Descriptions of Features and Specifications of Pulse Oximeters *(Continued)*

			MODEL						
	GETEMED	INVIVO	MASIMO RAINBOW SET	MASIMO RAINBOW SET	MASIMO RAINBOW SET	MASIMO RAINBOW SET	MASIMO RAINBOW SET	MASIMO RAINBOW SET	MASIMO SET
SPECIFICATIONS	VitaGuard VG 310	4500-MRI	2011 RADICAL-7	PRONTO	PRONTO-7	RAD-57	RAD-87	RADICAL-7	RAD-5
Printer-Recorder	No	No	External, standard serial printer	External, standard serial printer	External Bluetooth printer, external standard laser printer	External, standard serial printer	External, standard serial printer	External, standard serial printer	External, standard serial printer
Alarms									
Audiovisual	Yes	High/low pulse rate, probe off	SpO_2, SpHb, SpMet, SpCO, RRa, pulse rate, perfusion index, PVI, sensor, cable, system failure, low battery; optional advanced alarms (perfusion index and desaturation index)	Low battery, internal failure	NA	SpO_2, SpHb, SpMet, SpCO, pulse rate, sensor, cable, system failure, low battery	SpO_2, SpHb, SpMet, SpCO, RRa, pulse rate, perfusion index, PVI, sensor, cable, system failure, low battery; optional advanced alarms (perfusion index delta 3-D and desaturation index 3-D)	SpO_2, SpHb, SpMet, SpCO, RRa, pulse rate, perfusion index, PVI, sensor, cable, system failure, low battery; optional advanced alarms (perfusion index delta 3-D and desaturation index 3-D)	SpO_2, pulse rate, sensor, cable, system failure, low battery
Visual	Yes	Alarm conditions, system operating messages	SpO_2, SpHb, SpMet, SpCO, RRa, perfusion index, PVI, pulse rate, sensor, cable, system failure, low battery, alarms	No	No	SpO_2, SpHb, SpMet, SpCO, pulse rate, sensor, cable, system failure, low battery	SpO_2, SpHb, SpMet, SpCO, RRa, perfusion index, PVI, pulse rate, sensor, cable, system failure, low battery, 3-D alarms	SpO_2, SpHb, SpMet, SpCO, perfusion index, PVI, pulse rate, sensor, cable, system failure, low battery, 3-D alarms	SpO_2, pulse rate, sensor, cable, system failure, low battery
Alarm override	30–120 sec silence	Yes	Yes	No	No	Yes	Yes	Yes	Yes
Reactivation method	Automatic	Automatic	Automatic, manual	None	None	Automatic, manual	Automatic, manual	Automatic, manual	Automatic, manual
Volume control	Yes	Yes	4 levels and off	No	No	3 levels and off	4 levels and off	4 levels and off	3 levels and off

APPENDIX 7-A
Descriptions of Features and Specifications of Pulse Oximeters (Continued)

SPECIFICATIONS	GETEMED VitaGuard VG 310	INVIVO 4500-MRI	MASIMO RAINBOW SET 2011 RADICAL-7	MASIMO RAINBOW SET PRONTO	MASIMO RAINBOW SET PRONTO-7	MASIMO RAINBOW SET RAD-57	MASIMO RAINBOW SET RAD-87	MASIMO RAINBOW SET RADICAL-7	MASIMO SET RAD-5
Power									
VAC	100–240, 50/60 Hz, external power adapter	120–230 or 14–24 VDC	100–240, 47–63 Hz, 55 VA	Battery only	100–240, 50–60 Hz, 15 VA	Battery only	100–240, 50–60 Hz, 15 VA	100–240, 50–60 Hz, 55 VA	Battery only
Batteries	Rechargeable Ni-MH pack	Lead-acid	Ni-MH	AA alkaline	Rechargeable lithuim polymer	AA alkaline	Sealed lead-acid	Ni-MH	AA alkaline
Life, hr	8	5 continuous	4 handheld, 10 docking station	> 8	Not specified	> 8	4	4 handheld, 10 docking station	> 48
Rechargeable	Yes	Yes	Yes	No	Yes	No	Yes	Yes	No
Low battery notice	Yes	Displayed message	Yes	Yes	Yes	Yes	Yes	Yes	Yes
H × W × D, cm (in)	4.5 × 20.3 × 13.5 (1.8 × 8 × 5.3)	8.3 × 16.8 × 26 (3.3 × 6.6 × 10.3)	8.9 × 26.7 × 19.6 (3.5 × 10.5 × 7.7)	15.8 × 7.6 × 3.6 (6.2 × 3 × 1.4)	13 × 7.2 × 2.5 (5.1 × 2.8 × 1)	15.8 × 7.6 × 3.6 (6.2 × 3 × 1.4)	7.6 × 20.8 × 15.2 (3 × 8.2 × 6)	8.9 × 26.7 × 19.6 (3.5 × 10.5 × 7.7)	15.8 × 7.6 × 3.6 (6.2 × 3 × 1.4)
Weight, kg (lb)	0.75 (1.65)	2.5 (5.6); 3.4 (7.6) with battery	1.73 (3.8)	0.32 (0.7)	0.30 (0.7)	0.32 (0.7)	0.95 (2.1)	1.73 (3.8)	0.32 (0.7)
Green Features	None specified	None specified	Can be used with ReSposable Sensors	None specified	None specified	Can be used with ReSposable Sensors	Can be used with ReSposable Sensors	Can be used with ReSposable Sensors	Can be used with ReSposable Sensors
FDA Clearance	No	Yes	Yes	Yes	Yes	Yes	Yes	Yes	Yes
CE Mark	Yes	Yes	Yes	Yes	Yes	Yes	Yes	Yes	Yes

(continues)

APPENDIX 7-A
Descriptions of Features and Specifications of Pulse Oximeters (Continued)

SPECIFICATIONS	MASIMO SET RAD-5v	MASIMO SET RAD-8	MAXTEC PULSOX-300i	MEDIAID MODEL 100	MEDIAID MODEL 130	MEDIAID MODEL 30	MEDIAID MODEL 300	MEDIAID MODEL 305	MEDIAID MODEL 30B
Modular/ Stand-alone	Handheld	Stand-alone	Stand-alone, minipocket size	Stand-alone, minipocket size	Stand-alone, minipocket size	Stand-alone, palm size, rechargeable	Stand-alone, handheld	Stand-alone, handheld	Stand-alone, palm size, battery
MRI compatible	No	No	No	No	No	No	No	No	No
SpO$_2$ range, %	1–100	1–100	0–100%	20–100	20–100	20–100	20–100	20–100	0–100
Accuracy, %	± 2 (70–100), ± 3 (60–80)	± 2 (70–100), ± 3 (60–80)	± 2 (70–100)	± 2 (70–100), ± 3 (60–69)	± 2 (70–100), ± 3 (60–69)	± 2 (70–100), ± 3 (60–69)	± 2 (70–100), ± 3 (60–69)	± 2 (70–100), ± 3 (60–69)	± 2 (70–100), ± 3 (60–69)
Pulse rate, bpm	25–240	25–240	30–230	25–250	25–250	25–255	32–250	32–250	25–255
Accuracy	± 3 (no motion), ± 5 digits (motion)	± 3 (no motion), ± 5 digits (motion)	± 2 (30–100), ± 2% (100–230)	2 bpm or 2%, whichever is greater	2 bpm or 2%, whichever is greater	2 bpm or 2%, whichever is greater	None specified	None specified	2 bpm or 2%, whichever is greater
Probe Types									
Disposable	Digit, hand, foot, toe	Digit, hand, foot, toe	Not specified	Cable adapter for pediatric/adult use	Cable adapter for pediatric/adult use	Yes	Multisite adhesive	Multisite adhesive	Yes
Reusable	Digit, hand, foot, ear, forehead	Digit, hand, foot, ear, forehead	Finger soft tip, finger clip, finger spot check	Integral finger, cable adapter for pediatric/adult use	Integral finger, cable adapter for pediatric/adult use	Yes	Universal hinged, tape-on, soft, pediatric, adjustable, great toe, ear clip, R-adhesive	Universal hinged, tape-on, soft, pediatric, adjustable, great toe, ear clip, R-adhesive	Yes
Patient range	Adult, pediatric, infant, neonate	Adult, pediatric, infant, neonate	Adult, pediatric	Adult, pediatric; small to large	Adult, pediatric; small to large	Adult, pediatric; small to large	Adult, pediatric; small to large	Adult, pediatric; small to large	Adult, pediatric; small to large
Perfusion Index and/or Signal Strength Indicator	Yes	Yes	Not specified	Not specified	Not specified	Yes	None specified	None specified	Yes
Response Time, sec	Every second	Every second	1 sec	Every pulse	Every pulse	Every pulse	Every pulse	Every pulse	Every pulse
Start-Up Time, sec or pulses	10 sec	10 sec	Not specified	3 pulses	3 pulses	3 pulses	3 pulses	3 pulses	3 pulses
Averaging Time, sec	8	2, 4, 6, 8, 10, 12, 14, or 16	Not specified	Not specified	Not specified	Not specified	Not specified	Not specified	Not specified
Data Management									
Data stored	No	Yes	Yes	Not specified	Yes	Not specified	Not specified	Not specified	Not specified
Data storage, hr	NA	72 at 2-sec resolution	300	Not specified	11.5	Not specified	Not specified	Not specified	Not specified
External output	NA	Serial, ASCII 1, ASCII 2	NA	No	Yes	No	No	No	No

APPENDIX 7-A
Descriptions of Features and Specifications of Pulse Oximeters (Continued)

SPECIFICATIONS	MASIMO SET RAD-5v	MASIMO SET RAD-8	MAXTEC PULSOX-300i	MEDIAID MODEL 100	MEDIAID MODEL 130	MEDIAID MODEL 30	MEDIAID MODEL 300	MEDIAID MODEL 305	MEDIAID MODEL 30B
Displays	SpO$_2$, pulse rate, perfusion index, Signal IQ, status message, Fast Sat, low battery life, alarm status	SpO$_2$, pulse rate, perfusion index, Signal IQ, sensitivity, status message, Fast Sat, battery life, alarm status, trauma	SpO$_2$, pulse rate, strength indicator, battery life	SpO$_2$, pulse rate	SpO$_2$, pulse rate	SpO$_2$, pulse rate	SpO$_2$, pulse rate	SpO$_2$, pulse rate	SpO$_2$, pulse rate
Printer-Recorder	No	External, standard serial printer	No	No	Optional	No	No	No	No
Alarms									
Audiovisual	SpO$_2$, pulse rate, sensor, cable, system failure, low battery	SpO$_2$, pulse rate, sensor, cable, system failure, low battery	No	No	No	No	No	No	No
Visual	High/low SpO$_2$ and pulse, sensor off, loss of pulse, system failure, low battery, service	SpO$_2$, pulse rate, sensor, cable, system failure, low battery	Yes	No	No	No	No	No	No
Alarm override	Yes	Yes	No	No	No	No	No	No	No
Reactivation method	Automatic, manual	Automatic, manual	Automatic	NA	NA	NA	NA	NA	NA
Volume control	3 levels and off	3 levels and off	No	NA	NA	NA	NA	NA	NA
Power									
VAC	Battery only	100–240, 50–60 Hz, 15 VA	No	Battery only	Battery only	Yes	Battery only	AC adapter	Battery only
Batteries	AA alkaline	Sealed lead-acid	AAA	AA alkaline	AA alkaline	Lithium ion	AA alkaline	Ni-Cd	AA alkaline
Life, hr	> 48	≤ 7	30	14	14	18	8	12	18
Rechargeable	No	Yes	No	Not specified	Not specified	Yes	Not specified	Yes	No
Low battery notice	Yes	Yes	Yes	No	No	Yes	Yes	Yes	Yes
H × W × D, cm (in)	15.8 × 7.6 × 3.6 (6.2 × 3 × 1.4)	7.6 × 20.8 × 15.2 (3 × 8.2 × 6)	5.8 × 6.8 × 1.5 (2.28 × 2.68 × 0.59)	11.4 × 4.6 × 2.5 (4.5 × 1.8 × 1)	11.9 × 4.6 × 2.5 (4.7 × 1.8 × 1)	14 × 7.6 × 2.7 (5.5 × 3 × 1.1)	19.1 × 8.9 × 3.5 (7.5 × 3.5 × 1.4)	19.1 × 8.9 × 3.5 (7.5 × 3.5 × 1.4)	14 × 7.6 × 2.7 (5.5 × 3 × 1.1)
Weight, kg (lb)	0.32 (0.7)	0.95 (2.1)	0.056 (0.125)	0.095 (0.21) with batteries	0.098 (0.22) with batteries	0.2 (0.44)	0.44 (0.97)	0.45 (0.99)	0.2 (0.44)
Green Features	Can be used with ReSposable Sensors	Can be used with ReSposable Sensors	None specified	None specified	None specified	None specified	None specified	None specified	None specified
FDA Clearance	Yes	Yes	Yes	Yes	Yes	Yes	Yes	Yes	Yes
CE Mark	Yes	Yes	Yes	Yes	Yes	Yes	Yes	Yes	Yes

(continues)

APPENDIX 7-A
Descriptions of Features and Specifications of Pulse Oximeters (Continued)

SPECIFICATIONS	MEDIAID MODEL 31DT	MEDIAID MODEL 34	MEDIAID MODEL 340	MEDIAID MODEL 340DT	MEDIAID MODEL 34B	MEDIAID MODEL 5305	MEDIAID MODEL 5340	MEDIAID MODEL 900	MEDLAB CAPNOX
Modular/Stand-alone	Tabletop	Stand-alone, palm size, rechargeable	Stand-alone, handheld	Stand-alone	Stand-alone, palm size, battery	Stand-alone, handheld	Stand-alone, handheld	Stand-alone	Stand-alone
MRI compatible	No	No	No	No	No	No	No	No	No
SpO_2 range, %	0–100	0–100	0–100	0–100	0–100	0–100	0–100	0–100	0–100
Accuracy, %	± 2 (70–100), ± 3 (60–69)	± 2 (70–100), ± 3 (60–69)	± 2 (70–100), ± 3 (60–69)	± 2 (70–100), ± 3 (60–69)	± 2 (70–100), ± 3 (60–69)	± 2 (70–100), ± 3 (60–69)	± 2 (70–100), ± 3 (60–69)	± 2 (70–100), ± 3 (60–69)	± 2 (70–100)
Pulse rate, bpm	25–255	25–255	32–250	32–250	25–255	32–250	32–250	Not specified	30–250
Accuracy	2 bpm or 2%, whichever is greater	2 bpm or 2%, whichever is greater	Not specified	Not specified	2 bpm or 2%, whichever is greater	Not specified	Not specified	Not specified	1% or 1 digit
Probe Types									
Disposable	Yes	Yes	Multisite adhesive	Multisite adhesive	Yes	Multisite adhesive	Multisite adhesive	Multisite adhesive	Finger, foot (neonatal)
Reusable	Yes	Yes	Universal hinged, tape-on, soft, pediatric, adjustable, great toe, ear clip, R-adhesive	Universal hinged, tape-on, soft, pediatric, adjustable, great toe, ear clip, R-adhesive	Yes	Universal hinged, tape-on, soft, pediatric, adjustable, great toe, ear clip, R-adhesive	Universal hinged, tape-on, soft, pediatric, adjustable, great toe, ear clip, R-adhesive	Universal hinged, tape-on, soft, pediatric, adjustable, great toe, ear clip, R-adhesive	Finger, ear, multisite
Patient range	Adult, pediatric; small to large	Adult, pediatric; small to large	Adult, pediatric; small to large	Adult, pediatric; small to large	Adult, pediatric; small to large	Adult, pediatric; small to large	Adult, pediatric; small to large	Adult, pediatric; small to large	Adult, neonate
Perfusion Index and/or Signal Strength Indicator	Yes	Yes	Not specified	Not specified	Yes	Not specified	Not specified	Not specified	Pulse bar graph
Response Time, sec	Every pulse	Every pulse	Every pulse	Every pulse	Every pulse	Every pulse	Every pulse	Every pulse	1
Start-Up Time, sec or pulses	3 pulses	3 pulses	3 pulses	3 pulses	3 pulses	3 pulses	3 pulses	3 pulses	3–5 sec
Averaging Time, sec	Not specified	Not specified	Not specified	Not specified	Not specified	Not specified	Not specified	Not specified	4, 10, 20
Data Management	Yes	Yes	Not specified	Not specified	Yes	Not specified	Not specified	Not specified	Yes
Data stored	Yes	Yes	Not specified	Not specified	Yes	Not specified	Not specified	Not specified	SpO_2, pulse rate, $ETCO_2$, respiration rate
Data storage, hr	136	136	Not specified	Not specified	136	Not specified	Not specified	Not specified	17

APPENDIX 7-A
Descriptions of Features and Specifications of Pulse Oximeters *(Continued)*

SPECIFICATIONS	MEDIAID MODEL 31DT	MEDIAID MODEL 34	MEDIAID MODEL 340	MEDIAID MODEL 340DT	MEDIAID MODEL 34B	MEDIAID MODEL 5305	MEDIAID MODEL 5340	MEDIAID MODEL 900	MEDLAB CAPNOX
External output	Yes	Yes	Analog/serial	Analog/serial	Yes	No	Analog/serial	Analog/serial	Optical
Displays	SpO_2, pulse rate	SpO_2, pulse rate	SpO_2, pulse rate	SpO_2, pulse rate, blood perfusion	SpO_2, pulse rate, blood perfusion	SpO_2, pulse rate	SpO_2, pulse rate	SpO_2, pulse rate, waveform	SpO_2, pulse rate, $ETCO_2$, respiration rate, plethysmogram/capnogram, trends
Printer-Recorder	Optional	Optional	No	No	Optional	No	No	No	Optional
Alarms									
Audiovisual	Yes	Yes	High/low SpO_2, pulse rate	High/low SpO_2, pulse rate	Yes	No	High/low SpO_2, pulse rate	High/low SpO_2, pulse rate	High/low SpO_2, $ETCO_2$, respiration rate
Visual	Lights	Lights	Lights, high, low	Lights, high, low	Lights	No	Lights, high, low	Lights, high, low	High/low SpO_2, $ETCO_2$, respiration rate, pulse rate
Alarm override	Yes	Yes	Yes	Yes	Yes	No	Yes	Yes	Audible
Reactivation method	Yes	Yes	Press button for 3 sec	Press button for 3 sec	Yes	NA	Press button for 3 sec	Press button for 3 sec	Automatic
Volume control	Yes	Yes	Yes	Yes	Yes	NA	Yes	Yes	Yes
Power									
VAC	Yes	Yes	AC adapter	AC adapter	Battery only	AC adapter	AC adapter	AC adapter	NA (rechargeable battery pack)
Batteries	Lithium ion	Lithium ion	Ni-Cd	Ni-Cd	AAA	Ni-Cd	Ni-Cd	Ni-Cd	Ni-MH 4.8 V 2,700 mAh
Life, hr	18	18	12	10	18	12	12	3–6	12
Rechargeable	Yes	Yes	Yes	Yes	No	Yes	Yes	Yes	Yes
Low battery notice	Yes	Yes	Yes	Yes	Yes	Yes	Yes	Yes	Yes
H × W × D, cm (in)	14 × 7.6 × 2.7 (5.5 × 3 × 1.1)	14 × 7.6 × 2.7 (5.5 × 3 × 1.1)	19.1 × 8.9 × 3.5 (7.5 × 3.5 × 1.4)	30 × 20 × 9.8 (11.8 × 7.9 × 3.9)	14 × 7.6 × 2.7 (5.5 × 3 × 1.1)	19.1 × 8.9 × 3.5 (7.5 × 3.5 × 1.4)	19.1 × 8.9 × 3.5 (7.5 × 3.5 × 1.4)	30 × 20 × 9.8 (11.8 × 7.9 × 3.9)	18 × 10 × 4 (7.1 × 4 × 1.4)
Weight, kg (lb)	0.2 (0.44)	0.2 (0.44)	0.49 (1.1)	1.6 (3.6)	0.2 (0.44)	0.45 (1)	0.49 (1.1)	2.5 (5.6)	0.4 (0.9)
Green Features	None specified	None specified	None specified	None specified	None specified	None specified	None specified	None specified	Power consumption > 1 W operating
FDA Clearance	Yes	Yes	Yes	Yes	Yes	Yes	Yes	No	No
CE Mark	Yes	Yes	Yes	Yes	Yes	Yes	Yes	Yes	Yes

(continues)

APPENDIX 7-A
Descriptions of Features and Specifications of Pulse Oximeters (Continued)

SPECIFICATIONS	MEDLAB NANOX10	MEDLAB NANOX10C	MEDLAB NANOX Echo	MEDLAB PEARL 10	MEDLAB PEARL 100	MEDLAB P-OX 100	MINOLTA MD300 C2	MINOLTA MD300 C5	MINOLTA PULSOX-2
Modular/Stand-alone	Stand-alone	Stand-alone	Stand-alone	Stand-alone	Stand-alone	Stand-alone	Stand-alone	Stand-alone	Stand-alone
MRI compatible	No	No	No	No	No	No	Not specified	Not specified	Not specified
SpO_2 range, %	0–100	0–100	0–100	0–100	0–100	0–100	70–99	70–100	0–100
Accuracy, %	± 2 (70–100)	± 2 (70–100)	± 2 (70–100)	± 2 (70–100)	± 2 (70–100)	± 2 (70–100)	± 2 (80–99), ± 3 (70–80)	± 2 (80–100), ± 3 (70–79), unspecified (0–69)	± 2 (70–100)
Pulse rate, bpm	30–250	30–250	30–250	30–250	30–250	30–250	30–235	30–235	20–250
Accuracy	1% or 1 digit	1% or 1 digit	1% or 1 digit	1% or 1 digit	1% or 1 digit	1% or 1 digit	2	30–100 ± 2, 101–235 ± 2%	± 2
Probe Types									
Disposable	Finger, foot (neonatal)	Finger, foot (neonatal)	Finger, foot (neonatal)	Finger, foot (neonatal)	Finger, foot (neonatal)	Finger, foot (neonatal)	Finger	Finger	Finger, multisite
Reusable	Finger, ear, multisite	Finger, ear, multisite	Finger, ear, multisite	Finger, ear, multisite	Finger, ear, multisite	Finger, ear, multisite	Finger	Finger	Finger, multisite
Patient range	Adult, neonate	Adult, neonate	Adult, neonate	Adult, neonate	Adult, neonate	Adult, neonate	Adult, pediatric	Pediatric, infant	Adult
Perfusion Index and/or Signal Strength Indicator	Pulse bar graph	Pulse bar graph	Pulse bar graph	Perfusion index bar, pulse bar graph	Perfusion index bar, pulse bar graph	Perfusion index bar, pulse bar graph	Not specified	Not specified	Not specified
Response Time, sec	1	1	1	1	1	1	Not specified	Not specified	Not specified
Start-Up Time, sec or pulses	3–5 sec	3–5 sec	3–5 sec	3–5 sec	3–5 sec	3–5 sec	Not specified	Not specified	Not specified
Averaging Time, sec	4, 10, 20	4, 10, 20	8	4, 10, 20	4, 10, 20	4, 10, 20	Not specified	Not specified	Not specified
Data Management	Yes	Yes	No	Yes	Yes	Yes	Yes	Yes	Not specified
Data stored	SpO_2, pulse rate	SpO_2, pulse rate	NA	SpO_2, pulse rate, events	SpO_2, pulse rate	SpO_2, pulse rate	SpO_2	SpO_2	Not specified
Data storage, hr	26	26	NA	55 plus SD card interface, unlimited storage	110	110	Not specified	Not specified	Not specified
External output	Optical	RS232, USB	RS232, optical	Optical, Bluetooth	RS232, optical, Bluetooth	RS232, optical, Bluetooth	Not specified	Not specified	Not specified

APPENDIX 7-A
Descriptions of Features and Specifications of Pulse Oximeters (Continued)

SPECIFICATIONS	MEDLAB NANOX10	MEDLAB NANOX10C	MEDLAB NANOX Echo	MEDLAB PEARL 10	MEDLAB PEARL 100	MEDLAB P-OX 100	MINOLTA MD300 C2	MINOLTA MD300 C5	MINOLTA PULSOX-2
Displays	SpO_2, pulse rate	SpO_2, pulse rate	SpO_2, pulse rate	SpO_2, pulse rate, plethysmogram, alarms	SpO_2, pulse rate, plethysmogram, ECG, alarms	SpO_2, pulse rate, plethysmogram, ECG, alarms	SpO_2, pulse rate, pulse rate bar graph, low power indicator, SpO_2 wavelength	SpO_2, pulse rate, pulse bar	SpO_2, pulse rate, error messages
Printer-Recorder	Optional	Optional	Optional	Optional	Optional	Optional	No	No	No
Alarms									
Audiovisual	High/low SpO_2, $ETCO_2$, respiration rate	High/low SpO_2, $ETCO_2$, respiration rate	No	High/low SpO_2, $ETCO_2$, respiration rate	High/low SpO_2, $ETCO_2$, respiration rate	High/low SpO_2, $ETCO_2$, respiration rate	No	Visual	No
Visual	High/low SpO_2, $ETCO_2$, respiration rate	High/low SpO_2, $ETCO_2$, respiration rate	No	High/low SpO_2 and pulse rate	High/low SpO_2 and pulse rate	High/low SpO_2 and pulse rate	No	Low battery	Error messages
Alarm override	Audible	Audible	No	Audible	Audible	Audible	No	No	No
Reactivation method	Automatic	Automatic	NA	Automatic	Automatic	Automatic	NA	NA	NA
Volume control	Yes	No	NA	No	No	No	NA	NA	NA
Power									
VAC	Battery only	230, optional 115	Battery only	Battery only	115/230	115/230	Battery only	Battery only	Battery only
Batteries	Alkaline	Ni-MH	Alkaline, Ni-Cd, or Ni-MH	Alkaline, Ni-Cd, or Ni-MH	Ni-MH 7.2 V 1800 mAh	Ni-MH 7.2 V 1800 mAh	AAA	AAA alkaline or rechargeable	AAA
Life, hr	30	14	15	60	6	6	30	30	80
Rechargeable	No	Yes	Optional	Optional	Yes	Yes	No	No	No
Low battery notice	Yes	Yes	Yes	Yes	Yes	Yes	Yes	Yes	Yes
H × W × D, cm (in)	17 × 8 × 2.5 (6.7 × 3.1 × 1)	17 × 8 × 2.5 (6.7 × 3.1 × 1)	6 × 12 × 2.5 (2.4 × 4.7 × 1)	17 × 8 × 2.5 (6.7 × 3.1 × 1)	23 × 20 × 8 (9.1 × 7.9 × 3.1)	23 × 20 × 8 (9.1 × 7.9 × 3.1)	5.8 × 3.2 × 3.4 (2.3 × 1.3 × 1.3)	5 × 2.8 × 2.8 (2 × 1.1 × 1.1)	6 × 6.9 × 2.8 (2.4 × 2.7 × 1.1)
Weight, kg (lb)	0.2 (0.44)	0.2 (0.44)	0.15 (0.3)	0.25 (0.45)	1.5 (3.3)	1.5 (3.3)	0.05 (0.1) including batteries	0.03 (0.06) without batteries	0.06 (0.13) without batteries
Green Features	Power consumption > 0.2 W operating	Power consumption > 0.2 W operating	Power consumption > 0.2 W operating	Power consumption > 0.2 W operating	Power consumption > 0.2 W operating	Power consumption > 0.2 W operating	Auto-off function after 8 seconds of no use	None specified	None specified
FDA Clearance	No	No	No	No	No	No	Yes	Yes	Yes
CE Mark	Yes	Yes	Yes	Yes	Yes	Yes	Yes	Yes	Yes

(continues)

APPENDIX 7-A
Descriptions of Features and Specifications of Pulse Oximeters (Continued)

SPECIFICATIONS	MINOLTA PULSOX-300	MINOLTA PULSOX-300i	NELLCOR/ COVIDIEN OxiMax N-560	NELLCOR/ COVIDIEN OxiMax N-600x	NELLCOR/ COVIDIEN OxiMax N-65	NELLCOR/ COVIDIEN OxiMax N-85	NIHON KOHDEN OLV-2700K	NIHON KOHDEN OLV-3100K	NONIN MEDICAL 2500 PalmSAT
Modular/ Stand-alone	Stand-alone	Stand-alone	Stand-alone	Stand-alone	Handheld	Handheld	Stand-alone	Stand-alone	Stand-alone
MRI compatible	Not specified	Not specified	No	No	No	No	No	No	No
SpO$_2$ range, %	0–100	0–100	1–100	1–100	1–100	1–100	1–100	1–100	0–100
Accuracy, %	± 2 (70–100)	± 2 (70–100)	± 2 (70–100)	± 2 (70–100)	± 2 (70–100)	± 2 (70–100)	± 2 (80–100), ± 3 (70–80), not specified < 70	± 2 (80–100), ± 3 (70–80), not specified < 70	± 2 (70–100 no motion), ± 3 (70–100 motion, low perfusion)
Pulse rate, bpm	30–230	30–230	20–250	20–250	20–250	20–250	30–300	30–300	18–300
Accuracy	2	2	± 3 digits	± 3 digits	± 3 digits	± 3 digits	± 3% ± 1	± 3% ± 1	20–250 ± 3 digits (no motion); 40–240 ± 3 digits (low perfusion); 60 to 240 ± 5 digits (motion)
Probe Types									
Disposable	Finger, wrist	Finger, wrist	Nellcor OxiMax adhesives, reusables, and speciality	Nellcor OxiMax adhesives, reusables, and speciality	Nellcor OxiMax adhesives, reusables, and speciality	Nellcor OxiMax adhesives, reusables, and speciality	Finger, multisite	Finger, multisite	Repositionable comfort adhesive wrap
Reusable	Finger, wrist	Finger, wrist	Nellcor OxiMax adhesives, reusables, and speciality	Nellcor OxiMax adhesives, reusables, and speciality	Nellcor OxiMax adhesives, reusables, and speciality	Nellcor OxiMax adhesives, reusables, and speciality	Finger, multisite	Finger, multisite	Finger-clip, soft, flex, forehead, ear

APPENDIX 7-A
Descriptions of Features and Specifications of Pulse Oximeters *(Continued)*

			MODEL						
SPECIFICATIONS	MINOLTA PULSOX-300	MINOLTA PULSOX-300i	NELLCOR/COVIDIEN OxiMax N-560	NELLCOR/COVIDIEN OxiMax N-600x	NELLCOR/COVIDIEN OxiMax N-65	NELLCOR/COVIDIEN OxiMax N-85	NIHON KOHDEN OLV-2700K	NIHON KOHDEN OLV-3100K	NONIN MEDICAL 2500 PalmSAT
Patient range	Adult	Adult	Adult, pediatric, infant, neonate	Adult, pediatric, infant, neonate	Adult, pediatric, infant, neonate	Adult, pediatric, infant, neonate	Adult, pediatric, infant, neonate	Adult, pediatric, infant, neonate	Adult, pediatric, infant, neonate
Perfusion Index and/or Signal Strength Indicator	Not specified	Not specified	70–100% low perfusion	70–100% low perfusion	70–100% low perfusion	70–100% low perfusion	Not specified	Not specified	Tricolor pulse quality LED
Response Time, sec	Not specified	Not specified	Updated 1/sec	Updated 1/sec	Updated 1/sec	Updated 1/sec	4, 8, 16, user selectable	4, 8, 16, user selectable	1.5
Start-Up Time, sec or pulses	Not specified	Not specified	Typically 5–7, updated 1/sec	Typically 5–7, updated 1/sec	Typically 5–7, updated 1/sec	Typically 5–7, updated 1/sec	8 pulses	8 pulses	4 sec total, 3 heartbeats plus 0.5 sec
Averaging Time, sec	Not specified	Not specified	6–7 dynamic averaging, 2–3 fast SpO_2	6–7 dynamic averaging, 2–3 fast SpO_2	6–7 dynamic averaging, 2–3 fast SpO_2	6–7 dynamic averaging, 2–3 fast SpO_2	1	1	3, Smart Average
Data Management	Yes	Yes	Yes	Yes	Not specified	Yes	Not specified	Not specified	Yes
Data stored	SpO_2	SpO_2	Not specified	Not specified	Not specified	Not specified	Not specified	Not specified	SpO_2, pulse rate, pulse quality
Data storage, hr	4,000 spot measurements	Not specified	24	48	Not specified	8	Not specified	24	72
External output	Not specified	Yes	EIA-232	EIA-232 and RS422, analog	NA	RS232, optional analog	Not specified	Digital, analog, telemetry signals	RS232; USB adapter
Displays	SpO_2, pulse rate, error messages, battery indication	SpO_2, pulse rate, error messages, battery indication	SpO_2, pulse rate, pulse amplitude	SpO_2, pulse rate, pulse amplitude, plethysmogram	SpO_2, pulse rate, pulse amplitude	SpO_2, pulse rate, pulse amplitude, plethysmogram, $ETCO_2$, respiration rate	SpO_2, pulse rate, pulse-detection display, bar graph, measurement status indicator power status indicator	SpO_2, pulse rate, pulse-detection display, bar graph, measurement status indicator power status indicator	SpO_2, pulse rate, pulse quality

(continues)

APPENDIX 7-A
Descriptions of Features and Specifications of Pulse Oximeters *(Continued)*

SPECIFICATIONS	MINOLTA PULSOX-300	MINOLTA PULSOX-300i	NELLCOR/COVIDIEN OxiMax N-560	NELLCOR/COVIDIEN OxiMax N-600x	NELLCOR/COVIDIEN OxiMax N-65	NELLCOR/COVIDIEN OxiMax N-85	NIHON KOHDEN OLV-2700K	NIHON KOHDEN OLV-3100K	NONIN MEDICAL 2500 PalmSAT
Printer-Recorder	No	Yes	Optional	Optional	Optional Citizen via infrared link	Optional	No	Optional	No
Alarms									
Audiovisual	No	No	User configuration, high/low priority, SpO$_2$, pulse rate, SatSeconds, low battery, sensor off, sensor disconnected, alarms off reminder	User configuration, high/low priority, SpO$_2$, pulse rate, SatSeconds, low battery, sensor off, sensor disconnected, alarms off reminder	User configuration, high/low priority, SpO$_2$, pulse rate, loss of pulse, low battery, sensor off, sensor disconnected	High/low SpO$_2$ and pulse rate, ETCO$_2$, respiration, high FiCO$_2$, sensor disconnected (audio only)	High/low SpO$_2$, pulse rate, measurement condition, no pulse, connector off, no probe, check probe, battery empty, low battery, unit malfunction, probe failure	High/low SpO$_2$, pulse rate, high delta SpO$_2$, measurement condition, no pulse, check probe, connector off, no probe, battery empty, low battery, error/probe failure	NA
Visual	Error messages	Error messages	Pulse search, interference, alarms silenced	Pulse search, interference, alarms silenced	Pulse search, interference, alarms silenced	Alarm off or silenced, low battery	Blinking LED	Blinking LED	Pulse quality, low battery, finger removal
Alarm override	No	No	Yes	Yes	Yes	Yes	Yes	Yes	No
Reactivation method	NA	NA	Automatic, manual	Automatic, manual	Automatic, manual	Automatic, manual	Auto after 60, 90, 120 sec and user selectable or manual	Auto after 60, 90, 120 sec and user selectable or manual	NA
Volume control	NA	NA	Yes	Yes	Yes	Yes	8 steps	8 steps	NA
Power									
VAC	Battery only	Battery only	100–240	100–120, 200–240	Battery only	100–230	100–127, 220–240	100–127, 220–240	110/240 with optional charging stand

APPENDIX 7-A
Descriptions of Features and Specifications of Pulse Oximeters (Continued)

SPECIFICATIONS	MINOLTA	MINOLTA	NELLCOR/ COVIDIEN	NELLCOR/ COVIDIEN	NELLCOR/ COVIDIEN	NELLCOR/ COVIDIEN	NIHON KOHDEN	NIHON KOHDEN	NONIN MEDICAL
	PULSOX-300	PULSOX-300i	OxiMax N-560	OxiMax N-600x	OxiMax N-65	OxiMax N-85	OLV-2700K	OLV-3100K	2500 PalmSAT
Batteries	AAA	AAA	Ni-MH	Sealed lead-acid, internal	AA alkaline or lithium	Ni-MH	Ni-MH optional	Lead-acid	AA alkaline or Ni-MH rechargeable
Life, hr	80	30	8	7	19 (alkaline), 40 (lithium)	4–7	2	4	80
Rechargeable	No	No	Yes	Yes	No	Yes	Yes	Yes	Optional
Low battery notice	Yes	Yes	Yes	Yes	Yes	Yes	Yes	Yes	Yes
H × W × D, cm (in)	5.8 × 5.8 × 1.5 (2.3 × 2.3 × 0.6)	5.8 × 5.8 × 1.5 (2.3 × 2.7 × 0.6)	6.1 × 20.1 × 11.9 (2.4 × 7.9 × 4.7)	8.4 × 26.4 × 17.3 (3.3 × 10.4 × 6.8)	7.1 × 15.7 × 3.6 (2.8 × 6.2 × 1.4)	20.6 × 8.9 × 5.3 (8.1 × 3.5 × 2.1)	6.2 × 21 × 16.4 (2.4 × 8.3 × 6.5)	9.5 × 26 × 17.7 (3.7 × 10.2 × 7)	3.2 × 7 × 13.8 (1.3 × 2.8 × 5.4)
Weight, kg (lb)	0.06 (0.13)	0.06 (0.13) including batteries	1.1 (2.4)	2.6 (5.7)	0.3 (0.7)	0.82 (1.8)	1 (2.2)	2.8 (6.2)	0.23 (0.5)
Green Features	None specified	None specified	None specified	None specified	None specified	None specified	None specified	None specified	None specified
FDA Clearance	Yes	Yes	Yes	Yes	Yes	Yes	No	No	Yes
CE Mark	Yes	Yes	Yes	Yes	Yes	Yes	Yes	Yes	Yes

MODEL

(continues)

APPENDIX 7-A
Descriptions of Features and Specifications of Pulse Oximeters *(Continued)*

SPECIFICATIONS	NONIN MEDICAL 2500A PALMSAT	NONIN MEDICAL 7500	NONIN MEDICAL 7500FO (FIBEROPTIC)	NONIN MEDICAL AVANT 2120	NONIN MEDICAL AVANT 4000 (WIRELESS)	NONIN MEDICAL AVANT 9600	NONIN MEDICAL AVANT 9700	NONIN MEDICAL LIFESENSE	NONIN MEDICAL ONYX 9500 FINGERTIP
Modular/ Stand-alone	Stand-alone	Stand-alone	Stand-alone	Stand-alone	Stand-alone	Stand-alone	Stand-alone	Stand-alone	All-in-one
MRI compatible	No	No	No	No	No	No	No	No	No
SpO$_2$ range, %	0–100	0–100	0–100	0–100	0–100	0–100	0–100	0–100	0–100
Accuracy, %	± 2 (70–100 no motion), ± 3 (70–100 motion, low perfusion)	± 2 (70–100 no motion), ± 3 (70–100 motion, low perfusion)	± 2 (70–100 no motion), ± 3 (70–100 motion, low perfusion)	± 2 (70–100 no motion), ± 3 (70–100 motion, low perfusion)	± 2 (70–100 no motion), ± 3 (70–100 motion, low perfusion)	± 2 (70–100 no motion), ± 3 (70–100 motion, low perfusion)	± 2 (70–100 no motion), ± 3 (70–100 motion, low perfusion)	± 2 (70–100 no motion)	± 2 (70–100 no motion), ± 3 (70–100 motion, low perfusion)
Pulse rate, bpm	18–300	18–300	18–300	18–300	18–300	18–300	18–300	18–255	18–300
Accuracy	20–250 ± 3 digits (no motion); 40–240 ± 3 digits (low perfusion); 60 to 240 ± 5 digits (motion)	20–250 ± 3 digits (no motion); 40–240 ± 3 digits (low perfusion); 60 to 240 ± 5 digits (motion)	20–250 ± 3 digits (no motion); 40–240 ± 3 digits (low perfusion); 60 to 240 ± 5 digits (motion)	20–250 ± 3 digits (no motion); 40–240 ± 3 digits (low perfusion); 60 to 240 ± 5 digits (motion)	20–250 ± 3 digits (no motion); 40–240 ± 3 digits (low perfusion); 60 to 240 ± 5 digits (motion)	20–250 ± 3 digits (no motion); 40–240 ± 3 digits (low perfusion); 60 to 240 ± 5 digits (motion)	20–250 ± 3 digits (no motion); 40–240 ± 3 digits (low perfusion); 60 to 240 ± 5 digits (motion)	18–255 ± 3 digits (no motion); 40–240 ± 3 digits (low perfusion)	± 3 digits (no motion, low perfusion)
Probe Types									
Disposable	Repositionable comfort adhesive wrap	Repositionable comfort adhesive wrap	Not specified	Repositionable comfort adhesive wrap	Repositionable comfort adhesive wrap	Repositionable comfort adhesive wrap	Repositionable comfort adhesive wrap	Reposit onable comfort adhesive wrap	NA

APPENDIX 7-A
Descriptions of Features and Specifications of Pulse Oximeters (Continued)

SPECIFICATIONS	MODEL								
	NONIN MEDICAL 2500A PALMSAT	NONIN MEDICAL 7500	NONIN MEDICAL 7500FO (FIBEROPTIC)	NONIN MEDICAL AVANT 2120	NONIN MEDICAL AVANT 4000 (WIRELESS)	NONIN MEDICAL AVANT 9600	NONIN MEDICAL AVANT 9700	NONIN MEDICAL LIFESENSE	NONIN MEDICAL ONYX 9500 FINGERTIP
Reusable	Finger-clip, soft, flex, forehead, ear	Finger-clip, soft, flex, forehead, ear	Finger-clip, soft, flex, forehead, ear	Finger-clip, soft, flex, forehead, ear	Finger-clip, soft, flex, forehead, ear	Finger-clip, soft, forehead, ear	Finger-clip, soft, forehead, ear	Finger-clip, soft, forehead, ear	All-in-one
Patient range	Adult, pediatric, infant, neonate	Adult, pediatric, infant, neonate	Adult, pediatric, infant, neonate	Adult, pediatric, infant, neonate	Adult, pediatric, infant, neonate	Adult, pediatric, infant, neonate	Adult, pediatric, infant, neonate	Adult, pediatric, infant, neonate	Adult, pediatric
Perfusion Index and/or Signal Strength Indicator	Tricolor pulse quality LED	Tricolor bar graph	Tricolor bar graph	Tricolor bar graph	Tricolor bar graph	Tricolor bar graph	Tricolor bar graph	Plethysmograph waveform	Tricolor pulse quality
Response Time, sec	1.5	1.5	1.5	1.5	1.5	1.5	1.5	1.5	1.5
Start-Up Time, sec or pulses	4 sec total, 3 heartbeats plus 0.5 sec	4 sec total, 3 heartbeats plus 0.5 sec	4 sec total, 3 heartbeats plus 0.5 sec	4 sec total, 3 heartbeats plus 0.5 sec	4 sec total, 3 heartbeats plus 0.5 sec	4 sec total, 3 heartbeats plus 0.5 sec	4 sec total, 3 heartbeats plus 0.5 sec	4 sec total, 3 heartbeats plus 0.5 sec	4 sec total, 3 heartbeats plus 0.5 sec
Averaging Time, sec	3, Smart Average	3, Smart Average	6, Smart Average	3, Smart Average	3, Smart Average	3, Smart Average	3, Smart Average	3, Smart Average	3, Smart Average
Data Management	Yes	Yes	Yes	Yes	Yes	Yes	Yes	TrendSense memory module optional	No
Data stored	SpO$_2$, pulse rate, pulse quality	SpO$_2$, pulse rate, current time/date	SpO$_2$, pulse rate, current time/date	SpO$_2$, pulse rate, current time/date	SpO$_2$, pulse rate, current time/date	SpO$_2$, pulse rate, current time/date	SpO$_2$, pulse rate, current time/date	SpO$_2$, HR, ETCO$_2$, respiration	NA
Data storage, hr	72	70 continuous, nonvolatile	70 continuous, nonvolatile	70 continuous, nonvolatile	70 continuous, nonvolatile	115 continuous, nonvolatile	115 continuous, nonvolatile	72	NA
External output	RS232; USB adapter	RS232, analog, digital	RS232, analog, digital	RS232, analog, digital	RS232, analog, digital	RS232, optional analog	RS232, optional analog	RS232 and optional analog output	NA

(continues)

APPENDIX 7-A
Descriptions of Features and Specifications of Pulse Oximeters (Continued)

SPECIFICATIONS	NONIN MEDICAL 2500A PALMSAT	NONIN MEDICAL 7500	NONIN MEDICAL 7500FO (FIBEROPTIC)	NONIN MEDICAL AVANT 2120	NONIN MEDICAL AVANT 4000 (WIRELESS)	NONIN MEDICAL AVANT 9600	NONIN MEDICAL AVANT 9700	NONIN MEDICAL LIFESENSE	NONIN MEDICAL ONYX 9500 FINGERTIP
Displays	SpO_2, pulse rate, pulse quality	SpO_2, pulse rate, pulse quality, pulse strength, sensor indicator, alarm settings, AC power indicator	SpO_2, pulse rate, pulse quality, pulse strength, sensor indicator, alarm settings, AC power indicator	SpO_2, NIBP, pulse rate, pulse quality, pulse strength, sensor indicator, systolic, diastolic, MAP	SpO_2, pulse rate, pulse quality, pulse strength, sensor indicator, alarm settings, AC power indicator	SpO_2, pulse rate, pulse quality, pulse strength, sensor indicator, alarm settings, AC power indicator	SpO_2, pulse rate, color plethysmographic waveform, 24 hr trending, patient histogram, pulse quality, pulse strength, sensor indicator, alarm settings,	SpO_2, pulse rate, pulse strength, sensor indicator	SpO_2, pulse rate, pulse quality
Printer-Recorder	No	Optional	Optional	Optional	Optional	Optional	Optional	No	No
Alarms									
Audiovisual	High/low SpO_2 and pulse, sensor fault	High/low SpO_2 and pulse, sensor fault, self-test, low battery, variable pulse tone	High/low SpO_2 and pulse, sensor fault, low battery, variable pulse tone	High/low SpO_2 and pulse, sensor fault, self-test, low battery, variable pulse tone	High/low SpO_2 and pulse, sensor fault, self-test, low battery, variable pulse tone	High/low SpO_2 and pulse, low perfusion, sensor fault, self test, low battery	High/low SpO_2 and pulse, pulse quality, low perfusion, alarm silence, battery, sensor fault	High/low SpO_2 and pulse, sensor fault, self-test, low battery	No
Visual	Pulse quality, low battery, sensor fault, finger removal	High/low SpO_2 and pulse rate, pulse quality/low perfusion, alarm silence, battery, sensor fault	High/low SpO_2 and pulse rate, pulse quality/low perfusion, alarm silence, battery, sensor fault	High/low SpO_2 and pulse rate, pulse quality/low perfusion, alarm silence, battery, sensor fault	High/low SpO_2 and pulse rate, pulse quality/low perfusion, alarm silence, battery, sensor fault	High/low SpO_2 and pulse rate, pulse quality/low perfusion, alarm silence, battery, sensor fault	High/low SpO_2 and pulse rate, pulse quality/low perfusion, alarm silence, battery, sensor fault	High/low SpO_2 and pulse rate, pulse quality/low perfusion, alarm silence, battery, sensor fault	Pulse quality, low battery, finger removal
Alarm override	Yes	Yes	Yes	Yes	Yes	Yes	Yes	Yes	No
Reactivation method	Auto after 2 min or manual	Auto after 2 min or manual	Auto after 2 min or manual	Auto after 2 min	Auto after 2 min	Auto after 2 min or manual	Auto after 2 min or manual	Auto after 2 min or manual	NA
Volume control	Yes	Yes	Yes	Yes	Yes	Yes	Yes	Yes	NA

APPENDIX 7-A
Descriptions of Features and Specifications of Pulse Oximeters (Continued)

					MODEL				
	NONIN MEDICAL	NONIN MEDICAL	NONIN MEDICAL	NONIN MEDICAL	NONIN MEDICAL	NONIN MEDICAL	NONIN MEDICAL	NONIN MEDICAL	NONIN MEDICAL
SPECIFICATIONS	2500A PALMSAT	7500	7500FO (FIBEROPTIC)	AVANT 2120	AVANT 4000 (WIRELESS)	AVANT 9600	AVANT 9700	LIFESENSE	ONYX 9500 FINGERTIP
Power									
VAC	110/240 with optional charging stand	110/240	110/240	110/240	110/240	110/240	110/240	110/240	Battery only
Batteries	AA alkaline or Ni-MH rechargeable	Ni-MH	Ni-MH	Ni-MH	Ni-MH	Ni-MH	Ni-MH	Lithium ion	AAA alkaline
Life, hr	60	16	30 when 5 V supply is not used, 10 minimum when 250 mA5V supply is used	5	18	12	8–12	8	18 or 1,600 spot checks
Rechargeable	Optional	Yes	Yes	Yes	Yes	Yes	Yes	Yes	No
Low battery notice	Yes	Yes	Yes	Yes	Yes	Yes	Yes	Yes	Yes
H × W × D, cm (in)	3.2 × 7 × 13.8 (1.3 × 2.8 × 5.4)	21.9 × 9.2 × 14.2 (8.6 × 3.6 × 5.6)	21.9 × 9.2 × 14.2 (8.6 × 3.6 × 5.6)	18.4 × 14 × 11.4 (7.3 × 5 × 4.5)	18.4 × 14 × 11.4 (7.3 × 5 × 4.5)	18.4 × 14 × 11.4 (7.3 × 5 × 4.5)	18.4 × 14 × 11.4 (7.3 × 5 × 4.5)	20 × 13.5 × 5 (7.9 × 5.3 × 2)	5.7 × 3.3 × 3.3 (2.2 × 1.3 × 1.3)
Weight, kg (lb)	0.23 (0.5)	1 (2.2)	1 (2.2)	1.3 (2.8)	1 (2.2)	1 (2.2)	1.1 (2.4)	0.8 (1.8)	0.06 (0.13)
Green Features	None specified	None specified	None specified	None specified	None specified	None specified	None specified	None specified	None specified
FDA Clearance	Yes	Yes	Yes	Yes	Yes	Yes	Yes	Yes	Yes
CE Mark	Yes	Yes	Yes	Yes	Yes	Yes	Yes	Yes (Medair)	Yes

(continues)

APPENDIX 7-A
Descriptions of Features and Specifications of Pulse Oximeters (Continued)

SPECIFICATIONS	MODEL								
	NONIN MEDICAL ONYX II 9550 FINGERTIP	NONIN MEDICAL ONYX II 9560 WIRELESS FINGERTIP	NONIN MEDICAL PULSESENSE	NONIN MEDICAL WRISTOX 3100	NONIN MEDICAL WRISTOX2 MODEL 3150	PACE TECH VITALMAX 520	PACE TECH VITALMAX 530	PACE TECH VITALMAX 560	QRS DIAGNOSTIC SPIROXCARD
Modular/Stand-alone	All-in-one	All-in-one	Stand-alone	Stand-alone	Stand-alone	Stand-alone	Not specified	Not specified	Not specified
MRI compatible	No	No	No	No	No	No	No	No	No
SpO$_2$ range, %	0–100	0–100	0–100	0–100	0–100	0–100	0–100	0–100	0–100
Accuracy, %	± 2 (70–100 no motion), ± 3 (70–100 motion, low perfusion)	± 2 (70–100 no motion), ± 3 (70–100 motion, low perfusion)	± 2 (70–100 no motion)	± 2 (70–100)	± 2 (70–100)	± 2 (70–100), ± 3 (50–69), unspecified (0–49)	± 2 (70–100), ± 3 (50–69), unspecified (0–49)	± 2 (70–100), ± 3 (50–69), unspecified (0–49)	± 2 (70–100)
Pulse rate, bpm	18–300	18–300	18–255	18–300	18–300	30–254	30–254	30–254	18–300
Accuracy	± 3 digits (no motion, low perfusion)	± 3 digits (no motion, low perfusion)	18–255 ± 3 digits (no motion), 40–240 ± 3 digits (low perfusion)	± 3%	± 3%	± 2% at 30–100	± 2% at 30–100	± 2% at 30–100	3%
Probe Types									
Disposable	NA	NA	Repositionable comfort adhesive wrap	Repositionable comfort adhesive wrap	Repositionable comfort adhesive wrap	Universal Y with earlobe clip	Universal Y with earlobe clip	Universal Y with earlobe clip	Not specified
Reusable	All-in-one	All-in-one	Finger-clip, soft, flex, forehead, ear	Finger-clip, soft, flex, forehead, ear	Finger-clip, soft, flex, forehead, ear	Finger, flex	Finger, flex	Finger, flex	Adult
Patient range	Adult, pediatric	Adult, pediatric	Adult, pediatric, infant, neonate	Adult, pediatric, infant, neonate	Adult, pediatric, infant, neonate	Adult, pediatric, infant, neonate	Adult, pediatric, infant, neonate	Adult, pediatric, infant, neonate	Adult

APPENDIX 7-A
Descriptions of Features and Specifications of Pulse Oximeters (Continued)

SPECIFICATIONS	NONIN MEDICAL ONYX II 9550 FINGERTIP	NONIN MEDICAL ONYX II 9560 WIRELESS FINGERTIP	NONIN MEDICAL PULSESENSE	NONIN MEDICAL WRISTOX 3100	NONIN MEDICAL WRISTOX2 MODEL 3150	PACE TECH VITALMAX 520	PACE TECH VITALMAX 530	PACE TECH VITALMAX 560	QRS DIAGNOSTIC SPIROXCARD
Perfusion Index and/or Signal Strength Indicator	Tricolor pulse quality	Tricolor pulse quality	Plethysmograph waveform	Pulse quality bar graph	Pulse quality bar graph	Not specified	Not specified	Not specified	Not specified
Response Time, sec	1.5	1.5	1.5	1.5	1.5	1	1	1	< 2
Start-Up Time, sec or pulses	4 sec total, 3 heartbeats plus 0.5 sec	4 sec total, 3 heartbeats plus 0.5 sec	4 sec total, 3 heartbeats plus 0.5 sec	1, 2, or 4 sec total 3 heartbeats plus 0.5 sec	1, 2, or 4 sec total 3 heartbeats plus 0.5 sec	Not specified	Not specified	Not specified	4 pulses
Averaging Time, sec	3, Smart Average	3, Smart Average	3, Smart Average	3, Smart Average	3, Smart Average	8	8	8	5, 10, 30, or 60
Data Management	No	No	TrendSense memory module optional	Yes	Yes	Not specified	Not specified	Not specified	Yes
Data stored	NA	SpO$_2$, pulse rate	SpO$_2$, HR	SpO$_2$, pulse rate, pulse quality	SpO$_2$, pulse rate, pulse quality	Not specified	Not specified	Not specified	On host PCC or PPC
Data storage, hr	NA	Memory storage provides up to 20 single point measurements	72	33	1,080	Not specified	Not specified	Not specified	≤ 24
External output	NA	Bluetooth Serial Port Profile	RS232 and optional analog output	RS232, optional analog	USB	Optional RS232	Not specified	Optional RS232	Standard paper report
Displays	SpO$_2$, pulse rate, pulse quality	SpO$_2$, pulse rate, pulse quality	SpO$_2$, pulse rate, pulse quality, pulse strength, sensor indicator	SpO$_2$, pulse rate, perfusion amplitude	SpO$_2$, pulse rate, perfusion amplitude	SpO$_2$, pulse rate, pulse amplitude bar graph, time/date, system status	SpO$_2$, pulse rate, pulse amplitude bar graph, time/date, system status	SpO$_2$, pulse rate, pulse amplitude bar graph, time/date, system status	SpO$_2$, pulse rate, signal intensity, perfusion

(continues)

APPENDIX 7-A
Descriptions of Features and Specifications of Pulse Oximeters *(Continued)*

SPECIFICATIONS	NONIN MEDICAL ONYX II 9550 FINGERTIP	NONIN MEDICAL ONYX II 9560 WIRELESS FINGERTIP	NONIN MEDICAL PULSESENSE	NONIN MEDICAL WRISTOX 3100	NONIN MEDICAL WRISTOX2 MODEL 3150	PACE TECH VITALMAX 520	PACE TECH VITALMAX 530	PACE TECH VITALMAX 560	QRS DIAGNOSTIC SPIROXCARD
					MODEL				
Printer-Recorder	No	No	No	No	No	Optional 27-column thermal printer	Optional 27-column thermal printer	Not specified	Windows-based printer
Alarms									
Audiovisual	No	No	High/low SpO$_2$ and pulse, sensor fault, self-test, low battery	NA	NA	All parameters, full range, nonoverlapping	All parameters, full range, nonoverlapping	All parameters, full range, nonoverlapping	No
Visual	Pulse quality, low battery, finger removal	Pulse quality, low battery, finger removal	High/low SpO$_2$ and pulse rate, pulse quality/low perfusion, alarm silence, battery, sensor fault	Pulse quality, low battery, finger removal	Pulse quality, low battery, finger removal	Low battery, AC on, high/low, sensor off	Low battery, AC on, high/low, sensor off	Low battery, AC on, high/low, sensor off	No
Alarm override	No	No	Yes	No	NA	Yes	Yes	Yes	Not specified
Reactivation method	NA	NA	Automatic after 2 min or manual	NA	NA	Automatic after 2 min or manual	Automatic after 2 min or manual	Automatic after 2 min or manual	Not specified
Volume control	NA	NA	No	NA	NA	No	No	No	Not specified
Power									
VAC	Battery only	Battery only	110/240	Battery only	Battery only	110–120, 220–240; 50/60 Hz	110–250; 50/60 Hz	110–250; 50/60 Hz	5 VDC internal, < 80 mA, supplied by card slot
Batteries	AAA alkaline	AAA alkaline	Lithium ion	N-cell	AAA	6V 7.0 AH sealed acid	6V 3.3 AH sealed acid	6V 500 AH Ni-Cd	None

APPENDIX 7-A
Descriptions of Features and Specifications of Pulse Oximeters (*Continued*)

SPECIFICATIONS	MODEL								
	NONIN MEDICAL ONYX II 9550 FINGERTIP	NONIN MEDICAL ONYX II 9560 WIRELESS FINGERTIP	NONIN MEDICAL PULSESENSE	NONIN MEDICAL WRISTOX 3100	NONIN MEDICAL WRISTOX2 MODEL 3150	PACE TECH VITALMAX 520	PACE TECH VITALMAX 530	PACE TECH VITALMAX 560	QRS DIAGNOSTIC SPIROXCARD
Life, hr	21 or 2,500 spot checks	500 spot checks	12	24	24/48	8–10	2–2.5	2–2.5	NA
Rechargeable	No	No	Yes	No	No	No	Yes	Yes	NA
Low battery notice	Yes	Yes	Yes	Yes	Yes	Yes	Yes	Yes	
H × W × D, cm (in)	5.7 × 3.3 × 3.3 (2.2 × 1.3 × 1.3)	6.4 × 3.2 × 3.8 (2.5 × 1.3 × 1.5)	20 × 13.5 × 5 (7.9 × 5.3 × 2)	4.6 × 5.1 × 2 (1.8 × 2 × 0.8)	7.3 × 5.9 × 1.9 (2.9 × 2 × 0.75)	8.3 × 15.9 × 26 (3.3 × 6.3 × 10.3)	5.7 × 14 × 21 (2.3 × 5.5 × 8.3)	16.8 × 7.9 × 3.6 (6.6 × 3.1 × 1.4)	2.6 × 5.3 × 14 (1 × 2.1 × 5.5)
Weight, kg (lb)	0.06 (0.13)	0.06 (0.13)	0.7 (1.6)	0.03 (0.06)	0.03 (0.06)	3.33 (7.34)	1.7 (3.7)	0.5 (1.2)	0.08 (0.17)
Green Features	None specified	None specified	None specified	None specified	None specified	None specified	None specified	None specified	None specified
FDA Clearance	Yes	Yes	Yes	Yes	No	Yes	Yes	Yes	Yes
CE Mark	Yes	Yes	Yes (Medair)	Yes	Yes	Submitted	Submitted	Submitted	Yes

(continues)

240 CHAPTER 7 Patient Monitors

APPENDIX 7-A
Descriptions of Features and Specifications of Pulse Oximeters *(Continued)*

SPECIFICATIONS	RESPIORONICS NOVAMETRIX 512	RESPIORONICS NOVAMETRIX 513	RESPIORONICS NOVAMETRIX 515B	RESPIORONICS NOVAMETRIX OXYPLETH 520A	RGB MICROX	RGB MICROX BT	RGB OXYPRO	SHENZHEN MINDRAY PM-50	SHENZHEN MINDRAY PM-60
Modular/ Stand-alone	Handheld	Handheld	Stand-alone	Stand-alone	Handheld	Handheld	Stand-alone	Stand-alone	Stand-alone
MRI compatible	No	No	No	No	No	No	No	No	No
SpO$_2$ range, %	0–100	0–100	0–100	0–100	0–100	0–100	0–100	0–100	0–100
Accuracy, %	± 2 (70–100)	± 2 (70–100)	± 2 (80–100)	± 2 (80–100)	± 2 (70–100)	± 2 (70–100)	± 2 (70–100)	± 2 (70–100 adult/pediatric (± 3 70–100 neonatal)	± 2 (70–100 adult/ pediatric (± 3 70–100 neonatal)
Pulse rate, bpm	30–250	30–250	30–250	30–250	30–250	30–250	30–250	25–254	18–300
Accuracy	± 2	± 2	2	1% of full scale	3%	3%	3%	± 2 bpm	± 3 bpm (no motion), ± 5 bpm (motion)
Probe Types									
Disposable	NA	NA	NA	NA	Finger	Finger	Finger	Yes	Yes
Reusable	Finger, multisite Y-sensor	Finger, multisite Y-sensor	Finger, multisite Y-sensor	Finger, multisite Y-sensor	Finger, multisite Y-sensor	Finger, multisite Y-sensor	Finger, multisite Y-sensor	Finger, multisite	Finger, multisite
Patient range	Adult, pediatric, neonate	Adult, pediatric, neonate	Adult, pediatric, neonate	Adult, pediatric, neonate	Adult, pediatric, neonate	Adult, pediatric, neonate	Adult, pediatric, neonate	Adult, pediatric, neonate	Adult, pediatric, neonate
Perfusion Index and/or Signal Strength Indicator	Pulsatile signal strength bar	Pulsatile signal strength bar	Pulsatile signal strength bar	Pulsatile signal strength bar	Yes	Yes	Yes	Yes	Yes
Response Time, sec	Not specified	Not specified	Not specified	Not specified	2	2	2	Beat to beat	Beat to beat
Start-Up Time, sec or pulses	< 15 sec	< 15 sec	< 15 sec	< 15 sec	8 pulses	8 pulses	8 pulses	4–6 sec	4–6 sec

APPENDIX 7-A
Descriptions of Features and Specifications of Pulse Oximeters (Continued)

SPECIFICATIONS	RESPIORONICS NOVAMETRIX 512	RESPIORONICS NOVAMETRIX 513	RESPIORONICS NOVAMETRIX 515B	RESPIORONICS NOVAMETRIX OXYPLETH 520A	RGB MICROX	RGB MICROX BT	RGB OXYPRO	SHENZHEN MINDRAY PM-50	SHENZHEN MINDRAY PM-60
Averaging Time, sec	8	8	8	8	4, 8, 12, 16	4, 8, 12, 16	4, 8, 12, 16	Not specified	7, 9, 11
Data Management	No	Yes	Yes	Yes	Yes	Yes	Yes	Yes	Yes
Data stored	NA	SpO_2 and pulse rate	SpO_2 and pulse rate	SpO_2 and pulse rate	% saturation, pulse rate	% saturation, pulse rate	% saturation, pulse rate	100 patients' IDs, 200 data records	SpO_2 and pulse rate
Data storage, hr	NA	24	24	24	200	200	200	Not specified	96
External output	NA	RS232 optional	RS232, optional analog	RS232, optional analog	Yes, Bluetooth	Yes, Bluetooth	Serial RS232	Yes	Yes
Displays	SpO_2, pulse rate, pulse-activity bar, system status, messages, low-battery indicator	SpO_2, pulse rate, pulse-activity bar, system status, messages, low-battery indicator	SpO_2, pulse rate, pulse-activity bar, system status, messages, low-battery indicator	SpO_2, pulse rate, high/low alert limits, pulsatile signal-strength bar, system status/error messages, trends, plethysmogram, battery indicator	SpO_2, pulse rate, high/low alarm limits	SpO_2, pulse rate, high/low alarm limits, plethysmogram on computer screen	SpO_2, pulse rate, plethysmogram on computer screen, high/low alarm limits	SpO_2, pulse rate, pulse amplitude bar, system status	SpO_2, pulse rate, pulse amplitude bar, system status
Printer-Recorder	No	Data archive support	Data archive support	Data archive support	No	No	No	No	No
Alarms									
Audiovisual	High/low SpO_2 and pulse-rate alerts, system status and error messages	High/low SpO_2 and pulse-rate alerts, system status and error messages, low battery	High/low SpO_2 and pulse-rate alerts, system status and error messages, low battery	High/low SpO_2 and pulse-rate alerts, system status and error messages, low battery, alert icon	High/low SpO_2, sensor off, ambient-light interference, low signal strength, insufficient signal, noisy signal	High/low SpO_2, sensor off, ambient-light interference, low signal strength, insufficient signal, noisy signal	High/low SpO_2, sensor off, ambient-light interference, low signal strength, insufficient signal, noisy signal	NA	High/low SpO_2 and pulse rate, sensor off, technical alarm

(continues)

APPENDIX 7-A
Descriptions of Features and Specifications of Pulse Oximeters *(Continued)*

SPECIFICATIONS	RESPIRONICS NOVAMETRIX 512	RESPIRONICS NOVAMETRIX 513	RESPIRONICS NOVAMETRIX 515B	RESPIRONICS NOVAMETRIX OXYPLETH 520A	RGB MICROX	RGB MICROX BT	RGB OXYPRO	SHENZHEN MINDRAY PM-50	SHENZHEN MINDRAY PM-60
Visual	Status messages	Status messages	Flashing numerics upon violated limits and red Alert Bar	Flashing numerics upon violated limits and red Alert Bar	High/low SpO$_2$, sensor off, ambient-light interference, low signal strength, low/insufficient signal, noisy signal	High/low SpO$_2$, sensor off, ambient-light interference, low signal strength, low/insufficient signal, noisy signal	High/low SpO$_2$, sensor off, ambient-light interference, low signal strength, low/insufficient signal, noisy signal	Low battery	High/low SpO$_2$, and pulse rate, sensor off, sensor signal, low battery, technical alarm
Alarm override	Yes	Yes	Yes	Yes	Audible and visual	Audible and visual	Audible and visual	No	Yes
Reactivation method	Manual or automatic	Manual or automatic	2 min silence or audio off; automatic or manual	2 min silence or audio off; automatic or manual	Manual	Manual	Manual	NA	Manual
Volume control	No	No	Yes	Yes	Pulse and alarm (pulse pitch modulation with SpO$_2$ value)	Pulse and alarm (pulse pitch modulation with SpO$_2$ value)	Pulse and alarm (pulse pitch modulation with SpO$_2$ value)	NA	Yes
Power									
VAC	Battery only	Battery only	100–120, 200–240, 50–60 Hz	100–120, 200–240, 50–60 Hz	110/240, adapter to 5 V 1A	110/240, adapter to 5 V 1A	110/240	Battery only	Battery, DC power
Batteries	AA alkaline	AA alkaline	Sealed lead acid gel	Sealed lead acid gel	AA type	AA type	Sealed lead-acid	1.5 V AA alkaline or rechargeable	Lithium ion or AA
Life, hr	16	16	8	8	24, continuous	24, continuous	5, continuous	15	24 (lithium ion), 36 (AA)

APPENDIX 7-A
Descriptions of Features and Specifications of Pulse Oximeters (Continued)

SPECIFICATIONS	RESPIORONICS NOVAMETRIX 512	RESPIORONICS NOVAMETRIX 513	RESPIORONICS NOVAMETRIX 515B	RESPIORONICS NOVAMETRIX OXYPLETH 520A	RGB MICROX	RGB MICROX BT	RGB OXYPRO	SHENZHEN MINDRAY PM-50	SHENZHEN MINDRAY PM-60
Rechargeable	No	No	Yes	Yes	Disposable or rechargeable (recharge external)	Disposable or rechargeable (recharge external)	Yes	Yes	Yes
Low battery notice	Yes	Yes	Yes	Not specified	Yes	Yes	Yes	Yes	Yes
H × W × D, cm (in)	10.8 × 5.7 × 2.5 (4.3 × 2.3 × 1)	10.8 × 5.7 × 2.5 (4.3 × 2.3 × 1)	8.4 × 22.9 × 20.3 (3.3 × 9 × 8)	8.4 × 22.9 × 20.3 (3.3 × 9 × 8)	14.5 × 6 × 2.8 (5.7 × 2.4 × 1.1)	14.5 × 6 × 2.8 (5.7 × 2.4 × 1.1)	17.5 × 20 × 16 (6.9 × 7.9 × 6.3)	6.5 × 14 × 3.2 (2.6 × 5.5 × 1.3)	12 × 5.5 × 3 (4.7 × 2.2 × 1.2)
Weight, kg (lb)	0.16 (0.35)	0.16 (0.35)	2.72 (6)	3.32 (7.3)	0.21 (0.47)	0.21 (0.47)	3 (6.6)	0.13 (0.28) without battery and sensor	0.3 (0.67) with battery
Green Features	Automatic shut-off after 3.5 minutes if no data is received	Automatic shut-off after 3.5 minutes if no data is received	None specified	None specified	None specified	None specified	None specified	None specified	None specified
FDA Clearance	Yes	Yes	Yes	Yes	No	No	No	Yes	Yes
CE Mark	Yes	Yes	Yes	Yes	Yes	Yes	Yes	Yes	Yes

MODEL

(continues)

APPENDIX 7-A
Descriptions of Features and Specifications of Pulse Oximeters (*Continued*)

SPECIFICATIONS	SMITHS MEDICAL BCI 3180	SMITHS MEDICAL BCI 3301	SMITHS MEDICAL BCI SPECTRO2 10	SMITHS MEDICAL BCI SPECTRO2 20	SMITHS MEDICAL BCI SPECTRO2 30	SMITHS MEDICAL DIGIT	SMITHS MEDICAL FINGERPRINT	SMITHS MEDICAL PM AUTOCORR	SMITHS MEDICAL PM MINICORR
Modular/Stand-alone	Stand-alone	Not specified	Both	Both	Both	Not specified	Not specified	Not specified	Not specified
MRI compatible	Not specified	No	Not specified	Not specified	Not specified	No	No	No	Not specified
SpO$_2$ range, %	0–100	0–99	0–99 (1% increments)	0–100 (1% increments), display maximum 99%	0–100 (1% increments), display maximum 99%	0–99	0–99	0–100	0–99
Accuracy, %	± 2 (70–100 adult/pediatric (± 3 70–100 neonatal)	± 2 (70–100), ± 3 (50–69)	± 2 (70–99)	± 2 (70–100), ± 3 (70–100 neonate)	± 2 (70–100), ± 3 (70–100 neonate)	± 2 (70–99)	± 2 (70–99)	± 2 (70–100), ± 3 (50–69)	± 2 (70–99), ± 3 (50–69)
Pulse rate, bpm	Not specified	Not specified	30–254	20–300	20–300	Not specified	Not specified	Not specified	Not specified
Accuracy	Not specified	Not specified	± 2	± 2	± 2	Not specified	Not specified	Not specified	Not specified
Probe Types									
Disposable	Yes	Yes	Yes	Yes		Not specified	Not specified	Yes	Not specified
Reusable	Yes	Yes	Yes	Yes		Not specified	Not specified	Yes	Not specified
Patient range	Adult, pediatric, infant, neonate	Adult, pediatric, infant, neonate	Adult, pediatric, infant	Adult, pediatric, infant, neonate	Adult, pediatric, infant, neonate	Adult, pediatric	Adult, pediatric, infant, neonate	Adult, pediatric, infant, neonate	Adult, pediatric, infant, neonate
Perfusion Index and/or Signal Strength Indicator	Not specified	Not specified	SpO$_2$ and pulse rate; low perfusion accuracy	SpO$_2$ and pulse rate; low perfusion accuracy	SpO$_2$ and pulse rate; low perfusion accuracy	Not specified	Not specified	Not specified	Not specified
Response Time, sec	8	8	Not specified	Not specified	Not specified	Not specified	8	8, 16	Not specified

MODEL

APPENDIX 7-A
Descriptions of Features and Specifications of Pulse Oximeters *(Continued)*

SPECIFICATIONS	SMITHS MEDICAL BCI 3180	SMITHS MEDICAL BCI 3301	SMITHS MEDICAL BCI SPECTRO2 10	SMITHS MEDICAL BCI SPECTRO2 20	SMITHS MEDICAL BCI SPECTRO2 30	SMITHS MEDICAL DIGIT	SMITHS MEDICAL FINGERPRINT	SMITHS MEDICAL PM AUTOCORR	SMITHS MEDICAL PM MINICORR
Start-Up Time, sec or pulses	Not specified	8 pulses	Not specified	Not specified	Not specified	Not specified	8 pulses	4, 8, 16 pulses	Not specified
Averaging Time, sec	Not specified	Not specified	Not specified	Not specified	Not specified	Not specified	Not specified	Not specified	Not specified
Data Management									
Data stored	Not specified	Not specified	SpO$_2$ and pulse rate	SpO$_2$ and pulse rate	SpO$_2$ and pulse rate	Not specified	Not specified	Not specified	Not specified
Data storage, hr	Not specified	Not specified	144 at 4-sec intervals	144 at 4-sec intervals	144 at 4-sec intervals	Not specified	Not specified	Not specified	Not specified
External output	RS232	RS232	USB	USB	USB	No	RS232	RS232	RS232, infrared link
Displays	SpO$_2$, pulse rate, plethysmogram	SpO$_2$, pulse rate, quantitative pulse-strength bar	SpO$_2$, pulse rate, quantitative pulse-strength bar	SpO$_2$, pulse rate, quantitative pulse-strength bar	SpO$_2$, pulse rate, quantitative pulse-strength bar	SpO$_2$, pulse rate, pulse strength	SpO$_2$, pulse rate, quantitative pulse-strength bar	SpO$_2$, pulse rate, quantitative pulse-strength bar, low battery, alarm silence, probe, search, artifact	SpO$_2$, pulse rate, quantitative pulse-strength bar, low battery, audio disabled, sensor, artifact power
Printer-Recorder	Optional	Optional	Optional	Optional	Optional	No	Yes	Optional	Optional
Alarms									
Audiovisual	Alarms status, lost signal	No	No	No	High/low SpO$_2$, pulse rate	No	No	High/low SpO$_2$ and pulse rate, low battery, alarm, probe, sensor off, search, artifact	High/low SpO$_2$ and pulse rate

(continues)

APPENDIX 7-A
Descriptions of Features and Specifications of Pulse Oximeters (Continued)

SPECIFICATIONS	SMITHS MEDICAL BCI 3180	SMITHS MEDICAL BCI 3301	SMITHS MEDICAL BCI SPECTRO2 10	SMITHS MEDICAL BCI SPECTRO2 20	SMITHS MEDICAL BCI SPECTRO2 30	SMITHS MEDICAL DIGIT	SMITHS MEDICAL FINGERPRINT	SMITHS MEDICAL PM AUTCORR	SMITHS MEDICAL PM MINICORR
Visual	Low battery, lost signal	Low battery	Not specified	Not specified	Not specified	Not specified	Low battery	Low battery, probe, alarm silence, search, artifact, power	Low battery, audio disabled, sensor off, artifact, power off
Alarm override	Not specified	No	No	No	Yes	No	No	Yes	Yes
Reactivation method	Not specified	NA	Not specified	Not specified	Automatic	NA	NA	Automatic after 2 min or manual	Automatic
Volume control	No	NA	Not specified	Not specified	Yes	NA	NA	Yes	Yes
Power									
VAC	90–125, 200–240	Battery only	100–240	100–240	100–240	Battery only	Battery only	105–125, 100, 230	105–125, 100, 230
Batteries	Lead-acid	C	Alkaline or custom lithium ion rechargeable battery pack	Alkaline or custom lithium ion rechargeable battery pack	Alkaline or custom lithium ion rechargeable battery pack	AAA alkaline	AA alkaline or Ni-Cd	Ni-MH	Alkaline
Life, hr	4 with continuous use	24	32	26	17	Not specified	24 no printing, 14 continuous printing	4.5	24
Rechargeable	No	Not specified	54	31	30	Not specified	Not specified	Not specified	Not specified
Low battery notice	Yes	Yes	Not specified	Not specified	Not specified	Not specified	Yes	Yes	Yes

APPENDIX 7-A
Descriptions of Features and Specifications of Pulse Oximeters *(Continued)*

SPECIFICATIONS	SMITHS MEDICAL BCI 3180	SMITHS MEDICAL BCI 3301	SMITHS MEDICAL BCI SPECTRO2 10	SMITHS MEDICAL BCI SPECTRO2 20	SMITHS MEDICAL BCI SPECTRO2 30	SMITHS MEDICAL DIGIT	SMITHS MEDICAL FINGERPRINT	SMITHS MEDICAL PM AUTOCORR	SMITHS MEDICAL PM MINICORR
H × W × D, cm (in)	16.5 × 20.3 × 12.7 (6.5 × 8 × 5)	16 × 8.3 × 3.2 (6.3 × 3.3 × 1.3)	15.5 × 8.4 × 4.3 (6.1 × 3.3 × 1.7)	15.5 × 8.4 × 4.3 (6.1 × 3.3 × 1.7)	15.5 × 8.4 × 4.3 (6.1 × 3.3 × 1.7)	5.7 × 4.3 × 3.8 (2.3 × 1.7 × 1.5)	17.2 × 7.6 × 3.8 (6.8 × 3 × 1.5)	21.6 × 8.2 × 14 (8.5 × 3.2 × 5.5)	16.7 × 7 × 3.6 (6.6 × 2.8 × 1.4)
Weight, kg (lb)	2 (4.5)	0.47 (1)	0.34 (0.75) with batteries	0.34 (0.75) with batteries	0.34 (0.75) with batteries	0.09 (0.2)	1.1 (2.4)	0.85 (1.87)	0.5 (1.1) with batteries
Green Features	None specified	Automatic 2 min shutoff	None specified	None specified	None specified	Auto power shutdown after 8 seconds	Auto power shutdown when disconnected from patient	None specified	None specified
FDA Clearance	Yes	Yes	Yes	Yes	Yes	Yes	Yes	Yes	Yes
CE Mark	Yes	Yes	Yes	Yes	Yes	Yes	Yes	Yes	Yes

MODEL

(continues)

APPENDIX 7-A
Descriptions of Features and Specifications of Pulse Oximeters (Continued)

SPECIFICATIONS	MODEL				
	SPACELABS HEALTHCARE 91496-M ULTRAVIEW SL COMMAND MODULE (MASIMO SET SpO2)	**SPACELABS HEALTHCARE** 91496-N ULTRAVIEW SL COMMAND MODULE (NELLCOR OxiMax SpO2)	**SPACELABS HEALTHCARE** 91496-U ULTRAVIEW SL COMMAND MODULE (SPACELABS SpO2)	**WEINMANN** OXYCOUNT MINI	**WEINMANN** SmartOx
Modular/Stand-alone	Modular	Modular	Modular	Not specified	Stand-alone
MRI compatible	No	No	No	No	No
SpO$_2$ range, %	1–100	1–100	30–100	0–99	45–100
Accuracy, %	± 2 (70–100)	± 2 (70–100)	± 3 (70–100)	± 1.5 (86–100), ± 2 (75–85), ± 3 (50–74)	± 2 (70–100)
Pulse rate, bpm	25–240	25–300	30–250	30–250	20–300
Accuracy	Not specified	Not specified	Not specified	± 1%	± 1 (< 100 bpm), ± 1% (> 100 bpm)
Probe Types					
Disposable	Masimo LNCS or LNOP (various types)	Nellcor OxiMax and OxiCliq (various types)	Spacelabs TruLink finger or multisite, Masimo, Nellcor	Finger clip, universal Y-sensor	No
Reusable	Masimo LNCS or LNOP (various types)	Masimo LNCS or LNOP (various types)	Spacelabs TruLink finger or multisite, Masimo, Nellcor	Finger clip, universal Y-sensor	Finger clip, soft tip
Patient range	Adult, pediatric, infant, neonate	Adult, pediatric, infant, neonate	Adult, pediatric, infant, neonate	Adult, pediatric, infant, neonate	Adult, pediatric, infant, neonate
Perfusion Index and/or Signal Strength Indicator	Yes	Yes	Yes	Signal quality indicator (bar graph)	Not specified
Response Time, sec	3 (numeric update)	3 (numeric update)	3 (numeric update)	2	2
Start-Up Time, sec or pulses	Not specified	Not specified	Not specified	Depends on pulse signal	Depends on pulse signal
Averaging Time, sec	2–4, 4–6, 8, 10, 12, 14, 16	Normal 4–6, fast 2–4	4, 8, 16	Depends on signal quality	Depends on signal quality
Data Management	Yes	Yes	Yes	Yes, with MULTIBASE 2	No

APPENDIX 7-A
Descriptions of Features and Specifications of Pulse Oximeters (Continued)

	MODEL				
	SPACELABS HEALTHCARE	SPACELABS HEALTHCARE	SPACELABS HEALTHCARE	WEINMANN	WEINMANN
SPECIFICATIONS	91496-M ULTRAVIEW SL COMMAND MODULE (MASIMO SET SpO2)	91496-N ULTRAVIEW SL COMMAND MODULE (NELLCOR OxiMax SpO2)	91496-U ULTRAVIEW SL COMMAND MODULE (SPACELABS SpO2)	OXYCOUNT MINI	SmartOx
Data stored	% saturation, pulse rate, waveform, perfusion index	% saturation, pulse rate, waveform, perfusion index	% saturation, pulse rate, waveform, perfusion index	Yes	NA
Data storage, hr	24	24	24	7 (SpO$_2$, pulse, pulse quality)	NA
External output	No	No	No	RS232	NA
Displays	SpO$_2$, pulse rate, plethysmogram, high/low alarm limits, Sensorwatch signal-strength indicator	SpO$_2$, pulse rate, plethysmogram, high/low alarm limits, Sensorwatch signal-strength indicator, SatSeconds	SpO$_2$, pulse rate, plethysmogram, high/low alarm limits, Sensorwatch signal-strength indicator	SpO$_2$, pulse rate with heart beat symbol	SpO$_2$, pulse rate with bar graph
Printer-Recorder	Yes, function of the monitor/network	Yes, function of the monitor/network	Yes, function of the monitor/network	Optional with MULTIBASE 2	No
Alarms					
Audiovisual	High/low SpO$_2$, sensor off, ambient-light interference, low signal strength, insufficient signal, noisy signal	High/low SpO$_2$, sensor off, ambient-light interference, low signal strength, insufficient signal, noisy signal, SatSeconds	High/low SpO$_2$, sensor off, ambient-light interference, low signal strength, insufficient signal, noisy signal	High/low SpO$_2$ and pulse rate, sensor off, finger off, signal low/signal quality, sensor failure, out of set alarms	Sensor off, finger off, signal low, sensor failure
Visual	High/low SpO$_2$, sensor off, ambient-light interference, low signal strength, insufficient signal, noisy signal	High/low SpO$_2$/PR, sensor off, ambient-light interference, low signal strength, insufficient signal, noisy signal, SatSeconds	High/low SpO$_2$, sensor off, ambient-light interference, low signal strength, insufficient signal, noisy signal	Low battery, signal quality, system failure	Low battery, signal quality, system failure, sensor failure

(continues)

APPENDIX 7-A
Descriptions of Features and Specifications of Pulse Oximeters (Continued)

SPECIFICATIONS	MODEL				
	SPACELABS HEALTHCARE	SPACELABS HEALTHCARE	SPACELABS HEALTHCARE	WEINMANN	WEINMANN
	91496-M ULTRAVIEW SL COMMAND MODULE (MASIMO SET SpO2)	91496-N ULTRAVIEW SL COMMAND MODULE (NELLCOR OxiMax SpO2)	91496-U ULTRAVIEW SL COMMAND MODULE (SPACELABS SpO2)	OXYCOUNT MINI	SmartOx
Alarm override	Pause audio, pause alarm presentation	Pause audio, pause alarm presentation	Pause audio, pause alarm presentation	Audible	Audible
Reactivation method	Manual/auto recovery	Manual/auto recovery	Manual/auto recovery	Automatic after 30 sec or manual	Automatic after 30 sec or manual
Volume control	Yes	Yes	Yes	No	No
Power					
VAC	110/240 (for host monitor)	110/240 (for host monitor)	110/240 (for host monitor)	110/220 with charging/main station or 12 V in car	Battery only
Batteries	None	None	None	9 V alkaline; 7.2 V Ni-MH packs	AAA alkaline
Life, hr	NA	NA	NA	24 (9 V), 30 (Ni-MH)	> 2C continuous
Rechargeable	NA	NA	NA	Yes, with MULTIBASE 2	No
Low battery notice	NA	NA	NA	Yes	Yes
H × W × D, cm (in)	11.3 × 5.7 × 18 (4.5 × 2.2 × 7.1)	11.3 × 5.7 × 18 (4.5 × 2.2 × 7.1)	11.3 × 5.7 × 18 (4.5 × 2.2 × 7.1)	12.8 × 6.5 × 2.7 (5 × 2.6 × 1.1)	3.2 × 13.6 × 2.4 (1.3 × 5.4 × 0.9)
Weight, kg (lb)	0.8 (1.8)	0.8 (1.8)	0.8 (1.8)	0.3 (0.6) with battery, 0.16 (0.4) with no battery or sensor	0.07 (0.14) with battery, no sensor
Green Features	None specified	None specified	None specified	None specified	None specified
FDA Clearance	Yes	Yes	Yes	No	Yes
CE Mark	Yes	Yes	Yes	Yes	Yes

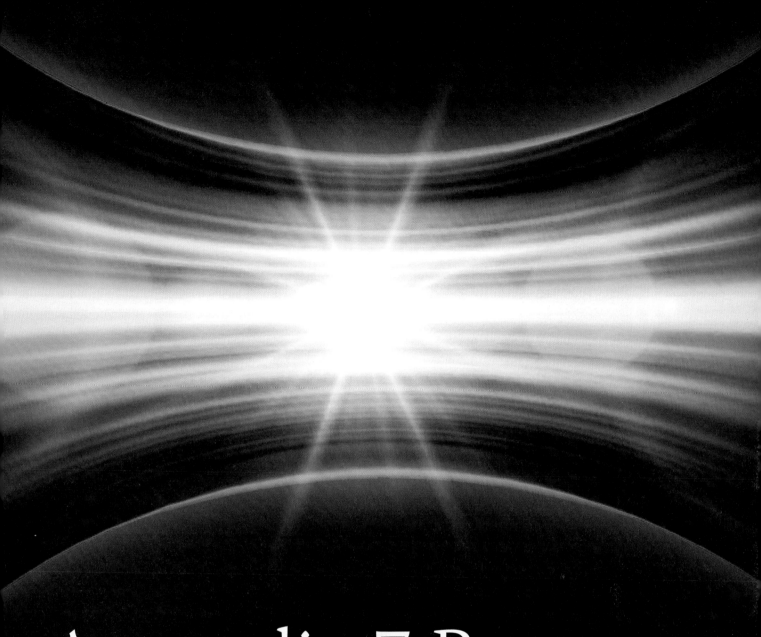

Appendix 7-B

APPENDIX 7-B
Technical Features and Specifications of Transcutaneous Oxygen and Carbon Dioxide Monitors

SPECIFICATIONS	DRAEGER MEDICAL INFINITY tpO2/tpCO2 SMARTPOD	PERIMED PERIFLUX SYSTEM 5000	PHILIPS INTELLIVUE TCG10	PHILIPS M1018A	RADIOMETER TCM COMBIM	RADIOMETER TCM TOSCA	RADIOMETER TCM4:TCM40	RADIOMETER TCM400	RADIOMETER TOSCA 500	SENTEC DIGITAL MONITORING SYSTEM
Patient Population	Neonates	Adult, neonates	Adults, pediatrics, neonates	Neonates	Adults, pediatrics, neonates	Adults, pediatrics	Adults, neonates	Adults	Adults, pediatrics	Adults, pediatrics, neonates
Modular/ Stand-alone	Modular	Stand-alone	Modular	Modular	Stand-alone	Stand-alone	Stand-alone	Stand-alone	Stand-alone	Stand-alone
Measured Parameters	$tcPCO_2$, $tcPO_2$	$tcPCO_2$, $tcPO_2$	$tcPCO_2$, $tcPO_2$	$tcPCO_2$, $tcPO_2$	$tcPCO_2$, $tcPO_2$	$tcPCO_2$, SpO_2, Pulse rate	$tcPCO_2$, $tcPO_2$	$tcPO_2$	$tcPCO_2$, SpO_2	$tcPCO_2$, SpO_2, Pulse rate; neonates: only $tcPCO_2$
Monitor										
PCO_2 measurement range, mm Hg	0–200	0–200	5–200	5–200	0–200	0–200	Not specified	N/A	0–200	0–200
PO_2 measurement range, mm Hg	0–800	0–2,000	0–800	0–750	0–800/0–99.9	0–800/0–99.9 (SpO_2)	0–800/0–99.9	0–2,000/ 0–266.7	N/A	N/A
Temperature range	37–45, user selectable	37–45	37–45	37, 41–45	37–45	37–45	37, 41–45	37–45	37–45	39–43.5
Increments, °C	0.1	0.5	0.5	0.5	0.5	0.5	0.5	0.5	0.5	0.5
Accuracy, °C	± 10%	0.1	0.1	0.1	0.2	0.2	0.1	0.1	0.2	0.1
Site change, hr	When site timer expires	4	12	Not specified	12 at 42°C	12 at 24°C	4	4	12 at 42°C	When site timer expires
Site timer, hr	0–8 or off, user selectable	User selectable	0.5–12, step wide 0.5 hr	0.5–8, off	≤ 25	≤ 25	0–8, 0.5 increments	0–99	≤ 24	0.5–12, user selectable; recommended 8 hours at 42°C for adults, 41°C for neonates

APPENDIX 7-B
Technical Features and Specifications of Transcutaneous Oxygen and Carbon Dioxide Monitors (Continued)

SPECIFICATIONS	MODEL									
	DRAEGER MEDICAL INFINITY tpO2/tpCO2 SMARTPOD	PERIMED PERIFLUX SYSTEM 5000	PHILIPS INTELLIVUE TCG10	PHILIPS M1018A	RADIOMETER TCM COMBIM	RADIOMETER TCM TOSCA	RADIOMETER TCM4:TCM40	RADIOMETER TCM400	RADIOMETER TOSCA 500	SENTEC DIGITAL MONITORING SYSTEM
Sensor	$tcPO_2$/$tcPCO_2$ solid state, dual thermistor electrode	Combination/single	tc Sensor 84 (Radiometer)	Combination (M1918A)	Combination/single, solid-state, Clark and Severinghaus	Combination/single	Single/combination, solid-state, Clark and Severinghauss	Single, solid-state, Clark	Combination/single	Digital Stow-Severinghaus PCO_2 combined with reflectance 2 wavelength pulse oximetry
$tcPCO_2$	CO_2 electrode, ceramic Severinghaus-type electrode	Yes	N/A	N/A	Stow-Severinghaus	Stow-Severinghaus	pH solid state glass electrode	N/A	Stow-Severinghaus	Yes
$tcPO_2$	O_2 platinum Clark-type electrode	Yes	N/A	N/A	Yes	SpO_2	Yes	Yes	SpO_2	N/A
Anode	O_2 electrode platinum Clark-type electrode	Ag	N/A	N/A	Ag/AgCl	N/A	Ag/AgCl	Ag	N/A	N/A
Cathode	Not specified	Platinum	N/A	N/A	Platinum	N/A	Platinum	Platinum	N/A	N/A
Combination $tcPCO_2$/$tcPO_2$	Yes	Yes	Yes	Yes	Yes	Yes (combined PCO_2/SpO_2)	Yes	N/A	Yes (combined PCO_2/SpO_2)	No (combined $tcPCO_2$/SpO_2)
Diameter × Height, mm (in)	Not specified	15 × 11 (0.6 × 0.43)	Not specified	11.3 × 15 (0.45 × 0.6)	15 × 8 (0.6 × 0.3)	15 × 8 (0.6 × 0.3)	15 × 11 (0.6 × 0.45)	15 × 11 (0.6 × 0.45)	15 × 8 (0.6 × 0.3)	14 × 9 (0.55 × 0.35)
Disposable/reusable	Not specified	Not specified	Not specified	Not specified	Not specified	Not specified	Not specified	Not specified	Not specified	Reusable
Membrane material	Fluorinated ethylene propylene/polypropylene	Fluorinated ethylene propylene/polypropylene combination, polypropylene $tcPO_2$	Gold shielded	Not specified	Mechanically protected	Mechanically protected	Fluorinated ethylene propylene/polypropylene	Polypropylene	Mechanically protected	N/A
Thickness, µm	12.5/15	12.5/15	Not specified	Not specified	N/A	N/A	12.5/15	15	N/A	N/A
Life, days	14	14	14	Approx. 7	14	14	14	14	14	42

(continues)

APPENDIX 7-B
Technical Features and Specifications of Transcutaneous Oxygen and Carbon Dioxide Monitors (Continued)

SPECIFICATIONS	DRAEGER MEDICAL INFINITY tpO2/tpCO2 SMARTPOD	PERIMED PERIFLUX SYSTEM 5000	PHILIPS INTELLIVUE TCG10	PHILIPS M1018A	RADIOMETER TCM COMBIM	RADIOMETER TCM TOSCA	RADIOMETER TCM4:TCM40	RADIOMETER TCM400	RADIOMETER TOSCA 500	SENTEC DIGITAL MONITORING SYSTEM
Response time, sec, T90	20 (O_2), 20 (CO_2)	20 (O_2), 20 (CO_2)	Not specified	Approx. 30 (O_2) and 60 (CO_2)	< 50 (CO_2)	< 50 (CO_2)	7–12 minmum (O_2), 5–7 minimum (CO_2), to equilibration; 20 sec O_2 and CO_2 change in status	< 11	< 50 (CO_2)	< 75
Drift										
pCO_2	± 10% over recommended calibration interval	1 mm Hg/hr	Not specified	< 2.5% per hour	< 0.5% per hour	< 0.5% per hour	1 mm Hg per hour	N/A	< 0.5% per hour	< 0.5% per hour
pO_2	± 5% over recommended calibration interval	1 mm Hg/hr	Not specified	< 1.25% per hour	N/A	N/A	1 mm Hg per hour	< 1% per hour	N/A	N/A
Temperature Thermistors, Number	Not specified	Not specified	Not specified	2	N/A	Not specified	Not specified	Not specified	Not specified	2, redundant design
Calibration										
Method	Reference gas cylinder (with 20.9% O_2, 5% CO_2)	1 point	Integrated and automated 1 point calibration with integrated calibration gas	1 point with calibration gas	Automatic 1 point, built-in calibrator with sensor storage chamber, 2 min calibration time	Automatic 1 point, built-in calibrator with sensor storage chamber, 2 min calibration time	1 point	1 point	Automatic, 1 point built-in calibrator with sensor storage chamber, 2 min calibration time	Automatic 1 point, intelligent
Interval, hr	Before monitoring and every 2 hours	4	Latest every 12 hr, automatically indicated	Every site change (recommended)	4 in storage mode, automatic, or between sensor site changes	4 in storage mode, automatic, or between sensor site changes	4	4	4 in storage mode, automatic, or between sensor site changes	≤ 12
Alarms										
High/low tcPCO2, mm Hg	10/150	N/A	10/195	10/195	0–99/5–200	0–99/5–200	0–200/0–99	N/A	0–99.5–200	0–200
High/low tcPO2, mm Hg	10/300	N/A	10/795	10/745	0–200/0–99	0–200/0–99	0–800/0–99	N/A	N/A	0–100% SpO_2

APPENDIX 7-B
Technical Features and Specifications of Transcutaneous Oxygen and Carbon Dioxide Monitors (Continued)

SPECIFICATIONS	MODEL									
	DRAEGER MEDICAL — INFINITY tpO2/tpCO2 SMARTPOD	PERIMED — PERIFLUX SYSTEM 5000	PHILIPS — INTELLIVUE TCG10	PHILIPS — M1018A	RADIOMETER — TCM COMBIM	RADIOMETER — TCM TOSCA	RADIOMETER — TCM4:TCM40	RADIOMETER — TCM400	RADIOMETER — TOSCA 500	SENTEC — DIGITAL MONITORING SYSTEM
Microprocessor										
Memory capacity, hr	24 (trends)	Unlimited with PC	4–48	4–48	72	72	48	24	72	≤ 288
Store interval, sec	0.5 (trend sample rate)	User selectable	12, 1 min, 5 min	12, 1 min, 5 min	Not specified	Not specified	24	10	Not specified	1–8, selectable
Recorder/Printer	From R50/R50N recorder or laser printer	Optional	Optional	Optional	Optional	Optional	Optional	Optional	Optional	Optional
Type	Thermal array	Thermal	Thermal	Thermal	Parallel port (IEEE-12-84)	Parallel port (IEEE-12-84)	Parallel port (IEEE-12-84)	Laser printer (external)	Not specified	Thermal, RS232 port
Channels	2	4	3	3	Not specified	Not specified	Not specified	N/A	Not specified	3
Chart speed, cm/min	150	0.2, 0.5, 1	1, 2, 3	1, 2, 3	Not specified	Not specified	Not specified	N/A	Not specified	0.56 cm/hr to 16.7 cm/hr
Accuracy, %	Not specified	1	2 mm Hg (0–200 mm Hg) for $tcPO_2$, 2 mm Hg (5–100 mm Hg) for $tcPCO_2$	2 mm Hg (0–200 mm Hg) for $tcPO_2$, 2 mm Hg (5–100 mm Hg) for $tcPCO_2$	Not specified	Not specified	Not specified	N/A	Not specified	NA
Formats	Records $tcPO_2$ and $tcPCO_2$ values on manual and alarm recordings; prints $tcPO_2$ trends	Records time, $tcPO_2$, $tcPCO_2$, trends, temperature, and calibration settings	Not specified	Not specified	Real time (fast or slow); memory 1, 12, 24, or 72 hours; graphics	Real time (fast or slow); memory 1, 12, 24, or 72 hours; graphics	Real time recordings and/or histograms, print from memory	Internal reporting software, memort export	Real time (fast or slow); memory 1, 12, 24, or 72 hours; graphics	Trendings, histograms, statistics
Parameters	Not specified	Not specified	Not specified	Not specified	Not specified	Not specified	Not specified	Not specified	Not specified	$tcPCO_2$, SpO_2, Pulse rate

(continues)

APPENDIX 7-B
Technical Features and Specifications of Transcutaneous Oxygen and Carbon Dioxide Monitors (Continued)

SPECIFICATIONS	DRAEGER MEDICAL INFINITY tpO2/tpCO2 SMARTPOD	PERIMED PERIFLUX SYSTEM 5000	PHILIPS INTELLIVUE TCG10	PHILIPS M1018A	RADIOMETER TCM COMBIM	RADIOMETER TCM TOSCA	RADIOMETER TCM4:TCM40	RADIOMETER TCM400	RADIOMETER TOSCA 500	SENTEC DIGITAL MONITORING SYSTEM
Auxiliary Output	Digital (from monitor)	Analog or digital RS232	Not specified	Not specified	EIA 232 or printer, USB, serial, and Ethernet port	EIA 232 or printer	EIA 232 or printer	RS232, Centronics interface	Analog, RS423, volt status signals, Centronics interface, nurse call	Analog, LAN port, serial
Power Requirements										
VAC, Hz	Powered from monitor	115–230, 50–60	100–240, 50–60	100–240, 50–60	100/120/220/240, 50–60	100/120/220/240, 50–60	100/120/220/240, 50–60	90–264, 47–63	100–120/200–240, 50–60	100–240/50–60
Battery, type	Sealed lead-acid (in monitor)	None	None	Optional with IntelliVue models MP40 and MP50; module powered through monitor	Lead	Lead	Lead	None	Lead	Sealed lithium-ion
Operating time, hr	Depends on monitor load	N/A	N/A	> 4, MP40 and MP50	1	1	1	N/A	0.5–2	≤ 16, if sleep mode
Recharge time, hr	Not specified	N/A	N/A	> 4 (monitor off), 5–12 (monitor on)	8	8	8	N/A	18	7
H × W × D, cm (in)	5.2 × 13.2 × 15.3 (2 × 5.2 × 6)	10.5 × 30 × 32 (4.1 × 11.8 × 12.6)	92 × 305 × 234 (3.6 × 11.9 × 9.3)	10.3 × 7.2 × 12.3 (4.1 × 2.9 × 3.9) module	16 × 30.8 × 23 (6.3 × 12.1 × 9)	16 × 30.8 × 23 (6.3 × 12.1 × 9)	16 × 30.8 × 23 (6.3 × 12.1 × 9)	16 × 30 × 23 (6.3 × 12.1 × 1)	13.5 × 26.6 × 30 (5.3 × 10.5 × 11.8)	10.2 × 27 × 23 (4 × 10.6 × 9.1)
Weight, kg (lb)	0.45 (1)	4.5 (9.9)	3.8 (6.6)	0.33 (0.73)	4 (8.8)	4 (8.8)	4 (8.8)	2.27 (5)	5.3 (11.6) with gas cylinder	2.5 (5.5)
Green Features	None specified	Latex free	None specified	None specified	Latex free	Not specified	Not specified	Not specified	Not specified	Reloadable membrane charger, display sleep mode
FDA Clearance	Yes	Yes	Yes	Yes	Yes	Yes	Yes	Yes	Yes	Yes
CE Mark	Yes	Yes	Yes	Yes	Yes	Yes	Yes	Yes	Yes	Yes

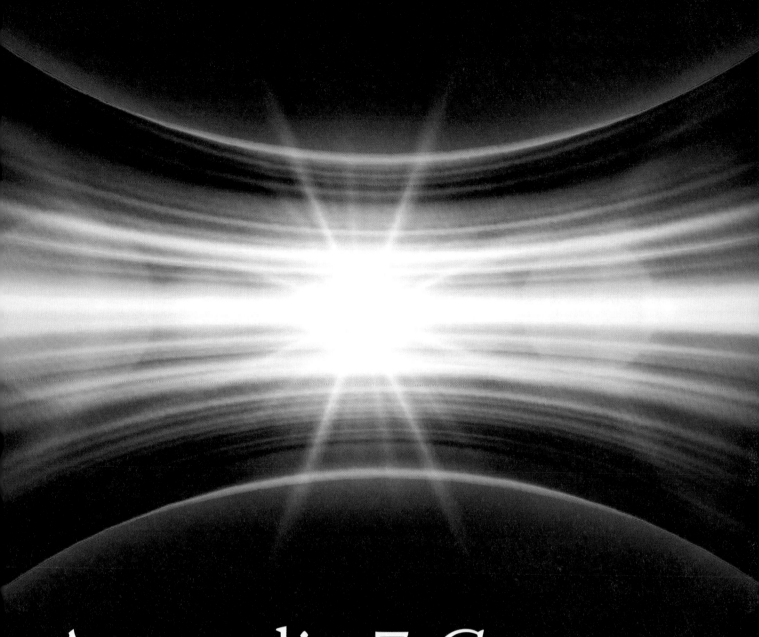

Appendix 7-C

APPENDIX 7-C
Features and Specifications of Indirect Calorimeters

SPECIFICATIONS	GE HEALTHCARE — DELATRAC II	CAREFUSION — MASTERSCREEN CPX	CAREFUSION — OXYCON MOBILE	CAREFUSION — OXYCON PRO	CAREFUSION — VMAX	MEDGRAPHICS — CCM EXPRESS	MEDGRAPHICS — CPX EXPRESS	MEDGRAPHICS — ULTIMA CardiO2	MEDGRAPHICS — ULTIMA SERIES	MEDGRAPHICS — VO2000	VACUMED — VISTA-MX/REE	VACUMED — VO2 LAB
Method	Open-system indirect calorimeter	Breath-by-breath indirect calorimetry	Breath-by-breath indirect calorimetry	Breath-by-breath indirect calorimetry	Breath-by-breath indirect calorimetry	Breath-by-breath indirect calorimetry	Breath-by-breath indirect calorimetry	Breath-by-breath indirect calorimetry	Breath-by-breath indirect calorimetry	Breath-by-breath indirect calorimetry	Breath-by-breath indirect calorimetry	Breath-by-breath indirect calorimetry
Configuration	Spontaneous breathing/mechanical ventilation	Spontaneous breathing	Spontaneous breathing	Spontaneous breathing/mechanical ventilation	Spontaneous breathing/mechanical ventilation	Spontaneous breathing/mechanical ventilation	Spontaneous breathing	Spontaneous breathing	Spontaneous breathing/mechanical ventilation	Spontaneous breathing	Spontaneous breathing	Spontaneous breathing
Inspiratory O_2 Concentrations												
Respirator mode	21–85%	NA	NA	Not specified	Not specified	Not specified	NA	NA	Not specified	NA	Not specified	Not specified
Canopy mode	21–50%	Not specified	Not specified	Not specified	Not specified	Not specified	Not specified	Not specified	Not specified	Not specified	Not specified	Not specified
Measurements												
O_2 consumption	Yes	Yes	Yes	Yes	Yes	Not specified	Not specified	Not specified	Not specified	Not specified	Yes	Yes
Range	5–2,000 mL/min	0 to 7 L/min	0 to 7 L/min	0 to 7 L/min	Not specified	Not specified	Not specified	Not specified	Not specified	Not specified	Not specified	Not specified
Accuracy	Not specified	3% or 0.05 L/min	2% or 0.05 L/min	2% or 0.05 L/min	Not specified	Not specified	Not specified	Not specified	Not specified	Not specified	± 2%	Not specified
CO_2 production	Yes	Yes	Yes	Yes	Yes	Not specified	Not specified	Not specified	Not specified	Not specified	Yes	Yes
Range	5–2,000 mL/min	0 to 7 L/min	0 to 7 L/min	0 to 7 L/min	Not specified	Not specified	Not specified	Not specified	Not specified	Not specified	Not specified	Not specified
Accuracy	Not specified	3% or 0.05 L/min	3% or 0.05 L/min	3% or 0.05 L/min	Not specified	Not specified	Not specified	Not specified	Not specified	Not specified	± 2%	Not specified
Energy expenditure	Yes	Not specified	Not specified	Not specified	Not specified	Not specified	Not specified	Not specified	Not specified	Not specified	Yes	Yes
Respiratory quotient	Yes	Yes	Yes	Yes	Yes	Not specified	Not specified	Not specified	Not specified	Not specified	Yes	Yes
Range	Not specified	0.6–2.0	0.6–2.0	0.6–2.0	Not specified	Not specified	Not specified	Not specified	Not specified	Not specified	Not specified	Not specified
Accuracy	Not specified	4%	70 mL/s or 3%	4%	Not specified	Not specified	Not specified	Not specified	Not specified	Not specified	Not specified	Not specified

APPENDIX 7-C
Features and Specifications of Indirect Calorimeters (Continued)

						MODEL						
	GE HEALTHCARE	CAREFUSION	CAREFUSION	CAREFUSION	CAREFUSION	MEDGRAPHICS	MEDGRAPHICS	MEDGRAPHICS	MEDGRAPHICS	MEDGRAPHICS	VACUMED	VACUMED
SPECIFICATIONS	DELATRAC II	MASTERSCREEN CPX	OXYCON MOBILE	OXYCON PRO	VMAX	CCM EXPRESS	CPX EXPRESS	ULTIMA CardiO2	ULTIMA SERIES	VO2000	VISTA-MX/REE	VO2 LAB
Minute ventilation	Yes	Yes	4%	Yes	10–100	Not specified	Not specified	Not specified	Not specified	Not specified	Yes	Yes
Range	Not specified	0–300 L/min	0 to 300 L/min	0–300 L/min	Not specified	Not specified	Not specified	Not specified	Not specified	Not specified	Not specified	Not specified
Accuracy	Not specified	2% or 0.05 L/min	2% or 0.05 L/min	2% or 0.05 L/min	Not specified	Not specified	Not specified	Not specified	Not specified	Not specified	Not specified	Not specified
F_IO_2	Yes	Yes	Yes	Yes	Not specified	Yes	Not specified	Not specified	Not specified	Not specified	Not specified	Not specified
O_2 Analyzer												
Type	Differential paramagnetic sensor	Electrochemical cell	Electro-chemical	Chemical fuel cell	Electro-chemical cell	Galvanic cell	Galvanic	Galvanic	Galvanic	Galvanic fuel cell	Electro-chemical fuel cell	Baro-compensated fuel cell (to 12,000 feet)
Measurement range	0–10%	0–25%	0–25% (optionally 0–100%)	0–25%	0–100%	0–100%	0–100%	0–100%	0–100%	0–96%	0–100%	0–25%
Resolution	Not specified	0.01%	Not specified	0.05%	0.01%	± 0.1%	± 0.1%		Not specified	Not specified	± 0.03 %	± 0.03%
Time to 90% of value max	Not specified	80 ms (after filtering)	80 ms (after filtering)	80 ms (after filtering)	Not specified	(10–90%) < 130 msec	(10–90%) < 130 msec	< 130 msec	(10–90%) < 130 msec	Not specified	Not specified	Not specified
Accuracy	Not specified	0.05 vol %	0.05 vol %	0.05%	± 0.02%	Not specified	Not specified	± 0.03%	Not specified	± 0.1 %	± 0.01%	± 0.01%
Baseline drift	Automatically compensated	Not specified	Not specified	Not specified	Not specified	Not specified	Not specified	Not specified	Not specified	Not specified	± 0.3%/week	± 0.1%/week
Gain drift	2%/24 hours	Not specified	Not specified	Not specified	Not specified	Not specified	Not specified	Not specified	Not specified	Not specified	Not specified	Not specified
CO_2 Analyzer												
Type	Infrared senor	Thermal conductivity	Thermal conductivity	Infrared absorption	Nondispersive infrared, thermopile	Nondispersive infrared	Nondispersive infrared	Nondispersive infrared	Nondispersive infrared	Nondispersive infrared	Infrared	Not specified
Measurement range	0–10%	0–10%	0–10%	0–25%	0–16%	0–15%	0–15%	0–15%	0–15%	0–10%	0–10%	Not specified

(continues)

APPENDIX 7-C
Features and Specifications of Indirect Calorimeters (Continued)

SPECIFICATIONS	GE HEALTHCARE DELATRAC II	CAREFUSION MASTERSCREEN CPX	CAREFUSION OXYCON MOBILE	CAREFUSION OXYCON PRO	CAREFUSION VMAX	MEDGRAPHICS CCM EXPRESS	MEDGRAPHICS CPX EXPRESS	MEDGRAPHICS ULTIMA CardiO2	MEDGRAPHICS ULTIMA SERIES	MEDGRAPHICS VO2000	VACUMED VISTA-MX/REE	VACUMED VO2 LAB
Resolution	Not specified	0.01%	Not specified	0.01%	0.01%	± 0.1%	± 0.1%		± 0.1%		± 0.03%	Not specified
Time to 90% of value max	Not specified	80 ms (after filtering)	80 ms (after filtering)	80 ms (after filtering)	Not specified	(10–90%) < 130 msec	(10–90%) < 130 msec	< 130 msec	(10–90%) < 130 msec		Not specified	Not specified
Accuracy	Not specified	0.05 vol %	0.05 vol %	0.05%	±0.02% CO_2 across range of 0–10%; no accuracy above 10% CO_2		Not specified	± 0.1%	Not specified	± 0.2%	± 0.1%	Not specified
Baseline drift	Automatically compensated	Not specified	Not specified	Not specified	Not specified	Not specified	Not specified	Not specified	Not specified	Not specified	± 0.3%/week	Not specified
Gain drift	2% of full scale/4 days	Not specified	Not specified	Not specified	Not specified	Not specified	Not specified	Not specified	Not specified	Not specified	Not specified	Not specified
Linearity error	2% of full scale	Not specified	Not specified	Not specified	Not specified	Not specified	Not specified	Not specified	Not specified	Not specified	Not specified	Not specified
Flow/Volume Measurement												
Type	Direct measurement of CO_2 production with room air dilution using a constant flow generator	Bidirectional, digital sensor (TripleV flat fan)	Bidirectional, digital sensor (TripleV flat fan)	Bidirectional, digital sensor (TripleV flat fan)	Mass flow sensor	Bidirectional pitot tube flow sensor	Patented preVent flow sensor	Bidirectional pitot tube flow sensor	Bidirectional pitot tube flow sensor	Bidirectional pitot tube	Not specified	Bidirectional turbine ventilation meter, on-board temperature and barometric pressure sensors
Volume	Not specified	0–10 L	0 to 10 L	0 to 10 L	Not specified		Not specified	Not specified	Not specified	Not specified	Not specified	Not specified
Volume accuracy	Not specified	50 mL or 2%	50 mL or 2%	50 mL or 2%	± 3% of reading or 0.05 L, whichever is greater		Not specified	Not specified	Not specified	± 3% of absolute volume	± 1.5%	± 2%

APPENDIX 7-C
Features and Specifications of Indirect Calorimeters (Continued)

		MODEL										
	GE HEALTHCARE	CAREFUSION	CAREFUSION	CAREFUSION	CAREFUSION	MEDGRAPHICS	MEDGRAPHICS	MEDGRAPHICS	MEDGRAPHICS	MEDGRAPHICS	VACUMED	VACUMED
SPECIFICATIONS	DELATRAC II	MASTERSCREEN CPX	OXYCON MOBILE	OXYCON PRO	VMAX	CCM EXPRESS	CPX EXPRESS	ULTIMA CardiO2	ULTIMA SERIES	VO2000	VISTA-MX/REE	VO2 LAB
Resolution	Not specified	3 mL	3 mL	3 mL	0.003 L/sec from 0.20–16 L/sec		2.4 mL/sec	Not specified	Not specified	Not specified	Not specified	Not specified
Flow	Not specified	0–15 L/sec	0–15 L/sec	0–15 L/sec	0–16 L/sec		Not specified	Not specified	Not specified	2–200 + L/min	Not specified	Not specified
Flow accuracy	Not specified	70 mL/sec or 3%	70 mL/sec or 3%	70 mL/sec or 3%	± 3% of reading or 0.25 L, whichever is greater, across range of 0.2 to 12 L/sec	± 3% or 10 mL, whichever is greater	2.4 mL/sec	± 3% of reading or 0.05 L, whichever is greater	± 3% of reading or 0.05 L, whichever is greater (meets or exceeds ATS/ERS clinical performance standards)	Not specified	± 1.5%	± 2%
Resistance	Not specified	< 0.1 kPa/L/sec at 15 L/sec	< 0.1 kPa/L/sec at 15 L/sec	< 0.1 kPa/L/sec at 15 L/sec	< 1.5 cm H2O/L/sec @12 L/sec	Not specified	Not specified	Not specified	Not specified	Not specified	Not specified	Not specified
Dead space	Not specified	30 mL	Not specified	Not specified	Not specified	Not specified	Not specified	39 mL	39 mL	Not specified	Not specified	Not specified
Weight	Not specified	45g	950 g	10,000 g	Not specified	Not specified	Not specified	Not specified	Not specified	Not specified	Not specified	Not specified
Warm-up Time	30 min	Not specified	Not specified	Not specified	15 min	30 min	Not specified	Not specified	Not required between patients	Not specified	Not specified	Selectable
Display	9" green monochrome picture tube with graphics	Monitor	Monitor	Monitor	Dual Monitor	PC based	Touch screen	PC based	PC based	PC based	Color LCD	PC based
Operating Conditions												
Temperature	31–35°C	5 to 40°C	–10 to +50°C	10 to 40°C	5–40°C	Not specified	Not specified	Not specified	Not specified	0–35°C	Not specified	Not specified
Humidity	Not specified	15–95%, noncondensing	10–95%	10–95%	15–95%, noncondensing	Not specified	Not specified	Not specified	Not specified	0–98% noncondensing	Not specified	Not specified
Altitude	Not specified	Not specified	–1,400 to 5,500 m	–1,000 to +5,500 m (approximately)	Not specified	Not specified	Not specified	Not specified	Not specified	Not specified	Not specified	Not specified

(continues)

APPENDIX 7-C
Features and Specifications of Indirect Calorimeters (Continued)

SPECIFICATIONS	GE HEALTHCARE DELATRAC II	CAREFUSION MASTERSCREEN CPX	CAREFUSION OXYCON MOBILE	CAREFUSION OXYCON PRO	CAREFUSION VMAX	MEDGRAPHICS CCM EXPRESS	MEDGRAPHICS CPX EXPRESS	MEDGRAPHICS ULTIMA CardiO2	MEDGRAPHICS ULTIMA SERIES	MEDGRAPHICS VO2000	VACUMED VISTA-MX/REE	VACUMED VO2 LAB
External Output	Serial data output for graphics printer or for PC data collection; composite video output for slave display	Not specified	Not specified	Not specified	Not specified	Not specified	USB	Thermal printer option	Not specified	RS232	8 channel A/D interface	RS232
W × D × H, cm (in)	42 × 34 × 31 46 with printer on top (16.5 × 13.4 × 12.2) 18.1	80 × 55 (31.5 × 21.7)	2 units 12.6 × 9.6 × 4.1 (4.96 × 3.78 × 1.61) each	24 × 18.6 × 43 (9.4 × 7.1 × 16.9)	38.1 × 15.24 × 38.1 (15 × 16 × 15)	24 × 26.7 × 19 (9.5 × 10.5 × 7.5)	24 × 26.7 × 19 (9.5 × 10.5 × 7.5)	Not specified	15 × 30 × 22 (6 × 11 × 13)	10.5 × 14 × 5 (4.25 × 5.5 × 2)	34.3 × 34.3 × 8.9 (13.5 × 13.5 × 3.5)	30 × 22.5 × 10.2 (12 × 8 × 4-1/8)
Weight, kg (lb)	21 (26.5) without the graphics printer	Not specified	0.95 (2.09) battery, belt system and mask included	10	26.2 (31)	4.7 (9.2)	4.7 (9.2)	Not specified	9.3 (20.5)	0.68 (1.5)	5.5 (12)	2.5 (6)
Power	100/110–120/220–240 V; 50/60 Hz; 120 W	100 VAC to 240 VAC	Lithium-ion battery	100–240 V, 50/60 Hz, 75 W	100 VAC to 240 VAC	100–240 V/ 50–60 Hz	100–240 V/50–60 Hz	Not specified	100–240 V/50–60 Hz	12 VDC @ 650 mA (peak)	Not specified	12 VDC
Green Features	Not specified	Not specified	Not specified	None specified	None specified	None specified	None specified	None specified	None specified	None specified	None specified	None specified
FDA Clearance	Yes	Yes	Yes	Yes	Yes	Yes	Yes	Yes	Yes	Yes	Yes	Yes
CE Mark	Yes	Yes	Yes	Yes	Yes	Yes	Yes	Yes	Yes	Yes	Yes	Yes

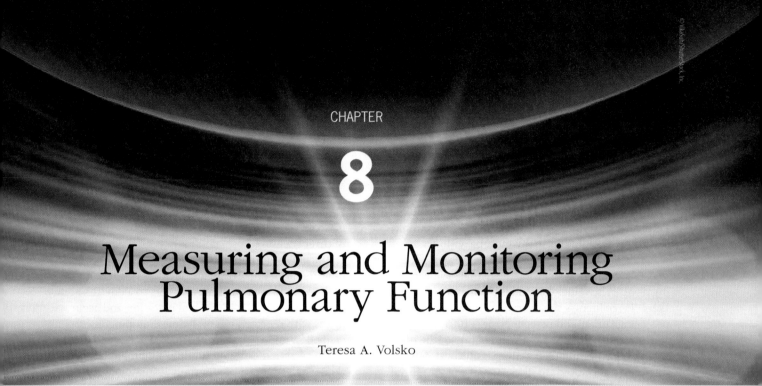

CHAPTER

8

Measuring and Monitoring Pulmonary Function

Teresa A. Volsko

CHAPTER OBJECTIVES

1. Explain measurement theory as it relates to the measurement of exhaled gas.
2. Describe the general characteristics of devices used to perform spirometry.
3. Differentiate between the types of pneumotachometers.
4. Discuss performance and quality control standards for spirometers.
5. Explain the role of a peak flowmeter in asthma disease management.

KEY TERMS

Accuracy
Body temperature and pressure, saturated (BTPS)
Capacity
Durability

Error
Linearity
Peak flowmeter
Pneumotachometer
Precision
Spirometer

Introduction

The measurement of lung volumes and flows is a primary diagnostic tool used to evaluate pulmonary health. Pulmonary diagnostic testing and spirometric screening can be accomplished with a variety of medical devices. Stationary instruments used in a laboratory, as well as portable devices used at the bedside and in ambulatory and home care settings, can be characterized by their measurement methods. Specifically, the three general measurement categories are (1) gas volumes, (2) gas flow rates, and (3) gas pressures.

These devices are useful in detecting airflow limitations,[1] physiological impairment of gas transfer,[2] volume limitations,[3] and respiratory muscle weakness.[4,5] In addition to detecting the presence and severity of pulmonary impairment, this group of medical devices can be used to monitor disease progression[6] and response to therapy.

Similar to the instruments used to analyze blood gases and analytes, this type of instrumentation has performance standards and requirements for training personnel and maintaining quality control.[7]

General Characteristics of Measuring Devices and Measurement Therapy

Devices used to perform pulmonary function measurement have characteristics of capacity, accuracy, error, precision, linearity, durability, operational complexity, and output. **Capacity** refers to the determination of how much or the range of limits an instrument can measure. Flow and volume measuring devices have volume, flow, and time capacity. The range of the largest and smallest volumes the device is capable of measuring is the volume capacity. The capacity of flow measuring devices is concerned with measuring airflow speed (slow or fast). Flow and volume measuring devices also have time capacity. An example of this would be how long a device can measure volume or flow during a specific test.

How well a device measures a known reference value is referred to as the instrument's **accuracy**. The American Thoracic Society (ATS) and European Respiratory Society (ERS) established guidelines for the standardization of spirometry, lung volume, and gas diffusion testing. These guidelines recommend a graduated 3-liter calibration syringe be used to provide the standard reference values for volume measurements.[8]

Reference values are also available for flow measuring devices. Calibration is required because it is unrealistic to expect that any instrument can perform perfect measurements. Typically an arithmetic difference between the known reference and the measured values exists and is known as **error**. Accuracy and error are opposite and complimentary terms. Highly accurate measurements have little error. To determine the percent accuracy and percent error, a series of measurements are taken and then entered into the equations found in **Table 8-1**. Performance standards for spirometers, for example, specify that volume accuracy must be within 3% when using the 3-liter syringe for reference.[7] When 3 liters are injected from the syringe into a volume or flow measuring device, the value obtained is the measured value in liters. Three liters is the reference value. The sum of the percent accuracy and percent error is 100%.

Precision, a measure of the reliability of the instrument's measurements, is synonymous with reproducibility. The standard deviation of the measured reference value is the statistic that is of most interest. The standard deviation shows how much variation or dispersion a measured value has from the average or mean. When measurements of reference values cluster together, even if that cluster is away from the mean (or target value), the measurements are precise. Perhaps the most widely used example demonstrating precision is a bull's-eye (**Figure 8-1**).

Linearity refers to the accuracy of the instrument over its capacity. Linearity will demonstrate discrepancies in accuracy along that continuum of values within the range. For example, a spirometer may have a capacity from 0.1 L to 6 L. **Figure 8-2** illustrates the linearity of three measured values.

Durability is an important characteristic of volume flow and pressure measuring devices. This feature, common to many medical devices, refers to a device's ability to operate within its functional precision and accuracy limits with repeated use over time. Equipment, especially flow and volume measuring devices, tend to have high utilization. Malfunctioning equipment is a particular safety concern, especially if treatment is based on incorrect diagnostic information. Broken equipment contributes to higher operational costs for respiratory

TABLE 8-1
Determining Percent Accuracy and Percent Error

To determine percent accuracy and percent error, measure several values, compute the mean of the measured values, and compare the mean measured value with the known reference value.	
Reference value = 3 L	Measured values 2.91 2.89 2.97 Mean of measured values = (2.91 + 2.98 + 2.97)/3 Mean of measured values = 2.92 L
$\text{Accuracy} = \dfrac{\text{Measured value}}{\text{Reference}}$	$\text{Accuracy} = \dfrac{2.92}{3} = 0.974444$
$\%\ \text{Accuracy} = \left[\dfrac{\text{Measured value}}{\text{Reference}}\right] \times 100$	$\%\ \text{Accuracy} = \left[\dfrac{2.92}{3}\right] \times 100$ $\%\ \text{Accuracy} = 0.97 \times 100$ $\%\ \text{Accuracy} = 97\%$
$\text{Error} = \dfrac{\text{Measured value} - \text{Reference}}{\text{Reference}}$	$\text{Error} = \dfrac{2.94 - 3}{3}$ $\text{Error} = \dfrac{-0.08}{3}$ $\text{Error} = -0.025555556$ The mean of the measured values is 0.02 lower than the measured
$\%\ \text{Error} = \left[\dfrac{\text{Measured value} - \text{Reference}}{\text{Reference}}\right] \times 100$	$\%\ \text{Error} = \left[\dfrac{2.94 - 3}{3}\right] \times 100$ $\%\ \text{Error} = -3\%$ The mean of the measured values is 3% lower than the measured

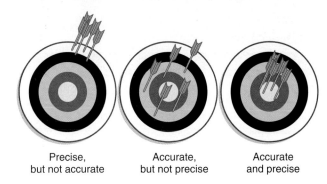

FIGURE 8-1 The bull's-eye target is a common analogy for accuracy. The three targets portray A. measurements that are precise (clustered together), but have a bias (did not reach the center of the target); B. measurements that are near the center of the target, but because they are scattered there is no bias and little precision; C. measurements that are accurate (located in the center of the target) and precise (clustered together).

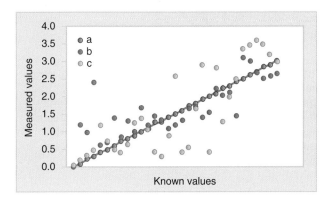

FIGURE 8-2 Three measured values are compared to a known standard. The linearity line (solid black line) is shown. Values for A are linear and are located on or near the linearity line throughout its capacity or range of values. Values for B and C are accurate at times, but are not consistent throughout all of the measured values.

care departments in terms of increased unplanned repair costs and/or the cost of rental equipment during the repair period. In addition to durability, the simplicity with which equipment operates is an important characteristic. Complex devices generally require additional operator training. When selecting a flow or volume measuring device, it may be worthwhile to consider the length of time it takes the machine to warm up, the frequency and complexity of the calibration procedures, the ease with which the operator can navigate through the setup and procedure screens, and how difficult it is to clean and disinfect the device.[9]

Spirometric Testing

Spirometry is a common diagnostic tool used along the continuum of care to evaluate the presence and severity of lung disease, monitor the effectiveness of therapy, and assess health risk and impairment or disability from pulmonary disease.[8,10,11] **Spirometers** are found not only in hospitals and outpatient pulmonary function laboratories, but also in physician offices and health clinics.[12,13] Historically, cumbersome cylindrical canisters, dry rolling or water seal models, were used to collect and measure a patient's volume. These devices were difficult to clean and operate. Spirometers used today measure flow. Flow measuring devices are smaller, lighter, and more portable than their volume measuring predecessors. This type of instrumentation directly measures gas flow rates and electronically integrates the flow rate to provide a calculated measurement of volume.

Pneumotachometers can be used to measure gas flow rates. There are a variety of different types of pneumotachometers available on the market. Electronic devices can also be used to measure spirometric values. Electronic devices are typically portable and used for point-of-care screening.

Pneumotachometers

This type of device measures the pressure created by breathing through a very low resistance. Modifications have been made to pneumotachometers over the years in terms of the materials used to create the resistance to flow. The principle of measurement that pneumotachometers use is based on Poiseuille's law of laminar flow and airflow resistance. If the resistance is constant, known, and low enough, the flow of gas during exhalation against that resistance will cause a small but measureable increase in pressure. During inspiration, the flow of gas across the resistance in the pneumotachometer will create a small but measureable decrease in pressure. This will occur on the proximal side of the resistance. A differential pressure transducer is used to measure the change in pressure across the resistance during inspiration and expiration. Flow rates are calculated by dividing the pressures by the value of the resistance. In accordance with Poiseuille's law, the viscosity of the gas and the radius and length of the pneumotachometer affect the accuracy and precision of the measurement.[14,15] The viscosity of the gases being measured is a factor that will impact clinical practice. The gas or gas mixture (e.g., helium/oxygen) and temperature affect viscosity. Therefore, it is important for the pneumotachometer to be calibrated with the same gas that is to be measured, and the temperature of that calibrating case should be similar to the temperature of the gas to be measured.[16] During normal spontaneous breathing, exhaled gas contains higher concentrations of carbon dioxide and water vapor and lower concentrations of oxygen, contributing to a lower viscosity than inspired air (**Table 8-2**).

The accuracy and precision of flow measurements taken with pneumotachometers are compromised when secretions or moisture clog the internal components, as well as when the flow through the device is turbulent. Laminar flow occurs at relatively low flows. Higher flows give rise to a turbulent flow pattern, when

TABLE 8-2
Gas Viscosity and Proportions During the Phases of the Respiratory Cycle

Gas	Viscosity (poise)	Proportion of Gas During Inspiration	Proportion of Gas During Expiration
Oxygen	206	Higher	Lower
Carbon dioxide	149	Lower	Higher
Water vapor	120	Higher	Lower

Poise = dyne sec/cm²

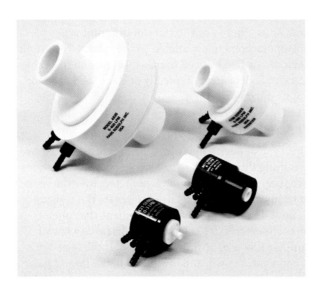

FIGURE 8-3 Examples of different sizes and types of pneumotachometers.

Courtesy of Hans Rudolph.

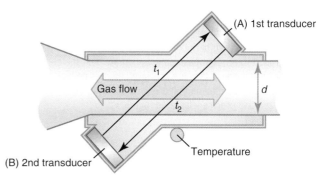

FIGURE 8-4 An ultrasonic flow sensing device. The transducers are located at opposite sides of the flow channel (A and B). Gas flow and molar mass are determined by the transit time of ultrasonic pulses (t_1 and t_2) traveling between the two transducers, bi-directionally and diagonally across the flow of gas from the patient. Flow is computed from the measured gas velocity and known cross-sectional area of the gas stream (d).

the pressure drop across the resistance changes more than proportionally with flow. Turbulent flow creates unpredictably high pressures and inaccurately high measurements. Accurate measurements are best performed when the flow pattern is laminar and the flow is linearly related to pressure drop. Therefore, pneumotachometers have been designed to minimize turbulence. **Figure 8-3** provides an example of pneumotachometers designed to minimize turbulent flow.

There are many types of pneumotachometers. The resistance to flow of a Fleisch pneumotachometer, for example, comes from an array of capillaries arranged in parallel with the direction of flow. Metal screen pneumotachometers allow gas to pass through three screens. The outer metal screen filters out particulate matter, the middle screen provides resistance, and the inner screen is used to laminarize flow. The screens may be heated to 98.6°F (37°C) to prevent condensation from occurring on the screens. Fibrous screens are used in disposable pneumotachometers and are commonly associated with portable spirometry equipment. Filter paper, Styrofoam, fabric, or nylon may be used to create resistance to flow. This type of pneumotachometer is designed to measure

only exhaled gas. It does not contain a heating element, and the fibrous material may absorb water vapor. Therefore, this single patient use device should be limited to a few exhalations before it is disposed of. Once the fibrous material becomes saturated with water vapor, the resistance this material provides will be altered, adversely affecting the accuracy of measurements. Ceramic pneumotachometers are larger and heavier than Fleisch pneumotachometers; however, the ceramic resistance element is porous and readily absorbs water vapor, and also has excellent heat conduction of gases, which ensures measurements at **body temperature and pressure, saturated (BTPS)** conditions.

Electronic Devices

Some electronic devices use an ultrasonic Doppler technique to measure flow. **Figure 8-4** illustrates how ultrasonic flow sensors are used to measure respired gas velocity. Two transducers are mounted at opposite sides of the flow channel. Figure 8-4 shows the two transducers, which are labeled as A and B. Gas flow and molar mass are determined by the transit time of bidirectional ultrasonic pulses (t_1 and t_2) that are directed diagonally across the flow of gas from the patient. Flow is computed from the measured gas velocity and known cross-sectional area of the gas stream (*d* in Figure 8-4).[17]

Performance Standards and Quality Control for Spirometers

The American Thoracic Society (ATS) established performance standards for spirometry. A 3-liter syringe must be used to perform daily equipment calibration checks. The accuracy of measured volume during the calibration checks must be within ± 3% of the calibration value (2.91–3.09 L). The forced vital capacity (FVC) and forced expiratory volume in 1 second (FEV_1) must be corrected for BTPS. Devices must be capable of measuring volumes up to 8 L and flows up to 14 L/sec. The ATS also has performance standards for reporting measured values obtained by spirometry. The report must contain two curves—a volume–time curve and a flow–volume loop. Additionally, when reporting values, the highest FEV_1 and FVC should be conveyed.

The ATS/ERS have quality control standards for spirometers as well. **Table 8-3** outlines the types of quality checks that should be performed and how frequently they should be completed.[8]

Currently Available Devices

There are a plethora of devices available on the market. When devices are selected for primary physician offices and/or outpatient primary care clinics, durability and ease of use are desirable features. Most office spirometers use the third National Health and Nutrition Examination Survey (NHANES III) reference equations for both FEV_1 and FEV_6. Vandevoorde et al. have demonstrated that an FEV_6 is easier to obtain and an acceptable surrogate for FVC in the detection of obstructive lung disease through spirometric assessment in physician offices and clinics.[18] The literature reports that the NHANES III prediction equations may overclassify obstruction, especially

in adults older than 40 years of age, underclassify obstruction in young adults, and underclassify restriction.[19] End users should be aware that there are limitations to office spirometry, and further diagnostic testing is needed when lung disease is suspected.

Flow Measuring Devices Used for Home Monitoring
Peak Flowmeters

Peak flowmeters are portable monitoring devices used for asthma management. There are many peak flow devices currently available on the market. These devices are generally inexpensive and manufactured for single patient use. The literature reports performance discrepancies between brands. In an evaluation of five different peak flowmeters, Takara et al. found no agreement between spirometric values and the peak flowmeters tested.[20] This report highlights the important differences in peak flows measured using different peak flowmeter brands and a spirometric device. Therefore, it is important to recognize that the value of peak flowmeters is in patient monitoring and disease management, rather than with the diagnosis of pulmonary disease.

The National Asthma Education and Prevention Program (NAEPP) Third Expert Panel (EPR-3) recommends the use of written asthma action plans. The EPR-3 recommends that written asthma action plans should be based on either symptoms or peak flow measurements.[21] Peak flow monitoring should be considered for individuals with moderate or severe persistent asthma. Although most predicted peak flow values are age, height, race, and gender adjusted,[22] the NAEPP recommends asthma action plans should incorporate the use of an individual's personal best peak flow value to direct care.[20] A three-zone approach to the management of asthma is used for symptom-based or peak flow monitoring asthma action plans. Zone management provides visual management mirroring that of a traffic light, with green signifying good control, yellow

TABLE 8-3
Quality Control Standards for Spirometers

Test	Minimum Interval	Action
Volume calibration	Daily	Verify accuracy with a 3-L syringe. Measured volumes should be within ± 3% of calibration volume.
Leak test	Daily	Assess for leaks with a pressure of 3 cm H_2O held constant for 1 minute.
Linearity (flow measuring)	Weekly	Verify accuracy of flow. Test three different flow ranges.
Linearity (volume measuring)	Quarterly	A calibrating syringe is used to verify volumes in 1-L increments over the range of volumes the device is capable of measuring.
Time	Quarterly	Assess timing mechanism by using a stopwatch to verify accuracy of time recorder.
Software	New versions	Record or log the date of new software installations. Perform a test using a known subject.

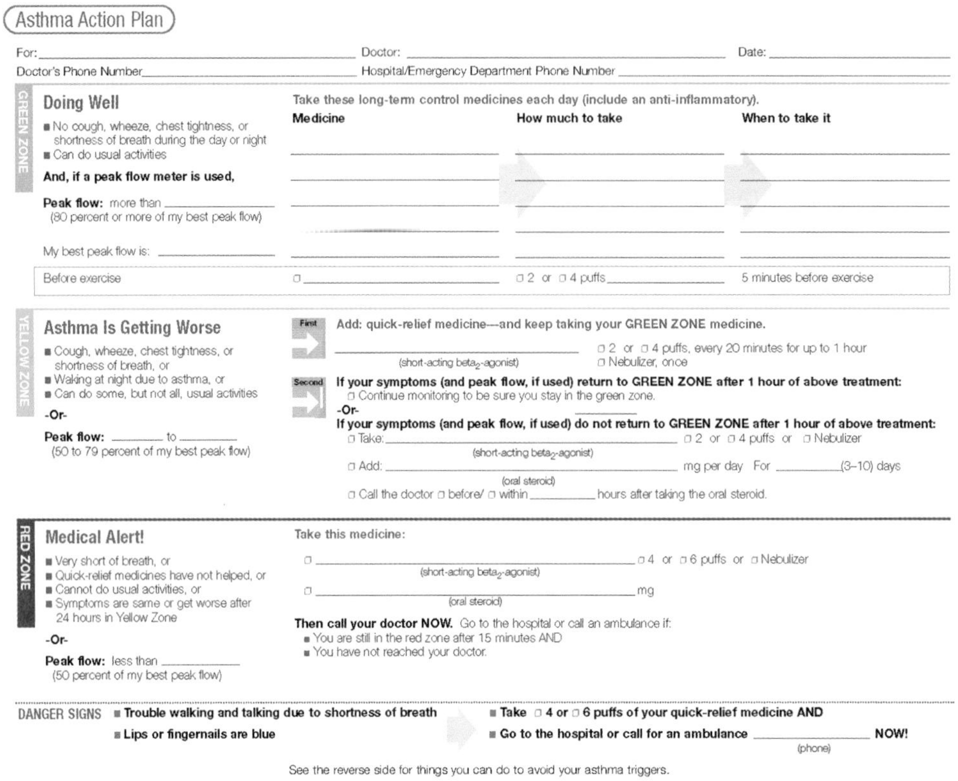

(Asthma Action Plan)

For:_____ Doctor:_____ Date:_____
Doctor's Phone Number_____ Hospital/Emergency Department Phone Number _____

GREEN ZONE

Doing Well
- No cough, wheeze, chest tightness, or shortness of breath during the day or night
- Can do usual activities

And, if a peak flow meter is used,

Peak flow: more than _____
(80 percent or more of my best peak flow)

My best peak flow is: _____

Take these long-term control medicines each day (include an anti-inflammatory).

Medicine	How much to take	When to take it
Before exercise	□ _____ □ 2 or □ 4 puffs_____	5 minutes before exercise

YELLOW ZONE

Asthma Is Getting Worse
- Cough, wheeze, chest tightness, or shortness of breath, or
- Waking at night due to asthma, or
- Can do some, but not all, usual activities

-Or-

Peak flow: _____ to _____
(50 to 79 percent of my best peak flow)

First Add: quick-relief medicine—and keep taking your GREEN ZONE medicine.

_____ □ 2 or □ 4 puffs, every 20 minutes for up to 1 hour
(short-acting beta₂-agonist)   □ Nebulizer, once

Second If your symptoms (and peak flow, if used) return to GREEN ZONE after 1 hour of above treatment:
□ Continue monitoring to be sure you stay in the green zone.

-Or- _____

If your symptoms (and peak flow, if used) do not return to GREEN ZONE after 1 hour of above treatment:
□ Take:_____ □ 2 or □ 4 puffs or □ Nebulizer
(short-acting beta₂-agonist)
□ Add:_____ _____ mg per day For _____(3–10) days
(oral steroid)
□ Call the doctor □ before/ □ within _____ hours after taking the oral steroid.

RED ZONE

Medical Alert!
- Very short of breath, or
- Quick-relief medicines have not helped, or
- Cannot do usual activities, or
- Symptoms are same or get worse after 24 hours in Yellow Zone

-Or-

Peak flow: less than _____
(50 percent of my best peak flow)

Take this medicine:

□ _____ □ 4 or □ 6 puffs or □ Nebulizer
(short-acting beta₂-agonist)
□ _____ mg
(oral steroid)

Then call your doctor NOW. Go to the hospital or call an ambulance if:
- You are still in the red zone after 15 minutes AND
- You have not reached your doctor.

DANGER SIGNS
- Trouble walking and talking due to shortness of breath
- Lips or fingernails are blue

- Take □ 4 or □ 6 puffs of your quick-relief medicine AND
- Go to the hospital or call for an ambulance _____ NOW!
  (phone)

See the reverse side for things you can do to avoid your asthma triggers.

FIGURE 8-5 An example of an asthma action plan developed by the National Heart, Lung, and Blood Institute and available as a free downloadable Web-based tool.

Reproduced from NHLBI Publication No. 07-5251. National Heart, Lung, and Blood Institute; National Institutes of Health; U.S. Department of Health and Human Services. 2007.

TABLE 8-4
An Example of Patient Instructions for Performing Home Peak Flow Monitoring

Step		Details
1	Prepare the device.	Move the marker to the bottom of the numbered scale.
2	Position patient.	Stand up or sit up straight.
3	Breathe in.	Take a deep breath in.
4	Position the device.	Place the peak flowmeter mouthpiece into your mouth. Position the mouthpiece between your teeth. Keep your tongue away from the inside portion of the mouthpiece. Close your lips around the mouthpiece.
5	Perform the maneuver.	Blow out through the mouthpiece as fast and hard as you can. Keep your lips tight around the mouthpiece.
6	Record the value.	Look at the indicator, and write down the value for the peak flow.
7	Repeat your steps.	Repeat steps 1–6 two more times.
8	Review your asthma action plan.	Check to see which treatment zone (green, yellow, or red) your value is in. Follow the asthma management listed in your action plan.

caution, and red medical alert. The patient's plan for controller or daily medications and quick relief (medications taken in the yellow and red zones) are specified on the plan and reviewed with the patient and family at each visit with the medical provider. There are a variety of free Web-based asthma action plans available for use. **Figure 8-5** provides an example of an asthma action plan from the National Heart, Lung, and Blood Institute that incorporates peak flow monitoring available.[23]

Patient instruction is paramount, and the technique for performing a peak flow maneuver should be reviewed periodically.[24] **Table 8-4** provides an outline for patient instruction of peak flowmeter use. Because measurement differences exist between devices, it is important to instruct the patient to always use the same brand of peak flowmeter. Patients should be informed to carry their device with them if peak flow monitoring is integrated into the asthma action plan, and to use values from their own personal portable monitoring device.

Summary

Flow sensing devices can be used for initial screening, diagnosis, and treatment of pulmonary disease. Devices used for home monitoring and office screening should conform to industry standards, be easy to use, and be durable. The ATS and ERS have established performance standards and quality control guidelines. It is essential for the patient to understand how to correctly operate screening, diagnostic, and monitoring devices and adhere to quality control guidelines so they can elicit the best technique to obtain optimal quality results.

References

1. Soriano JB, Zielinski J, Price D. Screening for and early detection of chronic obstructive pulmonary disease. *Lancet.* 2009;374 (9691):721-732.
2. Kaplan E, Bar-Yishay E, Prais D, et al. Encouraging pulmonary outcome for surviving, neurologically intact, extremely premature infants in the postsurfactant era. *Chest.* 2012;142(3):725-733.
3. Garfield JL, Marchetti N, Gaughan JP, Steiner RM, Criner GJ. Total lung capacity by plethysmography and high-resolution computed tomography in COPD. *Int J Chron Obstruct Pulmon Dis.* 2012;7:119-126.
4. Rochester DF, Esau SA. Assessment of ventilatory function in patients with neuromuscular disease. *Clin Chest Med.* 1994; 15(4):751-763.
5. Kabitz HJ, Lang F, Walterspacher S, Sorichter S, Müller-Quernheim J, Windisch W. Impact of impaired inspiratory muscle strength on dyspnea and walking capacity in sarcoidosis. *Chest.* 2006;130(5):1496-1502.
6. Hnizdo E. The value of periodic spirometry for early recognition of long-term excessive lung function decline in individuals. *J Occup Environ Med.* 2012;54(12):1506-1512.
7. Pellegrino R, Decramer M, van Schayck CP, et al. Quality control of spirometry: A lesson from the BRONCUS trial. *Eur Respir J.* 2005;26(6):1104-1109.
8. Miller MR, Hankinson J, Brusasco V, et al. ATS/ERS Task Force: Standardization of lung function testing. *Eur Respir J.* 2005;26: 319-338.
9. Hancock KL, Schermer TR, Holton C, Crockett AJ. Microbiological contamination of spirometers—an exploratory study in general practice. *Aust Fam Physician.* 2012;41(1-2):63-64.
10. Joo MJ, Sharp LK, Au DH, Lee TA, Fitzgibbon ML. Use of spirometry in the diagnosis of COPD: A qualitative study in primary care. *COPD.* 2013;10(4):444-449.
11. Ianiero L, Saranz RJ, Lozano NA, et al. Analysis of the flow-volume curve in children and adolescents with allergic rhinitis without asthma. *Arch Argent Pediatr.* 2013;111(4):322-327.
12. Cawley MJ, Moon J, Reinhold J, Willey VJ, Warning WJ II. Spirometry: Tool for pharmacy practitioners to expand direct patient care services. *J Am Pharm Assoc.* 2013;53(3): 307-315.
13. Coates AL, Graham BL, McFadden RG, et al. Spirometry in primary care. *Can Respir J.* 2013;20(1):13-21.
14. Zock JP. Linearity and frequency response of Fleisch type pneumotachometers. *Pflugers Arch.* 1981;391(4):345-352.
15. Francis G, Gelfand R, Peterson RE. Effects of gas density on the frequency response of gas-filled pressure transducers. *J Appl Physiol.* 1979; 47(3):631-637.
16. Miller MR, Pincock AC. Linearity and temperature control of the Fleisch pneumotachograph. *J Appl Physiol.* 1986;60(2): 710-715.
17. Walters JAE, Wood-Baker R, Walls J, Johns DP. Stability of the Easyone ultrasonic spirometer for use in general practice. *Respirology* 2006;11:306-310.
18. Vandevoorde J, Verbanck S, Schuermans D, Kartounian J, Vincken W. FEV_1/FEV_6 and FEV_6 as an alternative for FEV_1/FVC and FVC in the spirometric detection of airway obstruction and restriction. *Chest.* 2005;127(5):1560-1564.
19. Collen J, Greenburg D, Holley A, King CS, Hnatiuk O. Discordance in spirometric interpretations using three commonly used reference equations vs National Health and Nutrition Examination Study III. *Chest.* 2008;134(5):1009-1106.
20. Takara GN, Ruas G, Pessoa BV, Jamami LK, Di Lorenzo VA, Jamami M. Comparison of five portable peak flow meters. *Clinics (Sao Paulo).* 2010;65(5):469-474.
21. National Asthma Education Program, National Heart, Lung, and Blood Institute. *Expert Panel Report 3: Guidelines for the diagnosis and management of asthma.* NIH Publication 07-4051. Bethesda, MD: National Institutes of Health; 2007.
22. Wun YT, Chan MS, Wong NM, Kong AY, Lam TP. A curvilinear nomogram of peak expiratory flow rate for the young. *J Asthma.* 2013;50(1):39-44.
23. American Lung Association. Create an asthma management plan. Available at: http://www.lung.org/lung-disease/asthma/taking-control-of-asthma/create-an-asthma-management-plan.html. Accessed August 30, 2013.
24. Pruitt WC. Teaching your patient to use a peak flowmeter. *Nursing.* 2005;35(3):54-55.

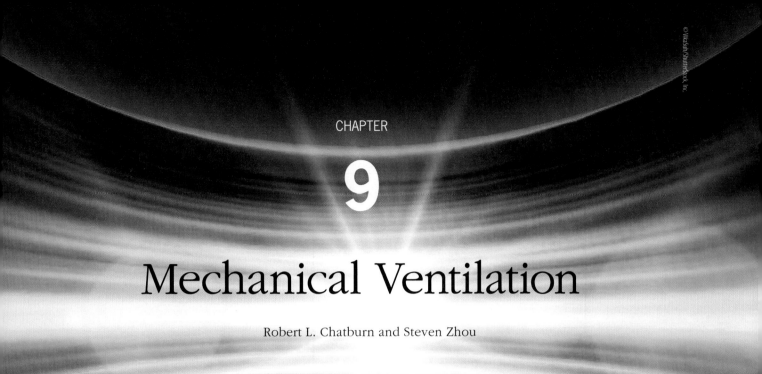

CHAPTER

9

Mechanical Ventilation

Robert L. Chatburn and Steven Zhou

CHAPTER OBJECTIVES

1. Define key terms related to mechanical ventilation.
2. Describe the basic components of ventilators including power inputs, power conversion subsystems, control valves, and output displays.
3. Explain the 10 basic concepts of ventilator technology that form the basis of a mode taxonomy.
4. Demonstrate how to find performance information for any ventilator of interest.

KEY TERMS

Adaptive targeting	Machine triggering
Assisted breath	Mandatory breath
Breath	Mechanical ventilator
Breath sequence	Optimal targeting
Compliance	Patient cycling
Continuous mandatory	Patient triggering
ventilation (CMV)	Pressure control
Continuous spontaneous	Pressure cycling
ventilation (CSV)	Pressure target
Cycle variable	Pressure triggering
Dual targeting	Resistance
Elastance	Sensitivity
Equation of motion for the	Servo targeting
respiratory system	Set-point targeting
Expiratory flow	Spontaneous breath
Expiratory time	Synchronized IMV (SIMV)
Flow cycling	Target
Flow target	Targeting scheme
Flow triggering	Taxonomy
Inspiratory flow time	Tidal volume
Inspiratory hold	Time constant
Inspiratory hold time	Time control
(pause time)	Time cycling
Inspiratory pressure	Time triggering
Inspiratory time	Ventilatory pattern
Intelligent targeting	Volume control
Intermittent mandatory	Volume cycling
ventilation (IMV)	Volume target
Machine cycling	

Section 1: Introduction to Ventilators

A **mechanical ventilator** is an automatic machine designed to provide all or part of the work required to move gas into and out of the lungs. The act of moving air into and out of the lungs is called breathing, or ventilation. Devices like resuscitation bags or (for infants) a T-piece resuscitator are certainly used to assist breathing, but these devices are not automatic; they require an operator to supply the energy to push the gas into the lungs through the mouth and nose or at least to control the flow direction. Thus, such devices are not considered mechanical ventilators.

Automating the ventilator requires three basic components:

1. A source of input energy to drive the device
2. A means of converting input energy into output energy in the form of pressure and flow waveforms to control the timing and size of breaths
3. A means of monitoring the output performance of the device and the condition of the patient

There was a time when you could do routine maintenance on your car engine yourself. About that time a clinician could also completely disassemble and reassemble a mechanical ventilator as a training exercise or to perform repairs. In those days (the late 1970s), textbooks[1,2] describing ventilators emphasized individual mechanical components and pneumatic schematics. Today, both cars and ventilators are incredibly complex mechanical devices controlled by multiple microprocessors running sophisticated software. All but the most rudimentary maintenance of ventilators is now the responsibility of specially trained biomedical

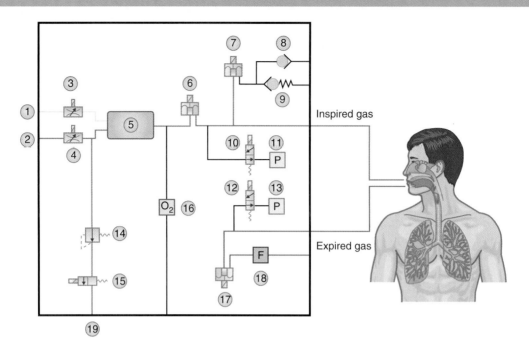

FIGURE 9-1 Simplified schematic of a modern intensive care ventilator. High pressure gas enters the ventilator through the gas inlet connections for oxygen and air (1, 2). Mixing takes place in a reservoir (5) and is controlled by two valves (3, 4). Inspiratory flow from the reservoir is controlled by a separate proportional valve (6). On the inspiratory circuit there is a safety valve (7) and two nonreturn valves (8, 9). In normal operation the safety valve is closed so that inspiratory flow is supplied to the patient's lungs. When the safety valve is open, spontaneous inspiration of atmospheric air is possible through the emergency breathing valve (8). The emergency expiratory valve (9) provides a second channel for expiration when the expiratory valve (17) is blocked. Also on the inspiratory circuit are an inspiratory pressure (P) sensor (11) and a pressure sensor calibration valve (10). The exhalation circuit consists of the expiratory valve (17), expiratory pressure sensor (13) with its calibration valve (12), and an expiratory flow (F) sensor (18). The expiratory valve is a proportional valve and is used to adjust the pressure in the patient circuit. Expiratory flow sensor. Conversion of mass flow to volume (barometric temperature and pressure saturated, BTPS) requires knowledge of ambient pressure, measured by another pressure sensor (20). Pressure in the patient circuit is measured with two independent pressure sensors (11, 13). Oxygen flow to the nebulizer port (19) is controlled by a pressure regulator (14) and a solenoid valve (15).

engineers. **Figure 9-1** shows a simplified pneumatic schematic of a current generation intensive care ventilator.

Our approach to describing ventilator design in this chapter is a major departure from previous equipment books. The focus of this book has changed from descriptions of individual components (valves, pistons, circuits, etc.) to a more generalized model of a ventilator as a "black box," a device for which we supply an input and expect a certain output.[3] The reason for the change is that the internal operations of the ventilator are largely unknowable and unimportant to most clinicians. What follows, then, is only a brief overview of the key design features of mechanical ventilators with an emphasis on input power requirements, transfer functions (pneumatic and electronic control systems), and outputs (pressure, volume, and flow waveforms). We will also discuss the interactions between the operator and the ventilator (the operator interface) and various types of ventilator output displays.

With this brief introduction to ventilator design, we then change the focus to the interaction between the ventilator and the patient. Ultimately, the application of mechanical ventilation involves selecting a mode of ventilation. The term *mode of ventilation* means a preset pattern of interaction between the ventilator and the patient. However, the word *mode* and many other words associated with mechanical ventilation are used without definition and often in illogical ways both in the research literature and in ventilator operators' manuals. Therefore, to understand the technology and terminology associated with modes, in Section 2 we will review 10 basic concepts starting with how a **breath** is defined and ending with a classification system for modes of ventilation.

Power Inputs

The input power for ventilators comes from electricity or compressed gas. Electricity, either from wall outlets (e.g., 110 to 240 volts A/C, at 50/60 Hz) or from batteries (e.g., 10 to 30 volts DC), is used to run compressors or blowers of various types. Batteries are a common power source for patient transport or emergency use in hospitals. Alternatively, the power to expand the lungs is supplied by compressed gas from tanks or from wall outlets in the hospital (e.g., 30 to 80 pounds per square inch, psi). Some transport and emergency ventilators use compressed gas to power both lung inflation and the control circuitry. For these ventilators, knowledge of gas consumption is critical when using cylinders of compressed gas to make sure the source is not depleted before the need for the ventilator (e.g., transport) is over.

Ventilators are powered by separate sources of compressed air and compressed oxygen. This permits the delivery of a range of oxygen concentrations to support the needs of sick patients. Hospital wall outlets supply air and oxygen at 50 psi, although most ventilators have internal regulators to reduce this pressure to a lower level (e.g., 20 psi). Because compressed gas has all moisture removed, the gas delivered to the patient must be warmed and humidified in order to avoid drying out the lung tissue.

Power Conversion Subsystems

Input power must be converted to get the desired outputs of pressure, volume, and flow. Electrically powered ventilators use a compressor or blower to generate the required pressure and flow. A compressor is a machine for moving a relatively low flow of gas at ambient pressure to a storage container at a higher level of pressure (e.g., 20 psi). Compressors are generally found on intensive care ventilators. A blower (sometimes called a turbine) is a machine for generating relatively larger flows of gas as the direct ventilator output (rather than filling a storage container) with a relatively moderate increase of pressure (e.g., 2 psi). Blowers are used on home care and transport ventilators. Compressors are typically larger and consume more electrical power than blowers, hence the use of blowers on small, portable devices.

Flow Control Valves

Ventilators use different kinds of flow control valves to manipulate the flow of gas from the ventilator to the patient. The simplest valve is a fixed orifice flow resistor that permits setting a constant flow to the external tubing that conducts the gas to the patient, called the "patient circuit." Manually adjusted variable orifice flowmeters allow the operator to set constant flows in a range of values. This provides a simple means, for example, of adjusting inspired volume during assisted ventilation. Fixed and adjustable flow valves are used in some transport ventilators and resuscitation devices. Inexpensive microprocessors became available in the 1980s and led to development of digital control of flow valves (**Figure 9-2**). Digital control allows a great deal of flexibility in shaping the ventilator's output pressure, volume, and flow.[4] Such valves are used in most of the current generation of intensive care ventilators.

Delivering flow to the patient requires the coordination of the output flow control valve and an expiratory valve or "exhalation manifold." When inspiration is triggered on, the output control valve opens (allowing flow from the source), the expiratory valve closes (so the gas does not escape to the atmosphere), and the only path left for gas is into the patient. When inspiration is cycled off, the output valve closes and flow from the ventilator ceases. At the same time, the exhalation valve opens and the patient exhales out through the expiratory valve (Figure 9-2). The exhalation valve also controls the level of positive end-expiratory pressure (PEEP). The most sophisticated ventilators employ a complex interaction between the output flow control valve and the exhalation valve such that many different pressure, volume, and

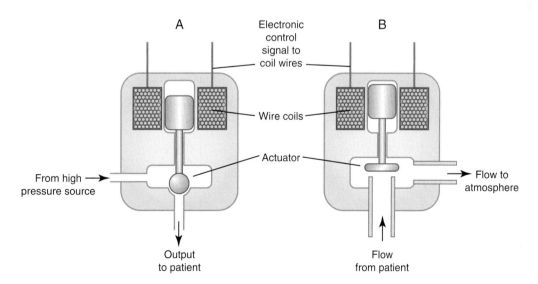

FIGURE 9-2 A. Simplified schematic of a general flow control valve, which is controlled by an electronic signal (usually a digital signal from a microcontroller). The signal energizes electrical coils comprising an electromagnet that moves the actuator. The movement of the actuator changes the diameter of the flow path from a high pressure source (e.g., air or oxygen) and thereby changes the flow waveform. B. Simplified schematic of a general exhalation valve, which also is controlled by an electronic signal. The movement of the actuator changes the diameter of the flow path from the patient's lungs and thereby allows exhalation and also the control of PEEP.

flow waveforms may be generated and coordinated with breathing efforts to promote patient safety and comfort.

Control System

A ventilator's control system generates the signals that operate the output valve and the exhalation manifold. Control systems may be based on mechanical, pneumatic, fluidic, or electronic components. Mechanical components include levers, pulleys, cams, and the like.[5] Pneumatic control circuits use gas pressure to operate diaphragms, jet entrainment devices, pistons, and so on. Fluidic circuits are like electronic logic circuits but they operate with gas instead of electricity.[6] Both pneumatic and fluidic control systems are immune to failure from electromagnetic interference, such as around magnetic resonance imaging equipment. Examples of simple pneumatic and fluidic ventilator control circuits have been illustrated elsewhere.[7] However, most ventilators use electronic control circuits with microprocessors and complex software algorithms to manage monitoring (e.g., from pressure and flow sensors) and control functions.

The differences among ventilators are due as much to the control system software as to the hardware. Software determines how the ventilator interacts with the patient (i.e., the modes available). Thus, a discussion about control systems is essentially a discussion about mode capabilities and classifications. But in order to understand modes, we must first discuss some fundamental concepts beyond the constructs of input and output. These concepts are described later in this chapter, in Section 2.

Pressure, Volume, and Flow Outputs

The outputs of a mechanical ventilator are the pressure, volume, and flow waveforms it generates in supporting the patient's work of breathing along with measured or calculated data it generates and displays to the operator. Note, first of all, that a waveform is simply a graphic representation of a variable function of time; that is, the variable (pressure, volume, or flow) is plotted on the vertical axis and time is plotted on the horizontal axis. We will discuss the waveforms here and the other data in the section on Ventilator Displays. The best way to approach this subject is to start with idealized waveforms, meaning the waveforms that would exist in an ideal world with perfect machines and no interferences from leaks or patient breathing efforts. Such waveforms can be generated for educational purposes by using graphs of mathematical models. With an understanding of idealized waveforms, one can more easily interpret waveforms displayed on ventilators in the real world.

Idealized Pressure, Volume, and Flow Waveforms

Many ventilators allow the display of pressure, volume, and flow waveforms. Some allow only two waveforms at a time. If only two are available at a time, the pressure and flow waveforms usually display the most useful information. The horizontal axis of all three graphs is the same and has the units of time. The vertical axes are in units of pressure, volume, and flow. When interpreting waveforms, pay attention to the relative magnitudes of each of the variables and how the value of one affects or is affected by the values of the others.

Typical waveforms available on modern ventilators are illustrated in **Figure 9-3**. These waveforms are defined by mathematical equations and are meant to characterize the operation of the ventilator's control system. They do not show the minor deviations,

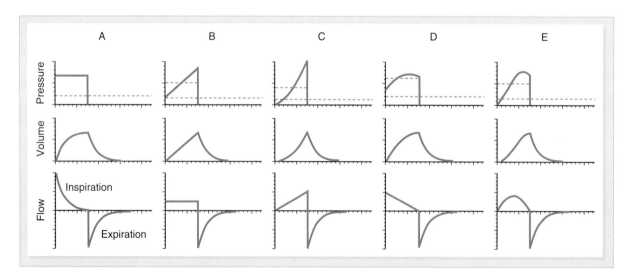

FIGURE 9-3 Idealized ventilator output waveforms. A. Pressure-controlled inspiration with a rectangular pressure waveform. B. Volume-controlled inspiration with a rectangular flow waveform. C. Volume-controlled inspiration with an ascending-ramp flow waveform. D. Volume-controlled inspiration with a descending-ramp flow waveform. E. Volume-controlled inspiration with a sinusoidal flow waveform. The short dashed lines represent mean inspiratory pressure, and the long dashed lines represent mean pressure for the complete respiratory cycle (i.e., mean airway pressure).

Reproduced with permission from Chatburn RL. *Fundamentals of mechanical ventilation*. Cleveland Heights, OH: Mandu Press Ltd; 2003:143.

or noise, often seen during actual ventilator use. This noise can be caused by extraneous factors such as vibration and flow turbulence. Of course, scaling of the horizontal and vertical axes can affect the appearance of actual waveforms considerably.

Interpretation of ventilator waveforms requires an in-depth understanding of a number of underlying concepts. These concepts are presented in Section 2.

Patient Circuit

The patient circuit is the tubing that connects the ventilator to the patient. There is an endless diversity of circuits but there are only three basic configurations (**Figure 9-4**). Homecare and transport ventilators often use only one tube, called a single-limb circuit (Figure 9-4, top). Near the end that connects to the patient is a pneumatically controlled exhalation valve connected inline with the flow to the patient. The exhalation valve is switched on and off by a pressure signal from the ventilator, conveyed through small-bore tubing. When the pressure signal goes high, the valve closes, and flow is directed from the ventilator to the patient. When the pressure signal goes low, the valve opens and the patient exhales to the atmosphere. Often there is a residual pressure in the valve that sets the PEEP level.

Most intensive care ventilators have the exhalation valve built into the ventilator and are connected to the patient with a double-limb circuit (Figure 9-4, middle). Ventilators designed for noninvasive ventilation, using a mask instead of an artificial airway, often have single-limb circuits that are used without an exhalation valve

(Figure 9-4, bottom). The circuit may have a small fitting that has a carefully sized opening or port. The port provides a known leak, and the relationship between circuit pressure and leak flow is programmed into the ventilator's microcontroller. Thus, by measuring the pressure in the circuit, calculating the leak flow, and deducting that from the total flow delivered by the blower, the ventilator can estimate the flow and hence volume delivered to the patient. Sometimes the leak port is in the mask instead of the patient circuit.

Some intensive care ventilators measure flow at the airway opening using a small, usually disposable sensor (**Figure 9-5**). Two basic types of flow sensors are used with ventilators. One is called a pneumotachometer. It has a flow-resistive element such as a screen or plastic flap in the flow path. The pressures on both sides of the resistor are conducted to pressure sensors in the ventilator through small-diameter tubing. The difference between the two pressures is proportional to flow. The second type of flow sensor is called a hot wire anemometer. Very thin wires are placed in the flow path and heated. The flow carries away the heat. Therefore, the amount of energy required to maintain the heat in the wires is proportional to flow.

Ventilator Alarm System

Ventilator alarms have increased in number and complexity. There is no generally agreed upon classification system for alarms, but MacIntyre and Branson[8] have proposed they be categorized by the events they are designed to detect. Level 1 events include life-threatening situations. This would be things like loss of input power or ventilator malfunction (e.g., excessive or no flow of gas to the patient). The alarms in this category

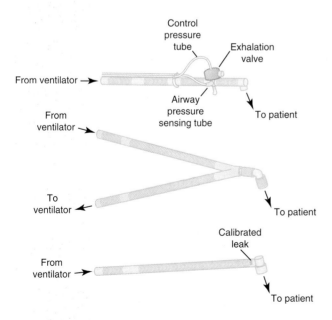

FIGURE 9-4 Three basic types of patient circuit. Top: Single-limb circuit with exhalation valve, often used on home care or transport ventilators. Middle: Double-limb circuit, usually used on intensive care ventilators. Bottom: Single-limb circuit without exhalation valve used on noninvasive ventilators.

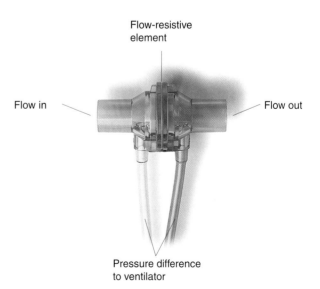

FIGURE 9-5 Example of a disposable flow sensor that uses the pressure difference across a flow-resistive element to generate a signal proportional to flow.

should be mandatory, redundant (using multiple sensors and circuits), and noncanceling. Noncanceling means that the alarm continues to be activated even if the event is corrected, and must be reset manually. Level 2 events can lead to life-threatening situations if not corrected quickly. These events include blender failure, high or low airway pressure, auto-triggering, and partial patient circuit occlusion. The alarm may also warn of suspicious ventilator settings such as an inspiratory time: expiratory time (I:E ratio) greater than 1:1. Alarms for level 2 events may be self-canceling, meaning that the alarm is automatically inactivated if the event ceases to occur. Level 3 events are those that may influence the level of support provided, such as changes in patient lung mechanics, changes in patient respiratory drive, and auto-PEEP. Alarm performance at this level is similar to that of level 2 alarms. Level 4 events reflect the patient condition alone rather than ventilator function. These events are usually detected by stand-alone monitors, such as oximeters, cardiac monitors, and blood gas analyzers. As ventilators have become more sophisticated, they have incorporated some stand-alone monitor functionality, such as esophageal pressure monitoring, pulse oximetry, and capnometry.

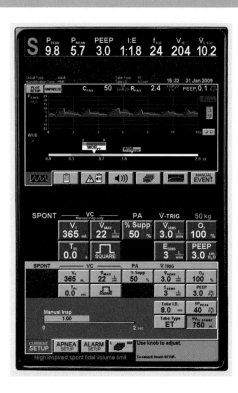

FIGURE 9-6 Example of an alphanumeric ventilator screen display.

Ventilator Displays

Ventilator output displays have advanced tremendously in the last 30 years. In this period displays have evolved from simple lights and dials to digital readouts to full graphic user interfaces with touch screens. There are four basic ways to present the monitored data: as numbers or text, as waveforms, as trend lines, and in the form of abstract graphic symbols.

Alphanumeric Values

Measured or calculated data are most commonly represented as numeric values such as F_IO_2, peak, plateau, mean and baseline airway pressures, inhaled/exhaled **tidal volume**, minute ventilation, and frequency. Depending on the ventilator, a wide range of calculated parameters may also be displayed including **resistance**, **compliance**, **time constant**, percent leak, I:E ratio, and peak inspiratory/expiratory flow, to name just a few. Text messages are now common on ventilator displays. They are used for explaining alarm conditions and also for giving brief instructions to the operator about settings. An example of an alphanumeric ventilator display is shown in **Figure 9-6**.

Trends

The basic display of all ventilators shows the current state of the device; however, we are often interested in how parameters related to mechanical support change

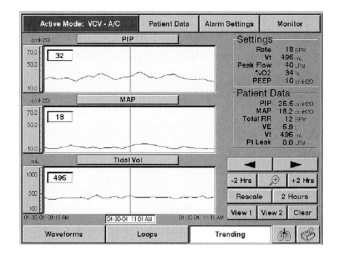

FIGURE 9-7 Example of a ventilator trend display.

over time. To satisfy this need, many ventilators provide trend graphs of just about any parameter they measure or calculate. These graphs show how the monitored parameters change over long periods of time (**Figure 9-7**). Significant events or gradual changes in patient condition can be easily identified. In addition, ventilators often provide an alarm log. This is usually a text-based list documenting such things as the date, time, alarm type, urgency level, and events associated with alarms including when activated and when canceled. Such a log could be invaluable in the event of a ventilator failure leading to a legal investigation.

Waveforms and Loops

Most ventilators display graphical depictions of pressure, volume, and flow waveforms. These waveforms are quite useful for adjusting ventilator settings or evaluating respiratory system mechanics.[9,10] They are essential for assessing sources of patient–ventilator asynchrony such as missed triggers, flow asynchrony, and delayed/premature cycling, and then making appropriate corrections.[11] Sometimes it is more useful to plot one variable against another as an X-Y or loop display. Pressure-volume loop displays are useful for identifying optimum PEEP levels (to avoid atelectrauma) and optimum tidal volume (to avoid volutrauma).[12] Ideally, loop displays for such usage should be made with patients who are paralyzed or heavily sedated (to avoid errors due to patient effort effects) and with very slow inflations (i.e., quasi-static curve). Caution must be exercised because ventilators display loops under any ventilating circumstances and hence the display may be meaningless. For example, loop displays for pressure control modes cannot be used to identify either optimum PEEP or optimum tidal volume. Loop displays for volume control modes (using constant inspiratory flow) can show overdistention and so may be used to adjust tidal volume. Flow-volume loops are useful for identifying the response to bronchodilators. An example of a composite display showing numeric values, waveforms, and loops is shown in **Figure 9-8**.

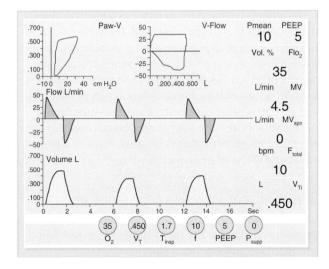

FIGURE 9-8 Example of a ventilator display with alphanumeric, waveform, and loop displays.

Reproduced with permission from Mandu Press Ltd., Cleveland, OH.

Section 2: Understanding Ventilator Technology

The main goal of a text on respiratory care equipment is to provide a source of technical information to supplement more general textbooks on respiratory care. One difficulty in creating such a reference is striking the proper balance between too much detail (as would be found in a ventilator operator's manual) and too little (as would be found in a ventilator specification sheet). Both manuals and spec sheets are readily available for most ventilators. However, as you read these documents you quickly realize an even bigger problem: there is no standardization in either vocabulary or format, making comparisons among devices difficult. This problem is particularly bothersome when it comes to understanding the modes of ventilation offered by the many different types of mechanical ventilators.

In the eighth edition of Mosby's *Respiratory Care Equipment* (2010), 174 unique mode *names* are mentioned on 34 different ventilators.[13] But they are certainly not 174 unique *modes*. There are many cases of different names for identical modes (e.g., Pressure-Control Ventilation Plus Adaptive Pressure Ventilation on the Hamilton Galileo is the same as Pressure Regulated Volume Control on the Siemens Servo 300) and a few cases of the same name used for very different modes (e.g., Assist/Control on the Puritan Bennett 840 is a form of volume control whereas Assist/Control on the Bear Cub infant ventilator is a form of pressure control).

The purpose of classifying modes of ventilation is the same as the purpose of classifying anything else—to make possible meaningful comparisons. By comparing and contrasting modes we are better able to match a given patient's immediate needs to the available technology. This is the same as matching a particular drug to a patient's disease. What is different is that up until now there has never been a standard reference for classifying modes of ventilation like there are for drugs. This chapter is, in part, an attempt to fill that need.

Despite the lack of a standardized classification system for modes, such a **taxonomy** has been described previously.[14,15] The basic principle of this system has been embraced by authors of ventilator textbooks.[16-18] What has been lacking, up until now, is a systematic approach for teaching this system. Indeed, a taxonomy can be viewed as the last step in a sequence of theoretical constructs that build the classification system. This section provides a detailed explanation of 10 fundamental constructs of ventilator design and function upon which a practical ventilator mode taxonomy can be based. These concepts build on one another to yield a practical framework for understanding, comparing, and contrasting the features of ventilators. This can provide the structural outline for a complete didactic course on mechanical ventilation. The ultimate purpose of these activities is to enable clinicians to select the most appropriate mode for a given clinical situation. The didactic approach described here is informed by the data from an international survey.[19] After describing these 10 concepts (stated as maxims or concise statements of scientific principles) we demonstrate how the resulting taxonomy can be used to guide selection of modes.

1. A Breath Is Defined in Terms of the Flow-Time Curve

The most basic function of a ventilator is to deliver a breath. The most basic definition of a breath is one cycle of inspiratory flow followed by a matching **expiratory flow** (**Figure 9-9**). These flows are paired by size, meaning approximately equal inspiratory and expiratory volumes. Inspiration is not necessarily followed immediately by the matching expiration. For example, during Airway Pressure Release Ventilation the transition from low pressure to high pressure results in a large **mandatory breath** inspiration. This is possibly followed by a few small **spontaneous breath** inspirations and expirations. Finally, the transition from high pressure to low pressure results in the matching mandatory exhalation. It is also possible to have many small mandatory breaths superimposed on larger spontaneous breaths, as during High Frequency Oscillatory Ventilation.

The two most basic definitions in reference to a breath are inspiratory time and expiratory time. **Inspiratory time** is the period from the start of inspiratory flow to the start of expiratory flow. Inspiratory time equals **inspiratory flow time** plus **inspiratory hold time (pause time)**. Inspiratory hold time or pause time is the period from the cessation of inspiratory flow (into the airway opening) to the start of expiratory flow during mechanical ventilation. On some ventilators, inspiratory hold time is set directly. On others, hold time is the difference between the preset inspiratory time and the inspiratory flow time due to the preset tidal volume at the preset inspiratory flow (i.e., Flow time = Tidal volume/ Inspiratory flow). Inspiratory hold time is often used to increase mean airway pressure and improve oxygenation and also to create a static airway pressure (called plateau pressure) that may be used to calculate respiratory system resistance and compliance. **Expiratory time** is the period from the start of expiratory flow to the start of inspiratory flow.

Figure 9-9 is the basis for several mathematical equations relevant to ventilator settings (**Table 9-1**).

2. A Breath Is Assisted If the Ventilator Provides Some or All of the Work of Breathing

The main purpose of a ventilator is to assist with the patient's work of breathing. Work is a function of pressure necessary to expand the volume of the respiratory system. Pressure is generated either by the patient's inspiratory muscles (P_{mus}) or the ventilator (P_{vent}). Either way, there is an increase in the pressure difference across the respiratory system (which we will refer to simply as **inspiratory pressure**; a detailed discussion of the subject is provided in a recent textbook[20]) so that its volume increases during inspiration. An **assisted breath** can be recognized on a ventilator graphic display by examining the pressure waveform during inspiration (i.e., positive flow). If airway pressure rises above baseline (end expiratory pressure) during inspiration (as defined in maxim 1 as a positive change in flow), then the breath is assisted. If airway pressure falls below baseline pressure during inspiration, the patient is doing some work on the ventilator and we say the breath is "loaded" rather than assisted. Some loading is unavoidable because ventilators cannot control airway pressure perfectly; some pressure drop is necessary for pressure triggering a breath and there are electrical/mechanical delays between sensing a patient effort and the start of inspiratory flow.[21]

3. A Ventilator Provides Assistance by Controlling Either the Pressure or Volume Waveform Based on the Equation of Motion for the Respiratory System

A ventilator provides assistance by maintaining a desired waveform for either inspiratory pressure (called **pressure control**) or inspiratory volume/flow (called **volume control**). The theoretical

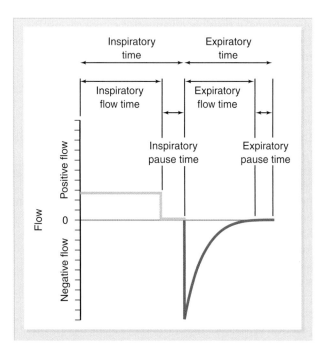

FIGURE 9-9 A breath is defined as one cycle of inspiratory flow followed by a matching expiratory flow, yielding approximately the same volumes.

Reproduced with permission from Mandu Press Ltd., Cleveland, OH.

TABLE 9-1
Equations for Breath Timing Based on Figure 9-9

Parameter	Symbol
Volume (L)	V
Flow (L/min)	$\dot{V}$
Time (sec)	t
Frequency (breaths/min)	f

Parameter	Symbol	Equation
Inspiratory time (sec)	T_I	$(60 / f) - T_E$ or $(60 \times I) / [f \times (I + E)]$
Expiratory time (sec)	T_E	$(60 / f) - T_I$ or $(60 \times E) / [f \times (I + E)]$
Total cycle time or period (sec)	T_{tot}	$T_I + T_E$ or $60/f$
Inspiratory to expiratory time ratio	I:E	$T_I : T_E$ or $D/(100\% - D)$
Duty cycle (%)	D	$(T_I / T_{tot}) \times 100\%$ or $100\% \times I/(I + E)$
Mean inspiratory flow	$\bar{\dot{V}}_I$	V_T / T_I
Tidal volume	V_T	$\bar{\dot{V}} \times T_I$

Reproduced with permission by Mandu Press Ltd., Cleveland, OH.

foundation for this assertion is a mathematical model of patient–ventilator interaction known as the **equation of motion for the respiratory system:**[22]

$$P_{vent}(t) = EV(t) + R\dot{V}(t)$$

where $P_{vent}(t)$ is inspiratory pressure generated by the ventilator as a function of time (see maxim 2), E is the **elastance** of the respiratory system (lungs and chest wall), $V(t)$ is volume as a function of time, R is respiratory-system resistance, and $\dot{V}(t)$ is flow as a function of time. *Note that all these variables are measured relative to their end expiratory values.* Under static (i.e., no flow) conditions these are P_{vent} = end expiratory pressure, usually set PEEP, V = end-expiratory lung volume (functional residual capacity if PEEP = 0), and $\dot{V} = 0$, assuming no autoPEEP.

In this equation, the term $EV(t)$ has the units of pressure and is called the *elastic load*. The term $R\dot{V}(t)$ also has the units of pressure and is called the *resistive load*. Hence, the term *breath unloading* means that the ventilator supplies some portion of the work to deliver volume and flow against these loads.

A plot of $P_{vent}(t)$ versus time gives the airway pressure waveform seen on ventilator displays. If the shape of this waveform is predetermined by the ventilator settings, we say that the ventilator is providing pressure control (PC). One very confusing issue with PC is that sometimes the operator sets the magnitude of the pressure waveform relative to atmospheric pressure (called peak inspiratory pressure) and other times the

magnitude is set relative to PEEP (in this case simply called inspiratory pressure).[23]

A plot of the $V(t)$ or $\dot{V}(t)$ yields the volume and flow waveforms. If the shape of these waveforms is predetermined by the ventilator settings, we say the ventilator is providing volume control (VC). Note that direct control of the flow waveform (e.g., with a flow control valve) implies indirect control of volume because volume is the integral of flow with respect to time. It is also true that direct control of the volume waveform (e.g., with a piston) implies indirect control of flow because flow is the derivative of volume with respect to time. We say "volume control" rather than "flow control" simply for historical reasons. We don't use both because that would lead to unnecessary complications when it comes to classifying modes.

Volume control (VC) means that *both* volume and flow are preset prior to inspiration. Setting tidal volume is a necessary but not sufficient criterion for declaring volume control because some modes of pressure control allow the operator to set a target tidal volume but allow the ventilator to determine the flow (see adaptive targeting schemes later in this chapter). Similarly, setting flow is also a necessary but not sufficient criterion; some pressure control modes allow the operator to set the maximum inspiratory flow but the tidal volume depends on the inspiratory pressure target and respiratory system mechanics.

Pressure control (PC) means that inspiratory pressure as a function of time is predetermined. In practice,

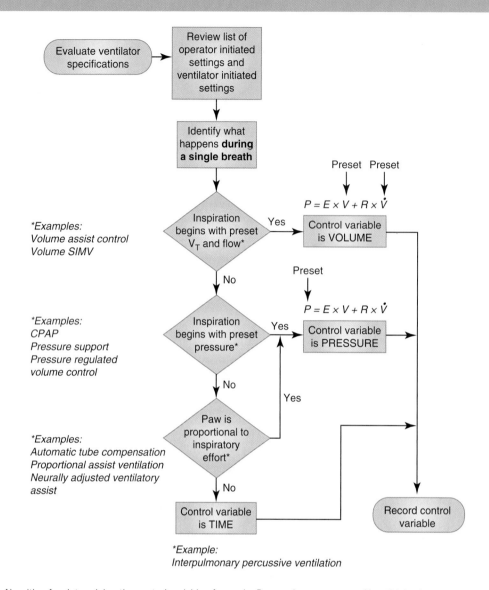

FIGURE 9-10 Algorithm for determining the control variable of a mode. Paw = airway pressure, V_T = tidal volume.
Reproduced with permission from Mandu Press Ltd., Cleveland, OH.

this currently means presetting a particular pressure waveform (e.g., $P(t)$ = constant), or inspiratory pressure is set to be proportional to patient inspiratory effort, measured by various means. For example, $P(t)$ = NAVA level × EAdi(t) where NAVA stands for Neurally Adjusted Ventilatory Assist and EAdi stands for electrical activity of the diaphragm (see servo targeting scheme later in this chapter). In a passive patient, after setting the form of the pressure function (i.e., the waveform), volume and flow depend on E and R.[24]

Time control (TC) is a general category of ventilator modes for which inspiratory flow, inspiratory volume, and inspiratory pressure are all dependent on respiratory system mechanics. As no parameters of the pressure, volume, or flow waveforms are preset, the only control of the breath is the timing (i.e., inspiratory and expiratory times). Examples of this are High Frequency Oscillatory Ventilation (CareFusion

3100 ventilator) and Volumetric Diffusive Respiration (Percussionaire).

The algorithm for determining the control variable for a given mode of ventilation is shown in **Figure 9-10**. Common pressure, volume, and flow waveforms produced by ventilators are shown in Figure 9-3. **Figures 9-11** and **9-12** show the relationships among factors that determine minute ventilation for volume control and pressure control.

4. Breaths Are Classified According to the Criteria That Trigger (Start) and Cycle (Stop) Inspiration

For unassisted breathing, the brain generates signals to start and stop inspiration. When a patient is connected to a ventilator, the ventilator requires a signal to start and stop the inspiratory flow. Starting inspiration

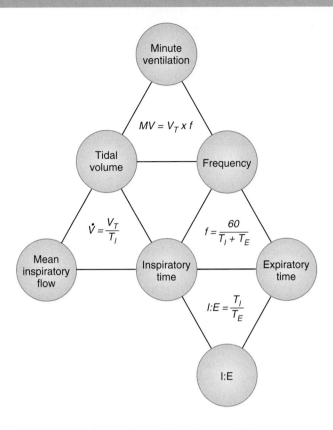

FIGURE 9-11 Influence diagram for volume control.
Reproduced with permission from Mandu Press Ltd., Cleveland, OH.

is called *triggering.* Common trigger signals include time, airway pressure, volume, flow, and the electrical signal from the diaphragm, but other signals are possible. Stopping inspiration is called *cycling.* Common cycle signals are the same as for triggering. The term **sensitivity** refers to the amount that the trigger or cycle signal must change before inspiration starts or stops.

As it turns out, *trigger* and *cycle* are key definitions in the development of a classification system for modes of ventilation. Some authors (including those who write standards and ventilator operator's manuals) tend to restrict the definition of *trigger* to only the act of the patient initiating inspiration, leaving machine starting of flow undefined. As a result, they have no convenient method of distinguishing machine trigger and cycle events from patient trigger and cycle events (see maxim 5) and no practical way to define mandatory and spontaneous breaths (see maxim 6). Without definitions for mandatory and spontaneous breaths, we cannot define ventilatory patterns (maxim 7) and there is no basis for the taxonomy built on all of the maxims (see maxim 10). The point is that each of the maxims is an important component of the theoretical foundation for this system of classifying modes. There may, of course, be other ways of developing a mode taxonomy; however, none has yet been described that is as practical and

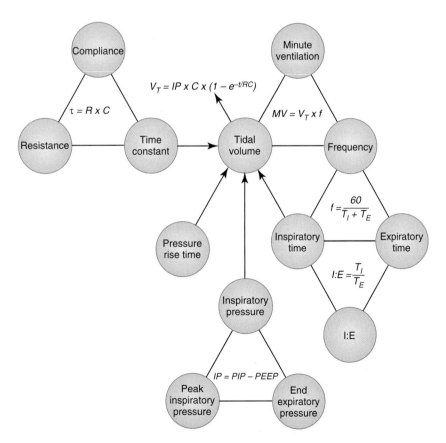

FIGURE 9-12 Influence diagram for pressure control.
Reproduced with permission from Mandu Press Ltd., Cleveland, OH.

consistent with current clinical and educational paradigms as the one described here.

5. Trigger or Cycle Events Can Be Either Patient or Ventilator Initiated

We normally want to keep the delivery of inspiratory flow in synchrony with the patient, assuming the patient is capable of generating trigger and cycle signals. Of course, if the patient is heavily sedated or paralyzed, we must rely on the ventilator to trigger and cycle on its own. In general, we don't usually specify whether the patient or the machine may trigger or cycle by using particular settings on the ventilator. Rather, these capabilities are built into the mode of ventilation. (A mode will be defined in maxim 10.) For now, we need to understand how we determine whether the patient or the machine has triggered or cycled an inspiration (or has the potential to do so). For this we again invoke the equation of motion described previously. Time (t) in the equation is a variable independent of the patient. Suppose inspiration starts after a preset time interval (e.g., because of a preset breathing frequency) or ends after a preset inspiratory time or a preset tidal volume (the integral of flow with respect to time). Clearly, inspiration has started or stopped regardless of any inspiratory or expiratory efforts made by the patient (i.e., changes in P_{mus}). Thus, we say that inspiration is machine triggered or cycled. Triggering due to a preset frequency is **time triggering**. Another signal the ventilator can use to trigger inspiration is if the minute ventilation (tidal volume divided by the time for one breath cycle) drops below a preset threshold. Cycling due to a preset tidal volume is called **volume cycling**; cycling due to a preset inspiratory time (or inspiratory pause time) is **time cycling**.

Conversely, **patient triggering** or **patient cycling** implies that inspiration starts or stops independent of any preset trigger or cycle signals generated by the ventilator. In the equation of motion, P_{mus}, elastance, and resistance are all patient determined. Thus, if inspiration starts or stops because of one or more of them, we say that inspiration is patient triggered or cycled. For example, it is easy to understand that if the patient makes an inspiratory effort (positive change in P_{mus}) then the ventilator may detect this by a change in airway pressure, volume, flow, or perhaps even electrical signals derived from the movement of the diaphragm (e.g., Neurally Adjusted Ventilatory Assist) or expansion of the chest wall (e.g., electrical impedance tomography). On detecting the signal, inspiration is triggered on. Similarly, if the patient makes an expiratory effort (negative change in P_{mus}), then inspiration may be cycled off. Thus, the patient can actively pressure, volume, or flow trigger and cycle inspiration.

The distinction between patient and **machine triggering** can also be based on the presence of a trigger or synchronization window. A *trigger window* is defined as the entire expiratory time, as determined by the preset frequency and inspiratory time (minus a short refractory period required to reduce the risk of triggering a breath before exhalation is complete). If a signal from the patient (indicating the need for inspiration) occurs within this trigger window, inspiration starts and is defined as a patient-triggered event that begins a mandatory breath. A *synchronization window* is defined as a short period at the end of the expiratory time. If a signal from the patient (indicating the need for inspiration) occurs within this synchronization window, inspiration starts and is defined as a machine-triggered event that begins a mandatory breath. This is because the mandatory breath would have been triggered regardless of whether the patient signal had appeared or not and because the distinction is necessary to avoid logical inconsistencies in defining mandatory and spontaneous breaths, which are the foundation of a mode taxonomy. Thus, patient efforts in continuous mandatory ventilation (CMV) may significantly increase the mandatory breath frequency above the set value (e.g., double or triple it) whereas those same efforts in synchronized intermittent mandatory ventilation (SIMV) affect frequency slightly or not at all (depending on the sophistication of the design of the ventilator).

Sometimes a synchronization window is used at the end of a pressure-controlled, time-cycled breath. For example, during Airway Pressure Release Ventilation, the patient is free to take spontaneous breaths during a mandatory breath. If a signal from the patient (the start of expiratory flow for a spontaneous breath) occurs within the synchronization window, inspiration stops and is defined as a machine-cycled event that ends a mandatory breath.

Respiratory system mechanics (i.e., elastance and resistance) play a role in triggering and cycling. These factors are easiest to understand in the passive patient ($P_{mus} = 0$). Consider the first cycling of inspiration. If the ventilator delivers a constant inspiratory flow then peak airway pressure is determined by not only the flow rate, but also the elastance and resistance. Now suppose the ventilator is set to cycle inspiration off when a preset pressure threshold is met. For a given preset inspiratory flow, the time it takes to meet this threshold is determined by elastance and resistance. If these patient-determined factors change, inspiratory time will change. Thus, cycling occurs independent of any preset machine-generated signal and we say that inspiration is patient cycled. Therefore, **pressure cycling** is a form of patient cycling. Of course, if the patient makes an expiratory effort, P_{mus} may also cause cycling, in which case patient cycling is obvious. Pressure cycling most often occurs as an alarm condition, but it is also a routine cycling mechanism used in automatic resuscitators.[25]

Another common example of routine patient cycling occurs for a mode of ventilation called Pressure Support. Pressure Support delivers pressure-controlled breaths.

Again we will consider a passive patient. During pressure control, inspiratory flow starts out at its peak value and decays exponentially (see Figure 9-3A). For Pressure Support, inspiration is cycled when the decaying flow signal meets a preset threshold (usually expressed as a percentage of the peak inspiratory flow). When this happens it determines the inspiratory time. If we set $P(t)$ in the equation of motion to be constant (i.e., set inspiratory pressure), we can solve for inspiratory flow as a function of time. This solution is

$$\dot{V}(t) = \frac{\Delta P}{R}(e^{-t/RC})$$

A plot of this equation will yield the flow waveform shown in Figure 9-3A. The term RC in the equation is called the time constant, which is the time at which an exponential function attains 63% of its steady state value in response to a step input (ΔP). In other words, in this case, it is the time necessary for inspiratory flow to drop 63% of its peak value. Thus, the time constant, for a passive patient, determines how long it takes to reach the cycle threshold, and thus it determines the inspiratory time independent of any cycle signal generated by the ventilator. So even a passive patient can cycle inspiration. Interestingly, inspiration can be triggered by the same mechanism in passive patients, except in this case the cycle threshold is based on the decay of expiratory pressure. (An exponential flow through a constant expiratory resistance gives an exponential pressure waveform.) This is the mechanism used in some automatic resuscitators.[25]

A detailed description of trigger and **cycle variables** has been presented elsewhere.[26]

6. Breaths Are Classified as Spontaneous or Mandatory Based on Both the Trigger and Cycle Events

Whether the ventilator or the patient triggers and cycles has clinical relevance because these events determine the extent to which the patient retains control over the timing of the breath. If the patient retains virtually full control over the timing (i.e., starting and stopping of inspiration independent of any machine settings) then we say the breath is *spontaneous* (i.e., occurring without external stimulus). This implies that the patient both triggers and cycles the breath. As a consequence, the patient also retains control over the size of the breath. Often the word *spontaneous* is used to refer to breathing without machine assistance. This is correct but a limited use of the word. The definition given here applies for assisted and unassisted breathing. For unassisted breathing, the brain provides the trigger and cycle signals. For assisted breathing, the signals may come from the brain or the ventilator.

If the machine triggers and/or cycles inspiration, the patient loses substantial control over timing and the breath is defined as *mandatory*. As mentioned previously, "synchronized" triggering is considered a form of machine triggering for the purposes of defining mandatory and spontaneous breaths.

7. Ventilators Deliver Three Basic Breath Sequences: Continuous Mandatory Ventilation (CMV), Intermittent Mandatory Ventilation (IMV), and Continuous Spontaneous Ventilation (CSV)

A simple way to describe a mode of ventilation is that it is a particular sequence of breath types delivered by the machine, similar to beads on a string. If there are only two categories of breath (mandatory and spontaneous) then there are only three possible sequences of breaths the ventilator can deliver: If mandatory breaths are delivered at a preset frequency and spontaneous breaths are permitted between mandatory breaths, then the sequence is called **intermittent mandatory ventilation (IMV)**. For most ventilators, a short window is opened before the scheduled machine triggering of mandatory breaths, to allow synchronization with any detected inspiratory effort on the part of the patient. This is referred to as **synchronized IMV (SIMV)**. Three common variations of IMV are: (1) mandatory breaths are always delivered at the set frequency; (2) mandatory breaths are delivered only when the spontaneous breath frequency falls below the set frequency; and (3) mandatory breaths are delivered only when the spontaneous minute ventilation (i.e., product of spontaneous breath frequency and spontaneous breath tidal volume) drops below a preset or computed threshold (also known as mandatory minute ventilation).

If all breaths are constrained to be spontaneous, then the sequence is called **continuous spontaneous ventilation (CSV)**.

Finally, if mandatory breaths are delivered at a preset rate and spontaneous breaths are not possible between mandatory breaths, the sequence is **continuous mandatory ventilation (CMV)** (commonly known as Assist/Control). Patient-triggered mandatory breaths may occur between machine-triggered breaths (i.e., the actual frequency is usually higher than the set frequency). The distinction between CMV and IMV can also be based on the trigger or synchronization window (see maxim 5).

Note that use of the definitions for mandatory and spontaneous breaths for determining the **breath sequence** (i.e., CMV, IMV, CSV) assumes normal ventilator operation. For example, coughing during VC-CMV may result in patient cycling for a patient-triggered breath due to the pressure alarm limit. Although inspiration for that breath is both patient triggered and patient cycled, this is not normal operation and the sequence does not turn into IMV.

The algorithm for determining the breath sequence of a given mode is shown in **Figure 9-13**.

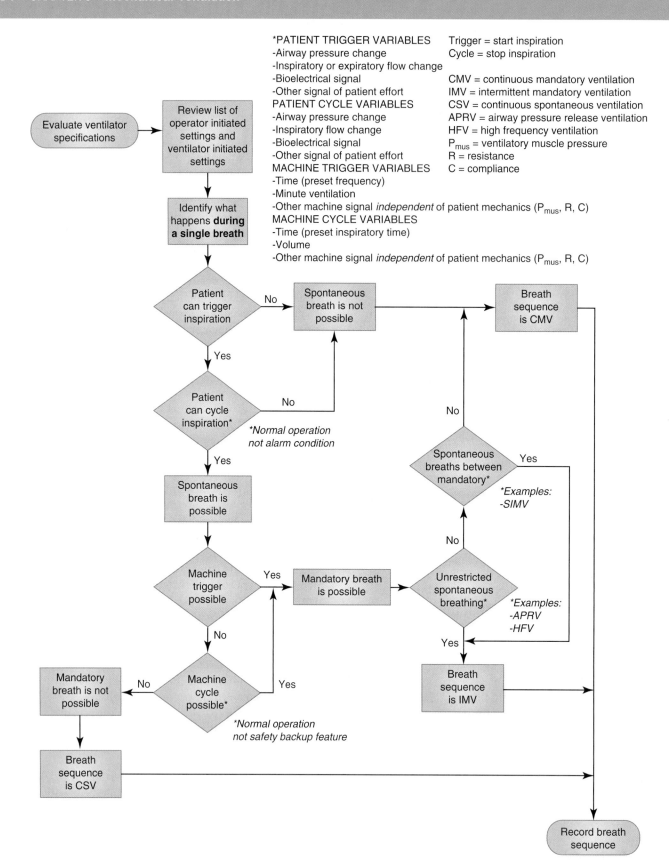

FIGURE 9-13 Algorithm for determining the breath sequence of a mode.

Reproduced with permission from Mandu Press Ltd., Cleveland, OH.

8. There Are Five Basic Ventilatory Patterns: VC-CMV, VC-IMV, PC-CMV, PC-IMV, and PC-CSV

There are two basic control variables and three breath sequences. Combining the two concepts results in a simple mode classification scheme we call a **ventilatory pattern**. These ventilatory patterns are VC-CMV, VC-IMV, PC-CMV, PC-IMV, and PC-CSV. Note that VC-CSV is not a valid pattern because presetting the tidal volume implies **machine cycling**, which makes spontaneous breaths (both triggered and cycled by the patient) impossible. Because any mode of ventilation can be associated with one and only one ventilatory pattern, the ventilatory pattern serves as a simple mode classification system.

This simple way of referring to modes frees us from having to use names coined by various ventilator manufacturers and offers practical advantages in clinical situations. For example, when a patient is anesthetized during surgery there may be no need to accommodate inspiratory efforts, and thus VC-CMV may be the most convenient mode. When the patient is in the recovery room, we may wish to switch to PC to allow unrestricted inspiratory flow with patient effort but still use CMV (i.e., PC-CMV) to assure adequate ventilation while allowing the patient some freedom over timing by permitting patient-triggered breaths. When the patient is ready for extubation, we may attempt a "spontaneous breathing trial" using PC-CSV (e.g., pressure support). Referring to modes in terms of breathing patterns instead of specific names on particular ventilators simplifies both verbal communication and documentation in the patient's record.

For completeness, we should also include the possibility of a time control (TC) ventilatory pattern such as TC-IMV. Although this is uncommon and nonconventional, it is possible as demonstrated by the modes like High Frequency Oscillatory Ventilation and Intrapulmonary Percussive Ventilation.

9. Within Each Ventilatory Pattern Are Several Variations That Can Be Distinguished by Their Targeting Scheme(s)

The five ventilatory patterns serve as simple but useful tags for classifying hundreds of mode names. However,

to distinguish among the fairly large number of modes within the same category we must have a deeper understanding of the feedback control schemes used by engineers to construct the mode. **Figure 9-14** illustrates a basic schematic of a closed loop or feedback control scheme. The operator sets a desired input (e.g., inspiratory pressure). The software reads the instruction and sends control signals to the hardware (e.g., flow control and exhalation valves). The manipulated variable (usually flow) is delivered to the "plant" (this is an engineering term that refers here to the patient). Various disturbances affect the result, such as patient circuit characteristics, leaks, patient ventilatory efforts, respiratory system mechanics, and so on. The resulting inspiratory pressure is measured as a feedback signal and compared to the input setting. If there is a difference, an error signal is sent to the ventilator to make adjustments to the manipulated variable, bringing the resultant inspiratory pressure closer to desired value. We call this system a targeting scheme when speaking of modes.

A **targeting scheme** is essentially a model of the relationship between operator inputs and ventilator outputs to achieve a specific ventilatory pattern. The targeting scheme is a key component of a mode description. Thus, a **target** is a predetermined goal of ventilator output. Targets can be viewed as the parameters of the targeting scheme. *Within-breath targets* are the parameters of the pressure, volume, and flow waveforms. Examples of within-breath targets include inspiratory pressure, inspiratory flow and rise time (**set-point targeting**), tidal volume (**dual targeting**), and the constant of proportionality between inspiratory pressure and patient effort (**servo targeting**). Note that preset values *within a breath* that end inspiration, such as tidal volume, inspiratory time, or percent of peak flow, are cycle variables, as well as target variables. *Between-breath targets* serve to modify the within-breath targets and/or the overall ventilatory pattern. Between-breath targets are used with more advanced targeting schemes, where targets act over multiple breaths. A simple example of a between-breath target is to compare actual exhaled volume to a preset between-breath tidal volume in order to automatically adjust the within-breath constant pressure or **flow target** for

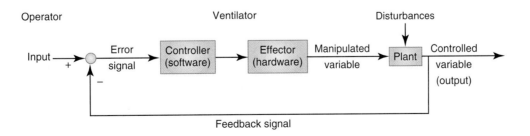

FIGURE 9-14 Schematic of closed loop or feedback control of a mechanical ventilator (i.e., the targeting scheme).

the next breath. Examples of between-breath targets and targeting schemes include average tidal volume (for adaptive targeting), percent minute ventilation (for **optimal targeting**), and combined pCO_2, volume, and frequency values describing a "zone of comfort" (for intelligent targeting).

Currently, there are at least seven different targeting schemes used on commercially available ventilators:[27]

- *Set-point:* The operator sets all parameters of the pressure waveform (pressure control modes) or volume and flow waveforms (volume control modes). The advantage is simplicity. The disadvantage is that changing patient condition may make the settings inappropriate, making frequent adjustment necessary. An example mode name is Assist/Control.
- *Dual:* The ventilator can automatically switch between volume control and pressure control during a single inspiration. The advantage is the ability to adjust to changing patient condition and assure either a preset tidal volume or peak inspiratory pressure, whichever is deemed most important. The disadvantage is that some forms are complicated, difficult to set, and need constant readjustment. The original mode using dual targeting was called Volume Assured Pressure Support. In this mode, inspiration started off in pressure control but changed to volume control if flow decayed to the preset value before the tidal volume was delivered.[28] An example of the opposite approach (i.e., switching from volume control to pressure control) is Flow Adaptive Volume Control on the Maquet Servo-i ventilator. If the patient makes little or no inspiratory effort the mode looks like VC-CMV (e.g., Assist/Control); however, if the patient makes strong enough efforts, the mode looks like PC-CSV (e.g., Pressure Support).[29]
- *Bio-variable:* Studies have shown that varying tidal volume breath by breath to mimic normal breathing improves gas exchange.[30,31] Currently this "biologically variable" targeting scheme is available in only one mode, Variable Pressure Support, on the Dräger V500 ventilator. The operator sets a target inspiratory pressure and a percent variability from 0% to 100%. A setting of 0% means the preset inspiratory pressure will be delivered for every breath. A 100% variability setting means that the actual inspiratory pressure varies randomly from PEEP/continuous positive airway pressure (CPAP) level to double the preset pressure support level.
- *Servo:* The output of the ventilator (pressure/volume/flow) automatically follows a varying input. In current modes, the varying input is some measure of the patient's inspiratory effort and inspiratory pressure is adjusted to be proportional to inspiratory effort. The advantage is that assistance is proportional to the patient's inspiratory effort; the more assistance the patient demands, the more the ventilator delivers. No other targeting scheme does this. The disadvantage is that it requires estimates of artificial airway and respiratory system mechanical properties or special equipment to monitor the respiratory effort signal. Example mode names include Automatic Tube Compensation, Proportional Assist Ventilation, and Neurally Adjusted Ventilatory Assist.
- *Adaptive:* The ventilator automatically sets target(s) between breaths in response to a varying patient condition. The advantage is that it can adjust to changing patient conditions. The disadvantage is that the automatic adjustment may be inappropriate if the algorithm assumptions are violated or they do not match the patient's actual physiology. The first mode to use this was called Pressure Regulated Volume Control.
- *Optimal:* The ventilator automatically adjusts the targets of the ventilatory pattern to either minimize or maximize some overall performance characteristic. The advantage is that it can adjust to a changing patient condition. The disadvantage is that the automatic adjustment may be inappropriate if the algorithm assumptions are violated or they do not match the patient's actual physiology. The only mode currently using this is Adaptive Support Ventilation, which attempts to minimize the work rate of breathing delivered by the ventilator based on respiratory system mechanics.
- *Intelligent:* This targeting scheme uses artificial intelligence programs such as fuzzy logic, rule-based expert systems, and artificial neural networks. The advantage is that it can adjust to a changing patient condition in a fashion that mimics human decision making. The disadvantage is that the automatic adjustment may be inappropriate if the algorithm assumptions are violated or they do not match the patient's actual physiology. The only modes currently using this are SmartCare/PS and IntelliVent-ASV.

Information for identifying the targeting schemes associated with various control variables is given in **Table 9-2**.

The reader can appreciate that as targeting schemes have evolved, they have become more automated and thus more complicated. However, more is not always better. Automation schemes rely on various assumptions, such as that compliance and resistance are linear or that a patient's carbon dioxide production is a particular number of milliliters per minute. If the underlying assumptions of a targeting scheme are violated, unexpected and possibly unwanted results may result. For example, set-point targeting assumes constant respiratory system mechanics. If mechanics change

TABLE 9-2
Identification of Control Variables and Targeting Schemes

#	Control Variable	Target Scheme	Explanation	Example Mode Name	Predetermined Inputs			Ventilator Output	
					WB Target	Cycle	BB Target	↓ impedance	↑ impedance
1	P	Set-point	Peak airway pressure is independent of impedance.	PC SIMV	**P**	**T**	None		
2	P	Set-point	Peak airway pressure is independent of impedance.	Pressure Support	**P**	**F**	None		
3	P	Set-point	Peak airway pressure is independent of impedance.	automatic resuscitator	**F**	**P**	None		
4	V	Set-point	Tidal volume is independent of impedance.	VC A/C	**F**	**T**	None		
5	P	Dual P-F	Same as #1 if secondary target not activated.	VAPS	**P,F**	**V**	None		
6	V	Dual F-P	Same as #4 if secondary target not activated.	CMV + Pressure Limited	**F,P**	**V**	None		
7	P	Servo	Pressure is automatically proportional to inspiratory effort. Effort is represented by patient: flow volume and flow	 ATC PAV+	**Percent Support**	**F**	None		
8	P	Servo	Pressure is automatically proportional to inspiratory effort represented by diaphgram EMG.	NAVA	$\dfrac{cm\,H_2O}{\mu v}$	**NA**	None		
9	P	Bio-variable	Pressure is automatically adjusted randomly using preset mean and % variability.	Variable Pressure Support	**P**	**F**	% variability of Pressure		

(continues)

TABLE 9-2
Identification of Control Variables and Targeting Schemes (*Continued*)

#	Control Variable	Target Scheme	Explanation	Example Mode Name	Predetermined Inputs			Ventilator Output	
					WB Target	Cycle	BB Target	↓ impedance	↑ impedance
10	P	Adaptive	Same as #1 within a breath plus volume target between breaths.	PRVC	NA	T	Volume		
11	P	Optimal	Same as #10 plus algorithm to minimize inspiratory work rate.	ASV	NA	F	% MV Frequency Volume		
12	P	Intelligent	Same as #10 plus volume, PCO_2, and frequency targets using artificial intelligence algorithms.	SmartCare/ PS	NA	NA	Frequency Volume $PetCO_2$		

P = pressure, V = volume, F = flow, T = time, R = resistance, E = elastance; red curves = pressure, blue curves = flow
MV = minute volume, Edi = electrical activity of diaphragm
WB Target = within-breath preset parameters of the pressure, volume, or flow waveform
BB Target = between breath targets modify WB targets or overall ventilatory pattern
Cycle = end of inspiration, NA = not available as operator preset, ventilator determines value if applicable
Targeting Scheme Abbreviations: s = set-point, d = dual, r = servo, b = bio-variable, a = adaptive, o = optimal, i = intelligent
low impedance = low resistance and/or elastance
high impedance = high resistance and/or elastance

rapidly, either peak airway pressure or tidal volume may become unstable and drift out of acceptable ranges. Dual targeting assumes that mechanics may change but may be useless without careful setting of the criteria for switching between volume and pressure control breaths. Servo control requires accurate data for respiratory system mechanical properties, such as resistance and elastance; if the data are unavailable, the mode cannot be used. Some forms of **adaptive targeting** assume that changes in respiratory system mechanics are only related to compliance. However, the ventilator cannot distinguish between patient inspiratory effort and an increase in compliance, thus fooling the targeting scheme into decreasing support when the patient needs it most. Optimal targeting is based on mathematical models (e.g., the relationships among power of breathing, lung mechanics, frequency, and tidal volume). When the models do not match the actual physiology of the patient, they may instruct the ventilator to do inappropriate things (e.g., hyper/hypoventilate the patient or increase risk of ventilator-induced lung damage). **Intelligent targeting** systems may rely on rules in the form of "if the patient does this, the ventilator should do this" derived from the consensus of clinical experts. Yet these rules, at present, cover a very small set of actual clinical scenarios. Hence, the assumptions upon which the artificial intelligence system is based may easily be violated by the actual conditions of the patient. For example, the targeting scheme might assume that the patient can be aggressively weaned when in fact the patient is not ready. These drawbacks of ventilator technology should alert the clinician to fully understand both the capabilities and the limitations of the modes used.

10. A Mode of Ventilation Is Classified According to Its Control Variable, Breath Sequence, and Targeting Scheme(s)

A *mode of ventilation* can be defined in the most general sense as a predefined pattern of interaction between the ventilator and the patient. Historically, modes have been referred to only by the names coined by their creators. As we discussed at the start of this section, there are now so many names that understanding and comparing all modes has become nearly impossible. The solution for this problematic complexity is to simplify with a classification system, or taxonomy. By doing this we gain at least four major benefits:

(1) research reports are easier to compare, making evidence for clinical practice more available; (2) educational programs will be more consistent regarding nomenclature and descriptions of how ventilators work; (3) clinicians will have the conceptual tools to select the most appropriate modes, making optimal ventilator management more likely; and (4) manufacturers can more easily communicate with clients, thus improving the effectiveness of both sales and training.

The taxonomy is based on the previous nine theoretical constructs.[14,15,32-34] It has four hierarchical levels:

1. Control variable (pressure or volume)
    A. Breath sequence (CMV, IMV, or CSV)
        i. Primary breath targeting scheme (for CMV or CSV)
            a. Secondary breath targeting scheme (for IMV)

The *primary breath* is either the only breath there is (mandatory for CMV and spontaneous for CSV) or it is the mandatory breath in IMV. The targeting schemes can be represented by single lowercase letters: set-point = s, dual = d, servo = r, bio-variable = b, adaptive = a, optimal = o, and intelligent = i. For example, on the Covidien PB 840 ventilator there is a mode called A/C Volume Control. This mode is classified as volume control, continuous mandatory ventilation with

set-point targeting, represented by VC-CMVs. A mode with the same functionality on the Dräger Evita XL ventilator is called Continuous Mandatory Ventilation. On that ventilator, you can alter the targeting scheme by activating a feature called AutoFlow. This changes the mode to pressure control continuous mandatory ventilation with adaptive targeting, PC-CMVa. Finally, some modes represent compound targeting schemes. For example, some ventilators offer Tube Compensation, a feature that increases inspiratory pressure in proportion to flow to support the resistive load of breathing through an artificial airway. This is a form of servo targeting. On the Dräger Evita XL, you can add Tube Compensation to CMV with AutoFlow to get a mode classified as PC-CMVar (ar represents the compound targeting scheme composed of servo added to set-point). A mode classified as pressure control intermittent mandatory ventilation with set-point control for both primary (mandatory) and secondary (spontaneous) breaths would have a tag that looks like this: PC-IMVs,s. If you added Tube Compensation to the spontaneous breaths (e.g., Covidien PB 840), the tag would change to PC-IMVs,sr. If you added it to both mandatory and spontaneous breaths (e.g., Dräger Evita XL), the tag would change to PC-IMVsr,sr.

An example of how this taxonomy can be used to compare the modes of two common intensive care ventilators is shown in Table 9-3.

TABLE 9-3
Comparison of Mode Names and Mode Tags for Two Leading Intensive Care Ventilators

Manufacturer	Model	Mode Name	Control Variable	Breath Sequence	Primary Breath Targeting Scheme	Secondary Breath Targeting Scheme	Tag
Covidien	PB 840	A/C Volume Control	volume	CMV	set-point	N/A	VC-CMVs
Covidien	PB 840	SIMV Volume Control with Pressure Support	volume	IMV	set-point	set-point	VC-IMVs,s
Covidien	PB 840	SIMV Volume Control with Tube Compensation	volume	IMV	set-point	servo	VC-IMVs,r
Covidien	PB 840	A/C Pressure Control	pressure	CMV	set-point	N/A	PC-CMVs
Covidien	PB 840	A/C Volume Control Plus	pressure	CMV	adaptive	N/A	PC-CMVa
Covidien	PB 840	SIMV-Pressure Control with Pressure Support	pressure	IMV	set-point	set-point	PC-IMVs,s
Covidien	PB 840	SIMV-Pressure Control with Tube Compensation	pressure	IMV	set-point	servo	PC-IMVs,r
Covidien	PB 840	Bilevel with Pressure Support	pressure	IMV	set-point	set-point	PC-IMVs,s

(continues)

TABLE 9-3
Comparison of Mode Names and Mode Tags for Two Leading Intensive Care Ventilators (*Continued*)

Manufacturer	Model	Mode Name	Mode Classification				Tag
			Control Variable	Breath Sequence	Primary Breath Targeting Scheme	Secondary Breath Targeting Scheme	
Covidien	PB 840	Bilevel with Tube Compensation	pressure	IMV	set-point	servo	PC-IMVs,r
Covidien	PB 840	SIMV Volume Control Plus with Pressure Support	pressure	IMV	adaptive	set-point	PC-IMVa,s
Covidien	PB 840	SIMV Volume Control Plus with Tube Compensation	pressure	IMV	adaptive	servo	PC-IMVa,r
Covidien	PB 840	Spont Pressure Support	pressure	CSV	set-point	N/A	PC-CSVs
Covidien	PB 840	Spont Tube Compensation	pressure	CSV	servo	N/A	PC-CSVr
Covidien	PB 840	Spont Proportional Assist	pressure	CSV	servo	N/A	PC-CSVr
Covidien	PB 840	Spont Volume Support	pressure	CSV	adaptive	N/A	PC-CSVa
Dräger	Evita XL	Continuous Mandatory Ventilation	volume	CMV	set-point	N/A	VC-CMVs
Dräger	Evita XL	Ventilation	volume	CMV	dual	N/A	VC-CMVd
Dräger	Evita XL	SIMV	volume	IMV	set-point	set-point	VC-IMVs,s
Dräger	Evita XL	SIMV with Automatic Tube Compensation	volume	IMV	set-point	set-point/ servo	VC-IMVs,sr
Dräger	Evita XL	SIMV with Pressure Limited Ventilation	volume	IMV	dual	set-point	VC-IMVd,s
Dräger	Evita XL	Compensation	volume	IMV	dual	set-point/ servo	VC-IMVd,sr
Dräger	Evita XL	Mandatory Minute Volume Ventilation	volume	IMV	adaptive	set-point	VC-IMVa,s
Dräger	Evita XL	Compensation	volume	IMV	adaptive	set-point/ servo	VC-IMVa,sr
Dräger	Evita XL	Mandatory Minute Volume with Pressure Limited Ventilation	volume	IMV	dual/adaptive	set-point	VC-IMVda,s

TABLE 9-3

Comparison of Mode Names and Mode Tags for Two Leading Intensive Care Ventilators (*Continued*)

Manufacturer	Model	Mode Name	Mode Classification				Tag
			Control Variable	Breath Sequence	Primary Breath Targeting Scheme	Secondary Breath Targeting Scheme	
Dräger	Evita XL	Automatic Tube Compensation	volume	IMV	dual/adaptive	set-point/ servo	VC-IMVda,sr
Dräger	Evita XL	Pressure Controlled Ventilation Plus Assisted	pressure	CMV	set-point	N/A	PC-CMVs
Dräger	Evita XL	Continuous Mandatory Ventilation with AutoFlow	pressure	CMV	adaptive	N/A	PC-CMVa
Dräger	Evita XL	Compensation	pressure	CMV	adaptive/ servo	N/A	PC-CMVa,r
Dräger	Evita XL	Pressure Controlled Ventilation Plus/ Pressure Support	pressure	IMV	set-point	set-pcint	PC-IMVs,s
Dräger	Evita XL	Airway Pressure Release Ventilation	pressure	IMV	set-point	set-point	PC-IMVs,s
Dräger	Evita XL	Mandatory Minute Volume with AutoFlow	pressure	IMV	adaptive	set-point	PC-IMVa,s
Dräger	Evita XL	Synchronized Intermittent Mandatory Ventilation with AutoFlow	pressure	IMV	adaptive	set-point	PC-IMVa,s
Dräger	Evita XL	Compensation	pressure	IMV	adaptive/ servo	set-point/ servo	PC-IMVar,sr
Dräger	Evita XL	and Tube Compensation	pressure	IMV	adaptive/ servo	set-point/ servo	PC-IMVar,sr
Dräger	Evita XL	Tube Compensation	pressure	IMV	set-point/ servo	set-point/ servo	PC-IMVsr,sr
Dräger	Evita XL	Airway Pressure Release Ventilation with Tube Compensation	pressure	IMV	set-point/ servo	set-point/ servo	PC-IMVsr,sr
Dräger	Evita XL	Continuous Positive Airway Pressure/ Pressure Support	pressure	CSV	set-point	N/A	PC-CSVs
Dräger	Evita XL	SmartCare	pressure	CSV	intelligent	N/A	PC-CSVi
Dräger	Evita XL	Tube Compensation	pressure	CSV	set-point/ servo	N/A	PC-CSVsr

This table is sorted by control variable, breath sequence, and targeting scheme. This illustrates how modes that are essentially the same or very similar are given very different names. Because of this, modes are most practically compared using their *tags* (taxonomic attribute groupings) rather than by their given names or ad-hoc pseudo-classifications (e.g., VC-CMV is often referred to as Assist/Control in the adult literature but it means PC-CMV in the pediatric literature).

Note that a four-level hierarchy does not distinguish among all possible modes. Minor differences can be accommodated by adding a fifth level that could be called "variety." As an example, there are three varieties of PC-CSV using servo targeting. One makes inspiratory pressure proportional to the square of inspiratory flow (Automatic Tube Compensation); one makes it proportional to the electrical signal from the diaphragm (Neurally Adjusted Ventilatory Support); and one makes it proportional to the patient's spontaneous volume and flow (Proportional Assist Ventilation). The first can only support the resistive load of breathing whereas the other two can support both the elastic and resistive loads.

Comparing Modes

As mentioned previously, the purpose of classifying modes of ventilation is to provide a means for comparing and contrasting the technological capabilities of the devices we use for life support. A taxonomy provides an important first step in this process. It allows us to distinguish the "tools in the toolbox." However, the ultimate goal is to appropriately match the technology to the patients' needs. For that we not only need to know what tool to use, but also when to use it. In other words, we need to understand the technological capabilities of a given mode of ventilation and how it facilitates the best patient care.

Our approach to this issue is to first postulate that there are only three main goals of mechanical ventilation: safety (adequate gas exchange while avoiding atelectrauma and volutrauma), comfort (optimum synchrony between patient and ventilator), and liberation (shortest duration of ventilation with fewest adverse events).[27] These general goals can be further refined into specific objectives and clinical aims that may be applied to individual patients. Goals, objectives, and aims are the product of clinical assessment. Having assessed the patient's needs, the next step is to match those needs to the technological capabilities of the available modes of ventilation. The framework for matching patient need with treatment options is shown in **Table 9-4**.

Table 9-5 is a list of the names and tags of the unique modes provided by current intensive care ventilators (only one name was selected from a group of

TABLE 9-4
Goals of Mechanical Ventilation

GOALS OF MECHANICAL VENTILATION

Objectives Serving Goals

Aims of Clinical Management

Capabilities of Ventilators

Features of Specific Modes

1. SAFETY

Optimize ventilation/perfusion of the lungs

Maximize alveolar ventilation

Automatic adjustment of minute ventilation target

Ventilator-set minute ventilation or CO_2 target
Example mode: INTELLiVENT (G5, Hamilton Medical)
Explanation: Clinician inputs patient condition. Ventilator monitors mechanics and end tidal CO_2 and automatically adjusts minute ventilation to keep end tidal CO_2 within target range.

Table 9-4
Goals of Mechanical Ventilation (*Continued*)

Example mode: VPAP Adapt (S9 VPAP Adapt, ResMed)
Explanation: VPAP Adapt algorithm adapts to the patient's ventilation needs on a breath-by-breath basis by automatically calculating a target ventilation (90% of the patient's recent average ventilation) and adjusting the pressure support to achieve it.

Automatic adjustment of support in response to changing respiratory mechanics

Ventilator-set inspiratory pressure to achieve target minute ventilation

Example mode: Automode with Pressure Regulated Volume Control and Volume Support (Servo-i, Maquet)
Explanation: Target minute ventilation is based on the set tidal volume and rate. It uses intermittent mandatory ventilation to synchronize mandatory breaths (PRVC) and spontaneous breaths (volume support). It uses an adaptive pressure targeting scheme in which the ventilator monitors tidal volume and automatically adjusts inspiratory pressure between breaths to achieve average exhaled tidal volume equal to the set target. If the spontaneous respiratory rate does not achieve the minimum minute ventilation, mandatory breaths are triggered.

Ventilator-set inspiratory pressure to achieve target tidal volume

Example mode: Pressure Regulated Volume Control (Servo-i, Maquet)
Explanation: PRVC is a pressure control mode but the clinician sets a target tidal volume. Ventilator monitors tidal volume and automatically adjusts inspiratory pressure between breaths to achieve average exhaled tidal volume equal to set target.

Automatic adjustment of minute ventilation parameters (f, V_T)

Ventilator-set mandatory breath frequency

Example modes: Volume Control Mandatory Minute Volume Ventilation (Evita Infinity V500, Dräger), AutoMode (Servo-i, Maquet)
Explanation: Clinician inputs minute ventilation target. If total minute ventilation created by mandatory and spontaneous breaths falls below the target, the ventilator triggers mandatory breaths.

Manual adjustment of minute ventilation parameters

Clinician-set tidal volume and frequency

Example mode: Volume Control (Servo 300, Maquet)
Explanation: Clinician sets tidal volume and frequency to meet predicted minute ventilation requirement.

Maximize oxygenation

Automatic adjustment of oxygen delivery

Ventilator-set F_IO_2

Example mode: INTELLiVENT (G5, Hamilton Medical)
Explanation: Operator inputs patient condition. Ventilator monitors SpO_2 and automatically adjusts F_IO_2 to keep oxygenation within target range.

Automatic adjustment of end expiratory lung volume

Ventilator-set PEEP

Example mode: INTELLiVENT (G5, Hamilton Medical)
Explanation: Clinician inputs patient condition. Ventilator automatically adjusts PEEP to keep SpO_2 within target range.

(continues)

Table 9-4
Goals of Mechanical Ventilation (*Continued*)

Optimize pressure/volume curve

Minimize risk of volutrauma

Automatic adjustment of lung-protective limits

Ventilator-set safety limits on ventilation parameters

Example mode: Adaptive Support Ventilation (G5, Hamilton Medical)
Explanation: Clinician inputs patient weight and % of predicted minute ventilation to support. Ventilator monitors mechanics and automatically sets minimum and maximum values for tidal volume, mandatory breath frequency, inspiratory pressure, and inspiratory/expiratory times.

Automatic adjustment of minute ventilation parameters (f, V_T)

Ventilator-set tidal volume and frequency

Example mode: Adaptive Support Ventilation (G5, Hamilton Medical)
Explanation: Clinician inputs patient weight and % of predicted minute ventilation to support. Ventilator monitors mechanics and then automatically adjusts tidal volume and frequency to minimize work rate. The effect is to decrease tidal volume as compliance decreases, consistent with a lung-protective ventilation strategy.

Minimize tidal volume

Ventilatory frequencies above 150/min

Example mode: High Frequency Jet Ventilation (LifePulse, Bunnell)
Explanation: High frequency modes allow the lowest possible tidal volume.

Minimize risk of atelectrauma

Automatic adjustment of end expiratory lung volume

Ventilator-set PEEP

Example mode: INTELLiVENT (G5, Hamilton Medical)
Explanation: Clinician inputs patient condition. Ventilator automatically adjusts PEEP to keep SpO_2 within target range.

Biologically variable tidal volume

Ventilator adjusts inspiratory pressure randomly

Example mode: Variable Pressure Support (Evita Infinity V500, Dräger)
Explanation: Clinician inputs the desired target Pressure Support level and the desired percent of pressure variation. Ventilator automatically adjusts Pressure Support level for individual breaths randomly within a range equal to the set Pressure Support plus or minus the set percentage.

Optimize alarm settings

Minimize time spent in unsafe conditions

Automatic selection of optimum alarm variables

Nothing available yet

Table 9-4
Goals of Mechanical Ventilation (*Continued*)

Minimize false alarms

Automatic adjustment of optimum alarm thresholds

Nothing available yet

2. COMFORT

Optimize patient–ventilator synchrony

Maximize trigger/cycle synchrony

All breaths are spontaneous with sufficient patient trigger effort

All breaths are patient triggered and patient cycled
Example mode: Pressure Support (Covidien PB 840)
Explanation: Pressure support delivers breaths that are pressure or flow triggered and flow cycled.

Trigger/cycle based on signal representing chest wall/diaphragm movement

Trigger/cycle based on diaphragm electromyogram
Example mode: Neurally Adjusted Ventilatory Support (Servo-i, Maquet)
Explanation: Ventilator monitors electrical activity of the diaphragm (Edi). Clinician sets Edi trigger threshold and ventilator sets default Edi cycle threshold.

Coordination of mandatory and spontaneous breaths

Spontaneous breaths suppress mandatory breaths
Example mode: Spont/T (V200, Philips)
Explanation: Clinician sets a breath frequency. Ventilator delivers time- or patient-triggered, pressure-limited, flow-cycled breaths. Breaths are machine triggered only if the spontaneous respiratory rate is below the set threshold.

Spontaneous breaths permitted between mandatory breaths
Example mode: Volume Control Synchronized Intermittent Mandatory Ventilation (PB 840, Covidien)
Explanation: Spontaneous breaths with or without pressure support are permitted between volume control mandatory breaths.

Pressure control mandatory breaths with unrestricted inspiration and expiration
Example mode: BiLevel (PB 840, Covidien)
Explanation: BiLevel is a form of pressure control synchronized intermittent mandatory ventilation. However, as opposed to conventional PC-SIMV, on this ventilator spontaneous breaths are allowed during mandatory breaths in BiLevel only.

Minimize autoPEEP

Automatic limitation of autoPEEP

(continues)

Table 9-4
Goals of Mechanical Ventilation (*Continued*)

Ventilator set minimum expiratory time

Example mode: Adaptive Support Ventilation (G5, Hamilton Medical)
Explanation: Clinician inputs patient weight and % of predicted minute ventilation to support. Ventilator monitors respiratory mechanics and automatically adjusts mandatory breath frequency, keeping expiratory time at least three time constants long to minimize autoPEEP.

Maximize flow synchrony

Unrestricted inspiratory flow

Pressure control mandatory breaths with unrestricted inspiration

Example mode: Pressure Control (Servo-i, Maquet)
Explanation: Inspiration is pressure controlled. Ventilator delivers flow to maintain the inspiratory pressure setting as the patient inhales.

Ventilator automatically switches from volume control to pressure control

Example mode: Volume Control (Servo-i, Maquet)
Explanation: During volume control modes, ventilator automatically switches from constant flow delivery to constant pressure delivery to meet the patient's inspiratory flow demand (i.e., dual targeting scheme). If inspiration was patient triggered, this action may turn a mandatory breath into a flow-cycled spontaneous breath, hence the breath sequence is intermittent mandatory ventilation (IMV).

Automatic adjustment of flow based on frequency

Ventilator maintains constant I:E ratio in volume control

Example mode: Adaptive Flow and I Time (iVent, Versamed)
Explanation: In volume control modes, ventilator automatically adjusts inspiratory flow and inspiratory time to deliver the preset tidal volume and maintain I:E ratio at 1:2.

Coordinate ventilator work output with patient demand

Automatic adjustment of support to maintain specified breathing pattern

Ventilator-set pressure support to keep patient in a predefined ventilatory pattern

Example mode: SmartCare/PS/PS (Evita XL, Dräger)
Explanation: SmartCare/PS/PS is a form of pressure control continuous spontaneous ventilation (e.g., Pressure Support). Ventilator automatically adjusts the level of pressure support to keep the patient within a "zone of comfort" based on end tidal CO_2, tidal volume, and frequency.

Ventilator-set pressure support to maintain frequency target

Example mode: Mandatory Rate Ventilation (Taema-Horus, Air Liquide)
Explanation: This mode is a form of pressure control continuous spontaneous ventilation (e.g., Pressure Support). Unlike conventional Pressure Support, the clinician sets a target frequency and the ventilator adjusts the pressure support in proportion to the difference between the target and actual frequencies. The assumption of the targeting scheme is that when the pressure support is correctly adjusted, the patient will have a "comfortable" ventilatory frequency (e.g., 15–25 breaths/min).

Table 9-4
Goals of Mechanical Ventilation (*Continued*)

Automatic adjustment of support to meet patient demand

Ventilator-set inspiratory pressure in proportion to inspiratory effort

Example mode: Proportional Assist Ventilation Plus (PB 840, Covidien)
Explanation: Clinician sets the percent support of total work of inspiration and ventilator delivers inspiratory pressure in proportion to both inspiratory volume and flow according to the equation of motion for the respiratory system.
Example mode: Automatic Tube Compensation (Evita XL, Dräger)
Explanation: Clinician sets the percent support of resistive work of breathing based on the size of the artificial airway. Ventilator delivers pressure in proportion to the square of spontaneous inspiratory flow.

3. LIBERATION

Optimize weaning experience

Minimize duration of ventilation

Ventilator-led weaning of support

Ventilator-initiated reduction of pressure support and evaluation of patient response

Example mode: SmartCare/PS (Evita XL, Dräger)
Explanation: SmartCare/PS is a form of pressure control continuous spontaneous ventilation (e.g., Pressure Support). Ventilator automatically adjusts the level of pressure support to keep the patient within a predefined ventilatory pattern based on end tidal CO_2, tidal volume, and frequency.

Ventilator recommends liberation

Ventilator-initiated spontaneous breathing trial

Example mode: SmartCare/PS (Evita XL, Dräger)
Explanation: SmartCare/PS is a form of pressure control continuous spontaneous ventilation (e.g., Pressure Support) with a rule-based expert system. Ventilator automatically conducts a spontaneous breathing trial and, if passed, recommends liberation.

Automatic reduction of support in response to increased patient effort

Ventilator reduces inspiratory pressure as inspiratory effort increases to maintain preset tidal volume target

Example mode: Continuous Mandatory Ventilation with AutoFlow (Evita XL, Dräger)
Explanation: Pressure control mode but clinician sets target tidal volume. Ventilator monitors tidal volume and automatically adjusts inspiratory pressure between breaths to achieve average exhaled tidal volume equal to set target. Increased patient effort results in reduced inspiratory pressure.

Minimize adverse events

Monitor probability of failure

Nothing available yet

Identify adverse event

Nothing available yet

TABLE 9-5
Technological Capabilities of Unique Modes of Ventilation

Mode Name	Mode Tag	Automatic adjustment of minute ventilation target	Automatic adjustment of support in response to changing respiratory mechanics	Automatic adjustment of minute ventilation parameters (f and V_t)	Manual adjustment of minimum minute ventilation parameters (f and V_t)	Automatic adjustment of oxygen delivery	Automatic adjustment of end expiratory lung volume	Automatic adjustment of ventilation parameters within lung protective limits	Minimize tidal volume	Safety Capabilities	All breaths are spontaneous with patient effort	Trigger/cycle based on signal representing chest wall/diaphragm movement	Coordination of mandatory and spontaneous breaths	Automatic limitation of autoPEEP	Unrestricted inspiratory flow	Automatic adjustment of flow based on frequency	Automatic adjustment of support to maintain specific breathing pattern	Automatic adjustment of support proportional to patient demand	Comfort Capabilities	Ventilator-initiated weaning of support	Ventilator recommends liberation	Automatic reduction of support in response to increased patient effort	Liberation Capabilities	Total Capabilities
INTELLiVENT-ASV	PC-IMVoi,oi	✓	✓	✓		✓	✓	✓		6	✓		✓	✓	✓				4	✓	✓	✓	3	13
Adaptive Support Ventilation	PC-IMVo,o oi,oi		✓	✓				✓		3	✓		✓	✓	✓				4			✓	1	8
SmartCare/PS	PC-CSVi		✓							1	✓				✓		✓		3	✓	✓	✓	3	7
Automode (Pressure Regulated Volume Control to Volume Support)	PC-IMVa,a		✓	✓	✓					3	✓		✓		✓				3			✓	1	7
Automode (Volume Control to Volume Support)	VC-IMVd,a		✓	✓	✓					3	✓		✓		✓				3			✓	1	7
Mandatory Minute Volume with Pressure Limited Ventilation	VC-IMVda,s			✓	✓					2	✓		✓		✓				3			✓	1	6
Adaptive Pressure Ventilation Synchronized Intermittent Mandatory Ventilation	PC-IMVa,s		✓		✓					2			✓		✓				2			✓	1	5
Mandatory Minute Volume Ventilation	VC-IMVa,s			✓	✓					2	✓		✓						2			✓	1	5
Neurally Adjusted Ventilatory Support	PC-CSVr									0	✓	✓			✓			✓	4				0	4
Volume Support	PC-CSVa		✓							1	✓				✓				2			✓	1	4
Mandatory Rate Ventilation	PC-CSVa			✓						1	✓				✓		✓		3				0	4
Pressure Regulated Volume Control	PC-CMVa		✓		✓					2					✓				1			✓	1	4
Synchronized Intermittent Mandatory Ventilation (Volume Control)	VC-IMVd,s				✓					1			✓		✓				2				0	3
Proportional Assist Ventilation	PC-CSVr									0	✓				✓			✓	3				0	3

TABLE 9-5
Technological Capabilities of Unique Modes of Ventilation (Continued)

Mode Name	Mode Tag	Automatic adjustment of minute ventilation target	Automatic adjustment of support in response to changing respiratory mechanics	Automatic adjustment of minute ventilation parameters (f and V_T)	Manual adjustment of minimum minute ventilation parameters (f and V_T)	Automatic adjustment of oxygen delivery	Automatic adjustment of end expiratory lung volume	Automatic adjustment of ventilation parameters within lung protective limits	Minimize tidal volume	Safety Capabilities	All breaths are spontaneous with patient effort	Trigger/cycle based on signal representing chest wall/diaphragm movement	Coordination of mandatory and spontaneous breaths	Automatic limitation of autoPEEP	Unrestricted inspiratory flow	Automatic adjustment of flow based on frequency	Automatic adjustment of support to maintain specific breathing pattern	Automatic adjustment of support proportional to patient demand	Comfort Capabilities	Ventilator-initiated weaning of support	Ventilator recommends liberation	Automatic reduction of support in response to increased patient effort	Liberation Capabilities	Total Capabilities
High Frequency Oscillatory Ventilation	PC-IMVs,s								✓	1			✓		✓				2				0	3
Volume Control Synchronized Intermittent Mandatory Ventilation (Adaptive Flow & I time)	VC-IMVa,s				✓					1			✓			✓			2				0	3
Volume Control Synchronized Intermittent Mandatory Ventilation	VC-IMVs,s				✓					1			✓						1				0	2
Pressure Support	PC-CSVs									0	✓				✓				2				0	2
Airway Pressure Release Ventilation	PC-IMVs,s									0			✓		✓				2				0	2
Pressure Control Synchronized Intermittent Mandatory Ventilation	PC-IMVs,s									0			✓		✓				2				0	2
Continuous Mandatory Ventilation with Pressure Limited	VC-CMVd				✓					1					✓				1				0	2
Pressure Control Assist Control	PC-CMVs									0					✓				1				0	1
Volume Control Assist/Control	VC-CMVs				✓					1									0				0	1

PC = pressure control, VC = volume control, CMV = continuous mandatory ventilation, IMV = intermittent mandatory ventilation, CSV = continuous spontaneous ventilation

Targeting scheme abbreviations: s = setpoint, d = dual, r = servo, a = adaptive, o = optimal, i = intelligent

Modified with permission from Mireles-Cabodevila E, Hatipoglu U, Chatburn RL. A rational framework for selecting modes of ventilation. *Respir Care*. 2013;58(2):348–366.

identical mode names identified by the taxonomy). These modes have been grouped according to the three goals of ventilation. The basic idea is that the available mode that has the most technological capabilities meeting the goals for a particular patient is the most appropriate mode to use. A full description of this system is beyond the scope of this chapter but has been explained in detail elsewhere.[35]

This system of matching patient needs to available technology should be applied cautiously. In order to compare modes we must consider the best case scenario, in which they are functioning under conditions that do not violate their underlying design assumptions (see the prior discussion about targeting schemes). *We thus take for granted that the clinician has appropriately diagnosed the patient's condition, assessed the needs, and ruled out any mode features that may be inappropriate.* Of course, the whole point of this chapter is to provide the conceptual tools that would allow the clinician to do this.

Section 3: Intensive Care Ventilators

Information in this section is taken from the ventilator operator's manuals, brochures, and Websites created by the manufacturers.

CareFusion Avea

The CareFusion Avea ventilator (**Figure 9-15**) is designed for intensive care ventilation of neonatal, pediatric, and adult patients.

Operator Interface

The Avea has an operator interface that uses a touch screen, buttons, and a control knob (**Figure 9-16**). Screen displays show ventilator settings, alarm settings, and monitored values using waveforms or digital values. Settings are entered by touching a virtual button on the screen to select the desired setting, turning the knob to select the setting value, and then pressing the ACCEPT button to finalize the setting. The real buttons provide various features related to menu navigation, alarm silencing, suctioning, temporary (2 minutes) 100% oxygen delivery, manual breath trigger, and expiratory hold.

Modes

Modes are selected by pressing the virtual button with the desired mode name. There are 10 basic mode names but a variety of "advanced settings" (**Table 9-6**). Some of these advanced settings actually change the mode (**Table 9-7**), resulting in many more modes by classification (**Table 9-8**).

The advanced settings increase both flexibility and confusion. For example, the mode named Volume Control A/C is classified as volume control continuous

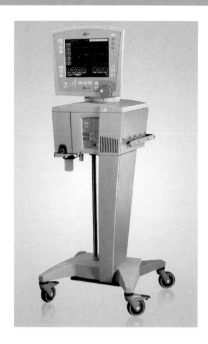

FIGURE 9-15 CareFusion Avea ventilator.
Reproduced with permission from CareFusion.

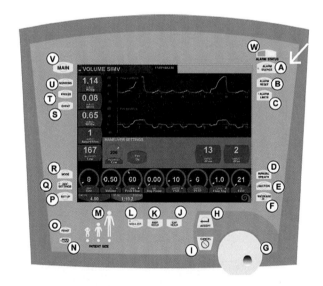

FIGURE 9-16 CareFusion Avea operator interface. A. Alarm silence (LED). B. Alarm reset. C. Alarm limits. D. Manual breath. E. Suction (LED). F. Increase O_2. G. Data dial. H. Accept. I. Cancel. J. Expiratory hold. K. Inspiratory hold. L. Nebulizer. M. Patient size. N. Panel lock (LED). O. Print. P. Set-up. Q. Advanced settings (LED). R. Mode. S. Event. T. Freeze. U. Screens. V. Main. W. Alarm status LEDs.
Reproduced with permission from CareFusion.

mandatory ventilation with set-point targeting (VC-CMVs). However, adding the Vsync and Flow Cycle advanced settings to this mode turns it into pressure control intermittent mandatory ventilation with adaptive and set-point targeting (PC-IMVa,s)—a very different mode indeed.

TABLE 9-6
Advanced Mode Settings for CareFusion Avea

Advanced Setting	Action
Volume Limit	For pressure control modes, this sets a volume cycle threshold. Note that volume cycling of a Pressure Support breath changes it from spontaneous to mandatory.
Machine Volume	For pressure control modes, this allows a volume target and flow and activates dual targeting. The operator sets the target volume and the ventilator calculates the target flow as the volume divided by the set inspiratory time. If flow decays to this flow target and the volume has not been delivered, then inspiration switches to volume control with constant flow until the volume has been delivered. Inspiratory time remains constant. Machine Volume overrides Flow Cycle setting, if activated.
Flow Cycle	For pressure control modes, this changes the cycle criterion from time to flow and sets the threshold for inspiratory flow termination as a percent of peak flow.
Demand Flow	For volume control modes, this sets a ventilator-determined pressure target and activates dual targeting. If inspiratory pressure decreases 2 cm H_2O (due to patient inspiratory effort), volume control switches to pressure control. If the set volume is delivered and flow is equal to the set flow, inspiration is volume cycled. Otherwise, inspiration is flow cycled at 25% of peak flow.
Vsync	Switches the mode from volume control to pressure control with adaptive targeting. Inspiratory pressure is automatically adjusted to maintain an average tidal volume equal to the set volume.

TABLE 9-7
Controls and Mode Names for CareFusion Avea Ventilator

Breath Type and Mode	Vol A/C	Vol SIMV	Pres A/C	Pres SIMV	PRVC A/C	PRVC SIMV	CPAP/ PSV	APRV/ Biphasic	TCPL A/C	TCPL SIMV
Primary Controls										
Rate bpm	*	*	*	*	*	*	* Apnea Mode	* Apnea Mode	*	*
Volume mL	*	*			*	*	* Apnea Mode	* Apnea Mode		
Insp pres cm H_2O			*	*			* Apnea Mode	* Apnea Mode	*	*
Peak flow L/min	*	*					* Apnea Mode	* Apnea Mode	*	*
Insp time sec			*	*	*	*	* Apnea Mode	* Apnea Mode	*	*
Insp pause sec	*	*					* Apnea Mode	* Apnea Mode		
PSV cm H_2O		*		*		*	*	*		*
PEEP cm H_2O	*	*	*	*	*	*	*	*	*	*
Flow trig L/min	*	*	*	*	*	*	*	*	*	*
% Oxygen % O_2	*	*	*	*	*	*	*	*	*	*
Pres high cm H_2O								*		

(continues)

TABLE 9-7
Controls and Mode Names for CareFusion Avea Ventilator (*Continued*)

Breath Type and Mode	Vol A/C	Vol SIMV	Pres A/C	Pres SIMV	PRVC A/C	PRVC SIMV	CPAP/ PSV	APRV/ Biphasic	TCPL A/C	TCPL SIMV
Time high sec								*		
Time low sec								*		
Pres high cm H₂O								*		
Advanced Settings Available Within Each Mode	Vsync,* Vsync rise,* Sigh,** Waveform, Bias flow, Pres trig, Vol limit (when Vsync = ON), Flow cycle,* Demand flow	Vsync,* Vsync rise,* Sigh,** Waveform, Vol limit, PSV rise, PSV cycle, PSV Tmax, Bias flow, Pres trig, Flow cycle,* Demand flow	Mach vol, Vol limit, Insp rise, Flow cycle, Bias flow, Pres trig	Mach vol, Vol limit, Insp rise, Flow cycle, PSV rise, PSV cycle, PSV Tmax, Bias flow, Pres trig	Insp rise, Bias flow, Pres trig, Vol limit, Flow cycle	Vol limit, PSV rise, PSV cycle, PSV Tmax, Bias flow, Pres trig, Flow cycle	Vol limit, PSV rise, PSV cycle, PSV Tmax, Bias flow, Pres trig	Vol limit, PSV rise, PSV cycle, PSV Tmax, Bias flow, Pres trig, T High sync, T High PSV, T Low Sync	Vol limit, Flow cycle, Bias flow, Pres trig	Vol limit, Flow cycle, PSV rise, PSV cycle, PSV Tmax, Bias flow, Pres trig

* Available only with Vsync activated for adult or pediatric patients only.
** Available for adult and pediatric patients only.

TABLE 9-8
Classification of Modes for CareFusion Avea

Mode Name	Mode Classification				Tag
	Control Variable	Breath Sequence	Primary Breath Targeting Scheme	Secondary Breath Targeting Scheme	
Volume A/C	volume	CMV	set-point	N/A	VC-CMVs
Volume SIMV	volume	IMV	set-point	set-point	VC-IMVs,s
Volume SIMV with Artificial Airway Compensation	volume	IMV	set-point	set-point/servo	VC-IMVs,sr
Volume A/C with Demand Flow	volume	IMV	dual	dual	VC-IMVd,d
Volume SIMV with Demand Flow	volume	IMV	dual	set-point	VC-IMVd,s
Volume SIMV with Demand Flow and Artificial Airway Compensation	volume	IMV	dual	set-point/servo	VC-IMVd,sr
Pressure A/C	pressure	CMV	set-point	N/A	PC-CMVs
Time Cycled Pressure Limited A/C	pressure	CMV	dual	N/A	PC-CMVs
Pressure A/C with Machine Volume	pressure	CMV	dual	N/A	PC-CMVd
Pressure A/C with Volume Guarantee	pressure	CMV	adaptive	N/A	PC-CMVa

TABLE 9-8
Classification of Modes for CareFusion Avea (*Continued*)

| Mode Name | Mode Classification | | | | |
	Control Variable	Breath Sequence	Primary Breath Targeting Scheme	Secondary Breath Targeting Scheme	Tag
Time Cycled Pressure Limited A/C with Volume Guarantee	pressure	CMV	adaptive	N/A	PC-CMVa
Volume A/C with Vsync	pressure	CMV	adaptive	N/A	PC-CMVa
Pressure Regulated Volume Control A/C	pressure	CMV	adaptive	N/A	PC-CMVa
Pressure A/C with Flow Cycle	pressure	IMV	set-point	set-point	PC-IMVs,s
Pressure A/C with Flow Cycle and Artificial Airway Compensation	pressure	IMV	set-point	set-point/servo	PC-IMVs,sr
Pressure SIMV	pressure	IMV	set-point	set-point	PC-IMVs,s
Pressure SIMV with Artificial Airway Compensation	pressure	IMV	set-point	set-point/servo	PC-IMVs,sr
CPAP/Pressure Support Ventilation with Volume Limit	pressure	IMV	set-point	set-point	PC-IMVs,s
CPAP/Pressure Support Ventilation with Volume Limit and Artificial Airway Compensation	pressure	IMV	set-point	set-point/servo	PC-IMVs,sr
Infant Nasal IMV	pressure	IMV	set-point	set-point	PC-IMVs,s
Infant Nasal IMV with Artificial Airway Compensation	pressure	IMV	set-point	set-point/servo	PC-IMVs,sr
Airway Pressure Release Ventilation/Biphasic	pressure	IMV	set-point	set-point	PC-IMVs,s
Time Cycled Pressure Limited A/C with Flow Cycle	pressure	IMV	set-point	set-point	PC-IMVs,s
Time Cycled Pressure Limited SIMV with Artificial Airway Compensation	pressure	IMV	set-point	set-point/servo	PC-IMVs,sr
Time Cycled Pressure Limited SIMV	pressure	IMV	dual	set-point	PC-IMVd,s
Pressure SIMV with Volume Guarantee	pressure	IMV	adaptive	set-point	PC-IMVa,s
Pressure SIMV with Volume Guarantee and Artificial Airway Compensation	pressure	IMV	adaptive	set-point/servo	PC-IMVa,sr
Time Cycled Pressure Limited A/C with Flow Cycle and Volume Guarantee	pressure	IMV	adaptive	set-point	PC-IMVa,s
Time Cycled Pressure Limited SIMV with Volume Guarantee	pressure	IMV	adaptive	set-point	PC-IMVa,s
Time Cycled Pressure Limited SIMV with Volume Guarantee and Artificial Airway Compensation	pressure	IMV	adaptive	set-point/servo	PC-IMVa,sr

(continues)

TABLE 9-8
Classification of Modes for CareFusion Avea *(Continued)*

Mode Name	Control Variable	Breath Sequence	Primary Breath Targeting Scheme	Secondary Breath Targeting Scheme	Tag
		Mode Classification			
Volume A/C with Vsync and Flow Cycle	pressure	IMV	adaptive	set-point	PC-IMVa,s
Volume SIMV with Vsync	pressure	IMV	adaptive	set-point	PC-IMVa,s
Volume SIMV with Vsync and Artificial Airway Compensation	pressure	IMV	adaptive	set-point/servo	PC-IMVa,sr
Pressure Regulated Volume Control A/C with Flow Cycle	pressure	IMV	adaptive	adaptive	PC-IMVa,a
Pressure Regulated Volume Control SIMV with Flow Cycle	pressure	IMV	adaptive	set-point	PC-IMVa,s
Pressure Regulated Volume Control SIMV	pressure	IMV	adaptive	set-point	PC-IMVa,s
Pressure Regulated Volume Control SIMV with Artificial Airway Compensation	pressure	IMV	adaptive	set-point/servo	PC-IMVa,sr
Time Cycled Pressure Limited A/C with Flow Cycle and Volume Guarantee and Artificial Airway Compensation	pressure	IMV	adaptive/servo	set-point/servo	PC-IMVas,sr
Volume A/C with Vsync and Flow Cycle and Artificial Airway Compensation	pressure	IMV	adaptive/servo	set-point/servo	PC-IMVar,sr
Pressure Regulated Volume Control A/C with Flow Cycle and Artificial Airway Compensation	pressure	IMV	adaptive/servo	set-point/servo	PC-IMVar,sr
Pressure Regulated Volume Control SIMV with Flow Cycle and Artificial Airway Compensation	pressure	IMV	adaptive/servo	set-point/servo	PC-IMVar,sr
Time Cycled Pressure Limited A/C with Flow Cycle and Artificial Airway Compensation	pressure	IMV	set-point/servo	set-point/servo	PC-IMVsr,sr
CPAP/Pressure Support Ventilation	pressure	CSV	set-point	N/A	PC-CSVs
CPAP/Pressure Support Ventilation and Artificial Airway Compensation	pressure	CSV	set-point/servo	N/A	PC-CSVsr

Reproduced with permission from Mandu Press Ltd., Cleveland, OH.

Airway Pressure Release Ventilation/Biphasic
- *Mandatory breaths:* Machine triggered (preset frequency) or patient synchronized (pressure or flow sensitivity) and machine cycled (inspiratory time or patient synchronized by flow sensitivity).

- Within-breath settings:
  - Operator-set PEEP (called Pres Low), peak inspiratory pressure (called Pres High), rise time, inspiratory time (called Time High), and expiratory time (called Time Low)

- *Spontaneous breaths:* Patient triggered (pressure or flow sensitivity) and patient cycled (% peak inspiratory flow). Spontaneous breaths are permitted both between and during mandatory breaths.
  - Within-breath settings:
    - Operator set inspiratory pressure and rise time
- *Between-breath targets:* None.

Artificial Airway Compensation

When Artificial Airway Compensation is turned on, the ventilator automatically calculates the pressure drop across the endotracheal tube and adjusts the airway pressure to deliver the set inspiratory pressure to the distal (carina) end of the endotracheal tube. This calculation takes into account flow, gas composition (heliox or nitrogen/oxygen), fraction of inspired oxygen (F_IO_2), tube diameter, length, and pharyngeal curvature based on patient size (neonatal, pediatric, or adult). This compensation occurs only during inspiration. Artificial Airway Compensation is active in all Pressure Support and Flow Cycled Pressure Control breaths.

- Within-breath settings:
  - Operator-set percent support (of resistive load) along with artificial airway tube diameter and tube type
  - Ventilator-set inspiratory pressure as a function of patient-generated inspiratory flow
- *Between-breath targets:* None

CPAP/Pressure Support
- *Mandatory breaths:* Not allowed
- *Spontaneous breaths:* Patient triggered (pressure or flow sensitivity) and patient cycled (% peak inspiratory flow)
  - Within-breath settings:
    - Operator-set inspiratory pressure, rise time, and cycle sensitivity (% peak inspiratory flow)
- *Between-breath targets:* None

CPAP/Pressure Support with Volume Limit
- *Mandatory breaths:* Patient triggered (pressure or flow sensitivity) and machine cycled (volume). Note that when a patient-triggered breath exceeds the set volume limit, inspiration is terminated. Thus, the breath is patient triggered but machine cycled and thus classified as mandatory because the patient has lost some control over timing and size. This condition is indicated by a yellow alarm status indicator.
  - Within-breath settings:
    - Operator-set PEEP, frequency, inspiratory pressure, rise time, inspiratory time, and volume limit
- *Spontaneous breaths:* Patient triggered (pressure or flow sensitivity) and patient cycled (% peak inspiratory flow).

- Within-breath settings:
  - Operator-set inspiratory pressure, rise time, and cycle sensitivity (% peak inspiratory flow)
- *Between-breath targets:* None.

Infant Nasal CPAP
- Available for neonatal patient size setting only
- Designed to work with standard two-limbed neonatal patient circuits and nasal prongs
- *Mandatory breaths:* Not allowed
- *Spontaneous breaths:* Patient triggered (pressure or flow sensitivity) and patient cycled (inspiratory flow)
  - Within-breath settings:
    - Operator-set CPAP
- *Between-breath targets:* None

Infant Nasal IMV
- Available for neonatal patient size setting only
- Designed to work with standard two-limbed neonatal patient circuits and nasal prongs
- *Mandatory breaths:* Machine triggered (preset frequency) and machine cycled (inspiratory time)
  - Within-breath settings:
    - Operator-set PEEP, frequency, inspiratory pressure, inspiratory rise time, and inspiratory time
- *Spontaneous breaths:* Patient triggered (pressure or flow sensitivity) and patient cycled (% peak inspiratory flow)
  - Within-breath settings:
    - Operator-set inspiratory pressure, rise time, and cycle sensitivity (% peak inspiratory flow)
- *Between-breath targets:* None

Pressure A/C
- *Mandatory breaths:* Machine triggered (preset frequency) or patient triggered (pressure or flow sensitivity) and machine cycled (inspiratory time)
  - Within-breath settings:
    - Operator-set PEEP, frequency, inspiratory pressure, rise time, and inspiratory time
- *Spontaneous breaths:* Not allowed
- *Between-breath targets:* None

Pressure A/C with Flow Cycle
- Activation of Flow Cycle makes this mode a form of IMV, not A/C. **Flow cycling** makes every breath patient cycled. Hence, every patient-triggered breath is spontaneous (i.e., patient triggered and cycled) whereas every machine-triggered breath is mandatory (i.e., machine triggered and patient cycled) by definition.

- *Mandatory breaths:* Machine triggered (preset frequency) and patient cycled (% peak inspiratory flow).
  - Within-breath settings:
    - Operator-set PEEP, frequency, inspiratory pressure, rise time, and cycle sensitivity (% peak flow)
- *Spontaneous breaths:* Patient triggered (pressure or flow sensitivity) and patient cycled (% peak inspiratory flow).
  - Within-breath settings:
    - Operator-set inspiratory pressure, rise time, and cycle sensitivity (% peak inspiratory flow)
- *Between-breath targets:* None.

Pressure A/C with Machine Volume

- *Mandatory breaths:* Machine triggered (preset frequency) or patient triggered (pressure or flow sensitivity) and machine cycled (inspiratory time)
  - Within-breath settings:
    - Operator-set PEEP, frequency, tidal volume, inspiratory pressure, rise time, and inspiratory time.
    - Ventilator switches from pressure control to volume control if inspiratory flow decays to a machine-determined threshold before preset tidal volume is reached. Inspiration continues at constant flow for preset inspiratory time.
- *Spontaneous breaths:* Not allowed
- *Between-breath targets:* None

Pressure A/C with Volume Guarantee

- Available for neonatal patient size setting only
- *Mandatory breaths:* Machine triggered (preset frequency) or patient triggered (pressure or flow sensitivity) and machine cycled (inspiratory time)
  - Within-breath settings:
    - Operator-set PEEP, frequency, rise time, and inspiratory time
    - Ventilator-set inspiratory pressure
- *Spontaneous breaths:* Not allowed
- Between-breath targets:
  - Operator-set tidal volume

Pressure Regulated Volume Control A/C

- *Mandatory breaths:* Machine triggered (preset frequency) or patient triggered (pressure or flow sensitivity) and machine cycled (inspiratory time)
  - Within-breath settings:
    - Operator-set PEEP, frequency, rise time, and inspiratory time
    - Ventilator-set inspiratory pressure
- *Spontaneous breaths:* Not allowed
- Between-breath targets:
  - Operator-set tidal volume

Pressure Regulated Volume Control A/C with Flow Cycle

- Activation of Flow Cycle makes this mode a form of IMV, not A/C. Flow cycling makes every breath patient cycled. Hence, every patient-triggered breath is spontaneous (i.e., patient triggered and cycled) whereas every machine-triggered breath is mandatory (i.e., machine triggered and patient cycled) by definition.
- *Mandatory breaths:* Machine triggered (preset frequency) or patient triggered (pressure or flow sensitivity) and machine cycled (inspiratory time).
  - Within-breath settings:
    - Operator-set PEEP, frequency, rise time, and inspiratory time
    - Ventilator-set inspiratory pressure
- *Spontaneous breaths:* Patient triggered (pressure or flow sensitivity) and patient cycled (% peak inspiratory flow).
  - Within-breath settings:
    - Operator-set rise time and cycle sensitivity (% peak inspiratory flow)
    - Ventilator-set inspiratory pressure
- Between-breath targets:
  - Operator-set tidal volume

Pressure Regulated Volume Control SIMV with Flow Cycle

- *Mandatory breaths:* Machine triggered (preset frequency) and patient cycled (% peak inspiratory flow)
  - Within-breath settings:
    - Operator-set PEEP, frequency, rise time, and cycle sensitivity (% peak flow)
    - Ventilator-set inspiratory pressure
- *Spontaneous breaths:* Patient triggered (pressure or flow sensitivity) and patient cycled (% peak inspiratory flow)
  - Within-breath settings:
    - Operator-set inspiratory pressure, rise time, and cycle sensitivity (% peak inspiratory flow)
- Between-breath targets:
  - Operator-set tidal volume

Pressure Regulated Volume Control SIMV

- *Mandatory breaths:* Machine triggered (preset frequency) or patient synchronized (pressure or flow sensitivity) and machine cycled (inspiratory time)
  - Within-breath settings:
    - Operator-set PEEP, frequency, rise time, and inspiratory time
    - Ventilator-set inspiratory pressure
- *Spontaneous breaths:* Patient triggered (pressure or flow sensitivity) and patient cycled (% peak inspiratory flow)

- Within-breath settings:
  - Operator-set inspiratory pressure, rise time, and cycle sensitivity (% peak inspiratory flow)
- Between-breath targets:
  - Operator-set tidal volume

Pressure SIMV

- *Mandatory breaths:* Machine triggered (preset frequency) or patient synchronized (pressure or flow sensitivity) and machine cycled (inspiratory time)
  - Within-breath settings:
    - Operator-set PEEP, frequency, inspiratory pressure, rise time, and inspiratory time
- *Spontaneous breaths:* Patient triggered (pressure or flow sensitivity) and patient cycled (% peak inspiratory flow)
  - Within-breath settings:
    - Operator-set inspiratory pressure, rise time, and cycle sensitivity (% peak inspiratory flow)
- *Between-breath targets:* None

Pressure SIMV with Volume Guarantee

- Available for neonatal patient size setting only
- *Mandatory breaths:* Machine triggered (preset frequency) or patient synchronized (pressure or flow sensitivity) and machine cycled (inspiratory time)
  - Within-breath settings:
    - Operator-set PEEP, frequency, rise time, and inspiratory time
    - Ventilator-set inspiratory pressure
- *Spontaneous breaths:* Patient triggered (pressure or flow sensitivity) and patient cycled (% peak inspiratory flow)
  - Within-breath settings:
    - Operator-set inspiratory pressure, rise time, and cycle sensitivity (% peak inspiratory flow)
- Between-breath targets:
  - Operator-set tidal volume

Time Cycled Pressure Limited A/C

- Available for neonatal patient size setting only
- *Mandatory breaths:* Machine triggered (preset frequency) or patient triggered (pressure or flow sensitivity) and machine cycled (inspiratory time)
  - Within-breath settings:
    - Operator-set PEEP, frequency, inspiratory pressure, peak inspiratory flow, rise time, and inspiratory time. Inspiration is delivered at the set inspiratory flow only until the inspiratory **pressure target** is reached. Flow decays exponentially after that.
- *Spontaneous breaths:* Not allowed
- *Between-breath targets:* None

Time Cycled Pressure Limited A/C with Flow Cycle

- Available for neonatal patient size setting only.
- Activation of Flow Cycle makes this mode a form of IMV, not A/C. Flow cycling makes every breath patient cycled. Hence, every patient-triggered breath is spontaneous (i.e., patient triggered and cycled) whereas every machine-triggered breath is mandatory (i.e., machine triggered and patient cycled) by definition.
- *Mandatory breaths:* Machine triggered (preset frequency) and patient cycled (% peak inspiratory flow).
  - Within-breath settings:
    - Operator-set PEEP, frequency, inspiratory pressure, peak inspiratory flow, and inspiratory time. Inspiration is delivered at the set inspiratory flow only until the inspiratory pressure target is reached. Flow decays exponentially after that.
- *Spontaneous breaths:* Patient triggered (pressure or flow sensitivity) and patient cycled (% peak inspiratory flow).
  - Within-breath settings:
    - Operator-set inspiratory pressure and cycle sensitivity (% peak inspiratory flow)
- *Between-breath targets:* None.

Time Cycled Pressure Limited A/C with Flow Cycle and Volume Guarantee

- Available for neonatal patient size setting only
- Activation of Flow Cycle makes this mode a form of IMV, not A/C. Flow cycling makes every breath patient cycled. Hence, every patient-triggered breath is spontaneous (i.e., patient triggered and cycled) whereas every machine-triggered breath is mandatory (i.e., machine triggered and patient cycled) by definition.
- *Mandatory breaths:* Machine triggered (preset frequency) and patient cycled (% peak inspiratory flow).
  - Within-breath settings:
    - Operator-set PEEP, frequency, inspiratory pressure, peak inspiratory flow, and inspiratory time. Inspiration is delivered at the set inspiratory flow only until the inspiratory pressure target is reached. Flow decays exponentially after that.
- *Spontaneous breaths:* Patient triggered (pressure or flow sensitivity) and patient cycled (% peak inspiratory flow).
  - Within-breath settings:
    - Operator-set cycle sensitivity (% peak inspiratory flow)
    - Ventilator-set inspiratory pressure
- Between-breath targets:
  - Operator-set average tidal volume

Time Cycled Pressure Limited A/C with Volume Guarantee
- Available for neonatal patient size setting only
- *Mandatory breaths:* Machine triggered (preset frequency) or patient triggered (pressure or flow sensitivity) and machine cycled (inspiratory time)
  - Within-breath settings:
    - Operator-set PEEP, frequency, inspiratory pressure, peak inspiratory flow, and inspiratory time. Inspiration is delivered at the set inspiratory flow only until the inspiratory pressure target is reached. Flow decays exponentially after that.
- *Spontaneous breaths:* Patient triggered (pressure or flow sensitivity) and patient cycled (% peak inspiratory flow)
  - Within-breath settings:
    - Operator-set cycle sensitivity (% peak inspiratory flow)
    - Ventilator-set inspiratory pressure
- *Between-breath targets:*
  - Operator-set average tidal volume

Time Cycled Pressure Limited SIMV
- Available for neonatal patient size setting only
- *Mandatory breaths:* Machine triggered (preset frequency) or patient synchronized (using pressure or flow sensitivity) and machine cycled (inspiratory time)
  - Within-breath settings:
    - Operator-set PEEP, frequency, inspiratory pressure, peak inspiratory flow, and inspiratory time. Inspiration is delivered at the set inspiratory flow only until the inspiratory pressure target is reached. Flow decays exponentially after that.
- *Spontaneous breaths:* Patient triggered (pressure or flow sensitivity) and patient cycled (% peak inspiratory flow)
  - Within-breath settings:
    - Operator-set inspiratory pressure and cycle sensitivity (% peak inspiratory flow)
- *Between-breath targets:* None

Time Cycled Pressure Limited SIMV with Volume Guarantee
- Available for neonatal patient size setting only
- *Mandatory breaths:* Machine triggered (preset frequency) or patient synchronized (pressure or flow sensitivity) and machine cycled (inspiratory time)
  - Within-breath settings:
    - Operator-set PEEP, frequency, and inspiratory time
    - Ventilator-set inspiratory pressure
- *Spontaneous breaths:* Patient triggered (pressure or flow sensitivity) and patient cycled (% peak inspiratory flow)

  - Within-breath settings:
    - Operator-set cycle sensitivity (% peak inspiratory flow)
    - Ventilator-set inspiratory pressure
- *Between-breath targets:*
  - Operator-set tidal volume

Volume A/C
- *Mandatory breaths:* Machine triggered (preset frequency) or patient triggered (pressure or flow sensitivity) and machine cycled (tidal volume or pause time)
  - Within-breath settings:
    - Operator-set PEEP, frequency, peak inspiratory flow, tidal volume, and pause time
- *Spontaneous breaths:* Not allowed
- *Between-breath targets:* None

Volume A/C with Demand Flow
- Activation of Demand Flow makes this mode a form of IMV, not A/C. See spontaneous breaths below.
- *Mandatory breaths:* Machine triggered (preset frequency) or patient triggered (pressure or flow sensitivity) and machine cycled (tidal volume or inspiratory pause time) or patient cycled (flow).
  - Within-breath settings:
    - Operator-set PEEP, frequency, inspiratory flow, tidal volume, and inspiratory pause time
    - Ventilator-set inspiratory pressure if inspiration switches from volume control to pressure control due to the dual targeting scheme (see spontaneous breaths below)
- *Spontaneous breaths:* Because this mode uses dual targeting, if the patient's inspiratory effort is large enough, inspiration will switch from volume control with time cycling to pressure control with flow cycling. If inspiration happened to also be patient triggered, the breath would be classified as spontaneous (i.e., patient triggered and cycled) and would be very similar to a breath in the Pressure Support mode. This possibility of spontaneous breaths appearing between mandatory breaths is the reason this mode is a form of IMV instead of CMV.
- *Between-breath targets:* None.

Volume A/C with Vsync and Flow Cycle
- Vsync is available only for adult and pediatric patients.
- Activation of Vsync makes this mode a form of pressure control, not volume control, because inspiratory pressure is preset within each breath. Vsync is a form of adaptive targeting that allows the ventilator to adjust inspiratory pressure between breaths to achieve an average preset tidal volume.

- Activation of Flow Cycle makes this mode a form of IMV, not A/C. Flow cycling makes every breath patient cycled. Hence, every patient-triggered breath is spontaneous (i.e., patient triggered and cycled) whereas every machine-triggered breath is mandatory (i.e., machine triggered and patient cycled) by definition.
- *Mandatory breaths:* Machine triggered (preset frequency) and patient cycled (% of peak inspiratory flow).
  - Within-breath settings:
    - Operator-set PEEP, frequency, peak flow, rise time, and cycle sensitivity (% peak flow)
    - Ventilator-set inspiratory pressure
- *Spontaneous breaths:* Patient triggered (pressure or flow sensitivity) and patient cycled (% peak inspiratory flow).
  - Within-breath settings:
    - Operator-set inspiratory pressure, rise time, and cycle sensitivity (% peak inspiratory flow)
- Between-breath targets:
  - Operator-set tidal volume

Volume A/C with Vsync
- Vsync is available only for adult and pediatric patients.
- Activation of Vsync makes this mode a form of pressure control, not volume control, because inspiratory pressure is preset within each breath. Vsync is a form of adaptive targeting that allows the ventilator to adjust inspiratory pressure between breaths to achieve an average preset tidal volume.
- *Mandatory breaths:* Machine triggered (preset frequency) or patient triggered (pressure or flow sensitivity) and machine cycled (volume or inspiratory pause time).
    - Operator-set PEEP, frequency, peak flow, rise time
    - Ventilator-set inspiratory pressure
- *Spontaneous breaths:* Not allowed.
- Between-breath targets:
  - Operator-set tidal volume

Volume IMV with Demand Flow
- *Mandatory breaths:* Machine triggered (preset frequency) or patient triggered (pressure or flow sensitivity) and machine cycled (tidal volume or inspiratory pause time).
  - Within-breath settings:
    - Operator-set PEEP, frequency, inspiratory flow, tidal volume, and inspiratory pause time

- Ventilator-set inspiratory pressure if inspiration switches from volume control to pressure control due to the dual targeting scheme (see spontaneous breaths below)
- *Spontaneous breaths:* Because this mode uses dual targeting, if the patient's inspiratory effort is large enough, inspiration will switch from volume control with time cycling to pressure control with flow cycling.
- *Between-breath targets:* None.

Volume SIMV
- *Mandatory breaths:* Machine triggered (preset frequency) or patient synchronized (pressure or flow sensitivity) and machine cycled (tidal volume or pause time)
  - Within-breath settings:
    - Operator-set PEEP, frequency, peak inspiratory flow, tidal volume, and pause time
- *Spontaneous breaths:* Patient triggered (pressure or flow sensitivity) and patient cycled (% peak inspiratory flow)
  - Within-breath settings:
    - Operator-set inspiratory pressure, rise time, and cycle sensitivity (% peak inspiratory flow)
- *Between-breath targets:* None

Volume SIMV with Vsync
- Vsync is available only for adult and pediatric patients.
- Activation of Vsync makes this mode a form of pressure control, not volume control, because inspiratory pressure is preset within each breath. Vsync is a form of adaptive targeting that allows the ventilator to adjust inspiratory pressure between breaths to achieve an average preset tidal volume.
- *Mandatory breaths:* Machine triggered (preset frequency) or patient synchronized (pressure or flow sensitivity) and machine cycled (tidal volume or pause time).
  - Within-breath settings:
    - Operator-set PEEP, frequency, peak inspiratory flow, tidal volume, and pause time
- *Spontaneous breaths:* Patient triggered (pressure or flow sensitivity) and patient cycled (% peak inspiratory flow).
  - Within-breath settings:
    - Operator-set inspiratory pressure, rise time, and cycle sensitivity (% peak inspiratory flow)
- *Between-breath targets:* None.

Special Features

Backup ventilation: Apnea Backup Ventilation is available in Assist Control, SIMV, CPAP/PSV and APRV/Biphasic modes.

Gas volume compensation: The Avea supports compensation for body temperature and pressure, saturated (BTPS) and atmospheric temperature and pressure, dry (ATPD) conditions. When the Circuit Compliance option is active, the volume of gas delivered during a volume-controlled or targeted breath is increased to include the set volume, plus the volume lost due to the compliance effect of the circuit. Circuit Compliance is active for the set tidal volume during volume control ventilation, the target tidal volume in PRVC mode, and machine volume. It is only active in adult and pediatric applications.

Leak compensation: The ventilator incorporates a leak compensation system. This system compensates for baseline leaks at the patient interface.

Miscellaneous: The Avea offers a port to allow independent lung ventilation (ILV). Independent lung ventilation allows two ventilators to be synchronized to the same breath rate (the rate control set on the master ventilator) while all other primary and advanced controls for each ventilator can be set independently. Master and slave ventilators need not operate in the same mode during ILV. This ventilator is unique in its ability to monitor esophageal pressure with an optional esophageal balloon and calculate related respiratory system mechanics from the signal. The Avea also allows volumetric capnography using an optional exhaled CO_2 monitor. The ventilator supports flow measurements at the airway using either a hot wire flow sensor or a pressure differential flow sensor. The Avea can deliver heliox blended gas instead of medical air. By simply changing a connector on the back panel, the ventilator identifies the gas input and adjusts to accommodate the change. All volumes (numeric and graphic) are automatically compensated for accurate display.

Nebulizer: The ventilator supplies blended gas to the nebulizer port for an inline jet nebulizer. Delivery of the nebulized gas is synchronized with the inspiratory phase of a breath and lasts for 20 minutes.

Neonatal ventilation: The Avea offers Infant Nasal CPAP, designed to work with standard two-limbed neonatal patient circuits and nasal prongs. There is also a Nasal Intermittent Mandatory Ventilation mode (PC-IMVs,s) that provides time-triggered, time-cycled mandatory breaths that are pressure controlled.

Noninvasive ventilation: The only explicitly noninvasive modes on the Avea are the neonatal modes Infant Nasal CPAP and a Nasal Intermittent Mandatory Ventilation mode (PC-IMVs,s).

Manufacturer's Specifications

The manufacturer's specifications are provided in Table 9-9.

CareFusion Vela

The Vela ventilator (Figure 9-17) is intended to provide continuous or intermittent ventilatory support for the care of adult and pediatric patients weighing at least 11 lb (5 kg). The ventilator is suitable for use in institutional and transport settings. It is not intended for use as an emergency medical transport ventilator or home care applications.

Operator Interface

The Vela has an operator interface that uses a touch screen, buttons, and a control knob (Figure 9-18). Screen displays show ventilator settings, alarm

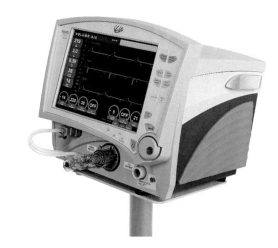

FIGURE 9-17 CareFusion Vela ventilator.
Reproduced with permission from CareFusion.

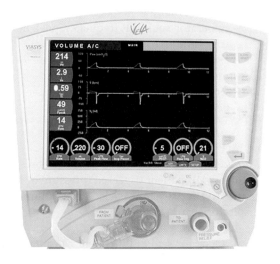

FIGURE 9-18 CareFusion Vela operator interface.
Reproduced with permission from CareFusion.

TABLE 9-9
Specifications for the CareFusion Avea Ventilator

Setting Category	Setting	Range
Pressure	Inspiratory Pressure	0–90 cm H_2O
	Pressure Support	0–90 cm H_2O
	PEEP	0–50 cm H_2O
Volume	Tidal Volume	0.025–2.50 L
Flow	Inspiratory Flow	3–150 L/min
	Waveform	Square/descending ramp
Time	Inspiratory Time	0.2–5.0 s
	Mandatory Breath Frequency	1–150/min
	Adjustable Rise Time	Yes
Sensitivity	Trigger Sensitivity (pressure)	0.1–20.0 cm H_2O
	Trigger Sensitivity (flow)	0.1–20.0 L/min
Alarm Category		
Pressure	High Peak Pressure	10–105 cm H_2O
	Low Peak Pressure	3–99 cm H_2O
	Low PEEP	0–60 cm H_2O
Volume	High Exhaled Tidal Volume	0.002–3.0 L
	Low Exhaled Tidal Volume	0–3.0 L
Flow	High Exhaled Minute Volume	0–75 L/min
	Low Exhaled Minute Volume	0–50 L/min
Time	Apnea Interval	6–60 s
	High Rate	1–200/min
Other	O_2 Sensor	Enabled/Disabled
Monitored Parameters	Exhaled Tidal Volume	
	Inspired Tidal Volume	
	Spontaneous Tidal Volume	
	Mandatory Tidal Volume	
	Delivered Machine Volume	
	% Leak	
	Minute Volume	
	Spontaneous Minute Volume	
	Breath Rate	

(continues)

TABLE 9-9
Specifications for the CareFusion Avea Ventilator (*Continued*)

Setting Category	Setting	Range
Monitored Parameters, cont.	Inspiratory Time	
	Exhalation Time	
	I:E Ratio	
	Rapid Shallow Breathing Index	
	Peak Inspiratory Pressure	
	Mean Airway Pressure	
	Plateau Pressure	
	PEEP	
	Air Inlet Gas Supply Pressure	
	Oxygen Inlet Gas Supply Pressure	
	Delivered % O_2	
	Dynamic Compliance	
	Respiratory System Compliance	
	Respiratory System Resistance	
	Peak Inspiratory Flow Rate	
	Peak Expiratory Flow Rate	
	Lung Compliance	
	Ccw	
	Total Inspiratory Resistance	
	Peak Expiratory Resistance	
	Airway Resistance	
	Rlung	
	dPaw	
	dPes	
	AutoPEEP	
	dAutoPEEP	
	AutoPEEPES	
	Ptp Plat	
	Ptp PEP	
	Maximum Negative Airway Pressure	
	WOBv	
	WOBp	
	WOBt	

settings, and monitored values using waveforms or digital values. Settings are entered by touching a virtual button on the screen to select the desired setting, turning the knob to select the setting value, and then pressing the ACCEPT button to finalize the setting. The real buttons provide various features related to menu navigation, alarm silencing, suctioning, temporary (2 minutes) 100% oxygen delivery, manual breath trigger, and expiratory hold.

Modes

Modes are selected by pressing the virtual button with the desired mode name. There are 11 basic mode names, but there are a variety of "advanced settings" (Table 9-10). Some of these advanced settings actually change the mode (Table 9-11), resulting in 17 different modes by classification (Table 9-12).

The advanced settings increase both flexibility and confusion. For example, the mode named Volume Control A/C is classified as volume control continuous mandatory ventilation with set-point targeting (VC-CMVs). However, adding the Vsync and Flow Cycle advanced settings to this mode turns it into pressure control intermittent mandatory ventilation with adaptive and set-point targeting (PC-IMVa,s)—a very different mode indeed.

Airway Pressure Release Ventilation/Biphasic
- *Mandatory breaths:* Machine triggered (preset frequency) or patient synchronized (pressure or flow sensitivity) and machine cycled (inspiratory time or patient synchronized by flow sensitivity).
  - Within-breath settings:
    - Operator-set PEEP (called Pres Low), peak inspiratory pressure (called Pres High), rise time, inspiratory time (called Time High), and expiratory time (called Time Low)
- *Spontaneous breaths:* Patient triggered (pressure or flow sensitivity) and patient cycled (% peak inspiratory flow). Spontaneous breaths are permitted both between and during mandatory breaths.
  - Within-breath settings:
    - Operator-set inspiratory pressure and rise time.
- *Between-breath targets:* None.

CPAP/Pressure Support
- *Mandatory breaths:* Not allowed
- *Spontaneous breaths:* Patient triggered (pressure or flow sensitivity) and patient cycled (% peak inspiratory flow)
  - Within-breath settings:
    - Operator-set inspiratory pressure, rise time, and cycle sensitivity (% peak inspiratory flow)
- *Between-breath targets:* None

Noninvasive Positive Pressure Ventilation A/C
- *Mandatory breaths:* Machine triggered (preset frequency) or patient triggered (pressure or flow sensitivity) and machine cycled (inspiratory time)
  - Within-breath settings:
    - Operator-set PEEP, frequency, inspiratory pressure, rise time, and inspiratory time
- *Spontaneous breaths:* Not allowed
- *Between-breath targets:* None

TABLE 9-10
Advanced Mode Settings for the CareFusion Vela

Advanced Setting	Action
Volume Limit	When the volume delivered in a pressure control mode exceeds the preset limit, inspiration is terminated.
Assured Volume	For pressure control modes, this sets a volume target and flow and activates dual targeting. The operator sets the target volume and the ventilator calculates the target flow as the volume divided by the set inspiratory time. If flow decays to this flow target and the volume has not been delivered, then inspiration switches to volume control with constant flow until the volume has been delivered. Inspiratory time remains constant.
Flow Cycle	For pressure control modes, this changes the cycle criterion from time to flow and sets the threshold for inspiratory flow termination as a percent of peak flow.
Demand Flow	For volume control modes, this sets a ventilator-determined pressure target and activates dual targeting. If inspiratory pressure decreases 2 cm H_2O (due to patient inspiratory effort), volume control switches to pressure control. If the set volume is delivered and flow is equal to the set flow, inspiration is volume cycled. Otherwise, inspiration is flow cycled at 25% of peak flow.
Vsync	Switches the mode from volume control to pressure control with adaptive targeting. Inspiratory pressure is automatically adjusted to maintain an average tidal volume equal to the set volume.

Reproduced with permission from Mandu Press Ltd.

TABLE 9-11
Controls and Mode Names for the CareFusion Vela

Breath Type and Mode	Vol A/C	Vol SIMV	Pres A/C	Pres SIMV	PRVC A/C	PRVC SIMV	CPAP/PSV	APRV/BIPHASIC	NPPV A/C	NPPV/SIMV	NPPV/CPAP/PS
Primary Controls											
Rate bpm	✓	✓	✓	✓	✓	✓			✓	✓	
Volume mL	✓	✓			✓	✓					
Insp pres cm H$_2$O			✓	✓							
NPPV Insp pres cm H$_2$O									✓	✓	
Peak flow L/min	✓	✓									
Insp time sec			✓	✓	✓	✓			✓	✓	
Insp pause sec	✓ (Not in Vsync)	✓ (Not in Vsync)									
PSV cm H$_2$O		✓		✓		✓	✓	✓			
NPPV PSV cm H$_2$O										✓	✓
PEEP cm H$_2$O	✓	✓	✓	✓	✓	✓	✓	✓	✓	✓	✓
Flow trig L/min	✓	✓	✓	✓	✓	✓	✓	✓	✓	✓	✓
% Oxygen % O$_2$	✓	✓	✓	✓	✓	✓	✓	✓	✓	✓	✓
Pres high cm H$_2$O								✓			
Time high sec								✓			
Time low sec								✓			
Pres low cm H$_2$O								✓			
Apnea (pressure and volume) settings							✓	✓			✓
Advanced Settings Available Within Each Mode	Vsync (Vol limit, Flow cycle), Sigh, Waveform, Bias flow	Vsync, Sigh, Waveform, PSV cycle, PSV Tmax, Bias flow, Vol limit,* Flow cycle*	Assured vol, PC flow cycle, Bias flow	Assured vol, PC flow cycle, PSV cycle, PSV Tmax, Bias flow	Bias flow, Vol limit, PC flow cycle	Vol limit, PC flow cycle, PSV cycle, PSV Tmax, Bias flow	PSV cycle, PSV Tmax, Bias flow	PSV cycle, PSV Tmax, Bias flow, T high sync, T high PSV, T low sync	PC flow cycle, Bias flow	PC flow cycle, PSV cycle, PSV Tmax, Bias flow	PSV cycle, PSV Tmax, Bias flow

TABLE 9-12
Classification of Modes for the CareFusion Vela

Mode Name	Mode Classification				
	Control Variable	Breath Sequence	Primary Breath Targeting Scheme	Secondary Breath Targeting Scheme	Tag
Volume A/C	volume	CMV	set-point	N/A	VC-CMVs
Volume SIMV	volume	IMV	set-point	set-point	VC-IMVs,s
Pressure A/C	pressure	CMV	set-point	N/A	PC-CMVs
Noninvasive Positive Pressure Ventilation A/C	pressure	CMV	set-point	N/A	PC-CMVs
Pressure A/C with Assured Volume	pressure	CMV	dual	N/A	PC-CMVd
Volume A/C with Vsync	pressure	CMV	adaptive	N/A	PC-CMVa
Pressure Regulated Volume Control A/C	pressure	CMV	adaptive	N/A	PC-CMVa
Pressure A/C with Flow Cycle	pressure	IMV	set-point	set-point	PC-IMVs,s
Pressure SIMV	pressure	IMV	set-point	set-point	PC-IMVs,s
Noninvasive Positive Pressure Ventilation SIMV	pressure	IMV	set-point	set-point	PC-IMVs,s
Airway Pressure Release Ventilation/Biphasic	pressure	IMV	set-point	set-point	PC-IMVs,s
Volume A/C with Vsync and Flow Cycle	pressure	IMV	adaptive	set-point	PC-IMVa,s
Volume SIMV with Vsync	pressure	IMV	adaptive	set-point	PC-IMVa,s
Pressure Regulated Volume Control A/C with Flow Cycle	pressure	IMV	adaptive	adaptive	PC-IMVa,a
Pressure Regulated Volume Control SIMV with Flow Cycle	pressure	IMV	adaptive	set-point	PC-IMVa,s
Pressure Regulated Volume Control SIMV	pressure	IMV	adaptive	set-point	PC-IMVa,s
CPAP/Pressure Support Ventilation	pressure	CSV	set-point	N/A	PC-CSVs
Noninvasive Positive Pressure Ventilation CPAP PS	pressure	CSV	set-point	N/A	PC-CSVs

Reproduced with permission from Mandu Press Ltd.

Noninvasive Positive Pressure Ventilation/CPAP/ Pressure Support
- *Mandatory breaths:* Not allowed
- *Spontaneous breaths:* Patient triggered (pressure or flow sensitivity) and patient cycled (% peak inspiratory flow)
  - Within-breath settings:
    - Operator-set inspiratory pressure, rise time, and cycle sensitivity (% peak inspiratory flow)
- *Between-breath targets:* None

Noninvasive Positive Pressure Ventilation SIMV
- *Mandatory breaths:* Machine triggered (preset frequency) or patient synchronized (pressure or flow sensitivity) and machine cycled (inspiratory time)
  - Within-breath settings:
    - Operator-set PEEP, frequency, inspiratory pressure, rise time, and inspiratory time
- *Spontaneous breaths:* Patient triggered (pressure or flow sensitivity) and patient cycled (% peak inspiratory flow)

- Within-breath settings:
  - Operator-set inspiratory pressure, rise time, and cycle sensitivity (% peak inspiratory flow)
- *Between-breath targets:* None

Pressure A/C

- *Mandatory breaths:* Machine triggered (preset frequency) or patient triggered (pressure or flow sensitivity) and machine cycled (inspiratory time)
  - Within-breath settings:
    - Operator-set PEEP, frequency, inspiratory pressure, rise time, and inspiratory time
- *Spontaneous breaths:* Not allowed
- *Between-breath targets:* None

Pressure A/C (with Assured Volume)

- *Mandatory breaths:* Machine triggered (preset frequency) or patient triggered (pressure or flow sensitivity) and machine cycled (inspiratory time)
  - Within-breath settings:
    - Operator-set PEEP, frequency, tidal volume, inspiratory pressure, rise time, and inspiratory time
    - Ventilator switches from pressure control to volume control if inspiratory flow decays to a machine-determined threshold before preset tidal volume is reached. Inspiration continues at constant flow for preset inspiratory time
- *Spontaneous breaths:* Not allowed
- *Between-breath targets:* None

Pressure A/C (with Flow Cycle)

- Activation of Flow Cycle makes this mode a form of IMV, not A/C. Flow cycling makes every breath patient cycled. Hence, every patient-triggered breath is spontaneous (i.e., patient triggered and cycled) whereas every machine-triggered breath is mandatory (i.e., machine triggered and patient cycled) by definition.
- *Mandatory breaths:* Machine triggered (preset frequency) and patient cycled (% peak inspiratory flow).
  - Within-breath settings:
    - Operator-set PEEP, frequency, inspiratory pressure, rise time, and cycle sensitivity (% peak flow)
- *Spontaneous breaths:* Patient triggered (pressure or flow sensitivity) and patient cycled (% peak inspiratory flow).
  - Within-breath settings:
    - Operator-set inspiratory pressure, rise time, and cycle sensitivity (% peak inspiratory flow)
- *Between-breath targets:* None.

Pressure Regulated Volume Control A/C

- *Mandatory breaths:* Machine triggered (preset frequency) or patient triggered (pressure or flow sensitivity) and machine cycled (inspiratory time)
  - Within-breath settings:
    - Operator-set PEEP, frequency, rise time, and inspiratory time
    - Ventilator-set inspiratory pressure
- *Spontaneous breaths:* Not allowed
- Between-breath targets:
  - Operator-set tidal volume

Pressure Regulated Volume Control (with Flow Cycle)

- *Mandatory breaths:* Machine triggered (preset frequency) and patient cycled (% peak inspiratory flow)
  - Within-breath settings:
    - Operator-set PEEP, frequency, rise time, and cycle sensitivity (% peak flow)
    - Ventilator-set inspiratory pressure
- *Spontaneous breaths:* Patient triggered (pressure or flow sensitivity) and patient cycled (% peak inspiratory flow)
  - Within-breath settings:
    - Operator-set inspiratory pressure, rise time, and cycle sensitivity (% peak inspiratory flow)
- Between-breath targets:
  - Operator-set tidal volume

Pressure Regulated Volume Control SIMV (with Flow Cycle)

- *Mandatory breaths:* Machine triggered (preset frequency) and patient cycled (% peak inspiratory flow)
  - Within-breath settings:
    - Operator-set PEEP, frequency, rise time, and cycle sensitivity (% peak flow)
    - Ventilator-set inspiratory pressure
- *Spontaneous breaths:* Patient triggered (pressure or flow sensitivity) and patient cycled (% peak inspiratory flow)
  - Within-breath settings:
    - Operator-set inspiratory pressure, rise time, and cycle sensitivity (% peak inspiratory flow)
- Between-breath targets:
  - Operator-set tidal volume

Pressure Regulated Volume Control SIMV

- *Mandatory breaths:* Machine triggered (preset frequency) or patient synchronized (pressure or flow sensitivity) and machine cycled (inspiratory time)
  - Within-breath settings:
    - Operator-set PEEP, frequency, rise time, and inspiratory time
    - Ventilator-set inspiratory pressure

- *Spontaneous breaths:* Patient triggered (pressure or flow sensitivity) and patient cycled (% peak inspiratory flow)
  - Within-breath settings:
    - Operator-set inspiratory pressure, rise time, and cycle sensitivity (% peak inspiratory flow)
- Between-breath targets:
  - Operator-set tidal volume

Pressure SIMV

- *Mandatory breaths:* Machine triggered (preset frequency) or patient synchronized (pressure or flow sensitivity) and machine cycled (inspiratory time)
  - Within-breath settings:
    - Operator-set PEEP, frequency, inspiratory pressure, rise time, and inspiratory time
- *Spontaneous breaths:* Patient triggered (pressure or flow sensitivity) and patient cycled (% peak inspiratory flow)
  - Within-breath settings:
    - Operator-set inspiratory pressure, rise time, and cycle sensitivity (% peak inspiratory flow)
- *Between-breath targets:* None

Volume A/C

- *Mandatory breaths:* Machine triggered (preset frequency) or patient triggered (pressure or flow sensitivity) and machine cycled (tidal volume or pause time)
  - Within-breath settings:
    - Operator-set PEEP, frequency, peak inspiratory flow, tidal volume, and pause time
- *Spontaneous breaths:* Not allowed
- *Between-breath targets:* None

Volume A/C (with Vsync and Flow Cycle)

- Vsync is available only for adult and pediatric patients.
- Activation of Vsync makes this mode a form of pressure control, not volume control, because inspiratory pressure is preset within each breath. Vsync is a form of adaptive targeting that allows the ventilator to adjust inspiratory pressure between breaths to achieve an average preset tidal volume.
- Activation of Flow Cycle makes this mode a form of IMV, not A/C. Flow cycling makes every breath patient cycled. Hence, every patient-triggered breath is spontaneous (i.e., patient triggered and cycled) whereas every machine-triggered breath is mandatory (i.e., machine triggered and patient cycled) by definition.
- *Mandatory breaths:* Machine triggered (preset frequency) and patient cycled (% of peak inspiratory flow).

- Within-breath settings:
  - Operator-set PEEP, frequency, peak flow, rise time, and cycle sensitivity (% peak flow)
  - Ventilator-set inspiratory pressure
- *Spontaneous breaths:* Patient triggered (pressure or flow sensitivity) and patient cycled (% peak inspiratory flow).
  - Within-breath settings:
    - Operator-set inspiratory pressure, rise time, and cycle sensitivity (% peak inspiratory flow)
- Between-breath targets:
  - Operator-set tidal volume

Volume A/C (with Vsync)

- Vsync is available only for adult and pediatric patients.
- Activation of Vsync makes this mode a form of pressure control, not volume control, because inspiratory pressure is preset within each breath. Vsync is a form of adaptive targeting that allows the ventilator to adjust inspiratory pressure between breaths to achieve an average preset tidal volume.
- *Mandatory breaths:* Machine triggered (preset frequency) or patient triggered (pressure or flow sensitivity) and machine cycled (volume or inspiratory pause time).
  - Within-breath settings:
    - Operator-set PEEP, frequency, peak flow, rise time
    - Ventilator-set inspiratory pressure
- *Spontaneous breaths:* Not allowed
- Between-breath targets:
  - Operator-set tidal volume

Volume SIMV

- *Mandatory breaths:* Machine triggered (preset frequency) or patient synchronized (pressure or flow sensitivity) and machine cycled (tidal volume or pause time)
  - Within-breath settings:
    - Operator-set PEEP, frequency, peak inspiratory flow, tidal volume, and pause time
- *Spontaneous breaths:* Patient triggered (pressure or flow sensitivity) and patient cycled (% peak inspiratory flow)
  - Within-breath settings:
    - Operator-set inspiratory pressure, rise time, and cycle sensitivity (% peak inspiratory flow)
- *Between-breath targets:* None

Volume SIMV (with Vsync)

- Vsync is available only for adult and pediatric patients.

- Activation of Vsync makes this mode a form of pressure control, not volume control, because inspiratory pressure is preset within each breath. Vsync is a form of adaptive targeting that allows the ventilator to adjust inspiratory pressure between breaths to achieve an average preset tidal volume.
- *Mandatory breaths:* Machine triggered (preset frequency) or patient synchronized (pressure or flow sensitivity) and machine cycled (tidal volume or pause time).
  - Within-breath settings:
    - Operator-set PEEP, frequency, peak inspiratory flow, tidal volume, and pause time
- *Spontaneous breaths:* Patient triggered (pressure or flow sensitivity) and patient cycled (% peak inspiratory flow).
  - Within-breath settings:
    - Operator-set inspiratory pressure, rise time, and cycle sensitivity (% peak inspiratory flow)
- *Between-breath targets:* None.

Special Features

Backup ventilation: Apnea ventilation is available when APRV/BiPhasic, CPAP/PSV, or NPPV/CPAP/PSV mode is selected. Apnea backup is active in all SIMV and CPAP modes.

Gas volume compensation: The Vela supports compensation for body temperature and pressure, saturated (BTPS).

Leak compensation: The NPPV Leak Compensation function ensures that any gas flow leakage around a mask (nonvented) or tracheal tube up to 40 L/min, in addition to the set bias flow, is automatically determined and compensated for. The determination of leakage amount is made during exhalation after all patient exhalation has occurred. Subsequently, leak compensation adjusts bias flow to maintain PEEP and establish a new baseline for patient triggering.

Miscellaneous: The Vela allows volumetric capnography using an optional exhaled CO_2 monitor.

Nebulizer: The ventilator supplies 100% oxygen to the nebulizer port when an inline jet nebulizer is attached. Delivery of the nebulized gas is synchronized with the inspiratory phase of a breath.

Manufacturer's Specifications

The manufacturer's specifications are provided in Table 9-13.

Covidien Newport e360T

The Covidien Newport e360T ventilator (Figure 9-19) is designed to provide invasive or noninvasive

TABLE 9-13
Specifications for the CareFusion Vela Ventilator

Setting Category	Setting	Range
Pressure	Inspiratory Pressure	1–100 cm H_2O
	Pressure Support	1–60 cm H_2O
	PEEP	0–35 cm H_2O
Volume	Tidal Volume	0.05–2.0 L
Flow	Inspiratory Flow	10–140 L/min
	Waveform	Square/descending ramp
Time	Inspiratory Time	0.3–10 s
	Mandatory Breath Frequency	2–80/min
	Adjustable Rise Time	Yes
Sensitivity	Trigger Sensitivity (pressure)	
	Trigger Sensitivity (flow)	1–20 L/min
	Cycle Sensitivity (flow)	
Alarm Category		
Pressure	High Pressure	5–120 cm H_2O
	Low Pressure	2–60 cm H_2O
Flow	Low Minute Volume	0.1–99.9 L/min
Time	High Breath Rate	3–150/min
	Apnea Interval	10–60 s

TABLE 9-13
Specifications for the CareFusion Vela Ventilator (*Continued*)

Setting Category	Setting	Range
Other	O_2 Sensor	Enabled/Disabled
	High $EtCO_2$	5–150 mm Hg
	Low $EtCO_2$	1 150 mm Hg
Monitored Parameters	Vte	
	Vti	
	Spontaneous Vt	
	Mandatory Vt	
	Ve	
	Spontaneous Ve	
	Spontaneous Rate	
	Rate	
	Inspiratory Time	
	Expiratory Time	
	I:E Ratio	
	Peak Presure	
	Mean Pressure	
	PEEP	
	O_2	

ventilatory support and monitoring for infant, pediatric, and adult patients with respiratory failure or respiratory insufficiency. It is electrically controlled and pneumatically powered (requires external gas sources).

Operator Interface

The e360T ventilator has an operator interface that uses a touch screen, buttons, and a control knob (**Figure 9-20**). Screen displays change according to the context of the operation, such as initial ventilator operation verification, entering ventilator settings, entering alarm settings, and reviewing monitored values including waveforms or digital values. Settings are entered by touching a real button on the face panel or a virtual button on the screen to select the desired setting, turning the knob to select the setting value, and then pressing the ACCEPT button to finalize the setting. The real buttons provide various functions such as selecting the modes, breath type, and basic settings, menu navigation, alarm silencing, temporary (3 minutes) 100% oxygen delivery, and manual breath trigger.

Modes

Modes are selected by pressing the Volume Control or Pressure Control buttons repeatedly until the desired ventilatory pattern is highlighted. Biphasic Pressure Release Ventilation is selected by choosing Pressure Control plus A/CMV or SIMV ventilatory pattern and then selecting Open Exhalation Valve from the Advanced Data Set screen (see D in Figure 9-20). **Volume Target** Pressure Control is selected by choosing a Volume Control or Pressure Control A/CMV or SIMV ventilatory pattern and then selecting Volume Target ON from the Advanced Data Set screen (see D in Figure 9-20). The modes available on the e360T are shown in **Table 9-14**.

Biphasic Pressure Release Assist Control Mandatory Ventilation

- *Mandatory breaths:* Machine triggered (preset frequency) or patient triggered (pressure or flow sensitivity) and machine cycled (inspiratory time)
  - Within-breath settings:
    - Operator-set PEEP, frequency, inspiratory pressure, slope rise, and inspiratory time

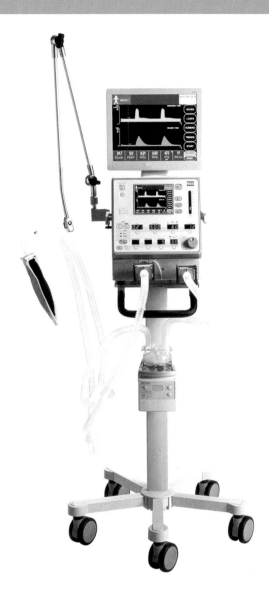

FIGURE 9-19 Covidien Newport e360T ventilator.

- *Spontaneous breaths:* Patient triggered (pressure or flow sensitivity) and patient cycled (% peak inspiratory flow) allowed during inflation period but not allowed between breaths
- *Between-breath targets:* None

Biphasic Pressure Release Synchronized Intermittent Mandatory Ventilation

- *Mandatory breaths:* Machine triggered (preset frequency), patient synchronized (pressure or flow sensitivity), and machine cycled (inspiratory time)
  - Within-breath settings:
    - Operator-set PEEP, frequency, inspiratory pressure, slope rise, and inspiratory time
- *Spontaneous breaths:* Patient triggered (pressure or flow sensitivity) and patient cycled (% peak inspiratory flow)

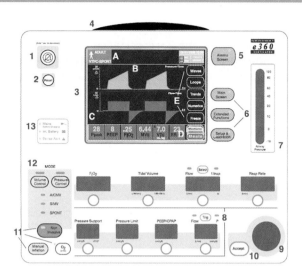

FIGURE 9-20 Covidien Newport e360T operator interface. 1. Alarm silence. 2. Alarm reset. 3. Graphical user interface. 4. Alarm lamp. 5. Alarms screen menu. 6. Graphical user interface screen buttons. 7. Pressure bar graph. 8. Ventilation controls 9. Adjustment knob. 10. Accept button. 11. Special functions. 12. Modes/breath types. 13. Power indicators. A. Graphical user interface status bar. B. Main display area. C. Data sets bar. D. Data set touch button. E. Graphical user interface touch buttons.

- Within-breath settings:
  - Operator-set inspiratory pressure, slope rise, and cycle sensitivity (% peak inspiratory flow or Auto)
- *Between-breath targets:* None

Pressure Control Assist Control Mandatory Ventilation

- *Mandatory breaths:* Machine triggered (preset frequency) or patient triggered (pressure or flow sensitivity) and machine cycled (inspiratory time)
  - Within-breath settings:
    - Operator-set PEEP, frequency, inspiratory pressure, slope rise, and inspiratory time
- *Spontaneous breaths:* Not allowed
- *Between-breath targets:* None

Pressure Control Spont

- *Mandatory breaths:* Not allowed
- *Spontaneous breaths:* Patient triggered (pressure or flow sensitivity) and patient cycled (% peak inspiratory flow or Auto)
  - Within-breath settings:
    - Operator-set inspiratory pressure, slope rise, and cycle sensitivity (% peak inspiratory flow or Auto)
- *Between-breath targets:* None

TABLE 9-14
Classification of Modes for the Covidien Newport e360T

Mode Name	Mode Classification				
	Control Variable	Breath Sequence	Primary Breath Targeting Scheme	Secondary Breath Targeting Scheme	Tag
Volume Control A/C Mandatory Ventilation	volume	CMV	set-point	N/A	VC-CMVs
Volume Control SIMV	volume	IMV	set-point	set-point	VC-IMVs,s
Pressure Control A/C Mandatory Ventilation	pressure	CMV	set-point	N/A	PC-CMVs
Biphasic Pressure Release A/C Mandatory Ventilation	pressure	CMV	set-point	N/A	PC-CMVs
Volume Target Pressure Control A/C Mandatory Ventilation	pressure	CMV	adaptive	N/A	PC-CMVa
Pressure Control SIMV	pressure	IMV	set-point	set-point	PC-IMVs,s
Biphasic Pressure Release SIMV	pressure	IMV	set-point	set-point	PC-IMVs,s
Volume Target Pressure Control SIMV	pressure	IMV	adaptive	adaptive	PC-IMVa,a
Pressure Control Spont	pressure	CSV	set-point	N/A	PC-CSVs
Volume Control Spont	pressure	CSV	set-point	N/A	PC-CSVs
Volume Target Pressure Control Spont	pressure	CSV	adaptive	N/A	PC-CSVa

Reproduced with permission from Mandu Press Ltd.

Pressure Control Synchronized Intermittent Mandatory Ventilation

- *Mandatory breaths:* Machine triggered (preset frequency), patient synchronized (pressure or flow sensitivity), and machine cycled (inspiratory time)
  - Within-breath settings:
    - Operator-set PEEP, frequency, inspiratory pressure, slope rise, and inspiratory time
- *Spontaneous breaths:* Patient triggered (pressure or flow sensitivity) and patient cycled (% peak inspiratory flow or Auto)
  - Within-breath settings:
    - Operator-set inspiratory pressure, slope rise, and cycle sensitivity (% peak inspiratory flow or Auto)
- *Between-breath targets:* None

Volume Control Assist Control Mandatory Ventilation

- *Mandatory breaths:* Machine triggered (preset frequency) or patient triggered (pressure or flow sensitivity) and machine cycled (tidal volume or inspiratory time plus pause time)
  - Within-breath settings:
    - Operator-set PEEP, frequency, peak inspiratory flow and flow waveform or inspiratory time, tidal volume, and pause time

- *Spontaneous breaths:* Not allowed
- *Between-breath targets:* None

Volume Control Spont

- *Mandatory breaths:* Not allowed
- *Spontaneous breaths:* Patient triggered (pressure or flow sensitivity) and patient cycled (% peak inspiratory flow or Auto)
  - Within-breath settings:
    - Operator-set inspiratory pressure, slope rise, and cycle sensitivity (% peak inspiratory flow or Auto)
- *Between-breath targets:* None

Volume Control Synchronized Intermittent Mandatory Ventilation

- *Mandatory breaths:* Machine triggered (preset frequency), patient synchronized (pressure or flow sensitivity), and machine cycled (tidal volume or pause time)
  - Within-breath settings:
    - Operator-set PEEP, frequency, peak inspiratory flow and flow waveform or inspiratory time, tidal volume, and pause time

- *Spontaneous breaths:* Patient triggered (pressure or flow sensitivity) and patient cycled (% peak inspiratory flow or Auto)
  - Within-breath settings:
    - Operator-set inspiratory pressure, slope rise, and cycle sensitivity (% peak inspiratory flow or Auto)
- *Between-breath targets:* None

Volume Target Pressure Control Assist Control Mandatory Ventilation

- *Mandatory breaths:* Machine triggered (preset frequency) or patient triggered (pressure or flow sensitivity) and machine cycled (inspiratory time)
  - Within-breath settings:
    - Operator-set PEEP, frequency, maximum inspiratory pressure, slope rise, and inspiratory time
    - Ventilator-set inspiratory pressure
- *Spontaneous breaths:* Not allowed
- Between-breath targets:
  - Operator-set tidal volume

Volume Target Pressure Control Spont

- *Mandatory breaths:* Not allowed
- *Spontaneous breaths:* Patient triggered (pressure or flow sensitivity) and patient cycled (% peak inspiratory flow or Auto)
  - Within-breath settings:
    - Operator-set maximum inspiratory pressure, slope rise, and cycle sensitivity (% peak inspiratory flow or Auto)
    - Ventilator-set inspiratory pressure
- Between-breath targets:
  - Operator-set tidal volume

Volume Target Pressure Control Synchronized Intermittent Mandatory Ventilation

- *Mandatory breaths:* Machine triggered (preset frequency, patient synchronized (pressure or flow sensitivity), and machine cycled (inspiratory time)
  - Within-breath settings:
    - Operator-set PEEP, frequency, maximum inspiratory pressure, slope rise, and inspiratory time
    - Ventilator-set inspiratory pressure
- *Spontaneous breaths:* Patient triggered (pressure or flow sensitivity) and patient cycled (% peak inspiratory flow or Auto)
  - Within-breath settings:
    - Operator-set maximum inspiratory pressure, slope rise, and cycle sensitivity (% peak inspiratory flow or Auto)
    - Ventilator-set inspiratory pressure
- Between-breath targets:
  - Operator-set tidal volume

Special Features

Backup ventilation: Backup ventilation is initiated when the low minute ventilation alarm threshold is reached. If the current mode is A/CMV or SIMV, backup ventilation employs the current Control Panel settings except for Respiratory Rate, which increases to 1.5 times the current setting (15 breaths/min minimum, 100 breaths/min maximum). If the current mode is SPONT, the ventilator delivers pressure control mandatory breaths with the following settings:

- *Inspiratory pressure:* 15 cm H_2O above PEEP setting
- *Inspiratory time:* 0.6 seconds Ped/Infant; 1.0 second Adult
- *Respiratory rate:* 20 breaths/min Ped/Infant; 12 breaths/min Adult

Backup ventilation terminates when the measured minute ventilation exceeds the set minute ventilation alarm threshold by more than 10%.

Gas volume compensation: Compliance Compensation for Volume Control mandatory breaths can be selected ON or OFF from the Patient Setup screen. When compensation is ON, inspiratory and expiratory tidal volumes are displayed as if they were being monitored at the patient's airway. When compensation is OFF, inspiratory and expiratory tidal volumes represent volumes monitored at the main flow outlet and exhalation valve. Inspiratory and expiratory tidal volume displayed values will not look any different with compensation ON or OFF even though inspiratory and expiratory tidal volume monitored values are different. Actual delivered/monitored values will be bigger with compensation ON, but you will not see it in the displayed value. The extra flow/volume that is added in and delivered to the patient in order to compensate for the volume that is "lost" in the tubing is subtracted from both the displayed values.

Leak compensation: The e360T provides 3 L/min of bias flow through the breathing circuit in between breaths (i.e., during the exhalation period). This flow facilitates both **flow triggering** and the stabilization of baseline pressure and flow in order to minimize auto-triggering of breaths. The Leak Comp (Automatic Leak Compensation/Baseline Pressure Management) function allows the user to select whether they want the e360 to compensate for leaks over and above the 3 L/min bias flow. Compensation is factory preset to ON and the selection is retained after power down. When compensation is ON, the e360 automatically adjusts the bias flow between 3 and 8 L/min for Ped/Infant selection and between 3 and 15 L/min for Adult selection, in order to maintain an end-expiratory base flow of 3 L/min. Flow triggering is automatically compensated for changes in bias flow delivery. When compensation is OFF, bias flow is 3 L/min regardless of leaks. If there is no leak, bias flow remains at 3 L/min whether compensation is ON or OFF.

Noninvasive ventilation: The e360 ventilator can be used for invasive (intubated patient) or noninvasive (mask) ventilation. When the Non Invasive button is activated, the ventilator automatically provides leak compensation/baseline pressure management with a bias flow range of 3 to 25 L/min in order to accommodate the potential for bigger airway leaks around the nonvented mask. (When Non Invasive is not activated and Leak Comp is ON, bias flow is only 3–8 L/min Ped/Infant and 3–15 L/min Adult.) The low minute ventilation and the disconnect alarms can be set to OFF while Non Invasive is activated. All other alarms such as the apnea alarm remain operative and cannot be set to OFF. If the low minute ventilation or disconnect alarm is OFF when Non Invasive is deactivated, the alarms are automatically turned back on and the low minute ventilation alarm is set to the lowest value while the disconnect alarm is set to the highest value. Non Invasive can be used with any mode of ventilation. It is factory preset to OFF and the setting returns to OFF after power down.

Manufacturer's Specifications

The manufacturer's specifications are provided in **Table 9-15**.

Covidien PB 840

The Covidien Puritan Bennett 840 ventilator (**Figure 9-21**) is designed for invasive and noninvasive ventilation of adult, pediatric, and neonatal patients. It is electrically controlled and pneumatically powered (requires external compressor).

Operator Interface

The PB 840 has an operator interface that uses a touch screen, buttons, and a control knob (**Figure 9-22**). Screen displays change according to the context of the operation, such as initial ventilator operation verification, entering ventilator settings, entering alarm settings, and reviewing monitored values including waveforms or digital values. Settings are entered by touching a virtual button on the screen to select the desired setting, turning the knob to select the setting value, and then pressing the ACCEPT button to finalize the setting. The real buttons provide various features related to menu navigation, alarm silencing, temporary

TABLE 9-15
Specifications for the Covidien Newport e360T Ventilator

Setting Category	Setting	Range	
Pressure	Inspiratory Pressure	0–80 cm H_2O	Pressure Limit
	Pressure Support	0–60 cm H_2O	
	PEEP	0–45 cm H_2O	
Volume	Tidal Volume	0–3.0 L	
Flow	Inspiratory Flow	1–180 L/min	
	Waveform	Square/descending ramp	
Time	Inspiratory Time	0.1–5.0 s	
	Mandatory Breath Frequency	1–120/min	
	Adjustable Rise Time	Yes	
Sensitivity	Trigger Sensitivity (pressure)	0–(–5) cm H_2O	
	Trigger Sensitivity (flow)	0.1–2.0 L/min	
	Cycle Sensitivity (flow)	5–55% and AUTO	
Alarm Category			
Pressure	High Airway Pressure	5–120 cm H_2O	
	Low Airway Pressure	3–95 cm H_2O	
Volume	Disconnect Threshold	20–95%	Percent of difference between inspiratory and expiratory tidal volumes

(continues)

TABLE 9-15
Specifications for the Covidien Newport e360T Ventilator (*Continued*)

Setting Category	Setting	Range	
Alarm Category, cont.			
Flow	High Expiratory Minute Volume	0.02–60 L/min	MVe
	Low Expiratory Minute Volume	0.01–50 L/min	
Time	Apnea	5–60 s	
	High Total Respiratory Rate	10–120/min or OFF	
Other	O_2 Sensor	Enabled/Disabled	
Monitored Parameters	Cdyn Effective		
	Static Compliance		
	F_IO_2		
	Inspiratory Flow		
	Expiratory Flow		
	I:E Ratio		
	Baseline Pressure		
	Peak Airway Pressure		
	Inspiratory Minute Volume		
	Expiratory Minute Volume	MV_E & MV_E spont	
	PEEP/CPAP		
	Total PEEP		
	Mean Pressure		
	Peak Pressure		
	Plateau Pressure		
	Expiratory Resistance		
	Compliance		
	Respiratory Rate	RR spont & RR tot	
	Inspiratory Resistance		
	Expiratory Resistance		
	Rapid Shallow Breathing Index (RSBI)		
	Inspiratory Time		
	Tidal Volume		
	Time Constant		
	Expiratory Tidal Volume		
	Inspiratory Tidal Volume		
	VTe %Var		
	WOBimp		
	$P_{0.1}$/NIF		

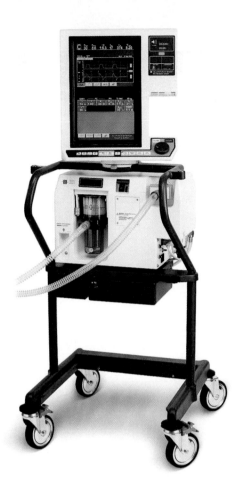

FIGURE 9-21 Covidien PB 840 ventilator.

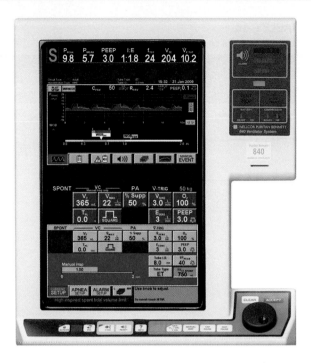

FIGURE 9-22 Covidien PB 840 operator interface. 1. Alarm messages. 2. Operator prompts. 3. Therapy status with ventilation mode. 4. Curves, loops, trends. 5. Ventilation parameters for current mode. 6. Measured ventilation values. 7. Humidification type and status. 8. Touch-sensitive screen keys for specific screen pages. 9. Power supply indication.

(2 minutes) 100% oxygen delivery, manual breath trigger, **inspiratory hold**, and expiratory hold.

Modes

Modes on the PB 840 are constructed by the operator by selecting the breath sequence and the control variables separately. The operator interface on the ventilator uses the term *mode* to refer to what we have described as the breath sequence (i.e., CMV, IMV, CSV). The operator may select from A/C (Assist/Control), SIMV (Synchronized Intermittent Mandatory Ventilation), SPONT (Spontaneous), CPAP (Continuous Positive Airway Pressure), and BILEVEL. Mandatory breath types available are PC (Pressure Control), VC (Volume Control), and VC+ (Volume Control Plus). Spontaneous breath types available are PS (Pressure Support), TC (Tube Compensation), VS (Volume Support), PA (Proportional Assist), and NONE. **Table 9-16** shows how these options can be combined to construct distinct modes.

An Apnea mode is available with default settings based on the patient's ideal body weight (entered during the setup routine), circuit type, and mandatory breath type. These settings can be changed.

The modes available on the PB 840 are shown in **Table 9-17**.

Tube Compensation
If Tube Compensation is selected as the spontaneous breath type, breath delivery during the inspiratory phase is determined by the settings for % support, expiratory sensitivity, tube ID, and tube type.

- Within-breath settings:
  - Operator-set Tube Compensation is set as a percent support (of resistive load) along with artificial airway tube diameter and tube type.
  - Ventilator-set inspiratory pressure as a function of patient-generated inspiratory flow.
- *Between-breath targets:* None

Assist/Control Pressure Control
- *Mandatory breaths:* Machine triggered (preset frequency) or patient triggered (pressure or flow sensitivity) and machine cycled (inspiratory time)
  - Within-breath settings:
  - Operator-set PEEP, frequency, inspiratory pressure, rise time, and inspiratory time
- *Spontaneous breaths:* Not allowed
- *Between-breath targets:* None

TABLE 9-16
Mode Options for the Covidien PB 840 Ventilator

Mode	Breath Category	
	Mandatory	**Spontaneous**
A/C	VC	NA
	PC	
	VC+	
SIMV	VC	PS
		TC
	PC	PS
		VS
		PA
		TC
	VC+	PS
		TC
Bilevel	PC	PS
		TC
Spont	NA	PS
		VS
		PA
		TC

A/C = assist/control, SIMV = synchronized intermittent mandatory ventilation, Spont = spontaneous, VC = volume control, PC = pressure control, VC+ = volume control plus, NA = not applicable, PS = pressure support, TC = tube compensation, VS = volume support, PA = proportional assist

TABLE 9-17
Classification of Modes for the Covidien PB 840 Ventilator

Mode Name	Mode Classification				
	Control Variable	**Breath Sequence**	**Primary Breath Targeting Scheme**	**Secondary Breath Targeting Scheme**	**Tag**
A/C Volume Control	volume	CMV	set-point	N/A	VC-CMVs
SIMV Volume Control with Pressure Support	volume	IMV	set-point	set-point	VC-IMVs,s
SIMV Volume Control with Tube Compensation	volume	IMV	set-point	servo	VC-IMVs,r
A/C Pressure Control	pressure	CMV	set-point	N/A	PC-CMVs
A/C Volume Control Plus	pressure	CMV	adaptive	N/A	PC-CMVa

TABLE 9-17
Classification of Modes for the Covidien PB 840 Ventilator *(Continued)*

| Mode Name | Mode Classification | | | | |
	Control Variable	Breath Sequence	Primary Breath Targeting Scheme	Secondary Breath Targeting Scheme	Tag
SIMV-Pressure Control with Pressure Support	pressure	IMV	set-point	set-point	PC-IMVs,s
SIMV-Pressure Control with Tube Compensation	pressure	IMV	set-point	servo	PC-IMVs,r
Bilevel with Pressure Support	pressure	IMV	set-point	set-point	PC-IMVs,s
Bilevel with Tube Compensation	pressure	IMV	set-point	servo	PC-IMVs,r
SIMV Volume Control Plus with Pressure Support	pressure	IMV	adaptive	set-point	PC-IMVa,s
SIMV Volume Control Plus with Tube Compensation	pressure	IMV	adaptive	servo	PC-IMVa,r
Spont Pressure Support	pressure	CSV	set-point	N/A	PC-CSVs
Spont Tube Compensation	pressure	CSV	servo	N/A	PC-CSVr
Spont Proportional Assist	pressure	CSV	servo	N/A	PC-CSVr
Spont Volume Support	pressure	CSV	adaptive	N/A	PC-CSVa

Reproduced with permission from Mandu Press Ltd.

Assist/Control Volume Control Plus

- *Mandatory breaths:* Machine triggered (preset frequency) or patient triggered (pressure or flow sensitivity) and machine cycled (inspiratory time)
  - Within-breath settings:
    - Operator-set PEEP, frequency, rise time, and inspiratory time
    - Ventilator-set inspiratory pressure
- *Spontaneous breaths:* Not allowed
- Between-breath targets:
  - Operator-set tidal volume

Assist/Control Volume Control

- *Mandatory breaths:* Machine triggered (preset frequency) or patient triggered (pressure or flow sensitivity) and machine cycled (tidal volume or pause time)
  - Within-breath settings:
    - Operator-set PEEP, frequency, flow waveform, peak inspiratory flow, tidal volume, and pause time
- *Spontaneous breaths:* Not allowed
- *Between-breath targets:* None

Bilevel (with Pressure Support)

- *Mandatory breaths:* Machine triggered (preset frequency) or patient synchronized (pressure or flow sensitivity) and machine cycled (inspiratory time or patient synchronized by flow sensitivity).
  - Within-breath settings:
    - Operator-set PEEP (called $PEEP_L$), peak inspiratory pressure (called $PEEP_H$), rise time, inspiratory time (called T_H), and expiratory time (called T_L)
- *Spontaneous breaths:* Patient triggered (pressure or flow sensitivity) and patient cycled (% peak inspiratory flow). Spontaneous breaths are permitted both between and during mandatory breaths.
  - Within-breath settings:
    - Operator-set inspiratory pressure and rise time
- *Between-breath targets:* None.

Bilevel (with Tube Compensation)

- *Mandatory breaths:* Machine triggered (preset frequency) or patient synchronized (pressure or flow sensitivity) and machine cycled (inspiratory time or patient synchronized by flow sensitivity).

- Within-breath settings:
  - Operator-set PEEP (called $PEEP_L$), peak inspiratory pressure (called $PEEP_H$), rise time, inspiratory time (called T_H), and expiratory time (called T_L).
- *Spontaneous breaths:* Patient triggered (pressure or flow sensitivity) and patient cycled (% peak inspiratory flow). Spontaneous breaths are allowed both during and between mandatory breaths.
  - Within-breath settings:
    - Tube Compensation as a percent support (of resistive load). Operator also sets artificial airway tube diameter, tube type, and humidification type.
    - Ventilator-set inspiratory pressure as a function of patient-generated inspiratory flow.
- *Between-breath targets:* None.

SIMV Pressure Control (with Pressure Support)

- *Mandatory breaths:* Machine triggered (preset frequency) or patient synchronized (pressure or flow sensitivity) and machine cycled (inspiratory time)
  - Within-breath settings:
    - Operator-set PEEP, frequency, inspiratory pressure, rise time, and inspiratory time
- *Spontaneous breaths:* Patient triggered (pressure or flow sensitivity) and patient cycled (% peak inspiratory flow)
  - Within-breath settings:
    - Operator-set inspiratory pressure, rise time, and cycle sensitivity (% peak inspiratory flow)
- *Between-breath targets:* None

SIMV Pressure Control (with Tube Compensation)

- *Mandatory breaths:* Machine triggered (preset frequency or patient synchronized using pressure or flow sensitivity) and machine cycled (inspiratory time)
  - Within-breath settings:
    - Operator-set PEEP, frequency, inspiratory pressure, rise time, and inspiratory time
- *Spontaneous breaths:* Patient triggered (pressure or flow sensitivity) and patient cycled (% peak inspiratory flow)
  - Within-breath settings:
    - Operator-set Tube Compensation is set as a percent support (of resistive load) along with artificial airway tube diameter, tube type, and humidification type.
    - Ventilator-set inspiratory pressure as a function of patient-generated inspiratory flow.
- *Between-breath targets:* None

SIMV Volume Control

- *Mandatory breaths:* Machine triggered (preset frequency) or patient synchronized (pressure or flow sensitivity) and machine cycled (tidal volume or pause time)
  - Within-breath settings:
    - Operator-set PEEP, frequency, flow waveform, peak inspiratory flow, tidal volume, and pause time
- *Spontaneous breaths:* Patient triggered (pressure or flow sensitivity) and patient cycled (% peak inspiratory flow)
  - Within-breath settings:
    - Operator-set inspiratory pressure, rise time, and cycle sensitivity (% peak inspiratory flow)
- *Between-breath targets:* None

SIMV Volume Control Plus (with Pressure Support)

- *Mandatory breaths:* Machine triggered (preset frequency or patient synchronized using pressure or flow sensitivity) and machine cycled (inspiratory time)
  - Within-breath settings:
    - Operator-set PEEP, frequency, rise time, and inspiratory time
    - Ventilator-set inspiratory pressure
- *Spontaneous breaths:* Patient triggered (pressure or flow sensitivity) and patient cycled (% peak inspiratory flow)
  - Within-breath settings:
    - Operator-set inspiratory pressure, rise time, and cycle sensitivity (% peak inspiratory flow)
- Between-breath targets:
  - Operator-set tidal volume

SIMV Volume Control Plus (with Tube Compensation)

- *Mandatory breaths:* Machine triggered (preset frequency) or patient synchronized (pressure or flow sensitivity) and machine cycled (inspiratory time)
  - Within-breath settings:
    - Operator-set PEEP, frequency, rise time, and inspiratory time
    - Ventilator-set inspiratory pressure
- *Spontaneous breaths:* Patient triggered (pressure or flow sensitivity) and patient cycled (% peak inspiratory flow)
  - Within-breath settings:
    - Operator-set Tube Compensation is set as a percent support (of resistive load) along with artificial airway tube diameter, tube type, and humidification type

- Ventilator-set inspiratory pressure as a function of patient-generated inspiratory flow
- Between-breath targets:
  - Operator-set tidal volume

Spont Pressure Support

- *Mandatory breaths:* Not allowed
- *Spontaneous breaths:* Patient triggered (pressure or flow sensitivity) and patient cycled (% peak inspiratory flow)
  - Within-breath settings:
    - Operator-set inspiratory pressure, rise time, and cycle sensitivity (% peak inspiratory flow)
- *Between-breath targets:* None

Spont Proportional Assist

- *Mandatory breaths:* Not allowed
- *Spontaneous breaths:* Patient triggered (pressure or flow sensitivity) and patient cycled (% peak inspiratory flow)
  - Within-breath settings:
    - Operator-set percent support (of inspiratory work)
    - Ventilator-set inspiratory pressure as a function of patient-generated inspiratory volume and flow according to the equation of motion for the respiratory system
- *Between-breath targets:* None

Spont Tube Compensation

- *Mandatory breaths:* Not allowed
- *Spontaneous breaths:* Patient triggered (pressure or flow sensitivity) and patient cycled (% peak inspiratory flow)
  - Within-breath settings:
    - Operator-set Tube Compensation is set as a percent support (of resistive load) along with artificial airway tube diameter, tube type, and humidification type.
    - Ventilator-set inspiratory pressure as a function of patient-generated inspiratory flow.
- *Between-breath targets:* None

Spont Volume Support

- *Mandatory breaths:* Not allowed
- *Spontaneous breaths:* Patient triggered (pressure or flow sensitivity) and patient cycled (% peak inspiratory flow)
  - Within-breath settings:
    - Operator-set rise time and cycle sensitivity (% peak inspiratory flow)
- Between-breath targets:
  - Operator-set average tidal volume

Special Features

Backup ventilation: A backup apnea ventilation mode starts if the patient fails to trigger inspiration for a time that exceeds the preset apnea interval. Apnea ventilation settings include rate, O_2%, volume

control (tidal volume, flow pattern, and peak inspiratory flow), or pressure control (inspiratory pressure and inspiratory time).

Gas volume compensation: For volume control modes, volume delivery is compensated for volume lost due to compression in the patient circuit. Compliance compensation does not change inspiratory time and is achieved by increasing flow. All volumes set or reported by the ventilator are at existing barometric pressure, 98.6°F (37°C), and fully saturated with water vapor (BTPS). Graphics data are not BTPS compensated.

Leak compensation: The leak compensation option is designed to compensate for leaks in the breathing circuit to maintain PEEP and prevent auto-triggering during noninvasive and invasive ventilation of neonatal, pediatric, and adult patients. It is available for Pressure Control, Pressure Support, Bilevel, and CPAP modes. A leak compensation option is designed to compensate for leaks in the patient circuit during invasive or noninvasive ventilation. This option "accurately quantifies instantaneous leak rates, therefore detecting patient respiratory phase transitions correctly and reducing patient work of breathing."[35]

Miscellaneous: In pressure control modes, four timing variables are interrelated: frequency, T_I, T_E, and I:E. The PB 840 display allows the operator to select which of these variables remains constant as frequency is changed.

Nebulizer: The PB 840 is designed to be used with an optional Aerogen Aeroneb vibrating mesh nebulizer. Unlike common jet nebulizers sometimes used with ventilators, this device does not increase the volume of inhaled gas.

Neonatal ventilation: A NeoMode option determines values for allowable settings based on patient circuit type and ideal body weight (range for neonates is 0.3 to 7.0 kg or 0.66 to 15 lb).

Noninvasive ventilation: An NIV (noninvasive ventilation) option allows ventilation with various noninvasive patient–ventilator interfaces including masks, infant nasal prongs, and uncuffed neonatal endotracheal tubes.

Manufacturer's Specifications

Table 9-18 lists specifications for the Covidien PB 840 ventilator.

Dräger Evita XL

The Dräger Evita XL ventilator (Figure 9-23) is designed for invasive and noninvasive ventilation of adult, pediatric, and neonatal patients. It is electrically controlled and pneumatically powered (requires external compressor).

TABLE 9-18
Specifications for the Covidien PB 840 Ventilator

Setting Category	Setting	Range
Pressure	Inspiratory Pressure	5–90 cm H_2O
	Pressure Support	0–70 cm H_2O
	PEEP	0–45 cm H_2O
Volume	Tidal Volume	0.005–2.5 L
Flow	Inspiratory Flow	1–150 L/min
	Waveform	Square/descending ramp
Time	Inspiratory Time	0.2–8.0 s
	Inspiratory Time—Bilevel	0.2–30 s
	Mandatory Breath Frequency	1–150/min
	Adjustable Rise Time	Yes
Sensitivity	Trigger Sensitivity (pressure)	0.1–20 cm H_2O
	Trigger Sensitivity (flow)	0.1–20 L/min
	Cycle Sensitivity (flow)	1–80%
Alarm Category		
Pressure	High Circuit Pressure	7–100 cm H_2O
	Low Circuit Pressure	PEEP–Ppeak
Volume	High Exhaled Tidal Volume	0.005–3 L
	Low Exhaled Tidal Volume	0.3–2.5 L
	Low Exhaled Spontaneous Tidal Volume	0–2.5 L
Flow	Minute Volume	25–75 L/min
	High Exhaled Minute Volume	10–100 L/min
	Low Exhaled Minute Volume	0.010–60 L/min
Time	Apnea Interval	10–60 s
	High Respiratory Rate	10–170/min
Other	O_2 Sensor	Enabled/Disabled
Monitored Parameters	Breath Type	
	Delivered O_2 %	
	End Expiratory Pressure (PEEP)	
	End Inspiratory Pressure	
	Exhaled Minute Volume	
	Exhaled Tidal Volume	

TABLE 9-18
Specifications for the Covidien PB 840 Ventilator (*Continued*)

Setting Category	Setting	Range
Monitored Parameters, cont.	I:E Ratio	
	Intrinsic PEEP	
	Peak Circuit Pressure	
	Mean Circuit Pressure	
	Plateau Pressure	
	Rapid Shallow Breathing Index	
	Spontaneous Inspiratory Time	
	Spontaneous Minute Volume	
	Spontaneous Percent Inspiratory Time	
	Static Compliance	
	Static Resistance	
	Total PEEP	
	Total Respiratory Rate	

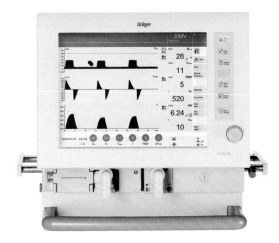

FIGURE 9-23 Dräger Evita XL ventilator.

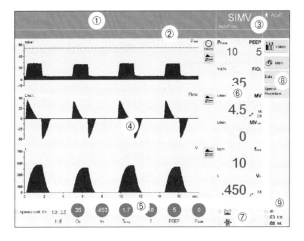

FIGURE 9-24 Dräger Evita XL operator interface. 1. Alarm messages. 2. Operator prompts. 3. Therapy status with ventilation mode. 4. Waveforms, loops, and trends visualizing ventilation. 5. Set ventilation parameters for the active ventilation mode and its extensions. 6. Measured values of ventilation (can be configured). 7. Humidification type and status. 8. Touch-sensitive screen keys for the specific screen pages (can be configured). 9. Power supply indicator.

Operator Interface

The Evita XL has an operator interface that uses a touch screen, buttons, and a control knob (**Figure 9-24**). Screen displays change according to the context of the operation, such as initial ventilator operation verification, entering ventilator settings, entering alarm settings, and reviewing monitored values including waveforms or digital values. Settings are entered by touching a virtual button on the screen to select the desired setting, turning the rotary knob to select the setting value, and then pressing the knob to finalize the setting. Other virtual buttons provide various features related to menu navigation, alarm silencing, temporary

(3 minutes) 100% oxygen delivery, manual breath trigger, inspiratory hold, and expiratory hold.

Modes

Modes on the Evita XL are selected by mode name (e.g., CMV, SIMV, etc.) using tabs on the touch screen. When the tab is selected, the relevant ventilator setting screens are displayed. The setting screens are also tabbed, giving access to basic settings (e.g., tidal volume for volume control modes and inspiratory pressure for pressure control modes) and additional settings. The additional settings include simple things like trigger sensitivity or automatic tube compensation, and complicated things such as activating AutoFlow. AutoFlow changes the mode from volume control to pressure control with adaptive targeting, essentially changing the mode classification in a major way. Table 9-19 shows the modes available on the Dräger Evita XL.

Automatic Tube Compensation

When automatic tube compensation is active, the ventilator controls airway pressure such that the resistive load of breathing through the artificial airway is supported. Compensation may be independently deactivated for the expiratory breathing cycle. Depending on the direction of the patient flow, the airway pressure is increased during inspiration or decreased during expiration. Tube compensation may be applied to spontaneous breaths and mandatory breaths in pressure control modes. Adding tube compensation

TABLE 9-19
Modes for Dräger Evita XL Ventilator

| Mode Name | Mode Classification | | | | Tag |
	Control Variable	Breath Sequence	Primary Breath Targeting Scheme	Secondary Breath Targeting Scheme	
Continuous Mandatory Ventilation	volume	CMV	set-point	N/A	VC-CMVs
Continuous Mandatory Ventilation with Pressure Limited Ventilation	volume	CMV	dual	N/A	VC-CMVd
SIMV	volume	IMV	set-point	set-point	VC-IMVs,s
SIMV with Automatic Tube Compensation	volume	IMV	set-point	set-point/servo	VC-IMVs,sr
SIMV with Pressure Limited Ventilation	volume	IMV	dual	set-point	VC-IMVd,s
SIMV with Pressure Limited Ventilation and Automatic Tube Compensation	volume	IMV	dual	set-point/servo	VC-IMVd,sr
Mandatory Minute Volume Ventilation	volume	IMV	adaptive	set-point	VC-IMVa,s
Mandatory Minute Volume Ventilation with Automatic Tube Compensation	volume	IMV	adaptive	set-point/servo	VC-IMVa,sr
Mandatory Minute Volume with Pressure Limited Ventilation	volume	IMV	dual/adaptive	set-point	VC-IMVda,s
Mandatory Minute Volume with Pressure Limited Ventilation and Automatic Tube Compensation	volume	IMV	dual/adaptive	set-point/servo	VC-IMVda,sr
Pressure Controlled Ventilation Plus Assisted	pressure	CMV	set-point	N/A	PC-CMVs
Continuous Mandatory Ventilation with AutoFlow	pressure	CMV	adaptive	N/A	PC-CMVa
Continuous Mandatory Ventilation with AutoFlow and Tube Compensation	pressure	CMV	adaptive/servo	N/A	PC-CMVar

TABLE 9-19
Modes for Dräger Evita XL Ventilator *(Continued)*

| Mode Name | Mode Classification | | | | |
	Control Variable	Breath Sequence	Primary Breath Targeting Scheme	Secondary Breath Targeting Scheme	Tag
Pressure Controlled Ventilation Plus/Pressure Support	pressure	IMV	set-point	set-point	PC-IMVs,s
Airway Pressure Release Ventilation	pressure	IMV	set-point	set-point	PC-IMVs,s
Mandatory Minute Volume with AutoFlow	pressure	IMV	adaptive	set-point	PC-IMVa,s
Synchronized Intermittent Mandatory Ventilation with AutoFlow	pressure	IMV	adaptive	set-point	PC-IMVa,s
Mandatory Minute Volume with AutoFlow and Tube Compensation	pressure	IMV	adaptive/servo	set-point/servo	PC-IMVar,sr
Synchronized Intermittent Mandatory Ventilation with AutoFlow and Tube Compensation	pressure	IMV	adaptive/servo	set-point/servo	PC-IMVar,sr
Pressure Controlled Ventilation Plus/Pressure Support and Tube Compensation	pressure	IMV	set-point/servo	set-point/servo	PC-IMVsr,sr
Airway Pressure Release Ventilation with Tube Compensation	pressure	IMV	set-point/servo	set-point/servo	PC-IMVsr,sr
Continuous Positive Airway Pressure/Pressure Support	pressure	CSV	set-point	N/A	PC-CSVs
SmartCare	pressure	CSV	intelligent	N/A	PC-CSVi
Continuous Positive Airway Pressure/Pressure Support with Tube Compensation	pressure	CSV	set-point/servo	N/A	PC-CSVsr

(a servo targeting scheme) to a mode changes its classification by making the targeting scheme compound. For example, Continuous Mandatory Ventilation with AutoFlow is classified as PC-CMVa because the primary breath targeting scheme is adaptive (a). Adding Tube Compensation, a servo targeting scheme (r), changes it to PC-CMVar.

- Within-breath settings:
  - Operator-set percent support (of resistive load) along with artificial airway tube diameter and tube type
  - Ventilator-set inspiratory pressure as a function of patient-generated inspiratory flow
- *Between-breath targets:* None

Airway Pressure Release Ventilation
- *Mandatory breaths:* Machine triggered (preset frequency) and machine cycled (inspiratory time).
  - Within-breath settings:
    - Operator-set PEEP (called P_{low}), peak inspiratory pressure (called P_{high}), rise time, inspiratory time (called T_{high}), and expiratory time (called T_{low})
- *Spontaneous breaths:* Patient triggered (flow sensitivity) and patient cycled (% peak inspiratory flow). Spontaneous breaths are permitted both between and during mandatory breaths.
  - Within-breath settings:
    - Automatic tube compensation
- *Between-breath targets:* None.

Continuous Mandatory Ventilation

- *Mandatory breaths:* Machine triggered (preset frequency) or patient triggered (flow sensitivity) and machine cycled (inspiratory time)
  - Within-breath settings:
    - Operator-set PEEP, frequency, peak inspiratory flow, inspiratory time, and tidal volume
- *Spontaneous breaths:* Not allowed
- *Between-breath targets:* None

Continuous Mandatory Ventilation with AutoFlow

- *Mandatory breaths:* Machine triggered (preset frequency) or patient triggered (flow sensitivity) and machine cycled (inspiratory time)
  - Within-breath settings:
    - Operator-set PEEP, frequency, rise time, and inspiratory time
    - Ventilator-set inspiratory pressure
- *Spontaneous breaths:* Not allowed
- Between-breath targets:
  - Operator-set tidal volume

Continuous Mandatory Ventilation with Pressure Limited Ventilation

- *Mandatory breaths:* Machine triggered (preset frequency) or patient triggered (flow sensitivity) and machine cycled (inspiratory time)
  - Within-breath settings:
    - Operator-set PEEP, frequency, inspiratory flow, inspiratory time, tidal volume, and inspiratory pressure (Pmax)
    - Ventilator-set inspiratory flow if inspiration switches from volume control to pressure control when inspiratory pressure meets the inspiratory pressure target (Pmax setting)
- *Spontaneous breaths:* None
- *Between-breath targets:* None

Continuous Positive Airway Pressure/Pressure Support

- *Mandatory breaths:* Not allowed
- *Spontaneous breaths:* Patient triggered (flow sensitivity) and patient cycled (% peak inspiratory flow)
  - Within-breath settings:
    - Operator-set inspiratory pressure, rise time, and % tube compensation
- *Between-breath targets:* None

Mandatory Minute Volume Ventilation

- *Mandatory breaths:* Machine triggered (preset frequency) and machine cycled (inspiratory time). Mandatory breaths are suppressed if minute ventilation from spontaneous breaths is above preset minute ventilation target (i.e., product of tidal volume and frequency).
  - Within-breath settings:

- Operator-set PEEP, frequency, peak inspiratory flow, inspiratory time, and tidal volume
- *Spontaneous breaths:* Patient triggered (flow sensitivity) and patient cycled (% peak inspiratory flow).
  - Within-breath settings:
    - Operator-set inspiratory pressure and rise time
- Between-breath targets:
  - The settings for tidal volume and frequency constitute a between-breath target for minimum minute ventilation. Mandatory breaths are suppressed if minute ventilation from spontaneous breaths is this target.

Mandatory Minute Volume Ventilation with AutoFlow

- *Mandatory breaths:* Machine triggered (preset frequency) or patient triggered (flow sensitivity) and machine cycled (inspiratory time). Mandatory breaths are suppressed if minute ventilation from spontaneous breaths is above preset minute ventilation target (i.e., product of tidal volume and frequency).
  - Within-breath settings:
    - Operator-set PEEP, frequency, rise time, inspiratory time, and % tube compensation
    - Ventilator-set inspiratory pressure
- *Spontaneous breaths:* Patient triggered (flow sensitivity) and patient cycled (% peak inspiratory flow).
  - Within-breath settings:
    - Operator-set inspiratory pressure, rise time, and % tube compensation
- Between-breath targets:
  - Operator-set tidal volume.
  - The settings for tidal volume and frequency constitute a between-breath target for minimum minute ventilation. Mandatory breaths are suppressed if minute ventilation from spontaneous breaths is this target.

Mandatory Minute Volume Ventilation with Pressure Limited Ventilation

- *Mandatory breaths:* Machine triggered (preset frequency) or patient triggered (flow sensitivity) and machine cycled (inspiratory time). Mandatory breaths are suppressed if minute ventilation from spontaneous breaths is above preset minute ventilation target (i.e., product of tidal volume and frequency).
  - Within-breath settings:
    - Operator-set PEEP, frequency, inspiratory flow, inspiratory time, tidal volume, and inspiratory pressure (Pmax)
    - Ventilator-set inspiratory flow if inspiration switches from volume control to pressure

control when inspiratory pressure meets the inspiratory pressure target (Pmax setting)
- *Spontaneous breaths:* Patient triggered (flow sensitivity) and patient cycled (% peak inspiratory flow).
  - Within-breath settings:
    - Operator-set inspiratory pressure and rise time
- Between-breath targets:
  - The settings for tidal volume and frequency constitute a between-breath target for minimum minute ventilation. Mandatory breaths are suppressed if minute ventilation from spontaneous breaths is this target.

Pressure Controlled Ventilation Plus Assisted
- *Mandatory breaths:* Machine triggered (preset frequency) or patient triggered (flow sensitivity) and machine cycled (inspiratory time)
  - Within-breath settings:
    - Operator-set PEEP, frequency, inspiratory pressure, rise time, and inspiratory time
- *Spontaneous breaths:* Permitted during mandatory breath but not between mandatory breaths
- *Between-breath targets:* None

Pressure Controlled Ventilation Plus/Pressure Support
- *Mandatory breaths:* Machine triggered (preset frequency) or patient synchronized (pressure or flow sensitivity) and machine cycled (inspiratory time). Spontaneous breaths are permitted both between and during mandatory breaths.
  - Within-breath settings:
    - Operator-set PEEP, frequency, inspiratory pressure, rise time, inspiratory time, and % tube compensation
- *Spontaneous breaths:* Patient triggered (low sensitivity) and patient cycled (% peak inspiratory flow).
  - Within-breath settings:
    - Operator-set inspiratory pressure, rise time, and % tube compensation
- *Between-breath targets:* None.

SmartCare/Pressure Support
- *Mandatory breaths:* Not allowed
- *Spontaneous breaths:* Patient triggered (flow sensitivity) and patient cycled (% peak inspiratory flow)
  - *Within-breath settings:* None
- Between-breath targets:
  - This mode is a specialized form of Pressure Support that is designed for true (i.e., ventilator-led) automatic weaning of patients. The targeting scheme uses artificial intelligence to determine acceptable ranges for spontaneous breathing frequency, tidal volume, and end-tidal carbon dioxide tension. These ranges are then used to automatically

adjust the inspiratory pressure to maintain the patient in a respiratory zone of comfort.

The SmartCare/PS system divides the control process into three steps. The first step is to stabilize the patient within the zone of respiratory comfort, defined as combinations of tidal volume, respiratory frequency, and end-tidal CO_2 values considered acceptable by the targeting scheme. These values depend on the operator-set patient diagnosis (i.e., chronic obstructive pulmonary disease or neuromuscular disorder). The second step is to progressively decrease the inspiratory pressure while making sure the patient remains in the "zone." The third step tests readiness for extubation by maintaining the patient at the lowest level of inspiratory pressure. The lowest level depends on the type of artificial airway (endotracheal tube vs. tracheostomy tube), the type of humidifier (heat and moisture exchanger vs. a heated humidifier) and the use of automatic tube compensation. Once the lowest level of inspiratory pressure is reached, a 1-hour observation period is started (i.e., a spontaneous breathing trial) during which the patient's breathing frequency, tidal volume, and end-tidal CO_2 are monitored. Upon successful completion of this step, a message on the screen suggests that the clinician "consider separation" of the patient from the ventilator.

Synchronized Intermittent Mandatory Ventilation
- *Mandatory breaths:* Machine triggered (preset frequency) or patient triggered (flow sensitivity) and machine cycled (inspiratory time)
  - Within-breath settings:
    - Operator-set PEEP, frequency, inspiratory flow, and tidal volume
    - Ventilator-set inspiratory flow if inspiration switches from volume control to pressure control when inspiratory pressure meets the inspiratory pressure target (Pmax setting)
- *Spontaneous breaths:* Patient triggered (low sensitivity) and patient cycled (% peak inspiratory flow)
  - Within-breath settings:
    - Operator-set inspiratory pressure and rise time
- *Between-breath targets:* None

Synchronized Intermittent Mandatory Ventilation with AutoFlow
- *Mandatory breaths:* Machine triggered (preset frequency) or patient triggered (flow sensitivity) and machine cycled (inspiratory time)
  - Within-breath settings:
    - Operator-set PEEP, frequency, rise time, inspiratory time, and % tube compensation
    - Ventilator-set inspiratory pressure

- *Spontaneous breaths:* Patient triggered (flow sensitivity) and patient cycled (% peak inspiratory flow)
  - Within-breath settings:
    - Operator-set inspiratory pressure, rise time, and % tube compensation
- Between-breath targets:
  - Operator-set tidal volume

Synchronized Intermittent Mandatory Ventilation with Pressure Limited Ventilation

- *Mandatory breaths:* Machine triggered (preset frequency) or patient triggered (flow sensitivity) and machine cycled (inspiratory time)
  - Within-breath settings:
    - Operator-set PEEP, frequency, inspiratory flow, tidal volume, and inspiratory pressure (Pmax)
    - Ventilator-set inspiratory flow if inspiration switches from volume control to pressure control when inspiratory pressure meets the inspiratory pressure target (Pmax setting)
- *Spontaneous breaths:* Patient triggered (low sensitivity) and patient cycled (% peak inspiratory flow)
  - Within-breath settings:
    - Operator-set inspiratory pressure and rise time
- *Between-breath targets:* None

Special Features

Backup ventilation: Apnea ventilation can be activated in the ventilation modes SIMV, PCV Plus, CPAP, and APRV. The apnea alarm is activated if either no expiratory flow is measured or insufficient inspiratory gas is delivered during the set apnea delay time. Apnea ventilation will then start volume-controlled ventilation with the set ventilation parameters for frequency and tidal volume. Inspiratory time for apnea ventilation is determined from the set apnea ventilatory frequency and a fixed I:E ratio of 1:2. As in SIMV, the patient can breathe spontaneously during apnea ventilation, and mandatory ventilator breaths will be synchronized with the patient's spontaneous breathing.

Gas volume compensation: The ventilator determines the compliance of the patient circuit during the operation verification procedure before the start of ventilation. It then compensates for the effect of this compliance on flow and volume measurement during ventilation. The ventilator increases output volume by the same amount that will be remaining in the ventilation circuit, depending on inspiratory pressure. Flow and volume measurements are also affected by temperature and humidity, as well as by leaks in the circuit system. The ventilator takes these effects into account and corrects set and measured values accordingly.

The volume of a gas entering the lungs depends on the gas conditions (i.e., temperature, pressure, and humidity). *Measured values for flow and volume are* characterized as Body Temperature (98.6°F/37°C) and ambient Pressure Saturated (47 mm Hg) with water vapor (BTPS). Medical gases from cylinders or from a central supply, on the other hand, are dry and are delivered from the ventilator at 68°F (20°C). Flow and volume measurements under these conditions are characterized as Normal Temperature, Pressure, Dry (NTPD). The difference between values measured as NTPD or BTPS is typically around 12%. For example, a 500 mL tidal volume NTPD becomes 564 mL BTPS when warmed to 98.6°F (37°C) and humidified to 100% relative humidity. The Evita XL controls tidal volume in such a way that the set value of tidal volume is applied under BTPS conditions in the lung. Measurement at the expiratory side is made with the assumption of saturated gas at 86°F (30°C).

Miscellaneous: Sigh is set with the parameter intermittent PEEP. When the sigh function is activated, end-expiratory pressure increases by the set value of intermittent PEEP for two ventilator breaths every 3 minutes. The ventilator determines the difference between the delivered flow on the inspiratory side and the flow measured on the expiratory side. This difference provides a measure of the amount of leakage and is displayed as the leakage minute volume. During volume-controlled ventilation, the ventilator can compensate for this leakage if the option is turned on.

The Low Flow PV-Loop measuring procedure records a quasi-static pressure-volume curve, which can be used to assess the mechanical properties of the lung.

An optional CO_2 sensor can be connected to the ventilator, which will allow both end-tidal and volumetric exhaled CO_2 measurements and calculations.

Nebulizer: For adults, nebulization is applicable in every ventilation mode. The ventilator applies nebulizer gas flow synchronized with inspiratory flow while maintaining a constant minute ventilation. Depending on the O_2 concentration set, the ventilator supplies the nebulizer with air, oxygen, or a mixture of air and oxygen. Deviations from the set O_2 concentration are thus kept as low as possible. For pediatric applications, nebulizer use is possible in pressure-controlled ventilation modes. In volume-controlled ventilation modes nebulizing is only possible while using the AutoFlow ventilation mode extension. In contrast to nebulizing for adults, aerosol is delivered continuously for pediatric applications.

Neonatal ventilation: The Evital XL can be used for ventilation of premature infants by using the NeoFlow option. This option offers flow measurement at the Y-piece, which provides precise volume monitoring independent from compliance of the patient circuit in addition to accurate triggering. The automatic compensation of leaks allows for direct adjustment of tidal volume down to 3 mL.

Noninvasive ventilation: All Evita XL ventilation modes are also available for use in noninvasive ventilation therapy. NIV Plus features an advanced, dynamic leak compensation system that provides adaptive responsiveness and reliable tidal volume delivery.

Manufacturer's Specifications

Table 9-20 lists specifications for the Dräger Evita XL ventilator.

Dräger Evita Infinity V500

The Dräger Evita Infinity V500 ventilator (**Figure 9-25**) is designed for invasive and noninvasive ventilation of adult, pediatric, and neonatal patients. It is electrically controlled and pneumatically powered (requires external compressor).

Operator Interface

The Infinity V500 has an operator interface that uses a touch screen, buttons, and a control knob (**Figure 9-26**). Screen displays change according to the context of the operation, such as initial ventilator operation verification, entering ventilator settings, entering alarm settings, and reviewing monitored values including waveforms or

TABLE 9-20
Specifications for the Dräger Evita XL Ventilator

Setting Category	Setting	Range
Pressure	Inspiratory Pressure	4–40 cm H_2O
	Pressure Support	5–40 cm H_2O
	PEEP	4–25 cm H_2O
Volume	Tidal Volume	0.2–2.0 L
Flow	Waveform	Not Specified
Time	Inspiratory Time	0.3–3.0 s
	Mandatory Breath Frequency	4–60/min
	Adjustable Rise Time	Yes
Alarm Category		
Pressure	Airway Pressure	10–100 cm H_2O
Volume	Volume	0.021–4 L
Flow	Expiratory Minute Volume	0.01–40 L/min
Time	Tachypnea Monitoring	5–120/min
	Apnea Alarm Delay Time	5–60 s
Other	O_2 Sensor	Enabled/Disabled
Monitored Parameters	Max Airway Pressure	
	Plateau Pressure	
	Positive End-Expiratory Pressure	
	Mean Airway Pressure	
	Minimum Airway Pressure	
	Inspiratory O_2	
	Spontaneously Breathed Minute Volume	
	Spontaneously Breathed Tidal Volume	
	Inspiratory Tidal Volume During PS	

(continues)

TABLE 9-20
Specifications for the Dräger Evita XL Ventilator (*Continued*)

Setting Category	Setting	Range
Monitored Parameters, cont.	Spontaneous Breathing Frequency	
	Breathing Gas Temperature	
	End-Expiratory CO_2 Concentration	
	CO_2 Production	
	Serial Dead Space	
	Dead Space Ventilation	
	Compliance	
	Resistance	
	Leakage Minute Volume	
	Rapid Shallow Breathing	
	Negative Inspiratory Force	
	Expiratory Minute Volume	
	Airway Pressure	
	Inspiratory O_2 Concentration	
	Tachypnea Monitoring	
	Volume	

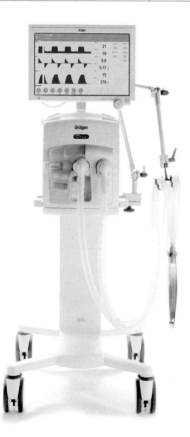

FIGURE 9-25 Dräger Evita V500 ventilator.

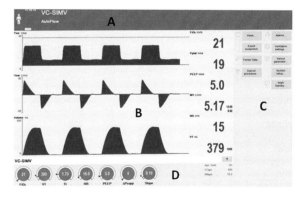

FIGURE 9-26 Dräger Evita V500 operator interface. A. Header bar (patient category, system data, therapy status, alarm status). B. Monitoring area (waveforms, loops, measured values). C. Main menu bar with buttons for opening dialog windows and activating functions. D. Therapy bar with controls for ventilation parameters.

digital values. Settings are entered by touching a virtual button on the screen to select the desired setting, turning the rotary knob to select the setting value, and then pressing the knob to finalize the setting. Other buttons provide various features related to menu navigation and alarm silencing.

The Infinity V500 has a unique interface for monitoring the patient's pulmonary status, called Smart Pulmonary View (**Figure 9-27**). This is a graphic display

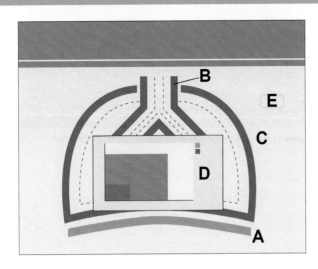

FIGURE 9-27 Dräger Smart Pulmonary View. A. The movement of the diaphragm indicates patient-triggered breaths. B. The blue line around the trachea indicates respiratory system resistance. The higher the resistance, the thicker the line. The value is also displayed. C. The blue line around the lungs indicates the respiratory system dynamic compliance. The higher the compliance, the thinner the line. The value is also displayed. D. Diagram displaying the relationship between spontaneous and mandatory ventilation. Values for tidal volume and respiratory rate are displayed for both spontaneous and mandatory breaths.

of the compliance and resistance as well as of the spontaneous and mandatory minute volume.

Modes

Modes on the Evita V500 are selected by mode name (e.g., VC-AC, VC-SIMV, etc.) using tabs on the touch screen. When the tab is selected, the relevant ventilator setting screens are displayed. The setting screens are also tabbed, giving access to basic settings (e.g., tidal volume for volume control modes and inspiratory pressure for pressure control modes) and additional settings. The additional settings include simple things like trigger sensitivity or automatic tube compensation, and complicated things such as activating AutoFlow. AutoFlow changes the mode from volume control to pressure control with adaptive targeting, essentially changing the mode classification in a major way. **Table 9-21** shows the modes available on the Dräger Evita V500.

Automatic Tube Compensation

When automatic tube compensation is active, the ventilator controls airway pressure such that the resistive load of breathing through the artificial airway is supported. Compensation may be

TABLE 9-21
Modes of Ventilation for the Dräger Evita V500

| Mode Name | Mode Classification | | | | |
	Control Variable	Breath Sequence	Primary Breath Targeting Scheme	Secondary Breath Targeting Scheme	Tag
Volume Control Continuous Mandatory Ventilation	volume	CMV	set-point	N/A	VC-CMVs
Volume Control Assist Control	volume	CMV	set-point	N/A	VC-CMVs
Volume Control Assist Control with Pressure Limited Ventilation	volume	CMV	dual	N/A	VC-CMVd
Volume Control Synchronized Intermittent Mandatory Ventilation	volume	IMV	set-point	set-point	VC-IMVs,s
Volume Control Synchronized Intermittent Mandatory Ventilation with Automatic Tube Compensation	volume	IMV	set-point	set-point/servo	VC-IMVs,sr
Volume Control Synchronized Intermittent Mandatory Ventilation with Pressure Limited Ventilation	volume	IMV	dual	set-point	VC-IMVd,s

(continues)

TABLE 9-21
Modes of Ventilation for the Dräger Evita V500 (*Continued*)

Mode Name	Mode Classification				
	Control Variable	Breath Sequence	Primary Breath Targeting Scheme	Secondary Breath Targeting Scheme	Tag
Volume Control Synchronized Intermittent Mandatory Ventilation with Pressure Limited Ventilation and Automatic Tube Compensation	volume	IMV	dual	set-point/servo	VC-IMVd,sr
Volume Control Mandatory Minute Volume Ventilation	volume	IMV	adaptive	set-point	VC-IMVa,s
Volume Control Mandatory Minute Volume Ventilation with Automatic Tube Compensation	volume	IMV	adaptive	set-point/servo	VC-IMVa,sr
Volume Control Mandatory Minute Volume with AutoFlow/Volume Guarantee	pressure	IMV	adaptive	set-point	PC-IMVa,s
Volume Control Mandatory Minute Volume with AutoFlow/Volume Guarantee and Automatic Tube Compensation	pressure	IMV	adaptive/servo	set-point/servo	PC-IMVa,sr
Volume Control Mandatory Minute Volume with Pressure Limited Ventilation	volume	IMV	dual/adaptive	set-point	VC-IMVda,s
Volume Control Mandatory Minute Volume with Pressure Limited Ventilation and Automatic Tube Compensation	volume	IMV	dual/adaptive	set-point/servo	VC-IMVda,sr
Pressure Control Assist Control	pressure	CMV	set-point	N/A	PC-CMVs
Pressure Control Assist Control with Automatic Tube Compensation	pressure	CMV	set-point/servo	N/A	PC-CMVsr
Volume Control Continuous Mandatory Ventilation with AutoFlow/Volume Guarantee	pressure	CMV	adaptive	N/A	PC-CMVa
Volume Control Continuous Mandatory Ventilation with AutoFlow/Volume Guarantee and Automatic Tube Compensation	pressure	CMV	adaptive/servo	N/A	PC-CMVar
Volume Control Assist Control with AutoFlow/Volume Guarantee	pressure	CMV	adaptive	N/A	PC-CMVa

TABLE 9-21
Modes of Ventilation for the Dräger Evita V500 (*Continued*)

Mode Name	Control Variable	Breath Sequence	Primary Breath Targeting Scheme	Secondary Breath Targeting Scheme	Tag
Volume Control Assist Control with AutoFlow/ Volume Guarantee and Automatic Tube Compensation	pressure	CMV	adaptive/servo	N/A	PC-CMVar
Pressure Control Continuous Mandatory Ventilation	pressure	CMV	set-point	N/A	PC-CMVs
Pressure Control Continuous Mandatory Ventilation with Automatic Tube Compensation	pressure	CMV	set-point/servo	N/A	PC-CMVsr
Pressure Control Synchronized Intermittent Mandatory Ventilation	pressure	IMV	set-point	set-point	PC-IMVs,s
Pressure Control Synchronized Intermittent Mandatory Ventilation with Automatic Tube Compensation	pressure	IMV	set-point/servo	set-point/servo	PC-IMVsr,sr
Pressure Control Biphasic Positive Airway Pressure	pressure	IMV	set-point	set-point	PC-IMVs,s
Pressure Control Biphasic Positive Airway Pressure with Automatic Tube Compensation	pressure	IMV	set-point/servo	set-point/servo	PC-IMVsr,sr
Pressure Control Airway Pressure Release Ventilation	pressure	IMV	set-point	set-point	PC-IMVs,s
Pressure Control Airway Pressure Release Ventilation with Automatic Tube Compensation	pressure	IMV	set-point/servo	set-point/servo	PC-IMVsr,sr
Pressure Control Pressure Support Ventilation	pressure	IMV	set-point	set-point	PC-IMVs,s
Pressure Control Pressure Support Ventilation with Automatic Tube Compensation	pressure	IMV	set-point/servo	set-point/servo	PC-IMVsr,sr
Volume Control Synchronized Intermittent Mandatory Ventilation with AutoFlow	pressure	IMV	adaptive	set-point	PC-IMVa,s
Volume Control Synchronized Intermittent Mandatory Ventilation with AutoFlow and Automatic Tube Compensation	pressure	IMV	adaptive/servo	set-point/servo	PC-IMVar,sr

(continues)

TABLE 9-21
Modes of Ventilation for the Dräger Evita V500 (*Continued*)

Mode Name	Control Variable	Breath Sequence	Mode Classification Primary Breath Targeting Scheme	Secondary Breath Targeting Scheme	Tag
Spontaneous Continuous Positive Airway Pressure/ Pressure Support	pressure	CSV	set-point	N/A	PC-CSVs
Spontaneous Continuous Positive Airway Pressure/ Pressure Support with Automatic Tube Compensation	pressure	CSV	set-point/servo	N/A	PC-CSVsr
Spontaneous Continuous Positive Airway Pressure/ Variable Pressure Support	pressure	CSV	bio-variable	N/A	PC-CSVb
Spontaneous Continuous Positive Airway Pressure/ Variable Pressure Support with Automatic Tube Compensation	pressure	CSV	bio-variable/servo	N/A	PC-CSVbr
Spontaneous Continuous Positive Airway Pressure/ Volume Support	pressure	CSV	adaptive	N/A	PC-CSVa
Spontaneous Continuous Positive Airway Pressure/ Volume Support with Automatic Tube Compensation	pressure	CSV	adaptive/servo	N/A	PC-CSVar
Spontaneous Proportional Pressure Support	pressure	CSV	servo	N/A	PC-CSVr
SmartCare	pressure	CSV	intelligent	N/A	PC-CSVi

Reproduced with permission from Mandu Press Ltd.

independently deactivated for the expiratory breathing cycle. Depending on the direction of the patient flow, the airway pressure is increased during inspiration or decreased during expiration. Tube compensation may be applied to spontaneous breaths and mandatory breaths in pressure control modes. Adding tube compensation (a servo targeting scheme) to a mode changes its classification by making the targeting scheme compound. For example, Continuous Mandatory Ventilation with AutoFlow is classified as PC-CMVa because the primary breath targeting scheme is adaptive (a). Adding Tube Compensation, a servo targeting scheme (r), changes it to PC-CMVar.

- Within-breath settings:
  - Operator-set Tube Compensation is set as a percent support (of resistive load) along with artificial airway tube diameter and tube type
  - Ventilator-set inspiratory pressure as a function of patient-generated inspiratory flow
- *Between-breath targets:* None

Pressure Control Airway Pressure Release Ventilation

- *Mandatory breaths:* Machine triggered (preset frequency) and machine cycled (inspiratory time). Patient triggering of mandatory breaths is possible using the AutoRelease feature. This triggers inspiration once a preset expiratory flow threshold is reached. When AutoRelease is turned on, the switch from P_{high} to P_{low} is synchronized with the patient's breathing. Thus, with AutoRelease, what were formerly machine-triggered and machine-cycled (mandatory) breaths are converted to patient-triggered and patient-cycled (spontaneous) breaths.
  - Within-breath settings:
    - Operator-set PEEP (called P_{low}), peak inspiratory pressure (called P_{high}), rise time, inspiratory time (called T_{high}), and expiratory time (called T_{low}). The inspiratory trigger sensitivity may also be set (using AutoRelease) as a percentage of peak expiratory flow.

- *Spontaneous breaths:* Patient triggered (flow sensitivity) and patient cycled (% peak inspiratory flow). Spontaneous breaths are permitted both between and during mandatory breaths.
  - Within-breath settings:
    - Automatic tube compensation
- *Between-breath targets:* None.

Pressure Control Assist Control

- *Mandatory breaths:* Machine triggered (preset frequency) or patient triggered (flow sensitivity) and machine cycled (inspiratory time)
  - Within-breath settings:
    - Operator-set PEEP, frequency, inspiratory pressure, rise time, and inspiratory time
- *Spontaneous breaths:* Permitted during mandatory breath but not between mandatory breaths
- *Between-breath targets:* None

Pressure Control Biphasic Positive Airway Pressure

- *Mandatory breaths:* Machine triggered (preset frequency) or patient synchronized (pressure or flow sensitivity) and machine cycled (inspiratory time) or patient cycled (synchronized with a spontaneous expiration after a spontaneous inspiration during the mandatory breath). Spontaneous breaths are permitted both between and during mandatory breaths.
  - Within-breath settings:
    - Operator-set PEEP, frequency, inspiratory pressure, rise time, and inspiratory time
- *Spontaneous breaths:* Patient triggered (flow sensitivity) and patient cycled (% peak inspiratory flow).
  - Within-breath settings:
    - Operator-set inspiratory pressure and rise time
- *Between-breath targets:* None.

Pressure Control Continuous Mandatory Ventilation

- *Mandatory breaths:* Machine triggered (preset frequency) and machine cycled (inspiratory time). Spontaneous breaths are permitted both between and during mandatory breaths. Because of this feature, the mode is classified as a form of intermittent mandatory ventilation, not continuous mandatory ventilation, despite the name given by Dräger.
  - Within-breath settings:
    - Operator-set PEEP, frequency, inspiratory pressure, rise time, and inspiratory time
- *Spontaneous breaths:* Patient triggered (flow sensitivity) and patient cycled (% peak inspiratory flow).
  - *Within-breath settings:* None
- *Between-breath targets:* None.

Pressure Control Pressure Support

- *Mandatory breaths:* Machine triggered (preset frequency) and patient cycled (% peak inspiratory flow). Spontaneous breaths triggered at a frequency higher than the set frequency suppress mandatory breaths.
  - Within-breath settings:
    - Operator-set PEEP, frequency, inspiratory pressure, rise time, and inspiratory time
- *Spontaneous breaths:* Patient triggered (flow sensitivity) and patient cycled (% peak inspiratory flow).
  - Within-breath settings:
    - Operator-set inspiratory pressure and rise time
- *Between-breath targets:* None.

Pressure Control Synchronized Intermittent Mandatory Ventilation

- *Mandatory breaths:* Machine triggered (preset frequency) or patient synchronized (flow sensitivity) and machine cycled (inspiratory time). Spontaneous breaths are permitted both between and during mandatory breaths.
  - Within-breath settings:
    - Operator-set PEEP, frequency, inspiratory pressure, rise time, and inspiratory time
- *Spontaneous breaths:* Patient triggered (flow sensitivity) and patient cycled (% peak inspiratory flow).
  - Within-breath settings:
    - Operator-set inspiratory pressure and rise time
- *Between-breath targets:* None.

SmartCare/Pressure Support

- *Mandatory breaths:* Not allowed
- *Spontaneous breaths:* Patient triggered (flow sensitivity) and patient cycled (% peak inspiratory flow)
  - *Within-breath settings*: None
- Between-breath targets:
  - This mode is a specialized form of Pressure Support that is designed for true (i.e., ventilator-led) automatic weaning of patients. The targeting scheme uses artificial intelligence to determine acceptable ranges for spontaneous breathing frequency, tidal volume, and end-tidal carbon dioxide tension. These ranges are then used to automatically adjust the inspiratory pressure to maintain the patient in a respiratory zone of comfort.

    The SmartCare/PS system divides the control process into three steps. The first step is to stabilize the patient within the zone of respiratory comfort, defined as combinations of tidal volume, respiratory frequency, and end-tidal CO_2

values considered acceptable by the targeting scheme. These values depend on the operator-set patient diagnosis (i.e., chronic obstructive pulmonary disease or neuromuscular disorder). The second step is to progressively decrease the inspiratory pressure while making sure the patient remains in the "zone." The third step tests readiness for extubation by maintaining the patient at the lowest level of inspiratory pressure. The lowest level depends on the type of artificial airway (endotracheal tube vs. tracheostomy tube), the type of humidifier (heat and moisture exchanger vs. a heated humidifier), and the use of Automatic Tube Compensation. Once the lowest level of inspiratory pressure is reached, a 1-hour observation period is started (i.e., a spontaneous breathing trial), during which the patient's breathing frequency, tidal volume, and end-tidal CO_2 are monitored. Upon successful completion of this step, a message on the screen suggests that the clinician "consider separation" of the patient from the ventilator.

Spontaneous Continuous Positive Airway Pressure/Pressure Support

- *Mandatory breaths:* Not allowed
- *Spontaneous breaths:* Patient triggered (flow sensitivity) and patient cycled (% peak inspiratory flow)
  - Within-breath settings:
    - Operator-set inspiratory pressure and rise time
- *Between-breath targets:* None

Spontaneous Continuous Positive Airway Pressure/Variable Pressure Support

- *Mandatory breaths:* Not allowed
- *Spontaneous breaths:* Patient triggered (flow sensitivity) and patient cycled (% peak inspiratory flow)
  - Within-breath settings:
    - Operator-set rise time
    - Ventilator-set inspiratory pressure
- Between-breath targets:
  - Operator-set average inspiratory pressure.
  - Operator-set percentage (0–100%) of set average inspiratory pressure that acts as the range of values for individual breaths. The ventilator varies the within-breath inspiratory pressure target randomly within this range to achieve randomly variable tidal volumes for individual breaths.

Spontaneous Continuous Positive Airway Pressure/Volume Support

- *Mandatory breaths:* Not allowed
- *Spontaneous breaths:* Patient triggered (pressure or flow sensitivity) and patient cycled (% peak inspiratory flow)
  - Within-breath settings:
    - Operator-set cycle sensitivity (% peak inspiratory flow)
    - Ventilator-set inspiratory pressure
- Between-breath targets:
  - Operator-set average tidal volume

Spontaneous Proportional Pressure Support

- *Mandatory breaths:* Not allowed
- *Spontaneous breaths:* Patient triggered (pressure or flow sensitivity) and patient cycled (% peak inspiratory flow)
  - *Within-breath settings:* None
- Between-breath targets:
  - Operator-set flow assist (amount of resistance to be supported) and volume assist (amount of elastance to be supported)

Volume Control Assist Control

- *Mandatory breaths:* Machine triggered (preset frequency) or patient triggered (flow sensitivity) and machine cycled (inspiratory time)
  - Within-breath settings:
    - Operator-set PEEP, frequency, peak inspiratory flow, inspiratory time, and tidal volume
- *Spontaneous breaths:* Not allowed
- *Between-breath targets:* None

Volume Control Assist Control with AutoFlow/Volume Guarantee

- *Mandatory breaths:* Machine triggered (preset frequency) or patient triggered (flow sensitivity) and machine cycled (inspiratory time)
  - Within-breath settings:
    - Operator-set PEEP, frequency, rise time, and inspiratory time
    - Ventilator-set inspiratory pressure
- *Spontaneous breaths:* Not allowed
- Between-breath targets:
  - Operator-set tidal volume

Volume Control Assist Control with Pressure Limited Ventilation

- *Mandatory breaths:* Machine triggered (preset frequency) or patient triggered (flow sensitivity) and machine cycled (inspiratory time)
  - Within-breath settings:
    - Operator-set PEEP, frequency, inspiratory flow, inspiratory time, tidal volume, and inspiratory pressure (Pmax)
    - Ventilator-set inspiratory flow if inspiration switches from volume control to pressure control when inspiratory pressure meets the inspiratory pressure target (Pmax setting)
- *Spontaneous breaths:* None
- *Between-breath targets:* None

Volume Control Continuous Mandatory Ventilation

- *Mandatory breaths:* Machine triggered (preset frequency) and machine cycled (inspiratory time). Patient-triggered breaths are not allowed.
  - Within-breath settings:
    - Operator-set PEEP, frequency, peak inspiratory flow, inspiratory time, and tidal volume
- *Spontaneous breaths:* Not allowed.
- *Between-breath targets:* None.

Volume Control Continuous Mandatory Ventilation with AutoFlow/Volume Guarantee

- *Mandatory breaths:* Machine triggered (preset frequency) and machine cycled (inspiratory time). Patient-triggered breaths are not allowed.
  - Within-breath settings:
    - Operator-set PEEP, frequency, rise time, and inspiratory time
    - Ventilator-set inspiratory pressure
- *Spontaneous breaths:* Not allowed.
- Between-breath targets:
  - Operator-set tidal volume

Volume Control Mandatory Minute Volume Ventilation

- *Mandatory breaths:* Machine triggered (preset frequency) and machine cycled (inspiratory time). Mandatory breaths are suppressed if minute ventilation from spontaneous breaths is above preset minute ventilation target (i.e., product of tidal volume and frequency).
  - Within-breath settings:
    - Operator-set PEEP, frequency, peak inspiratory flow, inspiratory time, and tidal volume
- *Spontaneous breaths:* Patient triggered (flow sensitivity) and patient cycled (% peak inspiratory flow).
  - Within-breath settings:
    - Operator-set inspiratory pressure and rise time
- Between-breath targets:
  - The settings for tidal volume and frequency constitute a between-breath target for minimum minute ventilation. Mandatory breaths are suppressed if minute ventilation from spontaneous breaths is this target.

Volume Control Mandatory Minute Volume Ventilation with AutoFlow/Volume Guarantee

- *Mandatory breaths:* Machine triggered (preset frequency) or patient triggered (flow sensitivity) and machine cycled (inspiratory time). Mandatory breaths are suppressed if minute ventilation from spontaneous breaths is above preset minute ventilation target (i.e., product of tidal volume and frequency).
  - Within-breath settings:
    - Operator-set PEEP, frequency, rise time, and inspiratory time
    - Ventilator-set inspiratory pressure

- *Spontaneous breaths:* Patient triggered (flow sensitivity) and patient cycled (% peak inspiratory flow).
  - Within-breath settings:
    - Operator-set inspiratory pressure and rise time
- Between-breath targets:
  - Operator-set tidal volume.
  - The settings for tidal volume and frequency constitute a between-breath target for minimum minute ventilation. Mandatory breaths are suppressed if minute ventilation from spontaneous breaths is this target.

Volume Control Mandatory Minute Volume Ventilation with Pressure Limited Ventilation

- *Mandatory breaths:* Machine triggered (preset frequency) or patient triggered (flow sensitivity) and machine cycled (inspiratory time). Mandatory breaths are suppressed if minute ventilation from spontaneous breaths is above preset minute ventilation target (i.e., product of tidal volume and frequency).
  - Within-breath settings:
    - Operator-set PEEP, frequency, inspiratory flow, inspiratory time, tidal volume, and inspiratory pressure (Pmax)
    - Ventilator-set inspiratory flow if inspiration switches from volume control to pressure control when inspiratory pressure meets the inspiratory pressure target (Pmax setting)
- *Spontaneous breaths:* Patient triggered (flow sensitivity) and patient cycled (% peak inspiratory flow).
  - Within-breath settings:
    - Operator-set inspiratory pressure and rise time
- Between-breath targets:
  - The settings for tidal volume and frequency constitute a between-breath target for minimum minute ventilation. Mandatory breaths are suppressed if minute ventilation from spontaneous breaths is this target.

Volume Control Synchronized Intermittent Mandatory Ventilation

- *Mandatory breaths:* Machine triggered (preset frequency) or patient triggered (flow sensitivity) and machine cycled (inspiratory time)
  - Within-breath settings:
    - Operator-set PEEP, frequency, inspiratory flow, and tidal volume
    - Ventilator-set inspiratory flow if inspiration switches from volume control to pressure control when inspiratory pressure meets the inspiratory pressure target (Pmax setting)

- *Spontaneous breaths:* Patient triggered (flow sensitivity) and patient cycled (% peak inspiratory flow)
  - Within-breath settings:
    - Operator-set inspiratory pressure and rise time
- *Between-breath targets:* None

Volume Control Synchronized Intermittent Mandatory Ventilation with AutoFlow/Volume Guarantee

- *Mandatory breaths:* Machine triggered (preset frequency) or patient triggered (flow sensitivity) and machine cycled (inspiratory time)
  - Within-breath settings:
    - Operator-set PEEP, frequency, rise time, and inspiratory time
    - Ventilator-set inspiratory pressure
- *Spontaneous breaths:* Patient triggered (flow sensitivity) and patient cycled (% peak inspiratory flow)
  - Within-breath settings:
    - Operator-set inspiratory pressure and rise time
- Between-breath targets:
  - Operator-set tidal volume

Volume Control Synchronized Intermittent Mandatory Ventilation with Pressure Limited Ventilation

- *Mandatory breaths:* Machine triggered (preset frequency) or patient triggered (flow sensitivity) and machine cycled (inspiratory time)
  - Within-breath settings:
    - Operator-set PEEP, frequency, inspiratory flow, tidal volume, and inspiratory pressure (Pmax)
    - Ventilator-set inspiratory flow if inspiration switches from volume control to pressure control when inspiratory pressure meets the inspiratory pressure target (Pmax setting)
- *Spontaneous breaths:* Patient triggered (flow sensitivity) and patient cycled (% peak inspiratory flow)
  - Within-breath settings:
    - Operator-set inspiratory pressure and rise time
- *Between-breath targets:* None

Special Features

Backup ventilation: If an adult patient is ventilated using a volume-controlled mode without AutoFlow, apnea ventilation is also volume-controlled without AutoFlow. In all other cases, apnea ventilation is volume-controlled with AutoFlow. The ventilator detects an apnea when no expiratory flow is measured or insufficient inspiratory gas is delivered during the set apnea alarm time. If apnea ventilation is activated, volume-controlled synchronized

intermittent mandatory ventilation starts with the preset apnea rate and tidal volume. The inspiratory time for apnea ventilation is determined from the set apnea ventilation rate and a fixed I:E ratio of 1:2. Apnea ventilation for neonates is Volume Guaranteed SIMV.

Gas volume compensation: The ventilator determines the compliance of the patient circuit during the operation verification procedure before the start of ventilation. It then compensates for the effect of this compliance on flow and volume measurement during ventilation. The ventilator increases output volume by the same amount that will be remaining in the ventilation circuit, depending on inspiratory pressure. Flow and volume measurements are also affected by temperature and humidity, as well as by leaks in the circuit system. The ventilator takes these effects into account and corrects set and measured values accordingly.

The volume of a gas entering the lungs depends on the gas conditions (i.e., temperature, pressure, and humidity). Measured values for flow and volume are characterized as body temperature (98.6°F/37°C) and ambient pressure saturated (47 mm Hg) with water vapor (BTPS). Medical gases from cylinders or from a central supply, on the other hand, are dry and are delivered from the ventilator at 68°F (20°C). Flow and volume measurements under these conditions are characterized as normal temperature and pressure, dry (NTPD). The difference between values measured as NTPD or BTPS is typically around 12%. For example, 500 mL tidal volume NTPD becomes 564 mL BTPS when warmed to 98.6°F (37°C) and humidified to 100% relative humidity. The Evita V500 controls tidal volume in such a way that the set value of tidal volume is applied under BTPS conditions in the lung. Measurement at the expiratory side is made with the assumption of saturated gas at 86°F (30°C).

Miscellaneous: The sigh function can be activated in all ventilation modes with mandatory breaths, except for PC-APRV. When the sigh function is activated, the end-expiratory pressure PEEP increases by the set value of the intermittent PEEP. In pressure-controlled ventilation, the inspiratory pressures increase by an amount equal to the intermittent PEEP. The time between the two sigh phases can be set. The operator can also set how many respiratory cycles are covered by the sigh phase.

The Low Flow PV-Loop measuring procedure records a quasi-static pressure–volume curve, which can be used to assess the mechanical properties of the lung.

An optional CO_2 sensor can be connected to the ventilator, which will allow both end-tidal and volumetric exhaled CO_2 measurements and calculations.

Nebulizer: For adults, nebulization is applicable in every ventilation mode. The ventilator applies nebulizer gas flow synchronized with inspiratory flow while maintaining a constant minute ventilation. Depending on the O_2 concentration set, the ventilator supplies the nebulizer with air, oxygen, or a mixture of air and oxygen. Deviations from the set O_2 concentration are thus kept as low as possible. For pediatric applications, nebulizer use is possible in pressure-controlled ventilation modes. In volume-controlled ventilation modes, nebulizing is possible only while using the AutoFlow ventilation mode extension. In contrast to nebulizing for adults, aerosol is delivered continuously for pediatric applications. The ventilator can also be used with the Aeroneb Pro vibrating mesh nebulizer.

Neonatal ventilation: The neonatal mode offers flow measurement at the Y-piece, which provides precise volume monitoring independent from compliance of the patient circuit in addition to accurate triggering. The measured values for minute ventilation and tidal volume are not leakage-corrected and are therefore lower than the actual minute and tidal volumes applied to the patient if a leakage occurs. When leakage compensation is activated, the measured volume and flow values as well as the curves for flow and volume are displayed with leakage correction. The Infinity V500 compensates leakages up to 100% of the set tidal volume.

Noninvasive ventilation: Noninvasive ventilation by mask is available for patients with spontaneous breathing. The ventilator compensates for mask leakages. The inspiratory trigger and the cycle criterion are automatically adapted to the measured leakage. This prevents auto-triggering due to a flow trigger that has been set too low. It also prevents delayed cycling due to a termination criterion that has been set too high. The inspiratory tidal volume is typically far higher than the patient's tidal volume. The expiratory tidal volume is slightly lower than the patient's tidal volume. The measured values for tidal volume are leakage-corrected and indicate the patient's actual tidal volume. In the ventilation modes with AutoFlow and Volume Guarantee, the corrected measured values are set when leakage compensation is selected. During volume-controlled ventilation, the inspiratory volume escaping through the leak is additionally supplied.

Manufacturer's Specifications

Table 9-22 lists specifications for the Dräger Infinity V500 ventilator.

GE Healthcare Engström Carestation

The Engström Carestation (Figure 9-28) is designed to be used with infant through adult patients with a body

TABLE 9-22
Specifications for the Dräger Infinity V500 Ventilator

Setting Category	Setting	Range
Pressure	Inspiratory Pressure	1–95 cm H_2O
	Pressure Support	0–95 cm H_2O
	PEEP	0–50 cm H_2O
Volume	Tidal Volume	0.002–3.0 L
Flow	Inspiratory Flow	2–120 L/min
	Waveform	Not Specified
Time	Inspiratory Time	0.1–10 s
	Mandatory Breath Frequency	0.5–150/min
	Adjustable Rise Time	Yes
Sensitivity	Trigger Sensitivity (flow)	0.2–15 L/min
	Cycle Sensitivity (flow)	1–80%

(continues)

TABLE 9-22
Specifications for the Dräger Infinity V500 Ventilator (*Continued*)

Setting Category	Setting	Range
Alarm Category		
Pressure	Airway Pressure	7–105 cm H_2O
Volume	Upper Tidal Volume	0.003–3.1 L
	Lower Tidal Volume	0.001–2.9 L
Flow	Upper Expiratory Minute Volume	0.03–60 L/min
	Lower Expiratory Minute Volume	0.02–40 L/min
Time	Upper Respiratory Rate	5–200/min
	Apnea Time	5–60 s
Other	O_2 Sensor	Enabled/Disabled
Monitored Parameters	Expiratory Minute Volume	
	Airway Pressure	
	Maximum Airway Pressure	
	Insp. O_2 Concentration	
	End-Expiratory CO_2 Concentration	
	Respiratory Rate	
	Tidal Volume	
	Occlusion Pressure (P0.1)	
	Intrinsic PEEP	
	Negative Inspiratory Force (NIF)	
	C20/C	

weight of 11 lb (5 kg) or greater. If the neonatal option is installed on the ventilator, patients weighing down to 0.55 lb (0.25 kg) may be ventilated with the Engström.

Operator Interface

The Engström has an operator interface that uses a touch screen, buttons, and a control knob (**Figure 9-29**). Screen displays change according to the context of the operation, such as initial ventilator operation verification, entering ventilator settings, entering alarm settings, and reviewing monitored values including waveforms or digital values. Settings are entered by touching a virtual button on the screen to select the desired setting, turning the rotary knob to select the setting value, and then pressing the knob to finalize the setting. Other buttons provide various features related to menu navigation, temporary increased oxygen delivery (2 minutes), and alarm silencing.

Modes

Modes on the Engström are selected by mode name (e.g., VCV, PCV, SIMV-VC, etc.) using a menu. Specific mode settings are selected using other menus. Available modes are shown in **Table 9-23**.

Airway Resistance Compensation

Airway Resistance Compensation (ARC) adjusts the target delivery pressure to compensate for the resistance caused by the endotracheal tube or tracheostomy tube used. The compensation is applied to the

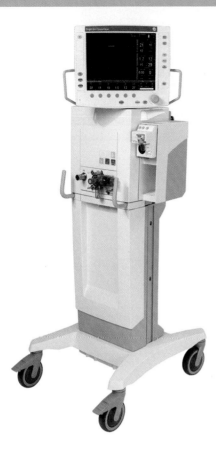

FIGURE 9-28 GE Healthcare Engström Carestation ventilator.

Used with permission of GE Healthcare.

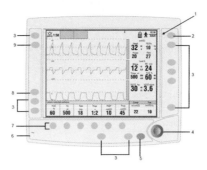

FIGURE 9-29 GE Healthcare Engström Carestation operator interface. 1. Alarm LEDs. 2. Silence Alarms key. 3. Menu keys. 4. ComWheel (turn to scroll menu or change settings; push to select menu item). 5. Normal Screen key. 6. AC mains indicator. 7. Quick keys (push to change corresponding ventilator setting). 8. O_2 key (delivers increased F_IO_2 for 2 minutes). 9. Lock/unlock.

Used with permission of GE Healthcare.

inspiratory phase of all pressure-controlled, CPAP, and pressure-supported breaths.

- Within-breath settings:
  - Operator-set percent support (of resistive load) along with artificial airway tube diameter and tube type
  - Ventilator-set inspiratory pressure as a function of patient-generated inspiratory flow
- *Between-breath targets:* None

TABLE 9-23

Classification of Modes for Engström Carestation Ventilator

Mode Name	Mode Classification				
	Control Variable	Breath Sequence	Primary Breath Targeting Scheme	Secondary Breath Targeting Scheme	Tag
Volume Controlled Ventilation	volume	CMV	set-point	N/A	VC-CMVs
Volume Controlled Ventilation with Pressure Limit	volume	CMV	dual	N/A	VC-CMVd
Synchronized Intermittent Mandatory Ventilation-Volume Controlled	volume	IMV	set-point	set-point	VC-IMVs,s
Synchronized Intermittent Mandatory Ventilation-Volume Controlled with Airway Resistance Compensation	volume	IMV	set-point	set-point/servo	VC-IMVs,sr
Synchronized Intermittent Mandatory Ventilation-Volume Controlled with Pressure Limit	volume	IMV	dual	set-point	VC-IMVd,s
Synchronized Intermittent Mandatory Ventilation-Volume Controlled with Pressure Limit and Airway Resistance Compensation	volume	IMV	dual	set-point/servo	VC-IMVd,sr

(continues)

TABLE 9-23

Classification of Modes for Engström Carestation Ventilator *(Continued)*

Mode Name	Mode Classification				Tag
	Control Variable	Breath Sequence	Primary Breath Targeting Scheme	Secondary Breath Targeting Scheme	
Pressure Controlled Ventilation	pressure	CMV	set-point	N/A	PC-CMVs
Pressure Controlled Ventilation with Airway Resistance Compensation	pressure	CMV	set-point/servo	N/A	PC-CMVsr
Pressure Controlled Ventilation-Volume Guaranteed	pressure	CMV	adaptive	N/A	PC-CMVa
Pressure Controlled Ventilation-Volume Guaranteed with Airway Resistance Compensation	pressure	CMV	adaptive/servo	N/A	PC-CMVar
Synchronized Intermittent Mandatory Ventilation-Pressure Controlled	pressure	IMV	set-point	set-point	PC-IMVs,s
Synchronized Intermittent Mandatory Ventilation-Pressure Controlled with Airway Resistance Compensation	pressure	IMV	set-point/servo	set-point/servo	PC-IMVsr,sr
Bilevel Airway Pressure Ventilation	pressure	IMV	set-point	set-point	PC-IMVs,s
Bilevel Airway Pressure Ventilation with Airway Resistance Compensation	pressure	IMV	set-point/servo	set-point/servo	PC-IMVsr,sr
Bilevel Airway Pressure Ventilation-Volume Guaranteed	pressure	IMV	adaptive	set-point	PC-IMVa,s
Bilevel Airway Pressure Ventilation-Volume Guaranteed with Airway Resistance Compensation	pressure	IMV	adaptive/servo	set-point/servo	PC-IMVar,sr
Synchronized Intermittent Mandatory Ventilation-Pressure Controlled Volume Guaranteed	pressure	IMV	adaptive	set-point	PC-IMVa,s
Synchronized Intermittent Mandatory Ventilation-Pressure Controlled Volume Guaranteed with Airway Resistance Compensation	pressure	IMV	adaptive/servo	set-point/servo	PC-IMVar,sr
Constant Positive Airway Pressure/Pressure Support	pressure	CSV	set-point	N/A	PC-CSVs
Constant Positive Airway Pressure/Pressure Support with Airway Resistance Compensation	pressure	CSV	set-point/servo	N/A	PC-CSVsr
Volume Guarantee Pressure Support	pressure	CSV	adaptive	N/A	PC-CSVa
Volume Guarantee Pressure Support with Airway Resistance Compensation	pressure	CSV	adaptive/servo	N/A	PC-CSVar

Bilevel Airway Pressure Ventilation

- *Mandatory breaths:* Machine triggered (preset frequency) or patient synchronized (pressure or flow sensitivity) and machine cycled (inspiratory time or patient synchronized by flow sensitivity).
  - Within-breath settings:
    - Operator-set PEEP (called $PEEP_{low}$), peak inspiratory pressure (called $PEEP_{high}$), rise time, inspiratory time, and frequency
- *Spontaneous breaths:* Patient triggered (pressure or flow sensitivity) and patient cycled (% peak inspiratory flow). Spontaneous breaths are permitted both between and during mandatory breaths.
  - Within-breath settings:
    - Operator-set inspiratory pressure and rise time
- *Between-breath targets:* None.

Bilevel Airway Pressure Ventilation-Volume Guaranteed

- *Mandatory breaths:* Machine triggered (preset frequency) or patient triggered (pressure or flow sensitivity) and machine cycled (inspiratory time)
  - Within-breath settings:
    - Operator-set PEEP, frequency, rise time, and inspiratory time
    - Ventilator-set inspiratory pressure
- *Spontaneous breaths:* Patient triggered (pressure or flow sensitivity) and patient cycled (% peak inspiratory flow)
  - Within-breath settings:
    - Operator-set inspiratory pressure and rise time
- Between-breath targets:
  - Operator-set tidal volume

Constant Positive Airway Pressure/Pressure Support

- *Mandatory breaths:* Not allowed
- *Spontaneous breaths:* Patient triggered (pressure or flow sensitivity) and patient cycled (% peak inspiratory flow)
  - Within-breath settings:
    - Operator-set inspiratory pressure and rise time
- *Between-breath targets:* None

Pressure Controlled Ventilation

- *Mandatory breaths:* Machine triggered (preset frequency) or patient triggered (pressure or flow sensitivity) and machine cycled (inspiratory time)
  - Within-breath settings:
    - Operator-set PEEP, frequency, inspiratory pressure, rise time, and I:E ratio
- *Spontaneous breaths:* Not allowed
- *Between-breath targets:* None

Pressure Controlled Ventilation-Volume Guarantee

- *Mandatory breaths:* Machine triggered (preset frequency) or patient triggered (pressure or flow sensitivity) and machine cycled (inspiratory time)
  - Within-breath settings:
    - Operator-set PEEP, frequency, rise time, and I:E ratio
    - Ventilator-set inspiratory pressure
- *Spontaneous breaths:* Not allowed
- Between-breath targets:
  - Operator-set tidal volume

Synchronized Intermittent Mandatory Ventilation-Pressure Controlled

- *Mandatory breaths:* Machine triggered (preset frequency or patient synchronized using pressure or flow sensitivity) and machine cycled (inspiratory time)
  - Within-breath settings:
    - Operator-set PEEP, frequency, rise time, and I:E ratio
    - Ventilator-set inspiratory pressure
- *Spontaneous breaths:* Patient triggered (pressure or flow sensitivity) and patient cycled (% peak inspiratory flow)
  - Within-breath settings:
    - Operator-set inspiratory pressure, rise time, and cycle sensitivity (% peak inspiratory flow)
- *Between-breath targets:* None

Synchronized Intermittent Mandatory Ventilation-Pressure Controlled Volume Guaranteed

- *Mandatory breaths:* Machine triggered (preset frequency or patient synchronized using pressure or flow sensitivity) and machine cycled (inspiratory time)
  - Within-breath settings:
    - Operator-set PEEP, frequency, rise time, and I:E ratio
    - Ventilator-set inspiratory pressure
- *Spontaneous breaths:* Patient triggered (pressure or flow sensitivity) and patient cycled (% peak inspiratory flow)
  - Within-breath settings:
    - Operator-set inspiratory pressure, rise time, and cycle sensitivity (% peak inspiratory flow)
- Between-breath targets:
  - Operator-set tidal volume

Synchronized Intermittent Mandatory Ventilation-Volume Controlled

- *Mandatory breaths:* Machine triggered (preset frequency) or patient synchronized (pressure or flow sensitivity) and machine cycled (tidal volume or pause time)

- Within-breath settings:
  - Operator-set PEEP, frequency, tidal volume, and inspiratory time
- *Spontaneous breaths:* Patient triggered (pressure or flow sensitivity) and patient cycled (% peak inspiratory flow)
  - Within-breath settings:
    - Operator-set inspiratory pressure, rise time, and cycle sensitivity (% peak inspiratory flow)
- *Between-breath targets:* None

Synchronized Intermittent Mandatory Ventilation-Volume Controlled with Pressure Limit

- *Mandatory breaths:* Machine triggered (preset frequency) or patient synchronized (pressure or flow sensitivity) and machine cycled (tidal volume or pause time)
  - Within-breath settings:
    - Operator-set PEEP, frequency, inspiratory flow, inspiratory time, tidal volume, and inspiratory pressure (P_{limit})
    - Ventilator-set inspiratory flow if inspiration switches from volume control to pressure control when inspiratory pressure meets the inspiratory pressure target (P_{limit} setting)
- *Spontaneous breaths:* Patient triggered (pressure or flow sensitivity) and patient cycled (% peak inspiratory flow)
  - Within-breath settings:
    - Operator-set inspiratory pressure, rise time, and cycle sensitivity (% peak inspiratory flow)
- *Between-breath targets:* None

Volume Controlled Ventilation

- *Mandatory breaths:* Machine triggered (preset frequency) or patient triggered (pressure or flow sensitivity) and machine cycled (tidal volume or pause time)
  - Within-breath settings:
    - Operator-set PEEP, frequency, inspiratory time, tidal volume, and pause time
- *Spontaneous breaths:* Not allowed
- *Between-breath targets:* None

Volume Controlled Ventilation with Pressure Limit

- *Mandatory breaths:* Machine triggered (preset frequency) or patient triggered (pressure or flow sensitivity) and machine cycled (tidal volume or pause time)
  - Within-breath settings:
    - Operator-set PEEP, frequency, inspiratory flow, inspiratory time, tidal volume, and inspiratory pressure (P_{limit})

- Ventilator-set inspiratory flow if inspiration switches from volume control to pressure control when inspiratory pressure meets the inspiratory pressure target (P_{limit} setting)
- *Spontaneous breaths:* Not allowed
- *Between-breath targets:* None

Special Features

Backup ventilation: Backup ventilation will be initiated if the Apnea alarm is triggered or if the patient's minute ventilation decreases to below 50% of the set low minute ventilation alarm. Backup settings may be changed for each patient. Any mode with mandatory breaths can be selected as the backup mode. The operator also may select the modes that will allow backup ventilation, such as SIMV-VC, SIMV-PC, BiLevel, CPAP/PSV, SIMV-PCVG, and VG-PS.

Gas volume compensation: The flow and volume values are adjusted based on the condition selected by the operator in the preferences menu.

- Use ambient temperature and pressure, dry (ATPD) when a humidifier is not added to the patient circuit.
- Use body temperature and pressure, saturated (BTPS) when an active humidifier is added to the inspiratory limb of the circuit.

  For example, if BTPS is selected and the tidal volume is set for 300 mL, the ventilator will deliver 266 mL (assuming ambient 68°F/20°C and 745 mm Hg). The humidifier will warm the tidal volume delivered and add water vapor. This results in a delivery of 300 mL to the patient because the temperature and humidity affect the flow and volume delivered.

Leak compensation: Leak compensation automatically adjusts ventilation delivery and monitoring for breathing circuit and patient airway leaks to maintain the desired tidal volume. Measured value for leak (%) indicates the amount of leak from the previous breath and is calculated as:

Leak % = (Measured inspired tidal volume − Measured expired tidal volume) × 100 / Measured inspired tidal volume.

Miscellaneous: The Engström is unique among ventilators in its ability to measure functional residual capacity (FRC). The FRC calculation is based on the nitrogen washout method using a step change in the oxygen/air concentration delivered to the patient by the ventilator. The ventilator's PEEP INview procedure can be used to see how a change in the PEEP value affects the FRC value.

  Another unique monitoring feature is called SpiroDynamics, which is a tracheal pressure measurement obtained through a catheter that provides true tracheal pressure and intrinsic PEEP measurements regardless of the ventilation settings. The measurements are obtained with an intratracheal pressure catheter that is guided down a standard endotracheal or tracheostomy tube. The catheter is connected to the auxiliary pressure port of the ventilator and attached to the patient airway. This catheter provides a more accurate measurement of pressure delivery to the lungs by removing the resistance of the endotracheal tube from the spirometry loop. After a breath, a dynostatic curve is calculated from the loop providing an estimate of the alveolar pressure and volume. An algorithm creates the dynostatic curve based on the two pressure and two flow values for a specific volume at several points along the breath loop. This curve is an estimate of the pulmonary compliance during a breath.

A Spontaneous Breathing Trial (SBT) feature will place the ventilator in CPAP/PSV mode at the settings defined in the SBT menu. If the minute volume, respiratory rate, or apnea alarm limits are exceeded during the SBT, the trial will immediately end and the ventilator will return to the previous mode and settings. The SBT Split Screen displays the minute ventilation, respiratory rate, and end-tidal CO_2 for the trial. A message appears while the SBT is running indicating the amount of time remaining. The trial will automatically end at the time set and the ventilator will return to the previous mode and settings.

Nebulizer: This ventilator is designed to be used with an optional Aerogen Aeroneb vibrating mesh nebulizer. Unlike common jet nebulizers sometimes used with ventilators, this device does not increase the volume of inhaled gas.

Neonatal ventilation: The neonatal option on the Engström Carestation provides ventilation for intubated neonatal patients weighing down to 0.55 lb (0.25 kg). This is accomplished by using a proximal flow sensor at the patient wye, which connects to the ventilator with a cable. This sensor allows the ventilator to deliver flows as low as 0.2 L/min and as high as 30 L/min.

Noninvasive ventilation: The Engström noninvasive ventilation (NIV) option is designed with two modes of noninvasive ventilation: NIV and neonatal nCPAP (nasal continuous positive airway pressure). NIV provides positive pressure ventilation without the need for an invasive artificial airway. NIV is accomplished by using a nasal or face mask and is delivered through a positive pressure support mode, such as CPAP/PSV.

Manufacturer's Specifications

Table 9-24 lists specifications for the GE Engström Carestation ventilator.

TABLE 9-24
Specifications for GE Engström Carestation Ventilator

Setting Category	Setting	Range
Pressure	Inspiratory Pressure	1–90 cm H_2O
	Pressure Support	0–60 cm H_2O
	PEEP	1–50 cm H_2O
Volume	Tidal Volume	0.02–2 L
Flow	Inspiratory Flow	2–160 L/min
	Waveform	Not Specified
Time	Inspiratory Time	0.25–15 s
	Mandatory Breath Frequency	3–150/min
	Adjustable Rise Time	Yes
Sensitivity	Trigger Sensitivity (pressure)	–10 to –0.25 cm H_2O
	Trigger Sensitivity (flow)	1–9 L/min
	Cycle Sensitivity (flow)	5–80%
Alarm Category		
Pressure	Pmax	7–100 cm H_2O
	Low Ppeak	1–97 cm H_2O

(continues)

TABLE 9-24
Specifications for GE Engström Carestation Ventilator (Continued)

Setting Category	Setting	Range
Pressure, cont.	High PEEPe	5–50 cm H_2O
	Low PEEPe	1–20 cm H_2O
	High PEEPi	1–20 cm H_2O
	Paux	12–100 cm H_2O
Volume	Low TVexp	0.005–1.95 L
	High Tvexp	0.01–2 L
Flow	Low MVexp	0.01–40 L/min
	High MVexp	0.4–99 L/min
Time	Apnea Time	10–60 s
	Low Respiratory Rate	1–99/min
	High Respiratory Rate	2–120/min
Other	O_2 Sensor	Enabled/Disabled
	Low EtCO$_2$	0.1–14.9%
	High EtCO$_2$	0.2–15%
	Low EtO$_2$	10–99%
	High EtO$_2$	11–100%
Monitored Parameters	Peak Pressure	
	Mean Pressure	
	Plateau Pressure	
	PEEPe	
	PEEPi	
	PEEPe+i	
	Peak Auxiliary Pressure	
	Mean Auxiliary Pressure	
	Min Auxiliary Pressure	
	Expiratory Minute Volume	
	Inspiratory Minute Volume	
	Spontaneous Minute Volume	
	MVmech	
	Expiratory Tidal Volume	
	Inspiratory Tidal Volume	
	Spontaneous Tidal Volume	
	TVmech	
	Respiratory Rate	

TABLE 9-24
Specifications for GE Engström Carestation Ventilator (*Continued*)

Setting Category	Setting	Range
Monitored Parameters, cont.	Spontaneous Respiratory Rate	
	RRmech	
	Compliance	
	Raw	
	F_IO_2	
	RSBI	

Used with permission of GE Healthcare.

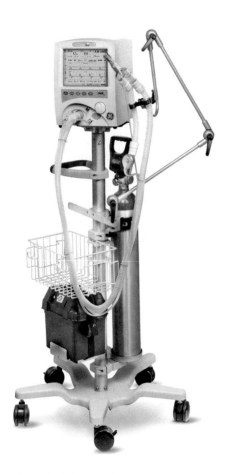

FIGURE 9-30 GE iVent201 ventilator.
Used with permission of GE Healthcare.

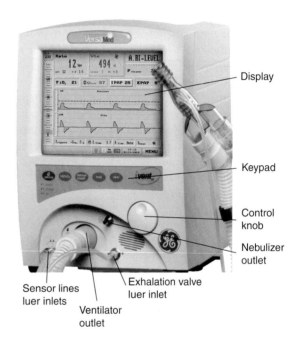

FIGURE 9-31 GE iVent201 operator interface.
Used with permission of GE Healthcare.

GE Healthcare iVent201

The iVent201 (**Figure 9-30**) is a compact, portable, full-featured, microprocessor-controlled ventilator offering the versatility and capability of larger and costlier ventilators. A turbine-powered air source and a rechargeable internal battery provide freedom from wall air and power outlets. The iVent201 ventilator (with or without the noninvasive Pulse Oximeter option) is suitable for use in the ICU and all other hospital areas, as well as all hospital-type facilities, alternate-care sites, during transport, emergency use, and in the home environment. The noninvasive Pulse Oximeter is intended for noninvasive monitoring of oxygen saturation and pulse rate and is suitable for use in all the above-mentioned areas.

Operator Interface

The iVent201 interface (**Figure 9-31**) consists of an LCD screen, a membrane keypad, and a selection knob. Turning the knob will change a value or move through a menu screen or a list of choices. Pressing the knob confirms the selection. Five dedicated keys below the screen are for alarm silence, 100% oxygen (3 minutes), manual breath, inspiratory/expiratory hold, and clear.

Modes

Modes on the iVent201 are selected by mode name (e.g., A/C Volume Control, SIMV Pressure Control, etc.) using a menu. Specific mode settings are selected using other menus. Available modes are shown in **Table 9-25**.

A/C Pressure Control

- *Mandatory breaths:* Machine triggered (preset frequency) or patient triggered (pressure or flow sensitivity) and machine cycled (inspiratory time)
  - Within-breath settings:
    - Operator-set PEEP, frequency, inspiratory pressure, rise time, and inspiratory time
- *Spontaneous breaths:* Not allowed
- *Between-breath targets:* None

A/C Volume Control

- *Mandatory breaths:* Machine triggered (preset frequency) or patient triggered (pressure or flow sensitivity) and machine cycled (tidal volume or pause time)
  - Within-breath settings:
    - Operator-set PEEP, frequency, peak inspiratory flow, inspiratory time, inspiratory pressure limit (ends inspiration but no alarm; high pressure alarm automatically set to pressure limit + 5 cm H_2O), and tidal volume
- *Spontaneous breaths:* Not allowed
- *Between-breath targets:* None

A/C Volume Control with Adaptive Flow and I-Time

- *Mandatory breaths:* Machine triggered (preset frequency) or patient triggered (pressure or flow sensitivity) and machine cycled (tidal volume)
  - Within-breath settings:
    - Operator-set PEEP, frequency, inspiratory pressure limit (high pressure alarm automatically set to pressure limit + 5 cm H_2O), and tidal volume. The Adaptive Peak Flow algorithm will adjust peak flow so that the tidal volume is delivered in the inspiratory time determined by the Adaptive I-Time algorithm to achieve an I:E ratio of 1:2.
- *Spontaneous breaths:* Not allowed
- *Between-breath targets:* None

Adaptive BiLevel

- *Mandatory breaths:* Machine triggered (preset frequency) or patient synchronized (pressure or flow sensitivity) and machine cycled (inspiratory time) or patient cycled (percent of peak flow). Spontaneous breaths are patient triggered (pressure or flow sensitivity) and patient cycled (percent of peak flow). Spontaneous breaths suppress mandatory breaths if they occur at a frequency higher than the set frequency.
  - Within-breath settings:
    - Operator set PEEP (called P-Low), peak inspiratory pressure (called P-High), rise time, inspiratory time, and frequency
- *Spontaneous breaths:* Patient triggered (pressure or flow sensitivity) and patient cycled (% peak inspiratory flow). Spontaneous breaths are permitted between mandatory breaths.
  - Within-breath settings:
    - Operator-set inspiratory pressure, rise time, and cycle sensitivity (% peak flow)
- *Between-breath targets:* None

TABLE 9-25
Classification of Modes for the iVent201

Mode Name	Mode Classification					
	Control Variable	Breath Sequence	Primary Breath Targeting Scheme	Secondary Breath Targeting Scheme	Tag
A/C Volume Control	volume	CMV	set-point	N/A	VC-CMVs
A/C Volume Control with Adaptive Flow and I-Time	volume	CMV	adaptive	N/A	VC-CMVa
SIMV Volume Control	volume	IMV	set-point	set-point	VC-IMVs,s
SIMV Volume Control with Adaptive Flow and I-Time	volume	IMV	adaptive	set-point	VC-IMVa,s
A/C Pressure Control	pressure	CMV	set-point	N/A	PC-CMVs
SIMV Pressure Control	pressure	IMV	set-point	set-point	PC-IMVs,s
Adaptive Bi-Level	pressure	IMV	set-point	set-point	PC-IMVs,s
CPAP/PSV	pressure	CSV	set-point	N/A	PC-CSVs

Reproduced with permission from Mandu Press Ltd.

CPAP/PSV

- *Mandatory breaths:* Not allowed
- *Spontaneous breaths:* Patient triggered (pressure or flow sensitivity) and patient cycled (% peak inspiratory flow)
  - Within-breath settings:
    - Operator-set inspiratory pressure, rise time, and cycle sensitivity (% peak flow)
- *Between-breath targets:* None

SIMV Pressure Controlled

- *Mandatory breaths:* Machine triggered (preset frequency or patient synchronized using pressure or flow sensitivity) and machine cycled (inspiratory time)
  - Within-breath settings:
    - Operator-set PEEP, inspiratory pressure, frequency, rise time, and I:E ratio
- *Spontaneous breaths:* Patient triggered (pressure or flow sensitivity) and patient cycled (% peak inspiratory flow)
  - Within-breath settings:
    - Operator-set inspiratory pressure, rise time, and cycle sensitivity (% peak inspiratory flow)
- *Between-breath targets:* None

SIMV Volume Controlled

- *Mandatory breaths:* Machine triggered (preset frequency) or patient synchronized (pressure or flow sensitivity) and machine cycled (tidal volume)
  - Within-breath settings:
    - Operator-set PEEP, frequency, peak inspiratory flow, inspiratory time, inspiratory pressure limit (ends inspiration but no alarm; high pressure alarm automatically set to pressure limit + 5 cm H_2O), and tidal volume
- *Spontaneous breaths:* Patient triggered (pressure or flow sensitivity) and patient cycled (% peak inspiratory flow)
  - Within-breath settings:
    - Operator-set inspiratory pressure, rise time, and cycle sensitivity (% peak inspiratory flow)
- *Between-breath targets:* None

SIMV Volume Controlled with Adaptive Flow and I-Time

- *Mandatory breaths:* Machine triggered (preset frequency) or patient synchronized (pressure or flow sensitivity) and machine cycled (tidal volume or pause time)
  - Within-breath settings:
    - Operator-set PEEP, frequency, peak inspiratory flow or Adaptive Flow, inspiratory time, and tidal volume. The Adaptive Peak Flow algorithm will adjust peak flow so that the tidal volume is delivered in the inspiratory time determined by the Adaptive I-Time algorithm to achieve an I:E ratio of 1:2.
- *Spontaneous breaths:* Patient triggered (pressure or flow sensitivity) and patient cycled (% peak inspiratory flow)
  - Within-breath settings:
    - Operator-set inspiratory pressure, rise time, and cycle sensitivity (% peak inspiratory flow)
- *Between-breath targets:* None

Special Features

Backup ventilation: Apnea backup ventilation will be activated if breathing has ceased for a period of time determined in the Alarms Settings window. (The default value is 20 seconds.) When apnea is detected the patient will be ventilated in the current ventilation mode except for CPAP. Rate is determined according to set Tidal volume for volume control; for all other modes the rate is based on an average of the previous inhaled tidal volumes. In CPAP the unit switches to SIMV volume control mode with rate and Tidal volume according to a look-up table.

Miscellaneous: In Volume control modes, the iVent201 permits sigh breaths, which are 1.5 times the set tidal volume. Easy Exhale is an advanced PEEP mode designed for use with severe obstructive airway flow. In situations where critical airway closure tends to create intrinsic PEEP, this feature introduces PEEP late in expiration in order to prevent airway pressure from falling below alveolar pressure. A pulse oximeter can be connected to the iVent201 ventilator with continuous monitoring of saturation on the iVent screen. Unique to the iVent201, Adaptive Flow and Adaptive Time automatically determine peak inspiratory flow and inspiratory time during breath delivery in volume control modes. When used together (the default state for SIMV Volume control mode) these two features maintain an I:E ratio of 1:2 by adapting to changes in breath rate. The Adaptive I-Time algorithm adjusts the inspiratory time over approximately 10 breaths in order to maintain the I:E ratio at 1:2. The Adaptive Flow algorithm reacts to changes in the inspiratory time and automatically adjusts the peak flow so that the delivery of the set tidal volume for the inspiratory time determined by the Adaptive I-Time algorithm is assured.

Nebulizer: A pneumatic nebulizer can be connected to the ventilator. During nebulization, the nebulizer flow will be synchronized with the inspiratory phase of each breath. Note that the nebulizer works during the inspiratory phase only.

Noninvasive ventilation: The Adaptive Bi-Level mode can accommodate high leak situations, such as when using a face mask (noninvasive ventilation) or pressure support for high leak ET tube ventilation (e.g., Passy Muir and cuffless applications).

Manufacturer's Specifications

Table 9-26 lists specifications for the GE iVent201.

Hamilton Medical Hamilton-C3

The Hamilton-C3 (**Figure 9-32**) is designed for intensive care ventilation of adult, pediatric, infant, and neonatal patients. This ventilator is an electronically controlled, pneumatically powered ventilation system with an integrated air compressing system. It is powered by AC or DC with battery backup to protect against power failure or unstable power and to facilitate intrahospital transport. The Hamilton-C3 receives inputs from a proximal flow sensor (required) and other sensors within the ventilator. Based on this monitored data, the device adjusts gas delivery to the patient. This sensor lets the ventilator sense even weak patient breathing efforts. The flow sensor is highly accurate even in the presence of secretions, moisture, and nebulized medications. There is an infant version of the flow sensor as well as a pediatric/adult version.

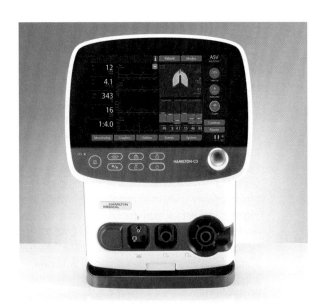

FIGURE 9-32 Hamilton Medical Hamilton-C3 ventilator. 1. Touch screen. 2. Alarm lamp. 3. Battery indicator. 4. Power/standby switch. 5. Screen lock/unlock. 6. Oxygen enrichment (2 min). 7. Manual breath/inspiratory hold. 8. Nebulizer on/off. 9. Print screen. 10. Alarm silence. 11. Press-and-turn knob to select and adjust settings. 12. Expiratory valve cover. 13. From patient port. 14. To patient port. 15. Flow sensor connection. 16. Pneumatic nebulizer output connector. 17. Oxygen cell.
Courtesy of Hamilton Medical.

Operator Interface

The operator provides inputs to the Hamilton-C3 microprocessor system through a touch screen, keys, and a press-and-turn knob (**Figure 9-33**). Turning the knob will change a value or move through a menu screen or a list of choices. Pressing the knob confirms the selection.

Modes

Modes on the C3 are selected by mode name (e.g., PCV+, PSIMV+, APRV, DuoPAP, etc.) using a menu. Specific mode settings are selected using other menus. Available modes are shown in **Table 9-27**.

For the C3 ventilator, spontaneous breathing is allowed at any time in any mode.

Adaptive Support Ventilation

- *Mandatory breaths:* Machine triggered (preset frequency) and machine cycled (inspiratory time). Spontaneous breaths suppress mandatory breaths if spontaneous minute ventilation is above target minute ventilation.
  - Within-breath settings:
    - Operator-set PEEP, maximum inspiratory pressure, patient height, and percent minute ventilation to support
    - Ventilator-set inspiratory pressure
- *Spontaneous breaths:* Patient triggered (flow sensitivity) and patient cycled (% peak inspiratory flow).
  - *Within-breath settings:* Rise time and cycle sensitivity (% peak flow)
- Between-breath targets:
  - Ventilator-set tidal volume and minute ventilation

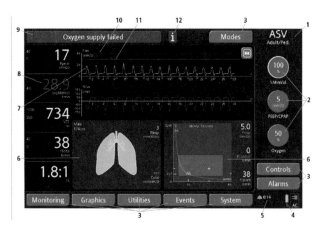

FIGURE 9-33 Hamilton Medical Hamilton-C3 operator interface. 1. Active mode, patient type, weaning, recruitment and apnea backup status. 2. Controller buttons for ventilation and oxygenation. 3. Window tabs (open the associated windows). 4. Shows all available power sources. 5. Alarm silence countdown. 6. Graphic display showing the pressure/time waveform plus one additional graphic, including another real-time waveform or an Intelligent Panel. 7. Trigger symbol. Indicates the patient is triggering a breath. 8. Main monitoring parameters. 9. Alarm message bar, 10. Maximum pressure indication line. 11. Pressure limitation indication line. 12. Inactive alarm indicator.
Courtesy of Hamilton Medical.

TABLE 9-26
Specifications for the GE iVent201

Setting Category	Setting	Range
Pressure	Inspiratory Pressure	5–80 cm H_2O
	Pressure Support	0–60 cm H_2O
	PEEP	0–40 cm H_2O
Volume	Tidal Volume	0.05–2.0 L
Flow	Inspiratory Flow	1–120 L/min
	Waveform	Not Specified
Time	Inspiratory Time	0.3–3.0 s
	Mandatory Breath Frequency	1–80/min
	Adjustable Rise Time	Yes
Sensitivity	Trigger Sensitivity (pressure)	–0.5 to –20 cm H_2O
	Trigger Sensitivity (flow)	1–20 L/min
	Cycle Sensitivity (flow)	10–90%
Alarm Category		
Pressure	High Inspiratory Pressure	4–80 cm H_2O
	Low Inspiratory Pressure	1–77 cm H_2O
Volume	Low Tidal Volume	15–85%
Flow	High Minute Volume	1–99 L/min
	Low Minute Volume	0–60 L/min
Time	High Respiratory Rate	4–80/min
	Low Respiratory Rate	1–77/min
	Apnea Time	5–120 s
Other	O_2 Sensor	Enabled/Disabled
	Leak	0–100%
Monitored Parameters	Airway Pressure	
	Total Breath Rate	
	I:E Ratio	
	Exhaled Tidal Volume	
	Exhaled Minute Volume	
	Peak Flow	
	Inspiratory Time	
	Compliance	
	Resistance	
	MAP	
	RR/Vt	
	SPO_2	

Used with permission of GE Healthcare.

Airway Pressure Release Ventilation

- *Mandatory breaths:* Machine triggered (preset frequency or patient synchronized using flow trigger sensitivity) and machine cycled (inspiratory time or patient synchronized using flow cycle sensitivity).
  - Within-breath settings:
    - Operator-set PEEP (called P_{low}), peak inspiratory pressure (called P_{high}), inspiratory time (called T_{high}), and expiratory time (called T_{low})

- *Spontaneous breaths:* Patient triggered (flow sensitivity) and patient cycled (% peak inspiratory flow). Spontaneous breaths are permitted both between and during mandatory breaths.
  - Within-breath settings:

TABLE 9-27
Classification of Modes for the Hamilton Medical Hamilton-C3 Ventilator

Mode Name	Control Variable	Breath Sequence	Primary Breath Targeting Scheme	Secondary Breath Targeting Scheme	Tag
Synchronized Controlled Mandatory Ventilation Plus	pressure	CMV	adaptive	N/A	PC-CMVa
Pressure Controlled Ventilation Plus	pressure	CMV	set-point	N/A	PC-CMVs
Pressure Controlled Synchronized Intermittent Mandatory Ventilation	pressure	IMV	set-point	set-point	PC-IMVs,s
Noninvasive Ventilation—Spontaneous Timed	pressure	IMV	set-point	set-point	PC-IMVs,s
Nasal Continuous Positive Airway Pressure—Pressure Support	pressure	IMV	set-point	set-point	PC-IMVs,s
Duo Positive Airway Pressure	pressure	IMV	set-point	set-point	PC-IMVs,s
Airway Pressure Release Ventilation	pressure	IMV	set-point	set-point	PC-IMVs,s
Synchronized Intermittent Mandatory Ventilation Plus	pressure	IMV	adaptive	set-point	PC-IMVa,s
Adaptive Support Ventilation	pressure	IMV	optimal/intelligent	optimal/intelligent	PC-IMVoi,oi
Spontaneous	pressure	CSV	set-point	N/A	PC-CSVs
Noninvasive Ventilation	pressure	CSV	set-point	N/A	PC-CSVs

Reproduced with permission from Mandu Press Ltd.

- Operator-set inspiratory pressure (pressure support) and cycle sensitivity (% peak flow)
- *Between-breath targets:* None.

Duo Positive Airway Pressure
- *Mandatory breaths:* Machine triggered (preset frequency or patient synchronized using flow trigger sensitivity) and machine cycled (inspiratory time or patient synchronized using flow cycle sensitivity).
  - Within-breath settings:
    - Operator-set PEEP (called P_{low}), peak inspiratory pressure (called P_{high}), frequency, and inspiratory time (called T_{high})
- *Spontaneous breaths:* Patient triggered (flow sensitivity) and patient cycled (% peak inspiratory flow). Spontaneous breaths are permitted both between and during mandatory breaths.

- Within-breath settings:
  - Inspiratory pressure (i.e., pressure support level) and cycle sensitivity (% peak flow)
- *Between-breath targets:* None.

Nasal Continuous Positive Airway Pressure/Pressure Support
This mode is designed to apply CPAP and intermittent positive pressure support with a nasal interface (mask or prongs).
- *Mandatory breaths:* Machine triggered (preset frequency or patient synchronized using flow sensitivity) and machine cycled (inspiratory time)
  - Within-breath settings:
    - Operator-set PEEP, frequency, inspiratory pressure and inspiratory time, and cycle sensitivity (% peak flow)

- *Spontaneous breaths:* Patient triggered (pressure or flow sensitivity) and patient cycled (% peak inspiratory flow)
  - *Within-breath settings:* None (inspiratory pressure set for mandatory breaths applies to spontaneous breaths automatically).
- *Between-breath targets:* None

Noninvasive Ventilation
Noninvasive ventilation (NIV) is an adaptation of the SPONT mode, whereas NIV-ST is an adaptation of the PSIMV+ mode. The primary difference is that NIV modes are designed to compensate for leaks when using a mask or other noninvasive patient interface.

- *Mandatory breaths:* Not allowed
- *Spontaneous breaths:* Patient triggered (flow sensitivity) and patient cycled (% peak inspiratory flow)
  - Within-breath settings:
    - Operator-set inspiratory pressure, cycle sensitivity (% peak inspiratory flow), and maximum inspiratory time
- *Between-breath targets:* None

Noninvasive Ventilation-Spontaneous Timed
Noninvasive ventilation (NIV) is an adaptation of the SPONT mode, whereas NIV-ST is an adaptation of the PSIMV+ mode. The primary difference is that NIV modes are designed to compensate for leaks when using a mask or other noninvasive patient interface.

- *Mandatory breaths:* Machine triggered (preset frequency or patient synchronized using flow sensitivity) and machine cycled (inspiratory time)
  - Within-breath settings:
    - Operator-set PEEP, inspiratory pressure, frequency, inspiratory time
- *Spontaneous breaths:* Patient triggered (pressure or flow sensitivity) and patient cycled (% peak inspiratory flow)
  - Within-breath settings:
    - Inspiratory pressure set for mandatory breaths applies to spontaneous breaths automatically, cycle sensitivity (% peak inspiratory flow), and maximum inspiratory time.
- *Between-breath targets:* None

Pressure Controlled Synchronized Intermittent Mandatory Ventilation
- *Mandatory breaths:* Machine triggered (preset frequency or patient synchronized using flow sensitivity) and machine cycled (inspiratory time)
  - Within-breath settings:
    - Operator-set PEEP, inspiratory pressure, frequency, and inspiratory time
- *Spontaneous breaths:* Patient triggered (flow sensitivity) and patient cycled (% peak inspiratory flow)

- Within-breath settings:
  - Operator-set inspiratory pressure, cycle sensitivity (% peak flow), and maximum inspiratory time
- *Between-breath targets:* None

Pressure Control Ventilation Plus
- *Mandatory breaths:* Machine triggered (preset frequency) or patient triggered (flow sensitivity) and machine cycled (inspiratory time)
  - Within-breath settings:
    - Operator-set PEEP, frequency, inspiratory pressure, rise time, and inspiratory time
- *Spontaneous breaths:* Not allowed
- *Between-breath targets:* None

Spontaneous
- *Mandatory breaths:* Not allowed
- *Spontaneous breaths:* Patient triggered (flow sensitivity) and patient cycled (% peak inspiratory flow)
  - Within-breath settings:
    - Operator-set inspiratory pressure, cycle sensitivity (% peak inspiratory flow), and maximum inspiratory time
- *Between-breath targets:* None

Synchronized Controlled Mandatory Ventilation Plus
- *Mandatory breaths:* Machine triggered (preset frequency) or patient triggered (flow sensitivity) and machine cycled (inspiratory time)
  - Within-breath settings:
    - Operator-set PEEP, frequency, rise time, and inspiratory time
    - Ventilator-set inspiratory pressure
- *Spontaneous breaths:* Not allowed
- Between-breath targets:
  - Operator-set tidal volume

Synchronized Intermittent Mandatory Ventilation Plus
- *Mandatory breaths:* Machine triggered (preset frequency) or patient triggered (flow sensitivity) and machine cycled (inspiratory time)
  - Within-breath settings:
    - Operator-set PEEP, frequency, rise time, and inspiratory time
    - Ventilator-set inspiratory pressure
- *Spontaneous breaths:* Patient triggered (flow sensitivity) and patient cycled (% peak inspiratory flow)
  - Within-breath settings:
    - Operator-set inspiratory pressure, rise time, and cycle sensitivity (% peak flow)
- Between-breath targets:
  - Operator-set tidal volume

Special Features

Backup ventilation: Backup ventilation is activated if no breath is detected during the set apnea delay time. The backup ventilation mode is either SIMV+ or PCV+, depending on the original mode in which the apnea occurred.

Gas volume compensation: Pressure, flow, and volume measurements are based on readings from the flow sensor, and they are expressed in BTPS (body temperature and pressure, saturated).

Miscellaneous: Sigh breaths delivered at a regular interval (every 50 breaths) at a pressure up to 10 cm H_2O higher than nonsigh breaths, as allowed by the Pressure alarm limit. Sigh breaths are available in all modes except Duo-PAP and APRV.

An optional CO_2 sensor can be connected to the ventilator, which will allow both end-tidal and volumetric exhaled CO_2 measurements and calculations.

Nebulizer: The C3's nebulization function powers a standard inline pneumatic nebulizer for delivery of medications in the ventilator circuit. The nebulizer flow is synchronized with the inspiratory phase of each breath for 30 min. Nebulization can be activated in all modes of ventilation. The ventilator may also be used with an optional Aerogen Aeroneb Pro vibrating mesh nebulizer.

Noninvasive ventilation: The C3 provides three modes of noninvasive ventilation: Noninvasive Ventilation, Noninvasive Ventilation—Spontaneous Timed, and Nasal Continuous Positive Airway Pressure—Pressure Support.

Manufacturer's Specifications

Table 9-28 lists specifications for the Hamilton-C3 ventilator.

Hamilton Medical Galileo

The Hamilton Galileo (**Figure 9-34**) is a full-function intensive care ventilator that offers conventional volume- and pressure-controlled modes. It is designed for ventilation of infant, pediatric, and adult patients up

TABLE 9-28

Specifications for the Hamilton Medical Hamilton-C3 Ventilator

Setting Category	Setting	Range
Pressure	Inspiratory Pressure	5–60 cm H_2O
	Pressure Support	0–60 cm H_2O
	PEEP	0–35 cm H_2O
Volume	Tidal Volume	0.02–2.0 L
Flow	Waveform	Square/descending ramp
	Inspiratory Time	0.1–12 s
Time	Mandatory Breath Frequency	1–80/min
	Trigger Sensitivity (flow)	1–20 L/min
	Adjustable Rise Time	Yes
Sensitivity	Cycle Sensitivity (flow)	5–80%
Alarm Category		
Pressure	High Pressure	15–70 cm H_2O
	Low Pressure	4–60 cm H_2O
Flow	High Expiratory Minute Volume	0.1–50 L/min
	Low Expiratory Minute Volume	0.1–50 L/min
Time	Apnea Time	15–60 s
	High Frequency	0–99/min
	Low Frequency	0–99/min
Other	High Oxygen	18–103%

TABLE 9-28
Specifications for the Hamilton-C3 Ventilator (*Continued*)

Setting Category	Setting	Range
Other, cont.	Low Oxygen	18–97%
	High EtCO$_2$	1–100 mm Hg
	Low EtCO$_2$	0–100 mm Hg
Monitored Parameters	Peak Pressure	
	Mean Pressure	
	PEEP/CPAP	
	AutoPEEP	
	Plateau Pressure	
	Inspiratory Flow	
	Expiratory Flow	
	Expiratory Tidal Volume	
	Inspiratory Tidal Volume	
	Expiratory Minute Volume	
	Spontaneous Minute Volume	
	Leak	
	I:E Ratio	
	Total Frequency	
	Spontaneous Frequency	
	Inspiratory Time	
	Expiratory Time	
	Cstat	
	Static Compliance	
	P0.1	
	PTP	
	RCexp	
	Inspiratory Resistance	
	IBW	
	VTES Spontaneous	
	Oxygen	
	Fractional End Tidal CO$_2$	
	Pet CO$_2$	
	Inspiratory Pressure	
	RSB	

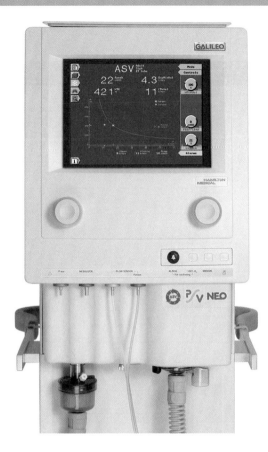

FIGURE 9-34 Hamilton Medical Galileo ventilator.
Courtesy of Hamilton Medical.

to 440 lb (200 kg). The Galileo is an electronically controlled pneumatic ventilator powered by AC with an internal battery backup to protect against power failure and to facilitate intrahospital transport. The ventilator's pneumatics deliver gas, and its electrical systems control pneumatics, monitor alarms, and distribute power. The Hamilton-Galileo receives inputs from a proximal flow sensor (required) and other sensors within the ventilator. Based on this monitored data, the device adjusts gas delivery to the patient. This sensor lets the ventilator sense even weak patient breathing efforts. The flow sensor is highly accurate even in the presence of secretions, moisture, and nebulized medications.

Operator Interface

The operator provides inputs to the Galileo microprocessor system through a touch screen, keys, and a press-and-turn knob (Figure 9-35). Turning the knob will change a value or move through a menu screen or a list of choices. Pressing the knob confirms the selection.

Modes

Modes on the Galileo are selected by mode name (e.g., SIMV, SPONT, ASV, DuoPAP, etc.) using a menu. Specific mode settings are selected using other menus. Available modes are shown in Table 9-29.

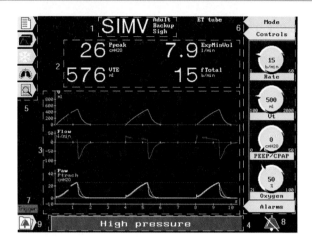

FIGURE 9-35 Hamilton Medical Galileo operator interface.
Courtesy of Hamilton Medical.

Adaptive Pressure Ventilation Continuous Mandatory Ventilation

- *Mandatory breaths:* Machine triggered (preset frequency) or patient triggered (pressure or flow sensitivity) and machine cycled (inspiratory time)
  - Within-breath settings:
    - Operator-set PEEP, frequency, rise time, and I:E or % inspiratory time
    - Ventilator-set inspiratory pressure
- *Spontaneous breaths:* Not allowed
- Between-breath targets:
  - Operator-set tidal volume

Adaptive Pressure Ventilation Synchronized Intermittent Mandatory Ventilation

- *Mandatory breaths:* Machine triggered (preset frequency) or patient triggered (pressure or flow sensitivity) and machine cycled (inspiratory time)
  - Within-breath settings:
    - Operator-set PEEP, frequency, rise time, and I:E or % inspiratory time
    - Ventilator-set inspiratory pressure
- *Spontaneous breaths:* Patient triggered (flow sensitivity) and patient cycled (% peak inspiratory flow)
  - Within-breath settings:
    - Operator-set inspiratory pressure, rise time, and cycle sensitivity (% peak flow)
- Between-breath targets:
  - Operator-set tidal volume

Adaptive Support Ventilation

- *Mandatory breaths:* Machine triggered (preset frequency) and machine cycled (inspiratory time).
  - Within-breath settings:
    - Operator-set PEEP, maximum inspiratory pressure, patient weight, and % minute ventilation to support
    - Ventilator-set inspiratory pressure

TABLE 9-29
Classification of Modes for the Hamilton Galileo Ventilator

Mode Name	Mode Classification				
	Control Variable	Breath Sequence	Primary Breath Targeting Scheme	Secondary Breath Targeting Scheme	Tag
Synchronized Controlled Mandatory Ventilation A/C	volume	CMV	set-point	N/A	VC-CMVs
SIMV	volume	IMV	set-point	set-point	VC-IMVs,s
SIMV with Tube Resistance Compensation	volume	IMV	set-point	set-point/servo	VC-IMVs,sr
Pressure Controlled Continuous Mandatory Ventilation A/C	pressure	CMV	set-point	N/A	PC-CMVs
Adaptive Pressure Ventilation Continuous Mandatory Ventilation	pressure	CMV	adaptive	N/A	PC-CMVa
Adaptive Pressure Ventilation Continuous Mandatory Ventilation with Tube Resistance Compensation	pressure	CMV	adaptive/servo	N/A	PC-CMVar
Pressure Controlled Continuous Mandatory Ventilation A/C with Tube Resistance Compensation	pressure	CMV	set-point/servo	N/A	PC-CMVsr
Pressure SIMV	pressure	IMV	set-point	set-point	PC-IMVs,s
Duo Positive Airway Pressure	pressure	IMV	set-point	set-point	PC-IMVs,s
Airway Pressure Release Ventilation	pressure	IMV	set-point	set-point	PC-IMVs,s
Adaptive Pressure Ventilation SIMV	pressure	IMV	adaptive	set-point	PC-IMVa,s
Adaptive Pressure Ventilation SIMV with Tube Resistance Compensation	pressure	IMV	adaptive/servo	set-point/servo	PC-IMVar,sr
Adaptive Support Ventilation	pressure	IMV	optimal/intelligent	optimal/intelligent	PC-IMVoi,oi
Adaptive Support Ventilation with Tube Resistance Compensation	pressure	IMV	optimal/intelligent/servo	optimal/intelligent/servo	PC-IMVois,ois
Pressure SIMV with Tube Resistance Compensation	pressure	IMV	set-point/servo	set-point/servo	PC-IMVsr,sr
Duo Positive Airway Pressure with Tube Resistance Compensation	pressure	IMV	set-point/servo	set-point/servo	PC-IMVsr,sr
Airway Pressure Release Ventilation with Tube Resistance Compensation	pressure	IMV	set-point/servo	set-point/servo	PC-IMVsr,sr
Spontaneous	pressure	CSV	set-point	N/A	PC-CSVs
Noninvasive Ventilation	pressure	CSV	set-point	N/A	PC-CSVs
Spontaneous with Tube Resistance Compensation	pressure	CSV	set-point/servo	N/A	PC-CSVs

Reproduced with permission from Mandu Press Ltd.

■ *Spontaneous breaths:* Patient triggered (pressure or flow sensitivity) and patient cycled (% peak inspiratory flow)
  • Within-breath settings:
    – Rise time and cycle sensitivity (% peak flow)
■ Between-breath targets:
  • Ventilator-set tidal volume and minute ventilation

Airway Pressure Release Ventilation

■ *Mandatory breaths:* Machine triggered (preset frequency or patient synchronized using pressure or flow trigger sensitivity) and machine cycled (inspiratory time or patient synchronized using flow cycle sensitivity).
  • Within-breath settings:
    – Operator-set PEEP (called P_{low}), peak inspiratory pressure (called P_{high}), rise time, inspiratory time (called T_{high}), and expiratory time (called T_{low})
■ *Spontaneous breaths:* Patient triggered (pressure or flow sensitivity) and patient cycled (% peak inspiratory flow). Spontaneous breaths are permitted both between and during mandatory breaths.
  • Within-breath settings:
    – Operator-set inspiratory pressure (i.e., pressure support), rise time, and cycle sensitivity (% peak flow)
■ *Between-breath targets:* None.

Duo Positive Airway Pressure

■ *Mandatory breaths:* Machine triggered (preset frequency or patient synchronized using pressure or flow trigger sensitivity) and machine cycled (inspiratory time or patient synchronized using flow cycle sensitivity).
  • Within-breath settings:
    – Operator-set PEEP (called P_{low}), peak inspiratory pressure (called P_{high}), rise time, frequency, and inspiratory time (called T_{high})
■ *Spontaneous breaths:* Patient triggered (pressure or flow sensitivity) and patient cycled (% peak inspiratory flow). Spontaneous breaths are permitted both between and during mandatory breaths.
  • Within-breath settings:
    – Inspiratory pressure (i.e., pressure support level), rise time, and cycle sensitivity (% peak flow)
■ *Between-breath targets:* None.

Noninvasive Ventilation

Noninvasive ventilation (NIV) is an adaptation of the SPONT mode. The primary difference is that NIV is designed to compensate for leaks when using a mask or other noninvasive patient interface.

■ *Mandatory breaths:* Not allowed
■ *Spontaneous breaths:* Patient triggered (pressure or flow sensitivity) and patient cycled (% peak inspiratory flow)
  • Within-breath settings:
    – Operator-set inspiratory pressure, rise time, cycle sensitivity (% peak flow), and maximum inspiratory time
■ *Between-breath targets:* None

Pressure Controlled Continuous Mandatory Ventilation Assist/Control

■ *Mandatory breaths:* Machine triggered (preset frequency) or patient triggered (pressure or flow sensitivity) and machine cycled (inspiratory time)
  • Within-breath settings:
    – Operator-set PEEP, frequency, inspiratory pressure, rise time, and I:E or % inspiratory time
■ *Spontaneous breaths:* Not allowed
■ *Between-breath targets:* None

Pressure Synchronized Intermittent Mandatory Ventilation

■ *Mandatory breaths:* Machine triggered (preset frequency or patient synchronized using pressure or flow sensitivity) and machine cycled (inspiratory time)
  • Within-breath settings:
    – Operator-set PEEP, inspiratory pressure, frequency, rise time, and I:E or % inspiratory time
■ *Spontaneous breaths:* Patient triggered (pressure or flow sensitivity) and patient cycled (% peak inspiratory flow)
  • Within-breath settings:
    – Operator-set PEEP, inspiratory pressure and maximum inspiratory time, rise time, and cycle sensitivity (% peak flow)
■ *Between-breath targets:* None

Spontaneous

■ *Mandatory breaths:* Not allowed
■ *Spontaneous breaths:* Patient triggered (pressure or flow sensitivity) and patient cycled (% peak inspiratory flow)
  • Within-breath settings:
    – Operator-set inspiratory pressure, rise time, cycle sensitivity (% peak flow), and maximum inspiratory time
■ *Between-breath targets:* None

Synchronized Controlled Mandatory Ventilation Assist/Control

■ *Mandatory breaths:* Machine triggered (preset frequency) or patient triggered (pressure or flow sensitivity) and machine cycled (tidal volume or pause time)

- Within-breath settings:
  - Operator-set PEEP, frequency, flow pattern, tidal volume, I:E and pause time, peak flow and inspiratory time, or % inspiration and pause time
- *Spontaneous breaths:* Not allowed
- *Between-breath targets:* None

Synchronized Intermittent Mandatory Ventilation

- *Mandatory breaths:* Machine triggered (preset frequency) or patient synchronized (pressure or flow sensitivity) and machine cycled (tidal volume or pause time)
  - Within-breath settings:
    - Operator-set PEEP, frequency, flow pattern, tidal volume, I:E and pause time, peak flow and inspiratory time, or % inspiration and pause time
- *Spontaneous breaths:* Patient triggered (pressure or flow sensitivity) and patient cycled (% peak inspiratory flow)
  - Within-breath settings:
    - Operator-set inspiratory pressure, rise time, and cycle sensitivity (% peak flow)
- *Between-breath targets:* None

Tube Resistance Compensation

To reduce the patient's work of breathing while on the ventilator, the Tube Resistance Compensation feature offsets the flow resistance imposed by the endotracheal or tracheostomy tube. Tube Resistance Compensation is active during exhalation in volume modes, and in both inspiration and exhalation in the other modes.

- Within-breath settings:
  - Operator-set percent support (of resistive load) along with artificial airway tube diameter and tube type
  - Ventilator-set inspiratory pressure as a function of patient-generated inspiratory flow
- *Between-breath targets:* None

Special Features

Backup ventilation: Backup ventilation is activated if no breath is detected during the set apnea delay time. The backup ventilation mode is SCMV A/C, P-CMVA/C, or APVcmv, depending on the original mode.

Gas volume compensation: Pressure, flow, and volume measurements are based on readings from the flow sensor, and they are expressed in BTPS (body temperature and pressure, saturated). The volume exhaled by the patient is determined

from the flow sensor measurement, so it does not show any volume added due to compression or lost due to leaks in the breathing circuit. If there is a gas leak at the patient end, the displayed exhaled tidal volume may be less than the tidal volume the patient actually receives.

Miscellaneous: In all modes except ASV, a sigh (if activated as an option) is delivered every 100 breaths. In volume control modes, sigh breaths are 50% higher than normal breaths, up to a maximum of 2,000 mL. In pressure control modes, sigh breaths are up to 10 cm H_2O higher than normal breaths, as allowed by the high pressure alarm setting. In ASV mode, the sigh is delivered every 50 breaths, at a pressure 10 cm H_2O higher than normal breaths.

The Galileo offers a unique feature (the P/V Tool) to record quasi-static pressure/ volume curves. The feature makes it possible to record both the inflation and deflation limbs of the P/V curve. The maneuver employs an adjustable pressure ramp in which airway pressure is slowly increased to an upper level and then decreased to a lower level. A cursor function permits graphical analysis of the curve, including identification of inflection points and "visual curve fitting" to determine the linear compliance.

Nebulizer: The Galileo's optional pneumatic nebulization function provides nebulization during the breath phases for the preset duration of treatment.

Noninvasive ventilation: The noninvasive ventilation (NIV) mode is the Galileo's implementation of noninvasive positive pressure ventilation. The patient interface for NIV may be a mask, mouthpiece, or helmet-type interface.

Manufacturer's Specifications

Table 9-30 lists specifications for the Hamilton Galileo ventilator.

Hamilton Medical Hamilton-G5

The Hamilton-G5 ventilator (Figure 9-36) is designed for intensive care ventilation of adult and pediatric patients, and optionally infant and neonatal patients. The device is intended for use in the hospital and institutional environment where healthcare professionals provide patient care. This ventilator has an electronically controlled pneumatic ventilation system with electrical power from an AC source with internal battery backup. The device's pneumatic system delivers gas, and its electrical systems control the pneumatics, monitor alarms, and distribute power. The Hamilton-G5 receives inputs from a disposable, proximal flow sensor (required) and other sensors within

TABLE 9-30
Specifications for the Hamilton Galileo Ventilator

Setting Category	Setting	Range
Pressure	Inspiratory Pressure	5–100 cm H_2O
	Pressure Support	0–100 cm H_2O
	PEEP	0–50 cm H_2O
Volume	Tidal Volume	0.02–2.0 L
Flow	Inspiratory Flow	1–180 L/min
	Waveform	Square/descending ramp
Time	Inspiratory Time	0.1–10 s
	Mandatory Breath Frequency	1–120/min
	Adjustable Rise Time	Yes
Sensitivity	Trigger Sensitivity (pressure)	0.1–10 cm H_2O
	Trigger Sensitivity (flow)	0.5–15 L/min
	Cycle Sensitivity (flow)	5–70%
Alarm Category		
Pressure	High Pressure	10–120 cm H_2O
	Low Pressure	2–119 cm H_2O
Volume	High Tidal Volume	0.001–3.0 L
	Low Tidal Volume	0–2.95 L
Flow	Air Trapping	1–10 L/min
	High Expiratory Minute Volume	0.03–50 L/min
	Low Expiratory Minute Volume	0.01–49 L/min
Time	Apnea Time	10–60 s
	High Rate	2–130/min
	Low Rate	0–128/min
Other	O_2 Sensor	Enabled/Disabled
Monitored Parameters	Peak Pressure	
	Mean Pressure	
	Minimum Pressure	
	Plateau Pressure	
	PEEP/CPAP	
	AutoPEEP	
	Inspiratory Flow	
	Expiratory Flow	
	Expiratory Tidal Volume	
	Expiratory Minute Volume	
	Leak Volume	

TABLE 9-30
Specifications for the Hamilton Galileo Ventilator *(Continued)*

Setting Category	Setting	Range
Monitored Parameters, cont.	I:E Ratio	
	Total Frequency	
	Spontaneous Frequency	
	Inspiratory Time	
	Expiratory Time	
	Cstat	
	P0.1	
	PTP	
	RCexp	
	RCinsp	
	Expiratory Resistance	
	Inspiratory Resistance	
	RSB	
	WOBimp	
	Oxygen	

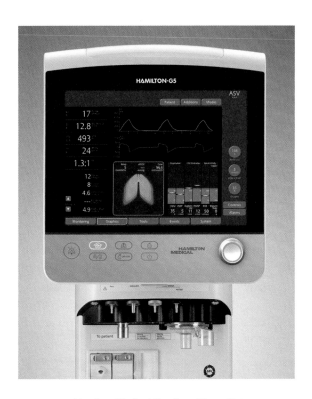

FIGURE 9-36 Hamilton Medical Hamilton-G5 ventilator.
Courtesy of Hamilton Medical.

the ventilator. Based on this monitored data, the device adjusts gas delivery to the patient. This sensor lets the ventilator sense even weak patient breathing efforts. The flow sensor is highly accurate even in the presence of secretions, moisture, and nebulized medications.

Operator Interface

The operator provides inputs to the G5 microprocessor system through a touch screen, keys, and a press-and-turn knob (**Figure 9-37**). Turning the knob will change a value or move through a menu screen or a list of choices. Pressing the knob confirms the selection.

Modes

Modes on the G5 are selected by mode name (e.g., SIMV, SPONT, ASV, DuoPAP, etc.) using a menu. Specific mode settings are selected using other menus. Available modes are shown in **Table 9-31**.

Adaptive Pressure Ventilation Continuous Mandatory Ventilation

- *Mandatory breaths:* Machine triggered (preset frequency) or patient triggered (pressure or flow sensitivity) and machine cycled (inspiratory time)
  - Within-breath settings:

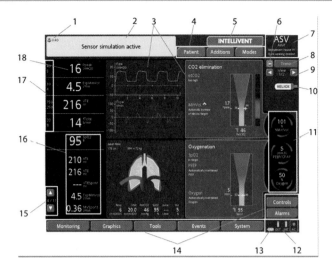

FIGURE 9-37 Hamilton Medical Hamilton-G5 operator interface. 1. Alarm silence countdown. 2. Message bar. Displays alarm and other messages. 3. Graphic display. Real-time waveforms (curves), loops, trend waveforms. 4. Access to Patient, Additions, and Mode windows. 5. INTELLiVENT tab. Opens the INTELLiVENT window. (Available as an option.) 6. Freeze or unfreeze graphics. 7. Active mode, patient type, weaning, recruitment, and apnea backup status. 8. Trend button. 9. View cursor. Changes between oxygenation and ventilation horizons, maps, and guides. 10. Indicates the heliox option is active. 11. Controller buttons for ventilation and oxygenation. 12. Input power. Shows all available power sources. 13. USB active. 14. Window tabs. Open the associated windows. 15. Secondary monitoring parameters, a group of numeric patient data accessed using the group scrolling arrows. 16. Secondary monitoring parameters. 17. Alarm limits. 18. Main monitoring parameters.

Courtesy of Hamilton Medical.

- – Operator-set PEEP, frequency, rise time, and I:E or % inspiratory time
- – Ventilator-set inspiratory pressure
- ■ *Spontaneous breaths:* Not allowed
- ■ Between-breath targets:
  - • Operator-set tidal volume

Adaptive Pressure Ventilation Synchronized Intermittent Mandatory Ventilation

- ■ *Mandatory breaths:* Machine triggered (preset frequency) or patient triggered (pressure or flow sensitivity) and machine cycled (inspiratory time)
  - • Within-breath settings:
    - – Operator-set PEEP, frequency, rise time, and I:E or % inspiratory time
    - – Ventilator-set inspiratory pressure
- ■ *Spontaneous breaths:* Patient triggered (flow sensitivity) and patient cycled (% peak inspiratory flow)
  - • Within-breath settings:
    - – Operator-set inspiratory pressure, rise time, and cycle sensitivity (% peak flow)
- ■ Between-breath targets:
  - • Operator-set tidal volume

Adaptive Support Ventilation

- ■ *Mandatory breaths:* Machine triggered (preset frequency) and machine cycled (inspiratory time)
  - • Within-breath settings:
    - – Operator-set PEEP, maximum inspiratory pressure, patient weight, and % minute ventilation to support
    - – Ventilator-set inspiratory pressure

TABLE 9-31
Classification of Modes for the Hamilton-G5 Ventilator

| Mode Name | Mode Classification | | | | | |
	Control Variable	Breath Sequence	Primary Breath Targeting Scheme	Secondary Breath Targeting Scheme	Tag
Synchronized Controlled Mandatory Ventilation	volume	CMV	set-point	N/A	VC-CMVs
SIMV	volume	IMV	set-point	set-point	VC-IMVs,s
SIMV with Tube Resistance Compensation	volume	IMV	set-point	set-point/servo	VC-IMVs,sr
Pressure Controlled Continuous Mandatory Ventilation	pressure	CMV	set-point	N/A	PC-CMVs
Adaptive Pressure Ventilation Continuous Mandatory Ventilation	pressure	CMV	adaptive	N/A	PC-CMVa
Adaptive Pressure Ventilation Continuous Mandatory Ventilation with Tube Resistance Compensation	pressure	CMV	adaptive/servo	N/A	PC-CMVar

TABLE 9-31
Classification of Modes for the Hamilton-G5 Ventilator (Continued)

Mode Name	Mode Classification				
	Control Variable	Breath Sequence	Primary Breath Targeting Scheme	Secondary Breath Targeting Scheme	Tag
Pressure Controlled Continuous Mandatory Ventilation with Tube Resistance Compensation	pressure	CMV	set-point/servo	N/A	PC-CMVsr
Pressure SIMV	pressure	IMV	set-point	set-point	PC-IMVs,s
Noninvasive Ventilation—Spontaneous Timed	pressure	IMV	set-point	set-point	PC-IMVs,s
Nasal Continuous Positive Airway Pressure—Pressure Support	pressure	IMV	set-point	set-point	PC-IMVs,s
Airway Pressure Release Ventilation	pressure	IMV	set-point	set-point	PC-IMVs,s
DuoPAP	pressure	IMV	set-point	set-point	PC-IMVs,s
Adaptive Pressure Ventilation SIMV	pressure	IMV	adaptive	set-point	PC-IMVa,s
Adaptive Pressure Ventilation SIMV with Tube Resistance Compensation	pressure	IMV	adaptive/servo	set-point/servo	PC-IMVar,sr
Adaptive Support Ventilation	pressure	IMV	optimal/intelligent	optimal/intelligent	PC-IMVoi,oi
IntelliVent-Adaptive Support Ventilation	pressure	IMV	optimal/intelligent	optimal/intelligent	PC-IMVoi,oi
Adaptive Support Ventilation with Tube Resistance Compensation	pressure	IMV	optimal/intelligent/servo	optimal/intelligent/servo	PC-IMVoir,oir
IntelliVent-Adaptive Support Ventilation with Tube Resistance Compensation	pressure	IMV	optimal/intelligent/servo	optimal/intelligent/servo	PC-IMVoir,oir
Pressure SIMV with Tube Resistance Compensation	pressure	IMV	set-point/servo	set-point/servo	PC-IMVsr,sr
Airway Pressure Release Ventilation with Tube Resistance Compensation	pressure	IMV	set-point/servo	set-point/servo	PC-IMVsr,sr
Spontaneous with Tube Resistance Compensation	pressure	IMV	set-point/servo	N/A	PC-IMVsr
Spontaneous	pressure	CSV	set-point	N/A	PC-CSVs
Noninvasive Ventilation	pressure	CSV	set-point	N/A	PC-CSVs

Reproduced with permission from Mandu Press Ltd.

- *Spontaneous breaths:* Patient triggered (pressure or flow sensitivity) and patient cycled (% peak inspiratory flow)
  - Within-breath settings:
    - Rise time and cycle sensitivity (% peak flow)
- Between-breath targets:
  - Ventilator-set tidal volume and minute ventilation

Airway Pressure Release Ventilation
- *Mandatory breaths:* Machine triggered (preset frequency or patient synchronized using pressure or flow trigger sensitivity) and machine cycled (inspiratory time or patient synchronized using flow cycle sensitivity).
  - Within-breath settings:

– Operator-set PEEP (called P_{low}), peak inspiratory pressure (called P_{high}), rise time, inspiratory time (called T_{high}), and expiratory time (called T_{low})
- *Spontaneous breaths:* Patient triggered (pressure or flow sensitivity) and patient cycled (% peak inspiratory flow). Spontaneous breaths are permitted both between and during mandatory breaths.
  - Within-breath settings:
    – Operator-set inspiratory pressure (i.e., pressure support), rise time, and cycle sensitivity (% peak flow)
- *Between-breath targets:* None.

Duo Positive Airway Pressure
- *Mandatory breaths:* Machine triggered (preset frequency or patient synchronized using pressure or flow trigger sensitivity) and machine cycled (inspiratory time or patient synchronized using flow cycle sensitivity).
  - Within-breath settings:
    – Operator-set PEEP (called P_{low}), peak inspiratory pressure (called P_{high}), rise time, frequency, and inspiratory time (called T_{high})
- *Spontaneous breaths:* Patient triggered (pressure or flow sensitivity) and patient cycled (% peak inspiratory flow). Spontaneous breaths are permitted both between and during mandatory breaths.
  - Within-breath settings:
    – Inspiratory pressure (i.e., pressure support level), rise time, and cycle sensitivity (% peak flow)
- *Between-breath targets:* None.

IntelliVent-Adaptive Support Ventilation (currently not available in the United States)
An optional mode, IntelliVent-ASV is a complete fully closed-loop ventilation algorithm for oxygenation and ventilation. It relies on ASV to select tidal volume and mandatory breath frequency. It uses a rule-based expert system in conjunction with volumetric CO_2 and SpO_2 measurements to select targets for minute ventilation, PEEP, and F_1O_2. It covers all applications from intubation until extubation with simplicity for an early weaning.

- *Mandatory breaths:* Machine triggered (preset frequency) and machine cycled (inspiratory time). Spontaneous breaths suppress mandatory breaths if spontaneous minute ventilation is above target minute ventilation.
  - Within-breath settings:
    – Operator maximum PEEP and inspiratory pressure, patient height, disease state, and weaning strategy
    – Ventilator-set inspiratory pressure
- *Spontaneous breaths:* Patient triggered (pressure or flow sensitivity) and patient cycled (% peak inspiratory flow)

- Within-breath settings:
  - Operator-set rise time and cycle sensitivity (% peak flow)
- Between-breath targets:
  - Ventilator-set tidal volume, minute ventilation, PEEP, and F_1O_2

Nasal Continuous Positive Airway Pressure/Pressure Support
This mode is designed to apply CPAP and intermittent positive pressure support with a nasal interface (mask or prongs).

- *Mandatory breaths:* Machine triggered (preset frequency or patient synchronized using pressure or flow sensitivity) and machine cycled (inspiratory time)
  - Within-breath settings:
    – Operator-set PEEP, frequency, inspiratory pressure, rise time, and inspiratory time
- *Spontaneous breaths:* Patient triggered (pressure or flow sensitivity) and patient cycled (% peak inspiratory flow)
  - Within-breath settings:
    – Operator-set cycle sensitivity (% peak flow). Inspiratory pressure and rise time set for mandatory breaths applies to spontaneous breaths automatically.
- *Between-breath targets:* None

Noninvasive Ventilation
Noninvasive ventilation (NIV) is an adaptation of the SPONT mode. The primary difference is that NIV is designed to compensate for leaks when using a mask or other noninvasive patient interface.

- *Mandatory breaths:* Not allowed
- *Spontaneous breaths:* Patient triggered (pressure or flow sensitivity) and patient cycled (% peak inspiratory flow)
  - Within-breath settings:
    – Operator-set inspiratory pressure, rise time, cycle sensitivity (% peak flow), and maximum inspiratory time
- *Between-breath targets:* None

Noninvasive Ventilation-Spontaneous Timed
Noninvasive ventilation (NIV) is an adaptation of the SPONT mode, whereas NIV-ST is an adaptation of the PSIMV+ mode. The primary difference is that NIV modes are designed to compensate for leaks when using a mask or other noninvasive patient interface.

- *Mandatory breaths:* Machine triggered (preset frequency or patient synchronized using flow sensitivity) and machine cycled (inspiratory time)
  - Within-breath settings:
    – Operator-set PEEP, inspiratory pressure, frequency, rise time, and inspiratory time
- *Spontaneous breaths:* Patient triggered (pressure or flow sensitivity) and patient cycled (% peak inspiratory flow)

- Within-breath settings:
  - Operator-set cycle sensitivity (% peak flow). Inspiratory pressure and rise time set for mandatory breaths applies to spontaneous breaths automatically.
- *Between-breath targets:* None

Pressure Controlled Continuous Mandatory Ventilation Assist/Control

- *Mandatory breaths:* Machine triggered (preset frequency) or patient triggered (pressure or flow sensitivity) and machine cycled (inspiratory time)
  - Within-breath settings:
    - Operator-set PEEP, frequency, inspiratory pressure, rise time, and I:E or % inspiratory time
- *Spontaneous breaths:* Not allowed
- *Between-breath targets:* None

Pressure Synchronized Intermittent Mandatory Ventilation

- *Mandatory breaths:* Machine triggered (preset frequency or patient synchronized using pressure or flow sensitivity) and machine cycled (inspiratory time)
  - Within-breath settings:
    - Operator-set PEEP, inspiratory pressure, frequency, rise time, and I:E or % inspiratory time
- *Spontaneous breaths:* Patient triggered (pressure or flow sensitivity) and patient cycled (% peak inspiratory flow)
  - Within-breath settings:
    - Operator-set PEEP, inspiratory pressure, rise time, cycle sensitivity (% inspiratory flow), and maximum inspiratory time
- *Between-breath targets:* None

Spontaneous

- *Mandatory breaths:* Not allowed
- *Spontaneous breaths:* Patient triggered (pressure or flow sensitivity) and patient cycled (% peak inspiratory flow)
  - Within-breath settings:
    - Operator-set PEEP, inspiratory pressure, rise time, cycle sensitivity (% inspiratory flow), and maximum inspiratory time
- *Between-breath targets:* None

Synchronized Controlled Mandatory Ventilation Assist/Control

- *Mandatory breaths:* Machine triggered (preset frequency) or patient triggered (pressure or flow sensitivity) and machine cycled (tidal volume or pause time)
  - Within-breath settings:

- Operator-set PEEP, frequency, flow pattern, tidal volume, I:E and pause time, peak flow and inspiratory time, or % inspiration and pause time
- *Spontaneous breaths:* Not allowed
- *Between-breath targets:* None

Synchronized Intermittent Mandatory Ventilation

- *Mandatory breaths:* Machine triggered (preset frequency) or patient synchronized (pressure or flow sensitivity) and machine cycled (tidal volume or pause time)
  - Within-breath settings:
    - Operator-set PEEP, frequency, flow pattern, tidal volume, I:E and pause time, peak flow and inspiratory time, or % inspiration and pause time
- *Spontaneous breaths:* Patient triggered (pressure or flow sensitivity) and patient cycled (% peak inspiratory flow)
  - Within-breath settings:
    - Operator-set PEEP, inspiratory pressure, rise time, cycle sensitivity (% inspiratory flow), and maximum inspiratory time
- *Between-breath targets:* None

Tube Resistance Compensation

To reduce the patient's work of breathing while on the ventilator, the Tube Resistance Compensation feature offsets the flow resistance imposed by the endotracheal or tracheostomy tube. Tube Resistance Compensation is active during exhalation in volume modes, and in both inspiration and exhalation in the other modes.

- Within-breath settings:
  - Operator-set percent support (of resistive load) along with artificial airway tube diameter and tube type
  - Ventilator-set inspiratory pressure as a function of patient-generated inspiratory flow
- *Between-breath targets:* None

Special Features

Backup ventilation: Backup ventilation is activated if no breath is detected during the set apnea delay time. The backup ventilation mode is SCMV A/C, PCMV A/C, or APVcmv depending on the original mode.

Gas volume compensation: Pressure, flow, and volume measurements are based on readings from the flow sensor, and they are expressed in BTPS (body temperature and pressure, saturated). The volume exhaled by the patient is determined from the flow sensor measurement, so it does not show any volume added due to compression or lost due to leaks in the breathing circuit. If there is a gas leak at the patient end, the displayed exhaled tidal volume may be less than the tidal volume the patient actually receives.

Miscellaneous: The sigh function delivers a sigh breath every 50 breaths, with a higher-than-normal pressure or volume. In volume-controlled modes, sigh breaths have a tidal volume 50% higher than nonsigh breaths, up to a maximum of 2,000 mL. In pressure-controlled modes, sigh breaths are delivered at a pressure up to 10 cm H_2O higher than nonsigh breaths, as permitted by the high pressure alarm setting.

Using the optional integrated humidifier it is possible to monitor and control humidifier settings directly from the ventilator screen. You can still use other humidifiers, without full system integration.

The ventilator has a feature called IntelliCuffR, which is an integrated automatic endotracheal tube cuff pressure controller. It provides the operator with continuous monitoring and the means to adjust the pressure of cuffed tracheal tubes and cuffed tracheostomy tubes.

The G5 can be used with integrated PetCO$_2$ and SpO$_2$ sensors.

The G5 offers a unique feature (the P/V Tool) to record quasi-static pressure/volume curves. The feature makes it possible to record both the inflation and deflation limbs of the P/V curve. The maneuver employs an adjustable pressure ramp in which airway pressure is slowly increased to an upper level and then decreased to a lower level. A cursor function permits graphical analysis of the curve, including identification of inflection points and "visual curve fitting" to determine the linear compliance.

The G5 has an advanced graphic interface feature called Dynamic Heart/Lung panel (**Figure 9-38**), which displays tidal volume, lung compliance, hemodynamic status, pulse, patient triggering, and resistance in real-time. The lungs expand and contract in synchrony with actual breaths. Numeric values for resistance, compliance, SpO$_2$, pulse, heart–lung interaction index, patient conditions, and PetCO$_2$ are also displayed.

Nebulizer: The G5's nebulization function powers a standard inline pneumatic nebulizer for delivery of medications in the ventilator circuit. The ventilator can compensate for the extra volume from the nebulizer so the set tidal volume is delivered. The ventilator may also be used with an optional Aerogen Aeroneb vibrating mesh nebulizer.

Noninvasive ventilation: The G5 provides three modes of noninvasive ventilation: Noninvasive Ventilation, Noninvasive Ventilation–Spontaneous Timed, and Nasal Continuous Positive Airway Pressure–Pressure Support.

Manufacturer's Specifications

Table 9-32 lists specifications for the Hamilton-G5 ventilator.

Maquet Servo-i

The Servo-i ventilator (**Figure 9-39**) is intended for invasive and noninvasive ventilation of neonates,

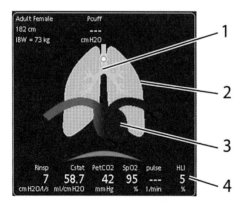

FIGURE 9-38 Hamilton Medical Hamilton-G5 dynamic heart/lung panel. 1. Bronchial tree (appearance changes to reflect changes in airway resistance. 2. Lungs (appearance changes to reflect changes in compliance. 3. Beating heart (appearance changes to reflect changes in hemodynamic stability). 4. Numeric display of parameters.
Courtesy of Hamilton Medical.

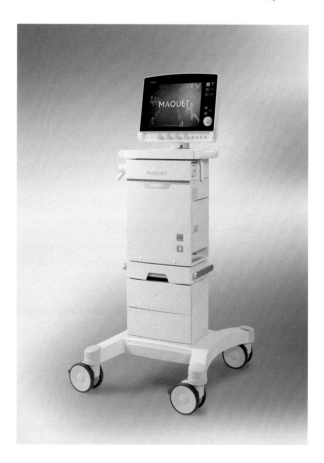

FIGURE 9-39 Maquet Servo-i ventilator.
Courtesy of Maquet Medical Systems.

TABLE 9-32
Specifications for the Hamilton Medical Hamilton-G5 Ventilator

Setting Category	Setting	Range
Pressure	Inspiratory Pressure	5–100 cm H_2O
	Pressure Support	0–100 cm H_2O
	PEEP	0–50 cm H_2O
Volume	Tidal Volume	0.02–2 L
Flow	Inspiratory Flow	1–180 L/min
	Waveform	Square/descending ramp
Time	Inspiratory Time	0.1–9.6 s
	Mandatory Breath Frequency	5–120/min
	Adjustable Rise Time	Yes
Sensitivity	Trigger Sensitivity (pressure)	0.5–10 cm H_2O
	Trigger Sensitivity (flow)	0.5–15 L/min
	Cycle Sensitivity (flow)	5–70%
Alarm Category		
Pressure	Pressure Low	2–119 cm H_2O
	Pressure High	10–120 cm H_2O
Volume	Tidal Volume Low	0–2.95 L
	Tidal Volume High	1–3 L
Flow	Expiratory Minute Volume Low	1–49 L/min
	Expiratory Minute Volume High	0.03–10 L/min
Time	Apnea Time	10–60 s
	Rate Low	0–128/min
	Rate High	2–130/min
Other	O_2 Sensor	Enabled/Disabled
	Leak	5–80%
Monitored Parameters	Peak Pressure	
	Mean Pressure	
	Min Pressure	
	Plateau Pressure	
	PEEP/CPAP	
	AutoPEEP	
	Inspiratory Flow	
	Expiratory Flow	
	Tidal Volume	
	Expiratory Minute Volume	
	Leak Volume	
	I:E	

TABLE 9-32
Specifications for the Hamilton Medical Hamilton-G5 Ventilator *(Continued)*

Setting Category	Setting	Range
Monitored Parameters, cont.	fTotal	
	fSpont	
	TI	
	TE	
	Cstat	
	P0.1	
	PTP	
	PCexp	
	RCinsp	
	Rexp	
	Rinsp	
	RSB	
	WOBimp	
	Oxygen	

infants, and adults with respiratory failure or respiratory insufficiency in hospitals or healthcare facilities and for in-hospital transport.

Operator Interface

The Servo-i operator interface (**Figure 9-40**) uses a touch screen, buttons, and knobs. The touch screen is used to select control variables and the main control knob allows adjustment of settings (by turning) and confirmation of settings (by pressing). The supplemental control knobs provide quick setting adjustments of O_2%, tidal volume, inspiratory pressure, and PEEP. The buttons provide for manual breath trigger, "O_2 breaths" (100% oxygen for 1 minute), inspiratory hold, and expiratory hold. Other buttons are related to alarms, system information, and navigation.

Modes

Mode names are selected by pressing buttons on the touch screen. Once a mode name is chosen, the screen changes to show the available setting options. The modes available on the Servo-i are shown in **Table 9-33**.

Automode (Pressure Control to Pressure Support)
- *Mandatory breaths:* Machine triggered (preset frequency) or patient synchronized (pressure or flow sensitivity) and machine cycled (inspiratory time).
  - Within-breath settings:
    - Operator-set PEEP, frequency, inspiratory rise time, and I:E or inspiratory time

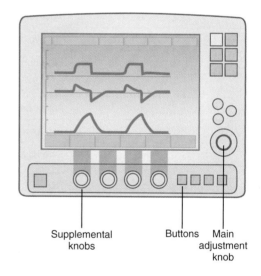

FIGURE 9-40 Maquet Servo-i operator interface.
Courtesy of Maquet Medical Systems.

- Operator-set inspiratory pressure
- *Spontaneous breaths:* Patient triggered (pressure or flow sensitivity) and patient cycled (% peak inspiratory flow). Spontaneous breaths suppress mandatory breaths if their frequency is at or above the set mandatory breath frequency.
  - Within-breath settings:
    - Operator-set inspiratory pressure (Pressure Support level), rise time, and cycle sensitivity (% peak inspiratory flow)
- *Between-breath targets:* None.

TABLE 9-33
Classification of Modes for the Maquet Servo-i

Mode Name	Control Variable	Breath Sequence	Primary Breath Targeting Scheme	Secondary Breath Targeting Scheme	Tag
Volume Control	volume	IMV	dual	dual	VC-IMVd,d
SIMV (Volume Control)	volume	IMV	dual	dual	VC-IMVd,d
Automode (Volume Control to Volume Support)	volume	IMV	dual	dual/adaptive	VC-IMVd,da
Pressure Control	pressure	CMV	set-point	N/A	PC-CMVs
Pressure Regulated Volume Control	pressure	CMV	adaptive	N/A	PC-CMVa
SIMV (Pressure Control)	pressure	IMV	set-point	set-point	PC-IMVs,s
Bi-Vent	pressure	IMV	set-point	set-point	PC-IMVs,s
Automode (Pressure Control to Pressure Support)	pressure	IMV	set-point	set-point	PC-IMVs,s
SIMV Pressure Regulated Volume Control	pressure	IMV	adaptive	set-point	PC-IMVa,s
Automode (Pressure Regulated Volume Control to Volume Support)	pressure	IMV	adaptive	adaptive	PC-IMVa,a
Spontaneous/CPAP	pressure	CSV	set-point	N/A	PC-CSVs
Pressure Support	pressure	CSV	set-point	N/A	PC-CSVs
Neurally Adjusted Ventilatory Assist	pressure	CSV	servo	N/A	PC-CSVr
Volume Support	pressure	CSV	adaptive	N/A	PC-CSVa

Reproduced with permission from Mandu Press Ltd.

Automode (Pressure Regulated Volume Control to Volume Support)
- *Mandatory breaths:* Machine triggered (preset frequency or patient synchronized using pressure or flow sensitivity) and machine cycled (inspiratory time).
  - Within-breath settings:
    - Operator-set PEEP, frequency, inspiratory rise time, and I:E or inspiratory time
    - Ventilator-set inspiratory pressure
- *Spontaneous breaths:* Patient triggered (pressure or flow sensitivity) and patient cycled (% peak inspiratory flow). Spontaneous breaths suppress mandatory breaths if their frequency is at or above the set mandatory breath frequency.
  - Within-breath settings:
    - Operator-set PEEP, inspiratory rise time, cycle sensitivity (% peak inspiratory flow)
    - Ventilator-set inspiratory pressure

- Between-breath targets:
  - Operator-set average tidal volume

Automode (Volume Control to Volume Support)
- *Mandatory breaths:* Machine triggered (preset frequency) or patient synchronized (pressure or flow sensitivity) and machine cycled (tidal volume or inspiratory time). Because this mode uses dual targeting, if the patient's inspiratory effort is large enough, inspiration will switch from volume control with time cycling (i.e., a mandatory breath) to pressure control with flow cycling. If inspiration happened to also be patient triggered, the breath would be classified as spontaneous (i.e., patient triggered and cycled) and would be very similar to a breath in the Pressure Support mode.
  - Within-breath settings:

- – Operator-set PEEP, frequency, peak inspiratory flow, tidal volume, and I:E or inspiratory time
    - – Ventilator-set inspiratory pressure if inspiration switches from volume control to pressure control due to the dual targeting scheme
- *Spontaneous breaths:* Patient triggered (pressure or flow sensitivity) and patient cycled (% peak inspiratory flow). Spontaneous breaths suppress mandatory breaths if their frequency is at or above the set mandatory breath frequency.
    - • Within-breath settings:
        - – Operator-set rise time and cycle sensitivity (% peak inspiratory flow)
        - – Ventilator-set inspiratory pressure
- *Between-breath targets:*
    - • Operator-set average tidal volume for spontaneous breaths

BiVent

- *Mandatory breaths:* Machine triggered (preset frequency) or patient synchronized (pressure or flow sensitivity) and machine cycled (inspiratory time or patient synchronized by flow sensitivity).
    - • Within-breath settings:
        - – Operator-set PEEP, peak inspiratory pressure (called P_{High}), rise time, inspiratory time (called T_{High}), and expiratory time (called T_{PEEP})
- *Spontaneous breaths:* Patient triggered (pressure or flow sensitivity) and patient cycled (% peak inspiratory flow). Spontaneous breaths are permitted both between and during mandatory breaths.
    - • Within-breath settings:
        - – Operator-set inspiratory pressure and rise time
- *Between-breath targets:* None.

Neurally Adjusted Ventilatory Assist (NAVA)

- *Mandatory breaths:* Not allowed
- *Spontaneous breaths:* Patient triggered (sensitivity based on electrical activity of diaphragm) and patient cycled (sensitivity based on electrical activity of diaphragm)
    - • Within-breath settings:
        - – Operator-set NAVA (constant of proportionality between electrical signal of the diaphragm and inspiratory pressure)
        - – Ventilator-set inspiratory pressure as a function of the electrical signal of the diaphragm.
        - – Note: If the diaphragm signal is lost, the ventilator switches to Pressure Support. It returns to NAVA if the signal is regained.
- *Between-breath targets:* None

Pressure Control

- *Mandatory breaths:* Machine triggered (preset frequency) or patient triggered (pressure or flow sensitivity) and machine cycled (inspiratory time)

- • Within-breath settings:
    - – Operator-set PEEP, frequency, inspiratory pressure, rise time, and inspiratory time
- *Spontaneous breaths:* Not allowed
- *Between-breath targets:* None

Pressure Regulated Volume Control

- *Mandatory breaths:* Machine triggered (preset frequency) or patient triggered (pressure or flow sensitivity) and machine cycled (inspiratory time)
    - • Within-breath settings:
        - – Operator-set PEEP, frequency, rise time, and inspiratory time
        - – Ventilator-set inspiratory pressure
- *Spontaneous breaths:* Not allowed
- Between-breath targets:
    - • Operator-set tidal volume

Pressure Support

- *Mandatory breaths:* Not allowed
- *Spontaneous breaths:* Patient triggered (pressure or flow sensitivity) and patient cycled (% peak inspiratory flow)
    - • Within-breath settings:
        - – Operator-set inspiratory pressure, rise time, and cycle sensitivity (% peak inspiratory flow)
- *Between-breath targets:* None

SIMV Pressure Control

- *Mandatory breaths:* Machine triggered (preset frequency) or patient synchronized (pressure or flow sensitivity) and machine cycled (inspiratory time)
    - • Within-breath settings:
        - – Operator-set PEEP, frequency, inspiratory pressure, rise time, and inspiratory time
- *Spontaneous breaths:* Patient triggered (pressure or flow sensitivity) and patient cycled (% peak inspiratory flow)
    - • Within-breath settings:
        - – Operator-set inspiratory pressure, rise time, and cycle sensitivity (% peak inspiratory flow)
- *Between-breath targets:* None

SIMV (Volume Control)

- *Mandatory breaths:* Machine triggered (preset frequency) or patient synchronized (pressure or flow sensitivity) and machine cycled (tidal volume or pause time)
    - • Within-breath settings:
        - – Operator-set PEEP, peak inspiratory flow, rise time, tidal volume, and I:E or inspiratory time
        - – Ventilator-set inspiratory pressure if inspiration switches from volume control to pressure control due to the dual targeting scheme (see spontaneous breaths below)

- *Spontaneous breaths:* Patient triggered (pressure or flow sensitivity) and patient cycled (% peak inspiratory flow)
  - Within-breath settings:
    - Operator-set inspiratory pressure and cycle sensitivity (% peak inspiratory flow)
  - In addition, this mode uses dual targeting (see the explanation of dual targeting above), so if the patient's inspiratory effort is large enough, inspiration will switch from volume control to pressure control with flow cycling. If inspiration happened to also be patient triggered, the breath would be classified as spontaneous (i.e., patient triggered and cycled) and would be very similar to a breath in the Pressure Support mode.
- *Between-breath targets:* None

SIMV Pressure Regulated Volume Control

- *Mandatory breaths:* Machine triggered (preset frequency) or patient synchronized (pressure or flow sensitivity) and machine cycled (inspiratory time)
  - Within-breath settings:
    - Operator-set PEEP, frequency, rise time, and inspiratory time
    - Ventilator-set inspiratory pressure
- *Spontaneous breaths:* Patient triggered (pressure or flow sensitivity) and patient cycled (% peak inspiratory flow)
  - Within-breath settings:
    - Operator-set inspiratory pressure, rise time, and cycle sensitivity (% peak inspiratory flow)
- Between-breath targets:
  - Operator-set tidal volume

Spontaneous/CPAP

- *Mandatory breaths:* Not allowed
- *Spontaneous breaths:* Patient triggered (pressure or flow sensitivity) and patient cycled (% peak inspiratory flow)
  - Within-breath settings:
    - Operator-set inspiratory pressure, rise time, and cycle sensitivity (% peak inspiratory flow)
- *Between-breath targets:* None

Volume Control

- *Mandatory breaths:* Machine triggered (preset frequency) or patient triggered (pressure or flow sensitivity) and machine cycled (tidal volume or inspiratory time).
  - Within-breath settings:
    - Operator-set PEEP, frequency, inspiratory rise time, tidal volume, and I:E or inspiratory time
    - Ventilator-set inspiratory pressure if inspiration switches from volume control to

pressure control due to the dual targeting scheme (see spontaneous breaths below)
- *Spontaneous breaths:* Because this mode uses dual targeting, if the patient's inspiratory effort is large enough, inspiration will switch from volume control with time cycling to pressure control with flow cycling. If inspiration happened to also be patient triggered, the breath would be classified as spontaneous (i.e., patient triggered and cycled) and would be very similar to a breath in the Pressure Support mode. This possibility of spontaneous breaths appearing between mandatory breaths is the reason Volume Control on this ventilator is a form of IMV instead of CMV.
- *Between-breath targets:* None

Volume Support

- *Mandatory breaths:* Not allowed
- *Spontaneous breaths:* Patient triggered (pressure or flow sensitivity) and patient cycled (% peak inspiratory flow)
  - Within-breath settings:
    - Operator-set rise time and cycle sensitivity (% peak inspiratory flow)
- Between-breath targets:
  - Operator-set average tidal volume

Special Features

Backup ventilation: Backup ventilation is available in all support modes (not applicable in Automode and NIV Pressure Support mode). The backup function switches Volume Support to Volume Control, and Pressure Support and CPAP to Pressure Control.

Gas volume compensation: Patient circuit compliance compensation may be turned on or off. Volumes are displayed as atmospheric temperature and pressure, dry (ATPD).

Leak compensation: During noninvasive ventilation (NIV) the ventilator automatically adapts to the variation of leakage in order to maintain the required inspiratory pressure and PEEP level. If the leakage is excessive, the ventilator will issue a high priority alarm, deliver a continuous flow, and pause breath cycling. Ventilation will resume automatically if the leakage decreases.

Miscellaneous: An optional CO_2 analyzer allows for continuous monitoring shown in a waveform indicating the exhaled CO_2 concentration. A numerical presentation of end-tidal CO_2 concentration (ETCO$_2$), CO_2 minute elimination, and CO_2 tidal elimination is also shown on the screen. Alarm limits for high and low ETCO$_2$ can be individually set.

The Open Lung Tool is a special display for graphically visualizing measured and calculated ventilation data. Three simultaneous graphical trends are presented with a fixed set of parameters as a function of a number of collected breaths. The user interface features an adjustable cursor that helps illustrate the opening and closing airway pressures. This alternative presentation may be used for immediate visualization of the effect of altered settings. The following parameters are presented:

- In the top window, measured end inspiratory pressure (EIP) and positive end-expiratory pressure (PEEP) are simultaneously presented, breath by breath.
- In the middle window, measured inspiratory tidal volume (V_T) and expiratory tidal volume are simultaneously presented, breath by breath.
- Dynamic compliance (C_{dyn}) is calculated breath by breath and filtered before presentation [$C_{dyn} = V_T/(EIP - PEEP)$].
- Tidal CO_2 elimination is shown in the lower window.

A special version of this ventilator can be used for magnetic resonance imaging (MRI).

There is an option for delivering heliox. When switching gas from air and O_2 to heliox and back, volume and CO_2 monitoring as well as flow delivery are adjusted automatically by the ventilator.

Nebulizer: The Servo Ultra (ultrasonic) Nebulizer is intended for nebulizing drugs to patients requiring mechanical ventilation or positive pressure breathing assistance via an endotracheal tube or face mask/prongs. The nebulizer operates continuously regardless of ventilation mode setting. No extra gas volume is added to the inspiratory Minute Volume and thus neither the ventilator settings nor the readings are affected.

Neonatal ventilation: An optional neonatal flow sensor is available with an airway adapter dead space of less than 0.75 mL and a weight of 4 grams. This allows flow readings as close to the patient as possible to maximize accuracy.

Noninvasive ventilation: The noninvasive (NIV) settings allow ventilation with various noninvasive patient–ventilator interfaces including masks, infant nasal prongs, and uncuffed neonatal endotracheal tubes. During NIV the ventilator automatically adapts to the variation of leakage in order to maintain the required pressure and PEEP level. If the leakage is excessive, the ventilator will issue a high priority alarm, deliver a continuous flow, and pause breath cycling. Ventilation will resume automatically if the leakage decreases.

Manufacturer's Specifications

Table 9-34 lists specifications for the Maquet Servo-i ventilator.

TABLE 9-34
Specifications for the Maquet Servo-i Ventilator

Setting Category	Setting	Range
Pressure	Inspiratory Pressure	0–120 cm H_2O
	Pressure Support	0–120 cm H_2O
	PEEP	0–50 cm H_2O
Volume	Tidal Volume	0.1–4 L
Flow	Inspiratory Flow	0–3.3 L/min
	Waveform	Not Specified
Time	Inspiratory Time	0.1–5 s
	Mandatory Breath Frequency	1–150/min
	Adjustable Rise Time	Yes
Sensitivity	Trigger Sensitivity (pressure)	–20–0 cm H_2O
	Trigger Sensitivity (flow)	0–100%
Alarm Category		
Pressure	Airway Pressure Upper Limit	16–120 cm H_2O
	CPAP High Limit	0–55 cm H_2O
	CPAP Lower Limit	0–47 cm H_2O

TABLE 9-34
Specifications for the Maquet Servo-i Ventilator (*Continued*)

Setting Category	Setting	Range
Pressure, cont.	End Expiratory Pressure High Limit	0–55 cm H_2O
	End Expiratory Pressure Lower Limit	0–47 cm H_2O
	$etCO_2$ Upper Limit	4–100 mm Hg
	$etCO_2$ Lower Limit	4–100 mm Hg
Flow	Expired Minute Volume Lower Limit	0.01–40.0 L/min
	Expired Minute Volume Upper Limit	0.01–60.0 L/min
Time	Apnea	2–45 s
	Respiratory Frequency Limit	1–160/min
Other	O_2 Sensor	Enabled/Disabled
Monitored Parameters	Breathing Frequency	
	Spontaneous Breaths per Minute	
	Peak Airway Pressure	
	Mean Airway Pressure	
	Pause Airway Pressure	
	End Expiratory Pressure	
	CPAP Pressure	
	Inspired Tidal Volume	
	Expired Tidal Volume	
	Inspired Minute Volume	
	Expired Minute Volume	
	Leakage Fraction in NIV	
	Ti/Ttotal	
	I:E Ratio	
	Total PEEP	
	Edi Peak	
	Edi Min	
	O_2 Concentration	
	CO_2 End Tidal Concentration	
	CO_2 Minute Elimination	
	Tidal CO_2 Elimination	
	MVe sp/MVe	
	Spontaneous Exp Minute Volume	

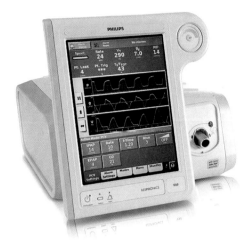

FIGURE 9-41 Philips Respironics V60 ventilator.
Reproduced with permission from Philips Healthcare.

Philips Respironics V60

The Philips Respironics V60 ventilator (**Figure 9-41**), formerly called the Vision, is a microprocessor-controlled, bilevel positive airway pressure (BiPAP) ventilatory assist system that provides noninvasive positive pressure ventilation (NPPV) and invasive ventilatory support for spontaneously breathing patients. The ventilator is intended to support adult patients and pediatric patients weighing 44 lb (20 kg) or greater. It is also intended for intubated patients meeting the same selection criteria as the noninvasive applications.

Operator Interface

The V60 operator interface (**Figure 9-42**) uses a touch screen, buttons, and knobs. The touch screen is used to select control variables and the main control knob allows adjustment of settings (by turning) and confirmation of settings (by pressing).

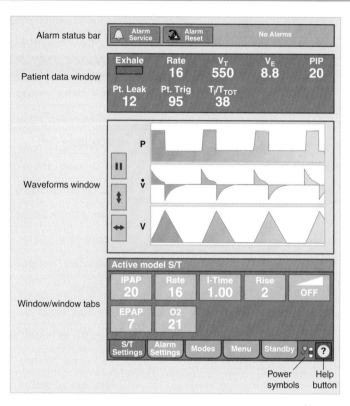

FIGURE 9-42 Philips Respironics V60 operator interface.
Reproduced with permission from Philips Healthcare.

Modes

Modes on the V60 are selected by mode name (e.g., CPAP, AVAPS, PCV, etc.) using a menu. Specific mode settings are selected using other menus. Available modes are shown in **Table 9-35**.

Unlike other ventilators, the Respironics V60 Ventilator does not require manual setting of triggering and cycling sensitivity for spontaneous breaths. The ventilator's unique Auto-Trak Sensitivity algorithm adjusts these automatically. Spontaneous breaths may

TABLE 9-35
Mode Classifications for the Philips Respironics V60 Ventilator

| Mode Name | Mode Classification | | | | |
	Control Variable	Breath Sequence	Primary Targeting Scheme	Secondary Targeting Scheme	Tag
Pressure Controlled Ventilation	pressure	CMV	set-point	set-point	PC-CMVs,s
Spontaneous/Timed	pressure	IMV	set-point	set-point	PC-IMVs,s
Average Volume-Assured Pressure Support	pressure	IMV	adaptive	adaptive	PC-IMVa,a
Proportional Pressure Support	pressure	IMV	set-point	servo	PC-IMVs,r
CPAP	pressure	CSV	set-point	N/A	PC-CSVs

Reproduced with permission from Mandu Press Ltd.

be patient (flow) triggered in all modes, typically when patient effort causes a certain volume of gas to accumulate above baseline flow (volume method). An inspiration is also triggered when the patient inspiratory effort distorts the expiratory flow waveform sufficiently (shape signal method). Cycling to exhalation occurs for spontaneous breaths in these cases:

- Patient expiratory effort distorts the inspiratory flow waveform sufficiently (shape signal method).
- Patient flow reaches the spontaneous exhalation threshold
- Flow reversal occurs, typically due to a mask or mouth leak

Breaths will also be time cycled after 3 seconds at the IPAP level (timed backup safety mechanism).

Average Volume Assured Pressure Support
- *Mandatory breaths:* Machine triggered (preset frequency) or patient triggered (Auto-Trak) and machine cycled (inspiratory time).
  - Within-breath settings:
    - Operator-set PEEP, frequency, rise time, and inspiratory time
    - Ventilator-set inspiratory pressure
- *Spontaneous breaths:* Patient triggered (Auto-Trak) and patient cycled (Auto-Trak). Spontaneous breaths suppress mandatory breaths if they occur at a frequency higher than the set mandatory rate.
  - Within-breath settings:
    - Operator-set rise time and cycle sensitivity (% peak inspiratory flow)
    - Ventilator-set inspiratory pressure
- Between-breath targets:
  - Operator-set tidal volume

Continuous Positive Airway Pressure
- *Mandatory breaths:* Not allowed
- *Spontaneous breaths:* Patient triggered (Auto-Trak) and patient cycled (Auto-Trak).
  - Within-breath settings:
    - Operator-set inspiratory CPAP, ramp time (an interval during which the ventilator linearly increases the target inspiratory and expiratory pressure, helping to reduce patient anxiety, and maximum inspiratory time), and C-Flex. C-Flex is a feature that reduces the pressure at the beginning of exhalation—a time when patients may be uncomfortable with CPAP—and returns it to the set CPAP pressure before the end of exhalation. The amount of pressure relief is determined by the C-Flex setting and the expiratory flow. The higher the setting number (1, 2, or 3) and the greater the expiratory flow, the greater the pressure relief (during the active part of exhalation only).
- *Between-breath targets:* None

Pressure Controlled Ventilation
- *Mandatory breaths:* Machine triggered (preset frequency) or patient triggered (Auto-Trak) and machine cycled (inspiratory time).
  - Within-breath settings:
    - Operator-set PEEP, frequency, inspiratory pressure, rise time, inspiratory time, and ramp time (see Continuous Positive Airway Pressure above).
- *Spontaneous breaths:* Not allowed
- *Between-breath targets:* None

Proportional Pressure Ventilation
- *Mandatory breaths:* Machine triggered (preset frequency) or patient triggered (Auto-Trak) and machine cycled (inspiratory time)
  - Within-breath settings:
    - Operator-set PEEP, frequency, inspiratory pressure, rise time, and inspiratory time
- *Spontaneous breaths:* Patient triggered (Auto-Trak) and patient cycled (Auto-Trak)
  - *Within-breath settings:* None
- Between-breath targets:
  - The delivery of a PPV breath is controlled by the maximum elastance (Max E), maximum resistance (Max R), and PPV % settings. The actual delivered assistance to overcome elastance (volume assist) is the product of PPV % and Max E. The actual delivered assistance to overcome resistance (flow assist) is the product of PPV % and Max R.

Spontaneous/Timed
- *Mandatory breaths:* Machine triggered (preset frequency) or patient triggered (Auto-Trak) and machine cycled (inspiratory time). Spontaneous breaths suppress mandatory breaths if they occur at a frequency higher than the set mandatory rate.
  - Within-breath settings:
    - Operator-set PEEP, inspiratory pressure, frequency, rise time, and ramp time (see Continuous Positive Airway Pressure above)
- *Spontaneous breaths:* Patient triggered (Auto-Trak) and patient cycled (Auto-Trak).
  - Within-breath settings:
    - Operator-set cycle sensitivity (% peak flow). Inspiratory pressure and rise time set for mandatory breaths apply to spontaneous breaths automatically.
- *Between-breath targets:* None.

Special Features

Backup ventilation: There is no backup mode in case of apnea, but there are alarms for low rate and low tidal volume.

Gas volume compensation: Exhaled tidal volume is compensated for body temperature and pressure, saturated (BTPS) conditions.

Noninvasive ventilation: The V60 is primarily designed for noninvasive ventilation.

Manufacturer's Specifications

Table 9-36 lists specifications for the Philips Respironics V60 ventilator.

Philips Respironics V200

The Philips Respironics V200 ventilator (Figure 9-43), formerly called the Esprit, is a microprocessor-controlled,

electrically powered mechanical ventilator intended to provide continuous or intermittent ventilatory support for adult, pediatric, and neonatal patients. The ventilator is designed for use in either invasive or noninvasive applications in institutional environments.

Operator Interface

The V200 operator interface (Figure 9-44) uses a touch screen, buttons, and knobs. The touch screen is used to select control variables and the main control knob

TABLE 9-36
Specifications for the Philips Respironics V60 Ventilator

Setting Category	Setting	Range
Pressure	Inspiratory Pressure	4–40 cm H_2O
	Pressure Support	6–40 cm H_2O
	PEEP	4–25 cm H_2O
Volume	Tidal Volume	0.2–2 L
Flow	Waveform	Not Specified
	Inspiratory Time	0.3–3.0 s
Time	Mandatory Breath Frequency	4–60/min
	Adjustable Rise Time	Yes
Alarm Category		
Pressure	High Inspiratory Pressure	5–50 cm H_2O
	Low Inspiratory Pressure	0–40 cm H_2O
Volume	High Tidal Volume	0.2–2.5 L
	Low Tidal Volume	0–1.5 L
Flow	Low Minute Ventilation	0.1 L–99 L
Time	Low Inspiratory Pressure Delay	5–60 s
	High Rate	5–90/min
	Low Rate	1–89/min
Other	O_2 Sensor	Enabled/Disabled
Monitored Parameters	PIP	
	Patient Leak	
	Patient Trigger	
	Rate	
	Tf/Ttot	
	Total Leak	
	Minute Ventilation	
	Tidal Volume	

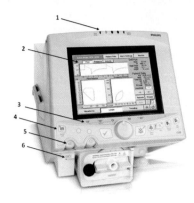

FIGURE 9-43 Philips Respironics V200 ventilator. 1. Alarm status indicators. 2. Touch display. 3. Power status indicators. 4. Front panel keys. 5. Level controls. 6. Power On/Off switch.

Reproduced with permission from Philips Healthcare.

allows adjustment of settings (by turning) and confirmation of settings (by pressing).

Modes

Modes on the V200 are set by first selecting a breath type (volume control ventilation, pressure control ventilation, or noninvasive positive pressure ventilation). Next, the operator selects a mode. In VCV or PCV, the choices are A/C, SIMV, or CPAP. In NPPV, the choices are Spont/T or Spont. The V200 has an optional feature called Flow-Trak. This is a form of dual targeting that is available in volume control modes. If the patient's inspiratory effort decreases inspiratory pressure sufficiently, Flow-Trak

increases flow above the set target enough to maintain pressure at 2 cm H_2O above the set PEEP. Once the preset tidal volume has been delivered, inspiration is cycled off when inspiratory flow decays to the preset value or to 20% of peak inspiratory flow, whichever is greater. In effect, Flow-Trak is capable of turning a mandatory volume control breath into a spontaneous pressure support breath. Therefore, when Flow-Trak is activated, the mode classification will change (i.e., from VC-CMVs or VC-IMVs,s to VC-IMVd,s) because of the possibility of a spontaneous breath occurring between two mandatory breaths. Once the mode and breath type are determined, specific target values are selected using context-specific menus. Available modes are shown in **Table 9-37**.

Respironics V200 has an optional feature, called Auto-Trak, that automatically sets the trigger and cycle thresholds for spontaneous breaths and patient-triggered mandatory breaths. Auto-Trak monitors changes in pressure and flow patterns throughout exhalation, applies compensation for circuit leaks, and triggers an inspiration when the criterion for one of the automatic triggering algorithms has been met. As a backup, Auto-Trak uses **pressure triggering** at a fixed level of 3 cm H_2O. Auto-Trak automatically cycles inspiration based on the pressure and flow patterns at the end of inspiration and beginning of expiration. The threshold used to cycle each breath changes with the patient's breathing pattern and lung dynamics. When Auto-Trak is selected in NPPV mode, the estimated exhaled tidal volume includes compensation for the estimated leak volume lost during exhalation. Therefore, all other

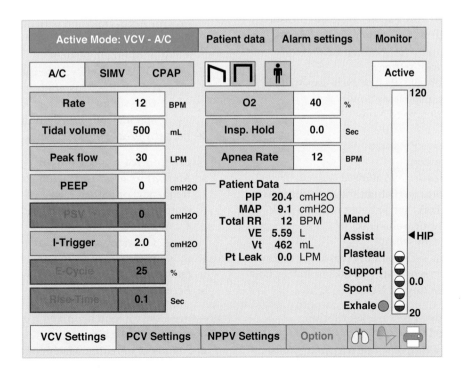

FIGURE 9-44 Philips Respironics V200 operator interface.

Reproduced with permission from Philips Healthcare.

TABLE 9-37
Mode Classifications for the Philips Respironics V200 Ventilator

Mode Name	Mode Classification				
	Control Variable	Breath Sequence	Primary Breath Targeting Scheme	Secondary Breath Targeting Scheme	Tag
Volume Control Ventilation Assist Control	volume	CMV	set-point	N/A	VC-CMVs
Volume Control Ventilation Assist Control with Flow-Trak	volume	CMV	dual	N/A	VC-CMVd
Volume Control Intermittent Mandatory Ventilation	volume	IMV	set-point	set-point	VC-IMVs,s
Volume Control Intermittent Mandatory Ventilation with Flow-Trak	volume	IMV	dual	set-point	VC-IMVd,s
Pressure Control Assist Control	pressure	CMV	set-point	N/A	PC-CMVs
Pressure Control Intermittent Mandatory Ventilation	pressure	IMV	set-point	set-point	PC-IMVs,s
Non-invasive Positive Pressure Ventilation Spontaneous/Timed	pressure	IMV	set-point	set-point	PC-IMVs,s
Continuous Positive Airway Pressure	pressure	CSV	set-point	N/A	PC-CSVs
Non-invasive Positive Pressure Ventilation Spontaneous	pressure	CSV	set-point	N/A	PC-CSVs

Reproduced with permission from Mandu Press Ltd.

parameters that depend on exhaled tidal volume also include this compensation (for example, minute ventilation and rapid-shallow breathing index).

Continuous Positive Airway Pressure
- *Mandatory breaths:* Not allowed
- *Spontaneous breaths:* Patient triggered (pressure, flow, or Auto-Trak) and patient cycled (% peak flow or Auto-Trak)
  - Within-breath settings:
    - Operator-set CPAP or cycle sensitivity (% peak inspiratory flow)
- *Between-breath targets:* None

Non-Invasive Positive Pressure Ventilation Spontaneous
- *Mandatory breaths:* Not allowed
- *Spontaneous breaths:* Patient triggered (pressure, flow or Auto-Trak) and patient cycled (% peak inspiratory flow or Auto-Trak)
  - Within-breath settings:
    - Operator-set inspiratory pressure, rise time, and cycle sensitivity (% peak inspiratory flow)
- *Between-breath targets:* None

Non-invasive Positive Pressure Ventilation Spontaneous/Timed
- *Mandatory breaths:* Machine triggered (preset frequency) or patient triggered (pressure, flow, or Auto-Trak) and machine cycled (inspiratory time or Auto-Trak). Spontaneous breaths suppress

mandatory breaths if they occur at a frequency higher than the set mandatory rate.
  - Within-breath settings:
    - Operator-set PEEP, inspiratory pressure, frequency, and rise time
- *Spontaneous breaths:* Patient triggered (pressure, flow, or Auto-Trak) and patient cycled (pressure, flow, or Auto-Trak)
  - Within-breath settings:
    - Operator-set cycle sensitivity (% peak inspiratory flow). Inspiratory pressure and rise time set for mandatory breaths apply to spontaneous breaths automatically.
- *Between-breath targets:* None

Pressure Control Assist Control
- *Mandatory breaths:* Machine triggered (preset frequency) or patient triggered (pressure, flow, or Auto-Trak) and machine cycled (inspiratory time)
  - Within-breath settings:
    - Operator-set PEEP, frequency, inspiratory pressure, rise time, and inspiratory time
- *Spontaneous breaths:* Not allowed
- *Between-breath targets:* None

Pressure Control Synchronized Intermittent Mandatory Ventilation
- *Mandatory breaths:* Machine triggered (preset frequency) or patient synchronized (pressure, flow, or Auto-Trak) and machine cycled (inspiratory time)

- Within-breath settings:
  - Operator-set PEEP, frequency, inspiratory pressure, rise time, and inspiratory time
- *Spontaneous breaths:* Patient triggered (pressure, flow, or Auto-Trak) and patient cycled (% peak inspiratory flow or Auto-Trak)
  - Within-breath settings:
    - Operator-set inspiratory pressure, rise time, and cycle sensitivity (% peak inspiratory flow)
- *Between-breath targets:* None

Volume Control Ventilation Assist/Control

- *Mandatory breaths:* Machine triggered (preset frequency) or patient triggered (pressure, flow, or Auto-Trak) and machine cycled (tidal volume or pause time)
  - Within-breath settings:
    - Operator-set PEEP, frequency, flow waveform, peak inspiratory flow, tidal volume, and pause time
- *Spontaneous breaths:* Not allowed
- *Between-breath targets:* None

Volume Control Ventilation Assist/Control with Flow-Trak

- *Mandatory breaths:* Machine triggered (preset frequency) or patient triggered (pressure, flow, or Auto-Trak) and machine cycled (tidal volume or pause time)
  - Within-breath settings:
    - Operator-set PEEP, frequency, flow waveform, peak inspiratory flow, tidal volume, and pause time
- *Spontaneous breaths:* Occur when Flow-Trak is active and inspiration is flow cycled
- *Between-breath targets:* None

Volume Control Synchronized Intermittent Mandatory Ventilation (With or Without Flow-Trak)

- *Mandatory breaths:* Machine triggered (preset frequency) or patient synchronized (pressure, flow, or Auto-Trak) and machine cycled (tidal volume or pause time)
  - Within-breath settings:
    - Operator-set PEEP, frequency, flow waveform, peak inspiratory flow, tidal volume, and pause time
- *Spontaneous breaths:* Patient triggered (pressure or flow sensitivity) and patient cycled (% peak inspiratory flow or Flow-Trak)
  - Within-breath settings:
    - Operator-set inspiratory pressure, rise time, and cycle sensitivity (% peak inspiratory flow)
- *Between-breath targets:* None

Special Features

Backup ventilation: When the apnea alarm is triggered in PCV and VCV, the ventilator will begin delivering breaths in Assist/Control, but with the operator-set

Apnea Rate. In NPPV, the ventilator will deliver only machine-controlled breaths either at the operator-set Apnea Rate or in response to patient effort.

Gas volume compensation: Displayed volumes are compensated for patient circuit compliance and body temperature and pressure, saturated (BTPS).

Leak compensation: Estimated patient leak is displayed in L/min and updated at each breath. Leak is estimated breath by breath as Delivered volume—Exhaled volume/Breath time. Bias flow through the patient circuit is automatically adjusted according to the estimated leak. Leaks that may occur during invasive ventilation are usually undesirable and are not compensated to allow easier leak detection.

Miscellaneous: The V200 has a unique Speaking Mode. This feature allows tracheostomized adult and pediatric patients to vocalize without the need for a speaking valve. The Speaking Mode software, when activated, closes the ventilator's exhalation valve, keeping it closed during the expiratory phase. This action redirects airflow around the deflated balloon cuff on the tracheostomy tube, through the larynx and pharynx, and out through the mouth. As the air flow passes through the vocal cords, speech is possible. Speaking Mode provides pressure control and volume control in A/C, SIMV, CPAP, Pressure Support, and the Flow-Trak ventilator option (if enabled). Speaking Mode is not available in NPPV mode, Respiratory Mechanics, and Neonatal options.

The V200 is designed to communicate with and display data from the Philips NICO respiratory profile monitor (i.e., cardiac output, O_2 saturation, and volumetric CO_2 measurements).

Neonatal ventilation: The Neonatal option allows the V200 to ventilate intubated neonatal patients with an ideal body weight range of 1.10–14.33 lb (0.5–6.5 kg) and an endotracheal tube ID range from 2.5 to 4.0 mm. The option provides pressure control in A/C, SIMV, and Apnea ventilation and also provides pressure support in SIMV and CPAP. The Neonatal Option is not available in VCV or NPPV modes.

Noninvasive ventilation: In Non-Invasive Ventilation, gas is delivered to the patient via a nasal mask, full face mask, nasal pillows, or mouthpiece with a lip seal. The operator determines whether the mode is totally spontaneous (Spont Ventilation Mode) or spontaneous with a backup rate (Spont/T Ventilation Mode).

Manufacturer's Specifications

Table 9-38 lists specifications for the Philips Respironics V200 ventilator.

Section 4: Portable Ventilators
Airon pNeuton

The pNeuton line of ventilators are small (less than 15 pounds), pneumatically controlled, and pneumatically powered (oxygen at 55 psi) ventilators capable of

TABLE 9-38
Specifications for the Philips Respironics V200 Ventilator

Setting Category	Setting	Range
Pressure	Inspiratory Pressure	5–100 cm H_2O
	Pressure Support	0–100 cm H_2O
	PEEP	0–35 cm H_2O
Volume	Tidal Volume	0.05–2.5 L
Flow	Inspiratory Flow	3–140 L/min
	Waveform	Square/descending ramp
Time	Inspiratory Time	0.1–9.9 s
	Mandatory Breath Frequency	1–80/min
	Adjustable Rise Time	Yes
Sensitivity	Trigger Sensitivity (pressure)	-20 to –0.1 cm H20
	Trigger Sensitivity (flow)	0.5–20 L/min
	Cycle Sensitivity (flow)	10–80%
Alarm Category		
Pressure	High Inspiratory Pressure	10–105 cm H_2O
	Low Inspiratory Pressure	3–105 cm H_2O
	Low PEEP/CPAP	0–35 cm H_2O
Volume	Low Expiratory Mandatory Tidal Volume	0–2.5 L
	Low Expiratory Spontaneous Tidal Volume	0–2.5 L
Flow	High Expiratory Minute Volume	0–60 L/min
	Low Expiratory Minute Volume	0–60 L/min
	High Leak	0–60 L/min
Time	High Respiratory Rate	0–150/min
	Apnea	10–60 s
Other	O_2 Sensor	Enabled/Disabled
Monitored Parameters	Peak Inspiratory Pressure	
	End Expiratory Pressure	
	End Inspiratory Pressure	
	Tidal Volume	
	I:E Ratio	
	Spontaneous Minute Ventilation	
	Minute Volume	
	Percent O_2	
	Spontaneous Respiratory Rate	
	Total Respiratory Rate	

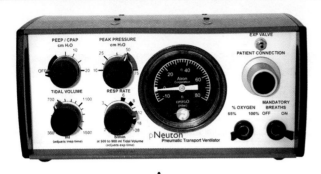

A

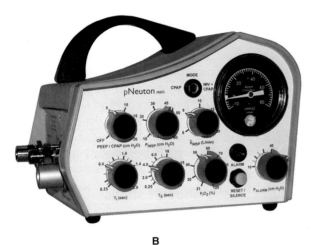

B

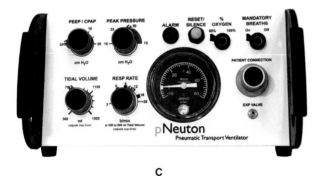

C

FIGURE 9-45 Airon pNeuton ventilators.

Photos courtesy of Airon Corporation.

invasive ventilation of patients from neonatal to adult size (**Figure 9-45**). **Table 9-39** shows the mode classifications for the pNeuton ventilators. A comparison of the different models is shown in **Table 9-40**.

Operator Interface

The operator interface for all three models of the pNeuton ventilator is composed of control knobs, switches, buttons, and a single aneroid pressure gauge for airway pressure.

Modes

Modes are selected using a mechanical switch.

pNeuton mini (neonatal–pediatric)
Continuous Positive Airway Pressure
- *Mandatory breaths:* Not allowed
- *Spontaneous breaths:* Patient triggered and patient cycled (demand flow only, not pressure supported)
  - Within-breath settings:
    - Operator-set inspiratory CPAP
- *Between-breath targets:* None

Intermittent Mandatory Ventilation + CPAP
- *Mandatory breaths:* Machine triggered (set expiratory time) and machine cycled (set inspiratory time)
  - Within-breath settings:
    - Operator-set PEEP, inspiratory pressure, bias flow, inspiratory time, and expiratory time. Inspiration is delivered at the set inspiratory flow only until the inspiratory pressure target is reached. Flow decays exponentially after that.
- *Spontaneous breaths:* Patient triggered and patient cycled (demand flow only, not pressure supported).
  - *Within-breath settings:* None (PEEP same as mandatory breaths)
- *Between-breath targets:* None

pNeuton A and B (pediatric–adult)
Continuous Positive Airway Pressure
- *Mandatory breaths:* Not allowed
- *Spontaneous breaths:* Patient triggered and patient cycled (demand flow only, not pressure supported)

TABLE 9-39
Classification of Modes for the Airon pNeuton Ventilators

Mode Name	Control Variable	Breath Sequence	Primary Breath Targeting Scheme	Secondary Breath Targeting Scheme	Tag
IMV + CPAP	volume	IMV	dual	set-point	VC-IMVd,s
CPAP	pressure	CSV	set-point	N/A	PC-CSVs
Volume Limited IMV + CPAP	volume	IMV	set-point	set-point	VC-IMVs,s
Pressure Limited IMV + CPAP	volume	IMV	dual	set-point	VC-IMVd,s

Reproduced with permission from Mandu Press Ltd.

TABLE 9-40
Different Models of pNeuton Ventilators

Model	Recommended Environment	Patient Population
pNeuton mini	hospital, EMS, MRI	0.4 to 25 Kg
pNeuton A	hospital, MRI	> 23 Kg
pNeuton S	hospital, EMS, MRI	> 23 Kg

Reproduced with permission from Mandu Press Ltd.

- Within-breath settings:
  - Operator-set inspiratory CPAP
- *Between-breath targets:* None

Pressure Limited Intermittent Mandatory Ventilation + CPAP

- *Mandatory breaths:* Machine triggered (set expiratory time) and machine cycled (inspiratory time, as determined by default flow setting and operator set tidal volume)
  - Within-breath settings:
    - Operator-set PEEP, inspiratory pressure, tidal volume, and frequency. Breath becomes pressure controlled if airway pressure reaches set peak pressure before inspiration is cycled off.
- *Spontaneous breaths:* Patient triggered and patient cycled (demand flow only, not pressure supported)
  - *Within-breath settings:* None (PEEP same as mandatory breaths)
- *Between-breath targets:* None

Special Features

Oxygen: F_1O_2 is selectable at either 100% or 65%.
Backup ventilation: None.
Gas volume compensation: None.
Leak compensation: None.
Nebulizer: The ventilator supplies blended gas to the nebulizer port for an inline jet nebulizer. Delivery of the nebulized gas is synchronized with the inspiratory phase of a breath and lasts for 20 minutes.
Neonatal ventilation: None.
Noninvasive ventilation: All three models of the pNeuton can be used for noninvasive ventilation.

Manufacturer's Specifications

Table 9-41 lists specifications for Airon pNeuton ventilators.

Bio-Med Devices Crossvent

The Bio-Med line of Crossvent ventilators are small (less than 10 lb/4.5 kg) microprocessor-controlled and

TABLE 9-41
Specifications for Airon pNeuton Ventilators

Setting Category	Setting	Range mini	Range A and B
Pressure	Inspiratory pressure	10–60 cm H_2O	15–75 cm H_2O
	PEEP	0–20 cm H_2O	0–20 cm H_2O
Volume	Tidal Volume	NA	0.36–1.5 L
Flow	Inspiratory Flow	6–20 L/min	36 L/min (default)
	Waveform	Square	Square
Time	Inspiratory Time	0.25–2.0 s	0.6–2.5 s
	Expiratory Time	0.25–2.0 s	
	Mandatory Breath Frequency		3–50/min
	Adjustable Rise Time		
Sensitivity	Trigger Sensitivity (pressure)		
	Trigger Sensitivity (flow)		
	Cycle Sensitivity (flow)		
Alarm Category			
Pressure		10–70 cm H_2O	Low inlet pressure
		Disconnect	Disconnect

TABLE 9-41
Specifications for Airon pNeuton Ventilators (Continued)

Setting Category	Setting	Range	
		mini	A and B
Volume			
Flow			
Time			
Other			
Monitored Parameters	Not specified		

TABLE 9-42
Different Models of Bio-Med Crossvent Ventilators

Modes	CV 4+	CV 3+	CV 2+	CV 2i+
Adult	✓	✓		
Pediatric	✓	✓	✓	
Neonatal	✓		✓	✓
A/C	✓	✓	✓	✓
IMV	✓		✓	✓
SIMV	✓	✓	✓	✓
PEEP	✓	✓	✓	✓
Sigh	✓	✓		✓
Pressure Support	✓	✓	✓	✓
Pressure Limit	✓	✓	✓	✓
Monitors/Alarms				
Pressure	✓	✓	✓	✓
Rate	✓	✓	✓	✓
Oxygen (%)	✓	✓	✓	✓
Mean Pressure	✓	✓	✓	✓
PEEP	✓	✓	✓	✓
Tidal Volume	✓	✓	✓	✓
Minute Ventilation	✓	✓	✓	✓
Low Battery	✓	✓	✓	✓
Low Supply Pressure	✓	✓	✓	
Functions				
Flow Trigger			✓	✓
Pressure Trigger	✓	✓	✓	
Nebulizer			✓	
Auto-Set Alarms			✓	✓

Courtesy of Bio-Med Devices, Inc.

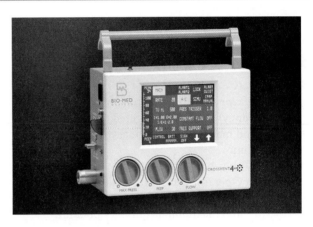

FIGURE 9-46 Bio-Med Crossvent-4+ ventilator.
Courtesy of Bio-Med Devices, Inc.

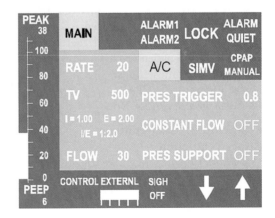

FIGURE 9-47 Bio-Med Crossvent-4+ operator interface.
Courtesy of Bio-Med Devices, Inc.

pneumatically powered ventilators capable of invasive and noninvasive ventilation of patients from neonatal to adult size (**Figure 9-46**). A comparison of the different models is shown in **Table 9-42**. **Table 9-43** shows the mode classifications for the Crossvent-4+ (neonatal–adult). These modes are described in the following section.

Operator Interface

The Crossvent-4+ uses a graphic LCD (liquid crystal display) with a touch screen keypad (**Figure 9-47**). There are also three knobs to adjust maximum inspiratory pressure, PEEP, and inspiratory flow.

TABLE 9-43
Classification of Modes for the Bio-Med Crossvent-4+

| Mode Name | Mode Classification | | | | |
	Control Variable	Breath Sequence	Primary Breath Targeting Scheme	Secondary Breath Targeting Scheme	Tag
A/C	volume	CMV	set-point	N/A	VC-CMVs
SIMV	volume	IMV	set-point	set-point	VC-IMVs,s
CPAP	pressure	CSV	set-point	N/A	PC-CSVs

Reproduced with permission from Mandu Press Ltd.

Modes

A/C (Assist/Control)

- *Mandatory breaths:* Machine triggered (preset frequency) or patient triggered (pressure sensitivity) and machine cycled (tidal volume or inspiratory time)
  - Within-breath settings:
    - Operator-set PEEP, frequency, peak inspiratory flow, tidal volume (or inspiratory time), and maximum inspiratory pressure
- *Spontaneous breaths:* Not allowed
- *Between-breath targets:* None

Continuous Positive Airway Pressure (CPAP)

- *Mandatory breaths:* Not allowed
- *Spontaneous breaths:* Patient triggered (pressure sensitivity) and patient cycled
  - Within-breath settings:
    - Operator-set CPAP
- *Between-breath targets:* None

SIMV (Synchronized Intermittent Mandatory Ventilation)

- *Mandatory breaths:* Machine triggered (preset frequency) or patient synchronized (pressure sensitivity) and machine cycled (tidal volume)
  - Within-breath settings:
    - Operator-set PEEP, frequency, peak inspiratory flow, tidal volume (or inspiratory time), and maximum inspiratory pressure
- *Spontaneous breaths:* Patient triggered (pressure sensitivity) and patient cycled
  - Within-breath settings:
    - Operator-set PEEP
- *Between-breath targets:* None

Special Features

Oxygen: When powered by compressed oxygen and equipped with the optional Air Entrainment Module, the Crossvent is able to supply either 100% or 50% (nominal) oxygen during transport, without the use of compressed air. The ventilator can be powered by an external blender.

Backup ventilation: A backup rate sets the rate at which backup breaths are delivered when in CPAP mode in the event of apnea. Backup breaths use preset tidal volume and flow.

Gas volume compensation: None. When equipped with the optional Air Entrainment Module, the Crossvent is able to supply either 100% or 50% (nominal) oxygen during transport, without the use of compressed air. A unique feature of the entrainment system is the ability to deliver repeatable volumes during volume-limited ventilation, with relatively constant oxygen concentration.

Leak compensation: None.

Nebulizer: None.

Neonatal ventilation: No specific modes, but the tidal volume can be set as low as 5 mL. An optional pneumotach can be used to accurately measure tidal volumes from 100 to 990 mL.

Noninvasive ventilation: No specific modes.

Manufacturer's Specifications

Table 9-44 lists specifications for the Bio-Med Crossvent-4+.

CareFusion EnVe and ReVel

The EnVe (Figure 9-48) and ReVel (Figure 9-49) are the same size, have very similar features, and can be used with the same accessories. The EnVe has a color LCD touch screen and is marketed as an ICU ventilator, whereas the ReVel has an interface with fixed buttons and an LED display and is marketed for transport applications. The EnVe ventilator is a high performance portable critical care ventilator that is pneumatically powered and electronically controlled. It is designed for adults and pediatric patients weighing at least 11 lb (5 kg). The pneumatic system is designed as

TABLE 9-44
Specifications for the Bio-Med Crossvent-4+

Setting Category	Setting	Range
Pressure	Inspiratory Pressure	0–120 cm H_2O
	Pressure Support	0–50 cm H_2O
	PEEP	0–35 cm H_2O
Volume	Tidal Volume	0.005–2.5 L
Flow	Inspiratory Flow	1–120 L/min
	Waveform	Not specified
Time	Inspiratory Time	0.1–3.0 s
	Mandatory Breath Frequency	5–150/min
Sensitivity	Trigger Sensitivity (pressure)	–0.2 to –10 cm H_2O
Alarm Category		
Pressure	Peak Pressure	0–125 cm H_2O
	PEEP	0-99 cm H_2O
	Mean Pressure	0–125 cm H_2O
Volume	Exhaled tidal volume	50–4,000 mL
Flow	Exhaled minute volume	0–200 L
Time	Rate	0–199 bpm
Other	O_2 Sensor	Enabled/Disabled
Monitored Parameters	Peak Pressure	
	Rate	
	Oxygen	
	PEEP/CPAP	
	Mean Pressure	
	Low Supply Pressure	
	Exhaled Tidal Volume	
	Exhaled Minute Ventilation	

a blower that draws in room air through a filter and delivers gas at the correct flow, volume, and/or pressure to the patient. The EnVe has an internal exhalation valve, supporting dual limb patient circuits. The ventilator delivers blended gases from an internal oxygen blender. The blended gas delivery can be monitored with an external F_IO_2 sensor and the values displayed on the user interface. When high pressure oxygen is attached to the O_2 Inlet port, the ventilator is able to drive a nebulizer to deliver aerosolized drugs to the patient while at the same time compensating for the added gas delivery. The ReVel is a simplified version of the EnVe designed for transport and home care. It differs from the EnVe in that it has an LED screen (versus LCD on EnVe) and uses a single limb circuit (versus double limb on EnVe). Also the EnVe has a waveform display and the ReVel does not. Both ventilators have the same modes.

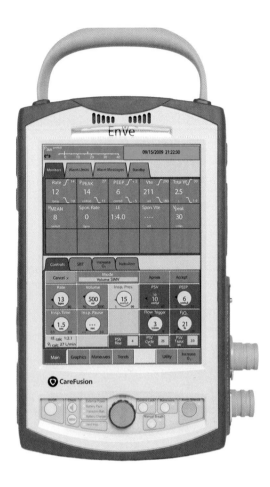
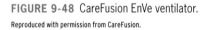

FIGURE 9-48 CareFusion EnVe ventilator.
Reproduced with permission from CareFusion.

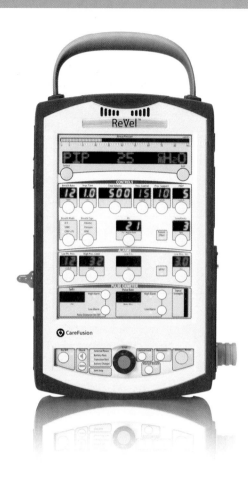

FIGURE 9-49 CareFusion ReVel ventilator.
Reproduced with permission from CareFusion.

Operator Interface

The EnVe uses a touch screen, buttons, and a scroll knob. Screen displays change according to the context of the operation, such as entering ventilator settings and alarm settings (**Figure 9-50**). Settings are entered by touching a virtual button on the screen to select the desired setting, turning the knob to select the setting value, and then touching the screen button again to finalize the setting. Graphic displays are available for scalar waveforms, loops, and trended values.

Modes

Modes are selected by pressing the virtual button with the desired mode name. There are nine basic mode names, but there is an option to set flow cycle instead of time cycle for terminating inspiration, resulting in more modes by classification (**Table 9-45**).

CPAP/Pressure Support Ventilation
- *Mandatory breaths:* Not allowed
- *Spontaneous breaths:* Patient triggered (pressure or flow sensitivity) and patient cycled (% peak inspiratory flow)
  - Within-breath settings:

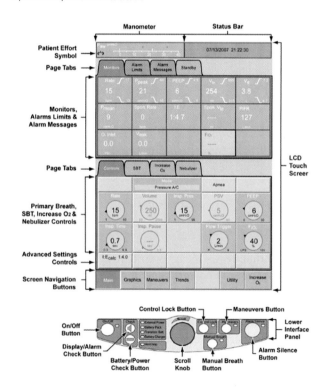

FIGURE 9-50 CareFusion EnVe operator interface.
Reproduced with permission from CareFusion.

TABLE 9-45
Modes for the CareFusion EnVe

| Mode Name | Mode Classification | | | | Tag |
	Control Variable	Breath Sequence	Primary Breath Targeting Scheme	Secondary Breath Targeting Scheme	
Volume A/C	volume	CMV	set-point	N/A	VC-CMVs
Volume SIMV	volume	IMV	set-point	set-point	VC-IMVs,s
Pressure A/C	pressure	CMV	set-point	N/A	PC-CMVs
Noninvasive Positive Pressure Ventilation Pressure	pressure	IMV	set-point	set-point	PC-IMVs,s
Pressure Regulated Volume Control A/C	pressure	CMV	adaptive	N/A	PC-CMVa
Pressure A/C with Flow Cycle	pressure	IMV	set-point	set-point	PC-IMVs,s
Pressure SIMV	pressure	IMV	set-point	set-point	PC-IMVs,s
Noninvasive Positive Pressure Ventilation Pressure with Flow Cycle	pressure	IMV	set-point	set-point	PC-IMVs,s
Pressure Regulated Volume Control A/C with Flow Cycle	pressure	IMV	adaptive	set-point	PC-IMVa,s
Pressure Regulated Volume Control SIMV	pressure	IMV	adaptive	set-point	PC-IMVa,s
CPAP/PSV	pressure	CSV	set-point	N/A	PC-CSVs
Noninvasive Positive Pressure Ventilation Pressure CPAP/PSV	pressure	CSV	set-point	N/A	PC-CSVs
CPAP + Volume Targeted Pressure Support Ventilation	pressure	CSV	adaptive	N/A	PC-CSVa

Reproduced with permission from Mandu Press Ltd.

– Operator-set inspiratory pressure, rise time, and cycle sensitivity (% peak inspiratory flow)
- *Between-breath targets:* None

CPAP/Volume Targeted Pressure Support Ventilation
- *Mandatory breaths:* Not allowed
- *Spontaneous breaths:* Patient triggered (pressure or flow sensitivity) and patient cycled (% peak inspiratory flow)
  • Within-breath settings:
    – Operator-set rise time and cycle sensitivity (% peak inspiratory flow)
    – Ventilator-set inspiratory pressure
- Between-breath targets:
  • Operator-set tidal volume

Noninvasive Positive Pressure Ventilation/Pressure Support Ventilation
- *Mandatory breaths:* Not allowed
- *Spontaneous breaths:* Patient triggered (pressure or flow sensitivity) and patient cycled (% peak inspiratory flow)
  • Within-breath settings:
    – Operator-set inspiratory pressure, rise time, and cycle sensitivity (% peak inspiratory flow)
- *Between-breath targets:* None

Noninvasive Positive Pressure Ventilation Pressure
- *Mandatory breaths:* Machine triggered (preset frequency) or patient synchronized (pressure or flow sensitivity) and machine cycled (inspiratory time)
  • Within-breath settings:

– Operator-set PEEP, frequency, inspiratory pressure, rise time, and inspiratory time
- *Spontaneous breaths:* Patient triggered (pressure or flow sensitivity) and patient cycled (% peak inspiratory flow)
  - Within-breath settings:
    – Operator-set inspiratory pressure, rise time, and cycle sensitivity (% peak inspiratory flow)
- *Between-breath targets:* None

Noninvasive Positive Pressure Ventilation Pressure with Flow Cycle
- Activation of Flow Cycle makes this mode a form of IMV, not A/C. Flow cycling makes every breath patient cycled. Hence, every patient-triggered breath is spontaneous (i.e., patient triggered and cycled) whereas every machine-triggered breath is mandatory (i.e., machine triggered and patient cycled) by definition.
- *Mandatory breaths:* Machine triggered (preset frequency) and patient cycled (% peak inspiratory flow).
  - Within-breath settings:
    – Operator-set PEEP, frequency, inspiratory pressure, rise time, and cycle sensitivity (% peak flow)
- *Spontaneous breaths:* Patient triggered (pressure or flow sensitivity) and patient cycled (% peak inspiratory flow)
  - Within-breath settings:
    – Operator-set inspiratory pressure, rise time, and cycle sensitivity (% peak inspiratory flow)
- *Between-breath targets:* None

Pressure A/C
- *Mandatory breaths:* Machine triggered (preset frequency) or patient triggered (pressure or flow sensitivity) and machine cycled (inspiratory time)
  - Within-breath settings:
    – Operator-set PEEP, frequency, inspiratory pressure, rise time, and inspiratory time
- *Spontaneous breaths:* Not allowed
- *Between-breath targets:* None

Pressure A/C with Flow Cycle
- Activation of Flow Cycle makes this mode a form of IMV, not A/C. Flow cycling makes every breath patient cycled. Hence, every patient-triggered breath is spontaneous (i.e., patient triggered and cycled) whereas every machine-triggered breath is mandatory (i.e., machine triggered and patient cycled) by definition.
- *Mandatory breaths:* Machine triggered (preset frequency) and patient cycled (% peak inspiratory flow).

- Within-breath settings:
    – Operator-set PEEP, frequency, inspiratory pressure, rise time, and cycle sensitivity (% peak flow)
- *Spontaneous breaths:* Patient triggered (pressure or flow sensitivity) and patient cycled (% peak inspiratory flow).
  - Within-breath settings:
    – Operator-set inspiratory pressure, rise time, and cycle sensitivity (% peak inspiratory flow)
- *Between-breath targets:* None.

Pressure SIMV
- *Mandatory breaths:* Machine triggered (preset frequency) or patient synchronized (pressure or flow sensitivity) and machine cycled (inspiratory time)
  - Within-breath settings:
    – Operator-set PEEP, frequency, inspiratory pressure, rise time, and inspiratory time
- *Spontaneous breaths:* Patient triggered (pressure or flow sensitivity) and patient cycled (% peak inspiratory flow)
  - Within-breath settings:
    – Operator-set inspiratory pressure, rise time, and cycle sensitivity (% peak inspiratory flow)
- *Between-breath targets:* None

Pressure Regulated Volume Control A/C
- *Mandatory breaths:* Machine triggered (preset frequency) or patient triggered (pressure or flow sensitivity) and machine cycled (inspiratory time)
  - Within-breath settings:
    – Operator-set PEEP, frequency, rise time, and inspiratory time
    – Ventilator-set inspiratory pressure
- *Spontaneous breaths:* Not allowed
- Between-breath targets:
  - Operator-set tidal volume

Pressure Regulated Volume Control A/C with Flow Cycle
- Activation of Flow Cycle makes this mode a form of IMV, not A/C. Flow cycling makes every breath patient cycled. Hence, every patient-triggered breath is spontaneous (i.e., patient triggered and cycled) whereas every machine-triggered breath is mandatory (i.e., machine triggered and patient cycled) by definition.
- *Mandatory breaths:* Machine triggered (preset frequency) or patient triggered (pressure or flow sensitivity) and machine cycled (inspiratory time).

- • Within-breath settings:
  - – Operator-set PEEP, frequency, rise time, and inspiratory time
  - – Ventilator-set inspiratory pressure
- ■ *Spontaneous breaths:* Patient triggered (pressure or flow sensitivity) and patient cycled (% peak inspiratory flow).
  - • Within-breath settings:
    - – Operator-set rise time and cycle sensitivity (% peak inspiratory flow)
    - – Ventilator-set inspiratory pressure
- ■ Between-breath targets:
  - • Operator-set tidal volume

Pressure Regulated Volume Control SIMV

- ■ *Mandatory breaths:* Machine triggered (preset frequency) or patient synchronized (pressure or flow sensitivity) and machine cycled (inspiratory time)
  - • Within-breath settings:
    - – Operator-set PEEP, frequency, rise time, and inspiratory time
    - – Ventilator-set inspiratory pressure
- ■ *Spontaneous breaths:* Patient triggered (pressure or flow sensitivity) and patient cycled (% peak inspiratory flow)
  - • Within-breath settings:
    - – Operator-set inspiratory pressure, rise time, and cycle sensitivity (% peak inspiratory flow)
- ■ Between-breath targets:
  - • Operator-set tidal volume

Volume A/C

- ■ *Mandatory breaths:* Machine triggered (preset frequency) or patient triggered (pressure or flow sensitivity) and machine cycled (tidal volume or pause time)
  - • Within-breath settings:
    - – Operator-set PEEP, frequency, inspiratory time, tidal volume, and pause time. Inspiratory flow is preset to be a descending ramp waveform.
- ■ *Spontaneous breaths:* Not allowed
- ■ *Between-breath targets:* None

Volume SIMV

- ■ *Mandatory breaths:* Machine triggered (preset frequency) or patient synchronized (pressure or flow sensitivity) and machine cycled (tidal volume or pause time)
  - • Within-breath settings:
    - – Operator-set PEEP, frequency, inspiratory time, tidal volume, and pause time. Inspiratory flow is preset to be a descending ramp waveform.

- ■ *Spontaneous breaths:* Patient triggered (pressure or flow sensitivity) and patient cycled (% peak inspiratory flow)
  - • Within-breath settings:
    - – Operator-set inspiratory pressure, rise time, and cycle sensitivity (% peak inspiratory flow)
- ■ *Between-breath targets:* None

Special Features

Oxygen: The EnVe can operate from either a high pressure (40–88 psi) or low pressure (less than 10 psi, e.g., flowmeter) oxygen source. F_IO_2 is adjustable from 21% to 100%.

Backup ventilation: When the set Apnea Interval (maximum time allowed between the beginning of one breath and the beginning of the next breath) is exceeded, the Apnea alarm is generated and the ventilator will enter Apnea Backup ventilation mode in Assist/Control mode at the previously set breath type and control settings.

Gas volume compensation: Exhaled tidal volume is calculated by integrating the flow from the patient through the patient circuit wye during the exhalation phase of the breath. Tidal volumes are displayed as body temperature and pressure, saturated (BTPS) compensated; however, volumes are not compensated for circuit compliance.

Leak compensation: Leak compensation is selectable and tracks steady state exhaled flow to improve monitored patient flow accuracy in the presence of a stable circuit leak.

Nebulizer: Nebulization can be performed during volume control breaths in Assist/Control mode only. When the Nebulizer is activated, a 6 L/min nominal flow is delivered to the nebulizer drive port. During nebulization, the ventilator decreases the flow to its inspiratory limb to compensate for the addition of the nebulization flow during inspiration. However, because the nebulizer is driven by 100% oxygen, the percentage of oxygen in the patient airway increases during nebulizer treatments. The nebulization can be set for continuous operation of synchronization with inspiration only.

Noninvasive ventilation: The ventilator is capable of performing noninvasive positive pressure ventilation (NPPV) with a standard dual-limb circuit. When either of the NPPV modes is selected, the leak compensation function is automatically enabled, and when either NPPV mode is exited the leak compensation function returns to its previous or default setting.

Manufacturer's Specifications

Table 9-46 lists specifications for the CareFusion EnVe.

TABLE 9-46
Specifications for the CareFusion EnVe

Setting Category	Setting	Range
Pressure	Inspiratory pressure	1–99 cm H_2O
	PEEP	0–30 cm H_2O
Volume	Tidal volume	50–2,000 mL
Flow		
Time	Inspiratory time	0.3–9.9 s
	Frequency	1–80 bpm
Sensitivity	Pressure trigger	1–20 cm H_2O
	Flow trigger	1–9 L/min
	Flow cycle	10–40%
Alarm Category		
Pressure	High inspiratory pressure	5–100 cm H_2O
	High PEEP	3–20 cm H_2O
	Low inspiratory pressure	1–60 cm H_2O
	Low PEEP	–3 to –20 cm H_2O
Volume	High tidal volume	50–2,000 mL
	High minute volume	0.1–99 L
	Low tidal volume	10–2,000 mL
	Low minute volume	0.1–99 L
Flow	N/A	
Time	High breath rate	1–120 bpm
	Low breath rate	1–99 bpm
Other	SBT high f/Vt	70–900 bpm/L
	SBT high breath rate	15–80 bpm
	SBT low f/Vt	5–90 bpm/L
	SBT low breath rate	1–40 bpm
Monitored Parameters	AutoPEEP	0–99 cm H_2O
	Delta pressure	1–99 cm H_2O
	Expiratory pressure	0–100 cm H_2O
	Plateau pressure	1–99 cm H_2O
	Static lung compliance	1–999 mL/cm H_2O

CareFusion LTV 1200

The LTV series (800–1200) includes small, portable ventilators, suitable for transport, that are electrically controlled and powered by blowers (Table 9-47). The latest model, the LTV 1200 ventilator (Figure 9-51), is intended to provide continuous or intermittent ventilatory support for individuals who require mechanical ventilation. The ventilator is applicable for adult and pediatric patients weighing at least 11 lb (5 kg) invasively or noninvasively (via mask or nasal prongs). The ventilator is suitable for use in institutional, home, or transport settings.

TABLE 9-47
Comparison of CareFusion LTV Series Ventilators

FEATURES	1200	MR Conditional 1200	1150	1000	950	900	800
Pressure Control	x	x	x	x	x		
Volume Control	x	x	x	x	x	x	x
Pressure Support	x	x	x	x	x	x	
Flow-Triggering	x	x	x	x	x	x	
Inspiratory & Expiratory Hold	x	x	x	x			
Leak Compensation	x	x	x	x	x	x	
Integral O_2 Blender	x	x		x			
O_2 Flush	x	x		x			
O_2 Cylinder Duration	x	x		x			
High Pressure & Low Pressure O_2 Inlet	x	x		x			
Multiple Power Sources	x	x	x	x	x	x	x
Noninvasive Ventilation	x	x	x	x	x	x	x
NPPV Mode	x	x	x				
Spontaneous Breathing Trial	x	x	x				
Patient Presets (Infant, Pediatric & Adult)	x	x	x				
Internal PEEP	x	x	x				
PEEP Compensation	x	x	x				
User-Replaceable Internal Battery	x	x	x				
Low PEEP Alarm	x	x	x				
Low Pressure O_2 Inlet			x		x	x	x
O_2 Conserve	x	x					
MR Conditional System Package		x					

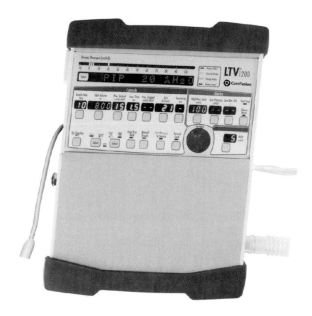

FIGURE 9-51 CareFusion LTV 1200 ventilator.
Reproduced with permission from CareFusion.

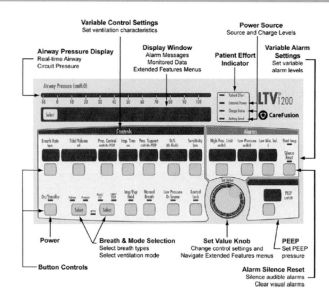

FIGURE 9-52 CareFusion LTV 1200 operator interface.
Reproduced with permission from CareFusion.

Operator Interface

The operator interface for the LTV 1200 is composed of LED displays, mechanical pushbuttons, and a rotary selection knob for adjusting settings (**Figure 9-52**). Settings are adjusted by pushing a button, turning the knob to get the desired setting, and pushing the button again to confirm. Buttons also permit manual breath triggering as well as inspiratory and expiratory hold maneuvers and alarm silencing.

Modes

Modes on the LTV 1200 are created by first selecting the control variable (volume or pressure button) and then the breath sequence (A/C button or SIMV/CPAP button). After that, the operator selects either the tidal volume or inspiratory pressure setting, along with inspiratory time and breath frequency. Flow termination is an optional setting that, when activated, may change the breath sequence (i.e., from CMV to IMV).

CPAP/Pressure Support Ventilation
- *Mandatory breaths:* Not allowed
- *Spontaneous breaths:* Patient triggered (pressure or flow sensitivity) and patient cycled (% peak inspiratory flow)
  - Within-breath settings:
    - Operator-set inspiratory pressure, rise time, and cycle sensitivity (% peak inspiratory flow)
- *Between-breath targets:* None

Noninvasive Positive Pressure Ventilation
- *Mandatory breaths:* Not allowed
- *Spontaneous breaths:* Patient triggered (pressure or flow sensitivity) and patient cycled (% peak inspiratory flow)

- Within-breath settings:
  - Operator-set inspiratory pressure, rise time, and cycle sensitivity (% peak inspiratory flow)
- *Between-breath targets:* None

Pressure A/C
- *Mandatory breaths:* Machine triggered (preset frequency) or patient triggered (pressure or flow sensitivity) and machine cycled (inspiratory time)
  - Within-breath settings:
    - Operator-set PEEP, frequency, inspiratory pressure, rise time, and inspiratory time
- *Spontaneous breaths:* Not allowed
- *Between-breath targets:* None

Pressure A/C with Flow Termination
- Activation of Flow Termination makes this mode a form of IMV, not A/C. Flow Termination makes every breath patient cycled. Hence, every patient-triggered breath is spontaneous (i.e., patient triggered and cycled) whereas every machine-triggered breath is mandatory (i.e., machine triggered and patient cycled) by definition.
- *Mandatory breaths:* Machine triggered (preset frequency) and patient cycled (% peak inspiratory flow).
  - Within-breath settings:
    - Operator-set PEEP, frequency, inspiratory pressure, rise time, and cycle sensitivity (% peak flow)
- *Spontaneous breaths:* Patient triggered (pressure or flow sensitivity) and patient cycled (% peak inspiratory flow).

- Within-breath settings:
  - Operator-set inspiratory pressure, rise time, and cycle sensitivity (% peak inspiratory flow)
- *Between-breath targets:* None.

Pressure SIMV

- *Mandatory breaths:* Machine triggered (preset frequency) or patient synchronized (pressure or flow sensitivity) and machine cycled (inspiratory time)
  - Within-breath settings:
    - Operator-set PEEP, frequency, inspiratory pressure, rise time, and inspiratory time
- *Spontaneous breaths:* Patient triggered (pressure or flow sensitivity) and patient cycled (% peak inspiratory flow)
  - Within-breath settings:
    - Operator-set inspiratory pressure, rise time, and cycle sensitivity (% peak inspiratory flow)
- *Between-breath targets:* None

Volume A/C

- *Mandatory breaths:* Machine triggered (preset frequency) or patient triggered (pressure or flow sensitivity) and machine cycled (tidal volume or pause time)
  - Within-breath settings:
    - Operator-set PEEP, frequency, inspiratory time, tidal volume, and pause time. Inspiratory flow is preset to be a descending ramp waveform.
- *Spontaneous breaths:* Not allowed
- *Between-breath targets:* None

Volume SIMV

- *Mandatory breaths:* Machine triggered (preset frequency) or patient synchronized (pressure or flow sensitivity) and machine cycled (tidal volume or pause time)
  - Within-breath settings:
    - Operator-set PEEP, frequency, inspiratory time, tidal volume, and pause time. Inspiratory flow is preset to be a descending ramp waveform.
- *Spontaneous breaths:* Patient triggered (pressure or flow sensitivity) and patient cycled (% peak inspiratory flow)
  - Within-breath settings:
    - Operator-set inspiratory pressure, rise time, and cycle sensitivity (% peak inspiratory flow)
- *Between-breath targets:* None

Special Features

Oxygen: Oxygen blending is available from a high pressure (40–80 psi) oxygen source or low pressure (less than 35 psi) oxygen bleed-in (e.g., oxygen concentrator or flowmeter). Using the high pressure source, F_IO_2 is adjustable from 21% to 100%. Using the low pressure source, the F_IO_2 is determined by the O_2 inlet flow and the total minute volume and is not regulated by the ventilator. (A chart is available for manual calculation of F_IO_2.)

Backup ventilation: When the set Apnea Interval (maximum time allowed between the beginning of one breath and the beginning of the next breath) is exceeded, the Apnea alarm is generated and the ventilator will enter Apnea Backup ventilation mode in Assist/Control mode at the previously set breath type and control settings.

Gas volume compensation: None.

Leak compensation: None.

Nebulizer: None.

Noninvasive ventilation: Noninvasive Positive Pressure Ventilation (NPPV) can be selected as the primary mode of ventilation. In the NPPV mode, the ventilator cycles between IPAP (Pressure Support) and EPAP (PEEP). When a patient trigger is detected, a Pressure Support patient breath is given.

Manufacturer's Specifications

Table 9-48 lists specifications for the CareFusion LTV 1200.

Dräger Carina

The Carina (**Figure 9-53**) is designed as a long-term care ventilator for ventilator-dependent patients in hospital or medical rooms. It can be used for invasive or noninvasive ventilation on patients with a tidal volume of at least 100 mL. The ventilator is electrically controlled and pneumatically powered with an internal blower.

Operator Interface

The Carina has an operator interface that uses an LCD screen, buttons, and a control knob (**Figure 9-54**). Settings are entered by pressing the menu button and then the settings, turning the rotary knob to select the setting value, and then pressing the knob to finalize the setting.

Modes

Modes are selected by name using push buttons and the rotary knob. Note that AutoFlow (i.e., pressure control with adaptive targeting, sometimes called volume targeted pressure control) is considered a form of volume control by Dräger. Hence what it calls VC-A/C and VC-SIMV are classified as PC-CMV and PC-IMV, respectively. **Table 9-49** shows the available modes.

Pressure Control Assist Control

- *Mandatory breaths:* Machine triggered (preset frequency) or patient triggered (flow sensitivity) and machine cycled (inspiratory time)

TABLE 9-48
Specifications for the CareFusion LTV 1200

Setting Category	Setting	Range
Pressure	Inspiratory Pressure	1–99 cm H_2O
	Pressure Support	1–60 cm H_2O
	PEEP	0–20 cm H_2O
Volume	Tidal Volume	0.005–2 L
Flow	Waveform	Not Specified
	Inspiratory Time	0.3–9.9 s
Time	Mandatory Breath Frequency	1–80/min
	Trigger Sensitivity (pressure)	1–9 cm H_2O
	Adjustable Rise Time	Yes
Alarm Category		
Pressure	High PEEP	–3 to –20 cm H_2O
	Low PEEP	–3 to –20 cm H_2O
	High Pressure Limit	5–100 cm H_2O
	Low Peak Pressure	1–60 cm H_2O
Flow	Low Minute Volume	0.1–99 L/min
Time	Apnea Interval	10–60 s
	High Breath Rate	5–80/min
	SBT High f	15–80/min
	SBT Low f	1–40/min
Other	O_2 Sensor	Enabled/Disabled
	SBT High f/Vt	70–900 f/Vt
	SBT Low f/Vt	5–90 f/Vt
	HP Alarm Delay	
Monitored Parameters	Peak Flow	
	Exhaled Tidal Volume	
	I:E Ratio	
	Mean Airway Pressure	
	O_2 Cylinder Duration	
	Peak Inspiratory Pressure	
	PEEP	
	Total Breath Rate	
	Total Minute Volume	
	SBT Minutes	
	f/Vt	
	Frequency	

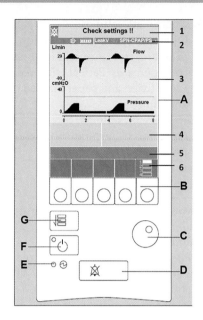

FIGURE 9-54 Dräger Carina operator interface. 1. Alarm line for display of suppressed acoustic alarm signal and alarm message. 2. Status line for current device settings. 3. Display for real-time waveforms of flow and pressure or bar graph for pressure and 4 measured values. 4. Display for 2 measured values. 5. Information line, e.g., for information when the limit of the setting range is reached. 6. Display of functions and ventilation parameters The display is activated by the associated key. A. Screen for displaying application-specific information for ventilation. B. Keys for selecting functions and ventilation parameters. C. Rotary knob for setting and confirming functions and parameters. D. Audio paused 2 min. key for suppressing the alarm tone for 2 minutes.

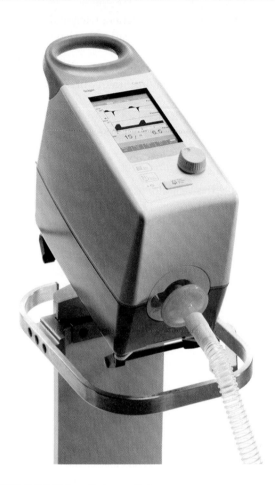

FIGURE 9-53 Dräger Carina ventilator.

TABLE 9-49
Modes for the Dräger Carina

Mode Name	Mode Classification				Tag
	Control Variable	Breath Sequence	Primary Breath Targeting Scheme	Secondary Breath Targeting Scheme	
PC-A/C	pressure	CMV	set-point	N/A	PC-CMVs
VC-A/C with Auto Flow	pressure	CMV	adaptive	N/A	PC-CMVa
PC-SIMV	pressure	IMV	set-point	set-point	PC-IMVs,s
VC-SIMV with Auto Flow	pressure	IMV	adaptive	set-point	PC-IMVa,s
SPN-CPAP/PS	pressure	CSV	set-point	N/A	PC-CSVs
SPN-CPAP/PS with Volume Guarantee	pressure	CSV	adaptive	N/A	PC-CSVa

Reproduced with permission from Mandu Press Ltd.

- Within-breath settings:
  - Operator-set PEEP, frequency, inspiratory pressure, rise time, and inspiratory time
- *Spontaneous breaths:* Permitted during mandatory breath but not between mandatory breaths
- *Between-breath targets:* None

Pressure Control Synchronized Intermittent Mandatory Ventilation

- *Mandatory breaths:* Machine triggered (preset frequency) or patient synchronized (pressure or flow sensitivity) and machine cycled (inspiratory time). Spontaneous breaths are permitted both between and during mandatory breaths.

- Within-breath settings:
  - Operator-set PEEP, frequency, inspiratory pressure, rise time, and inspiratory time
- *Spontaneous breaths:* Patient triggered (pressure or flow sensitivity) and patient cycled (% peak inspiratory flow).
  - Within-breath settings:
    - Operator-set inspiratory pressure and rise time
- *Between-breath targets:* None.

Spontaneous Continuous Positive Airway Pressure/ Pressure Support

- *Mandatory breaths:* Not allowed
- *Spontaneous breaths:* Patient triggered (pressure or flow sensitivity) and patient cycled (% peak inspiratory flow)
  - Within-breath settings:
    - Operator-set inspiratory pressure and rise time
- *Between-breath targets:* None

Spontaneous Continuous Positive Airway Pressure/ Volume Guarantee

- *Mandatory breaths:* Not allowed
- *Spontaneous breaths:* Patient triggered (pressure or flow sensitivity) and patient cycled (% peak inspiratory flow)
  - Within-breath settings:
    - Operator-set cycle sensitivity (% peak inspiratory flow)
    - Ventilator-set inspiratory pressure
- Between-breath targets:
  - Operator-set average tidal volume

Volume Control Assist Control with AutoFlow

- *Mandatory breaths:* Machine triggered (preset frequency) or patient triggered (pressure or flow sensitivity) and machine cycled (inspiratory time)
  - Within-breath settings:
    - Operator-set PEEP, frequency, rise time, and inspiratory time
    - Ventilator-set inspiratory pressure
- *Spontaneous breaths:* Not allowed
- Between-breath targets:
  - Operator-set tidal volume

Volume Control Synchronized Intermittent Mandatory Ventilation with AutoFlow

- *Mandatory breaths:* Machine triggered (preset frequency) or patient triggered (pressure or flow sensitivity) and machine cycled (inspiratory time)
  - Within-breath settings:
    - Operator-set PEEP, frequency, rise time, and inspiratory time
    - Ventilator-set inspiratory pressure

- *Spontaneous breaths:* Patient triggered (pressure or flow sensitivity) and patient cycled (% peak inspiratory flow)
  - Within-breath settings:
    - Operator-set inspiratory pressure and rise time
- Between-breath targets:
  - Operator-set tidal volume

Special Features

Oxygen: This ventilator uses ambient air for ventilation, which is delivered by means of an internal turbine. The O_2 supply is provided by a high pressure (40–87 psi) source or a low pressure (less than 7 psi) source (e.g., oxygen concentrator). Using the high pressure source, F_IO_2 is adjustable from 21% to 100%. Using the low pressure source, the F_IO_2 is determined by the O_2 inlet flow and the total minute volume.

Backup ventilation: Backup ventilation is available in the SPN-CPAP modes. If apnea occurs, backup ventilation starts in the VC-CMV with AutoFlow mode.

Gas volume compensation: The device does not include the compliance of the breathing circuit in the calculation of the displayed tidal volume. The ventilator measures the degree of leakage in the breathing system and defines a new trigger base. Tidal volume and minute ventilation displays are corrected for body temperature and pressure, saturated (BTPS).

Nebulizer: None.

Neonatal ventilation: None.

Noninvasive ventilation: Noninvasive ventilation is an option when selecting the modes. When selected, the device automatically adjusts the trigger thresholds to the current leakage situation. An alarm is triggered if the patient leakage exceeds 60 L/min.

Manufacturer's Specifications

Table 9-50 lists specifications for the Dräger Carina ventilator.

Dräger Oxylog 3000 Plus

The Oxylog 3000 plus (**Figure 9-55**) is an electronically controlled, pneumatically powered emergency and transport ventilator for patients with a tidal volume of at least 50 mL. It does not have an internal blower and thus requires an external source of compressed gas.

Operator Interface

The Oxylog 3000 plus has an operator interface that uses an LCD screen, buttons, and knobs (**Figure 9-56**). Settings are entered by pressing the menu button and turning the rotary knob to select the setting value, and

TABLE 9-50
Specifications for the Dräger Carina Ventilator

Setting Category	Setting	Range
Pressure	Inspiratory Pressure	5–50 cm H_2O
	PEEP	3–20 cm H_2O
Volume	Tidal Volume	0.1–2.0 L
Flow	Waveform	Not specified
Time	Inspiratory Time	0.3–8 s
	Mandatory Breath Frequency	5–50/min
	Adjustable Rise Time	Yes
Sensitivity		Sensitive/Normal
Alarm Category		
Pressure	High Inspiratory Pressure	10–55 cm H_2O
Volume		
Flow	Ventilation	2–60 L/min
	Low Minute Ventilation	0.1–39 L/min
Time	High Breath Frequency	10–74/min
	Apnea Time	5–60 s
	Disconnect Time	0–120 s

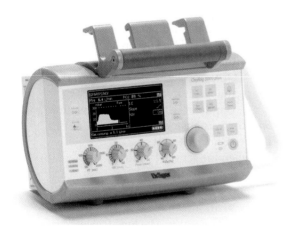

FIGURE 9-55 Dräger Oxylog 3000 plus ventilator.

then pressing the knob to finalize the setting. Some parameters (rate, tidal volume, Pmax, and F_IO_2) have dedicated knobs.

Modes

Modes are set by pressing dedicated buttons that name basic modes and then selecting options such as AutoFlow (for VC modes), Pressure Support (for IMV and CSV modes), and noninvasive ventilation. Modes are shown in **Table 9-51**.

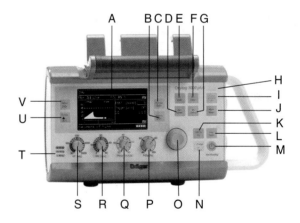

FIGURE 9-56 Dräger Oxylog 3000 plus operator interface. A. Screen with screen pages for the specific application. B. Alarms. C. Ventilation parameters. D. Key for ventilation mode SpnCPAP. E. Key for setting the ventilation modes VC-CMV/VC-AC. F. Key for setting the ventilation mode VC-SIMV. G. Key for setting the ventilation mode PC-SIMV+. H. Red and yellow alarm indicators. I. Key for suppressing the audible alarm for 2 minutes. J. Alarm reset key. K. Key for 100 % O_2 inhalation. L. Key for initiating a manual inspiration. N. Display symbols for the power supply. O. Rotary knob for making selections, changing and confirming settings. P. Control knob for setting the O_2 concentration. Q. Control knob for setting the maximum inspiratory pressure. R. Control knob for setting the respiratory rate. S. Control knob for setting the tidal volume. T. Key to change between the pressure, flow or CO_2 (optional) curve in small and large presentation. V. Key to change screen pages in the "Measured Values" window.

TABLE 9-51
Modes for the Dräger Oxylog 3000 Plus

Mode Name	Control Variable	Breath Sequence	Primary Breath Targeting Scheme	Secondary Breath Targeting Scheme	Tag
VC-A/C	volume	CMV	set-point	N/A	VC-CMVs
VC-SIMV	volume	IMV	set-point	set-point	VC-IMVs,s
VC-A/C with Auto Flow	pressure	CMV	adaptive	N/A	PC-CMVa
VC-SIMV with Auto Flow	pressure	IMV	adaptive	set-point	PC-IMVa,s
PC-IMV+	pressure	IMV	set-point	set-point	PC-IMVs,s
SpnCPAP/PS	pressure	CSV	set-point	N/A	PC-CSVs

Reproduced with permission from Mandu Press Ltd.

Pressure Control Synchronized Intermittent Mandatory Ventilation Plus

- *Mandatory breaths:* Machine triggered (preset frequency) or patient synchronized (flow sensitivity) and machine cycled (inspiratory time). Spontaneous breaths are permitted both between and during mandatory breaths. The + designation calls attention to the fact that patients are free to breath spontaneously during mandatory breaths.
  - Within-breath settings:
    - Operator-set PEEP, frequency, inspiratory pressure, rise time, and inspiratory time
- *Spontaneous breaths:* Patient triggered (flow sensitivity) and patient cycled (% peak inspiratory flow).
  - Within-breath settings:
    - Operator-set inspiratory pressure and rise time
- *Between-breath targets:* None.

Spontaneous Continuous Positive Airway Pressure/Pressure Support

- *Mandatory breaths:* Not allowed
- *Spontaneous breaths:* Patient triggered (flow sensitivity) and patient cycled (% peak inspiratory flow)
  - Within-breath settings:
    - Operator-set inspiratory pressure and rise time
- *Between-breath targets:* None

Volume Control Assist Control

This is called Volume Control Controlled Mandatory Ventilation if sensitivity is turned off.

- *Mandatory breaths:* Machine triggered (preset frequency) or patient triggered (flow sensitivity) and machine cycled (inspiratory time)
  - Within-breath settings:
    - Operator-set PEEP, frequency, peak inspiratory flow, inspiratory time, and tidal volume
- *Spontaneous breaths:* Not allowed
- *Between-breath targets:* None

Volume Control Assist/Control with AutoFlow

- *Mandatory breaths:* Machine triggered (preset frequency) and machine cycled (inspiratory time). Patient-triggered breaths are not allowed.
  - Within-breath settings:
    - Operator-set PEEP, frequency, rise time, and inspiratory time
    - Ventilator-set inspiratory pressure
- *Spontaneous breaths:* Not allowed.
- Between-breath targets:
  - Operator-set tidal volume

Volume Control Synchronized Intermittent Mandatory Ventilation

- *Mandatory breaths:* Machine triggered (preset frequency) or patient triggered (flow sensitivity) and machine cycled (inspiratory time)
  - Within-breath settings:
    - Operator-set PEEP, frequency, inspiratory flow, and tidal volume
    - Ventilator-set inspiratory flow if inspiration switches from volume control to pressure control when inspiratory pressure meets the inspiratory pressure target (P_{max} setting)
- *Spontaneous breaths:* Patient triggered (flow sensitivity) and patient cycled (% peak inspiratory flow)
  - Within-breath settings:
    - Operator-set inspiratory pressure and rise time
- *Between-breath targets:* None

Volume Control Synchronized Intermittent Mandatory Ventilation with AutoFlow

- *Mandatory breaths:* Machine triggered (preset frequency) or patient triggered (flow sensitivity) and machine cycled (inspiratory time)
  - Within-breath settings:
    - Operator-set PEEP, frequency, rise time, and inspiratory time
    - Ventilator-set inspiratory pressure
- *Spontaneous breaths:* Patient triggered (flow sensitivity) and patient cycled (% peak inspiratory flow)
  - Within-breath settings:
    - Operator-set inspiratory pressure and rise time
- Between-breath targets:
  - Operator-set tidal volume

Special Features

Oxygen: The O_2 supply is provided by a high pressure (39–87 psi) source. F_IO_2 is adjustable from 40% to 100%. The actual value depends on the inspiratory flow and mean airway pressure.

Backup ventilation: Apnea backup ventilation is applicable only when using the SpnCPAP mode. In the event of an apnea, the ventilator will automatically activate volume-controlled mandatory ventilation (VC-CMV).

Gas volume compensation: The tidal volume is applied regardless of ambient pressure under patient conditions BTPS for volume-controlled modes.

Miscellaneous: With installation of an optional CO_2 sensor, measurement and display of exhaled CO_2 values is possible.

Nebulizer: None.

Neonatal ventilation: None.

Noninvasive ventilation: NIV can be activated only as a supplementary function in the ventilation modes SpnCPAP, PC-SIMV+, VC-AC with AutoFlow, and VC-SIMV with AutoFlow. Mask leakages are detected and compensation applied. Therefore, the displayed measured values for tidal volume and minute ventilation do not include the leakage. The leakage alarm is inactive.

Manufacturer's Specifications

Table 9-52 lists specifications for the Dräger Oxylog 3000 plus.

TABLE 9-52
Specifications for the Dräger Oxylog 3000 Plus

Setting Category	Setting	Range
Pressure	Inspiratory Pressure	3–75 cm H_2O
	Pressure Support	0–35 cm H_2O
	PEEP	0–20 cm H_2O
Volume	Tidal Volume	0.05–2.0 L
Flow	Inspiratory Flow	39, 80, 100 L/min
	Waveform	Not specified
Time	Inspiratory Time	0.2–10 s
	Mandatory Breath Frequency	2–60/min
	Adjustable Rise Time	Yes
Sensitivity	Trigger Sensitivity (flow)	1–15 L/min
Alarm Category		
Pressure	High Airway Pressure	20–60 cm H_2O
Volume	None	
Flow	High Minute Ventilation	2–41 L/min
	Low Minute Ventilation	0.5–40 L/min
Time	High Respiratory Rate	10–100/min
Other	High etCO$_2$	1–100 mm Hg
	Low etCO$_2$	0–100 mm Hg

(continues)

TABLE 9-52
Specifications for the Dräger Oxylog 3000 Plus (*Continued*)

Setting Category	Setting	Range
Monitored Parameters	Airway Pressure	
	Leakage	
	Respiratory Rate	
	etCO$_2$	
	Expiratory Minute Volume	
	Supply Pressure	

Covidien Puritan Bennett 540

The Puritan Bennett (PB) 540 ventilator (**Figure 9-57**) is electronically controlled and pneumatically powered (internal blower). It is indicated for the continuous or intermittent mechanical ventilatory support of patients weighing at least 11 lb (5 kg).

Operator Interface

The operator interface of the PB 540 has an LCD screen and buttons (**Figure 9-58**). Settings are entered by selecting the parameter and then pressing the up or down arrows to adjust the value.

Modes

Modes are selected by name. **Table 9-53** lists the available modes.

Pressure Support Ventilation/CPAP
- *Mandatory breaths:* Not allowed
- *Spontaneous breaths:* Patient triggered (flow sensitivity) and patient cycled (% peak inspiratory flow)
  - Within-breath settings:
    - Operator-set inspiratory pressure, rise time, and cycle sensitivity (% peak inspiratory flow)
- *Between-breath targets:* None

Pressure Assist/Control
- *Mandatory breaths:* Machine triggered (preset frequency) or patient triggered (flow sensitivity) and machine cycled (inspiratory time)
  - Within-breath settings:
    - Operator-set PEEP, frequency, inspiratory pressure, rise time, and inspiratory time
- *Spontaneous breaths:* Not allowed
- *Between-breath targets:* None

Pressure SIMV
- *Mandatory breaths:* Machine triggered (preset frequency) or patient synchronized (flow sensitivity) and machine cycled (inspiratory time)
  - Within-breath settings:
    - Operator-set PEEP, frequency, inspiratory pressure, rise time, and inspiratory time

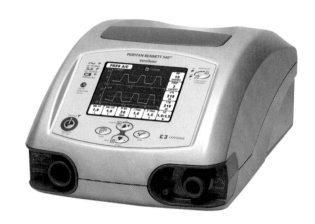

FIGURE 9-57 Covidien PB 540 ventilator.

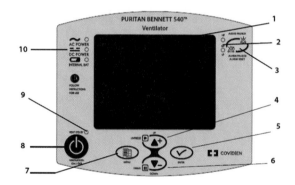

FIGURE 9-58 Covidien PB 540 operator interface. 1. Display screen showing modes, ventilation settings, patient data and waveforms, configuration of the ventilator and alarm management. 2. Alarm indicators. 3. Alarm control key. 4. Moves cursor up to increase setting values. 5. Enter key to confirm setting value. 6. Moves cursor down to decrease setting values. 7. Menu key changes between ventilation and alarm screens. 8. Ventilator on/off button. 9. Ventilation status indicator. 10. Electrical power source indicators.

- *Spontaneous breaths:* Patient triggered (pressure or flow sensitivity) and patient cycled (% peak inspiratory flow)
  - Within-breath settings:
    - Operator-set inspiratory pressure
- *Between-breath targets:* None

TABLE 9-53
Modes for the Covidien PB 540 Ventilator

Mode Name	Mode Classification				
	Control Variable	Breath Sequence	Primary Breath Targeting Scheme	Secondary Breath Targeting Scheme	Tag
Volume A/C	volume	CMV	set-point	N/A	VC-CMVs
Volume SIMV	volume	IMV	set-point	set-point	VC-IMVs,s
Pressure A/C	pressure	CMV	set-point	N/A	PC-CMVs
Pressure SIMV	pressure	IMV	set-point	set-point	PC-IMVs,s
Pressure Support Ventilation/CPAP	pressure	CSV	set-point	N/A	PC-CSVs

Volume Assist/Control

- *Mandatory breaths:* Machine triggered (preset frequency) or patient triggered (flow sensitivity) and machine cycled (inspiratory time)
  - Within-breath settings:
    - Operator-set PEEP, frequency, flow waveform, inspiratory time, and tidal volume
- *Spontaneous breaths:* Not allowed
- *Between-breath targets:* None

Volume SIMV

- *Mandatory breaths:* Machine triggered (preset frequency) or patient synchronized (flow sensitivity) and machine cycled (inspiratory time)
  - Within-breath settings:
    - Operator-set PEEP, frequency, inspiratory time, and tidal volume
- *Spontaneous breaths:* Patient triggered (pressure or flow sensitivity) and patient cycled (% peak inspiratory flow)
  - Within-breath settings:
    - Operator-set inspiratory pressure
- *Between-breath targets:* None

Special Features

Oxygen: Oxygen may be supplied from an external low pressure source, but the oxygen flow must be limited to 15 L/min at 7.25 psi. The ventilator automatically compensates for the extra flow created by the external oxygen supply. The external oxygen source must also have independent means of flow adjustment from the ventilator. The F_IO_2 must be measured or calculated by hand.

Backup ventilation: In SIMV mode, the ventilator delivers backup ventilation during apnea at a breath rate equal to the maximum of 8 and the breath rate setting. If the patient triggers a breath, the ventilator will stop the mandatory breaths and return to the previous operating parameters. In PSV mode, the backup rate is activated so that the ventilator will automatically begin to deliver breaths at the breath rate setting if no patient effort occurs for the apnea time setting. The pressure during a backup breath is equal to the Pressure Support setting before the apnea condition began. If the patient triggers a breath while the backup rate is in effect, the ventilator will return to the previous operating parameters. In CPAP, a backup rate is not set, but the operator must still set an apnea time. In that case, the ventilator will sound an APNEA alarm if no breath is triggered by the patient in the apnea time; however, no backup breaths will be generated.

Gas volume compensation: None.
Leak compensation: None.

Manufacturer's Specifications

Table 9-54 lists specifications for the Covidien PB 540 ventilator.

Covidien Newport HT70 Plus

The Newport HT70 family of ventilators is designed for infant, pediatric, and adult patients (greater than 11 lb/5 kg ideal body weight) in emergency care, transport, critical care, subacute care, and home care applications. The HT70 Basic is for use when Pressure Support is not needed. The HT70 Classic adds Pressure Support and related parameters. The HT70 Plus (Figure 9-59) adds oxygen cylinder use time estimator and alarms, real time battery use time estimator, graphics, trends, and the option of using the on-airway flow sensor, which provides flow triggering, exhaled volumes, and a high exhaled tidal volume alarm. The HT70 is electronically controlled but is unique in that the pneumatic power is provided by micro-pistons that use a fraction of the power consumed by conventional blowers.

TABLE 9-54
Specifications for the Covidien PB 540 Ventilator

Setting Category	Setting	Range
Pressure	Inspiratory Pressure	5–55 cm H_2O
	Pressure Support	5–55 cm H_2O
	PEEP	0.5–20 cm H_2O
Volume	Tidal Volume	0.05–2.0 L
Flow	Waveform	Square/descending ramp
	Inspiratory Time	0.3–6.0 s
Time	Mandatory Breath Frequency	1–60/min
	Adjustable Rise Time	Yes
Sensitivity	Cycle Sensitivity (flow)	5–95%
Alarm Category		
Pressure	High Peak Inspiratory Pressure	12–60 cm H_2O
	Low Peak Inspiratory Pressure	2–52 cm H_2O
Volume	High Inspired Tidal Volume	0.08–3.0 L
	Low Inspired Tidal Volume	0.03–1.99 L
	High Exhaled Tidal Volume	0.08–3.0 L
	Low Exhaled Tidal Volume	0.03–1.99 L
Flow	High Minute Volume	2–99 L
	Low Minute Volume	0.5–50.0 L
Time	High Respiratory Rate	10–70/min
	Maximum Inspiratory Time	0.8–3.0 s
	Minimum Inspiratory Time	0.1–3.0 s
Other	O_2 Sensor	Enabled/Disabled
Monitored Parameters	Peak Inspiratory Pressure	
	PEEP	
	Inspiratory Tidal Volume	
	Expiratory Tidal Volume	
	Inspiratory Minute Volume	
	Expiratory Minute Volume	
	Total Respiratory Rate	
	Mean Airway Pressure	
	I:E Ratio	
	Inspiratory Time	
	Expiratory Time	

Operator Interface

The operator interface of the HT70 Plus is based on a color-coded LCD touch screen (**Figure 9-60**). The buttons for accessing alarms and display screens as well as the buttons for selecting mode and breath type are consolidated along the left margin. Monitored values are displayed across the bottom margin and the pressure bar graph rises and falls along the right. Settings are entered by selecting the parameter and then pressing the up or down arrows to adjust the value and pressing the Accept button to confirm.

Modes

Modes on the Newport HT70 Plus are constructed by the operator by selecting the breath sequence (i.e., CMV, IMV, CSV) and the control variable separately. The operator may select from A/C (Assist/Control), SIMV (Synchronized Intermittent Mandatory Ventilation), or SPONT (Spontaneous). After selecting the breath sequence, the operator selects either pressure control or volume control to complete the mode selection. **Table 9-55** lists the available modes.

Pressure Control Assist Control Mandatory Ventilation
- *Mandatory breaths*: Machine triggered (preset frequency) or patient triggered (pressure or flow sensitivity) and machine cycled (inspiratory time)

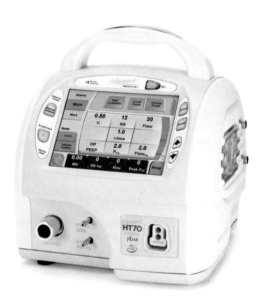

FIGURE 9-59 Covidien Newport HT70 Plus ventilator.

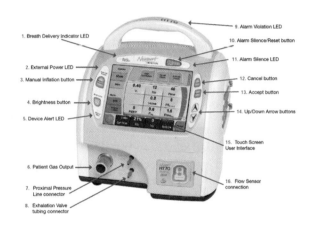

FIGURE 9-60 Covidien Newport HT70 Plus operator interface.

TABLE 9-55
Modes for the Covidien Newport HT70 Plus

Mode Name	Control Variable	Breath Sequence	Mode Classification Primary Breath Targeting Scheme	Secondary Breath Targeting Scheme	Tag
A/C Mandatory Ventilation Volume Control	volume	CMV	set-point	N/A	VC-CMVs
SIMV Volume Control	volume	IMV	set-point	set-point	VC-IMVs,s
A/C Mandatory Ventilation Pressure Control	pressure	CMV	set-point	N/A	PC-CMVs
SIMV Pressure Control	pressure	IMV	set-point	set-point	PC-IMVs,s
Spont	pressure	CSV	set-point	N/A	PC-CSVs

- Within-breath settings:
  - Operator-set PEEP, frequency, inspiratory pressure, slope rise, and inspiratory time
- *Spontaneous breaths*: Not allowed
- *Between-breath targets*: None

Pressure Control Synchronized Intermittent Mandatory Ventilation

- *Mandatory breaths*: Machine triggered (preset frequency), patient synchronized (pressure or flow sensitivity), and machine cycled (inspiratory time)
  - Within-breath settings:
    - Operator-set PEEP, frequency, inspiratory pressure, slope rise, and inspiratory time
  - *Between-breath targets*: None
- *Spontaneous breaths*: Patient triggered (pressure or flow sensitivity) and patient cycled (% peak inspiratory flow) or machine cycled (PS Max I Time)
  - Within-breath settings:
    - Operator-set inspiratory pressure, slope rise, and cycle sensitivity (% peak inspiratory flow and PS Max I Time)
  - *Between-breath targets*: None

Volume Control Assist Control Mandatory Ventilation

- *Mandatory breaths*: Machine triggered (preset frequency) or patient triggered (pressure or flow sensitivity) and machine cycled (tidal volume)
  - Within-breath settings:
    - Operator-set PEEP, frequency, peak inspiratory flow and flow waveform and flow waveform or inspiratory time, and tidal volume
- *Spontaneous breaths*: Not allowed
- *Between-breath targets*: None

Volume Control Synchronized Intermittent Mandatory Ventilation

- *Mandatory breaths*: Machine triggered (preset frequency), patient synchronized (pressure or flow sensitivity), and machine cycled (tidal volume)
  - Within-breath settings:
    - Operator-set PEEP, frequency, peak inspiratory flow and flow waveform or inspiratory time, and tidal volume
  - *Between-breath targets*: None
- *Spontaneous breaths*: Patient triggered (pressure or flow sensitivity) and patient cycled (% peak inspiratory flow) or machine cycled (PS Max I Time)
  - Within-breath settings:
    - Operator-set inspiratory pressure, slope rise, and cycle sensitivity (% peak inspiratory flow and PS Max I Time)
  - *Between-breath targets*: None

SPONT

- *Mandatory breaths*: Not allowed
- *Spontaneous breaths*: Patient triggered (pressure or flow sensitivity) and patient cycled (% peak inspiratory flow) or machine cycled (PS Max I Time)
  - Within-breath settings:
    - Operator set inspiratory pressure, slope rise, and cycle sensitivity (% peak inspiratory flow and PS Max I Time)
- *Between-breath targets*: None

Special Features

Oxygen: The ventilator may be used with optional devices for oxygen enrichment: an air/oxygen entrainment mixer or a low flow oxygen reservoir. Both fit on the ventilator's fresh gas intake port. The mixer is used to blend atmospheric air with oxygen from a 50 psi source. Using the mixer's control knob, F_IO_2 can be adjusted from .21–1.00. The low flow reservoir is used to blend atmospheric air with 1–10 L/min source oxygen (e.g., from a flowmeter). With the reservoir, delivered F_IO_2 will vary depending on the use of bias flow and PEEP, the delivered minute ventilation, and the O_2 concentration of the source gas (e.g., gas from an oxygen concentrator is usually around 93% oxygen). The operator's manual provides graphs for estimating the oxygen flow required for the desired F_IO_2. The ventilator has a built-in oxygen sensor, a display of monitored F_IO_2, and user-set high and low F_IO_2 alarms.

Backup ventilation: Backup ventilation activates when the currently linked alarm occurs. This function can be linked with the low minute volume alarm, the apnea alarm, or both alarms. Backup ventilation is functional in all modes and has customizable settings. In A/CMV and SIMV modes, backup ventilation maintains all breath delivery settings except respiratory rate. That setting is increased by a user-set value (default = 1.5) times the set rate, up to a maximum of 99 breaths/min. In the SPONT mode, backup ventilation changes the mode to SIMV pressure control mode, maintaining the spontaneous breath settings but adding mandatory breaths with a mandatory respiratory rate = user-set at ≥ 15 breaths/min, inspiratory pressure = user-set at a value above set PEEP, and inspiratory time = user-set. In all modes and breath types, the minimum breath rate delivered during backup ventilation is user-set at ≥ 15 breaths/min.

Gas volume compensation: None.

Neonatal ventilation: None.

Noninvasive ventilation: The HT70 can be used for noninvasive ventilation in all modes. When activated, the following features are applied: bias flow is increased to 10 L/min and can be adjusted as needed from 3 to 30 L/min; the low minute volume alarm can be turned off; the low pressure alarm can be set closer to the base pressure (1 cm H_2O above baseline); and the high minute volume alarm is expanded to 80 L/min.

Manufacturer's Specifications

Table 9-56 lists specifications for the Covidien Newport HT70 Plus.

GE Healthcare iVent 101

The iVent 101 (Figure 9-61) is a microprocessor-controlled ventilator, intended for use in home,

institutional, and portable environments. The iVent 101 ventilator (with single or dual limb configuration) is intended to provide continuous or intermittent ventilatory support for infants from 11 lb (5 kg) through adult patients who require invasive or noninvasive support.

Operator Interface

The iVent 101 interface (Figure 9-62) consists of an LCD touch screen. Pressure and flow waveforms are available.

Modes

Modes on the iVent 101 are selected by mode name (e.g., A/C Volume Control, SIMV Pressure Control, etc.) using

TABLE 9-56
Specifications for the Covidien Newport HT70 Plus

Setting Category	Setting	Range
Pressure	Inspiratory Pressure	5–60 cm H_2O
	Pressure Support	0–60 cm H_2O
	PEEP	0–30 cm H_2O
Volume	Tidal Volume	50–2,200 mL
Flow	Inspiratory Flow	6–100 L/min
	Waveform	Square/descending ramp
Time	Inspiratory Time	0.1–3.0 s
	Mandatory Breath Frequency	1–99/min
	Adjustable Rise Time	Yes
	PS Max i time	0.1–3.0 s
	PS % Exp. Threshold	5–85%
Sensitivity	Trigger Sensitivity (pressure)	–9.9 to 0 cm H_2O
	Trigger Sensitivity (flow) Flow trig w/flow sensor	0.0–10.0 L/min, Off
	Manual Inflation	3 s maximum
Other	NIV (noninvasive ventilation)	On/off in all modes
	O_2 (oxygen) w/mixer	21–100%
	Bias Flow	NIV off: 7 L/min w/PEEP; NIV on: 3–30 L/min w/PEEP
	Infant/Ped/Adult Presets	
	Custom BUV settings	
Alarm Category		
Pressure	High Pressure	4–99 cm H_2O
	Low Pressure	3–98 cm H_2O

(continues)

TABLE 9-56
Specifications for the Covidien Newport HT70 Plus (*Continued*)

Setting Category	Setting	Range
Flow	High Inspiratory/Expiratory (Exp w/flow sensor) Minute Volume	1.1–50.0 L/min
	Low Inspiratory/Expiratory (Exp w/flow sensor) Minute Volume	0.1–49.0 L/min
Time	Apnea	5–60 s
	High Respiratory Rate	30–100/min
Other	O$_2$ Sensor	Enabled/Disabled/Manually Adjustable High/Low Alarms
	Low/Empty Battery	
	Cylinder Use Time Estimator	Enabled/Disabled
Monitored Parameters	Inspiratory/Expiratory (Exp w/flow sensor) Minute Volume	
	Inspiratory/Expiratory (Exp w/flow sensor) Tidal Volume	
	Respiratory Rate Total	
	Peak Pressure	
	Mean Pressure	
	P Base (PEEP)	
	Peak Flow	
	F$_I$O$_2$	
	I:E Ratio	
	O$_2$ Cylinder Use Time Available	
	Battery Use Time Available	

a menu. Specific mode settings are selected using other menus. Special features are available that, when activated, actually change the mode classification (e.g., activation of Pressure Limit or Adaptive Peak Flow in volume control modes). Available modes are shown in Table 9-57.

A/C Pressure Control
- *Mandatory breaths:* Machine triggered (preset frequency) or patient triggered (pressure or flow sensitivity) and machine cycled (inspiratory time or tidal volume limit)
  - Within-breath settings:
    - Operator-set PEEP, frequency, inspiratory pressure, rise time, inspiratory time, tidal volume limit
- *Spontaneous breaths:* Not allowed
- *Between-breath targets:* None

A/C Pressure Regulated Volume Control
- *Mandatory breaths:* Machine triggered (preset frequency) or patient triggered (pressure or flow sensitivity) and machine cycled (inspiratory time)

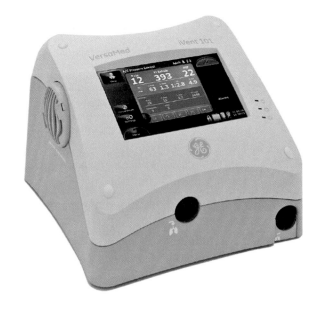

FIGURE 9-61 GE iVent 101 ventilator.
Used with permission of GE Healthcare.

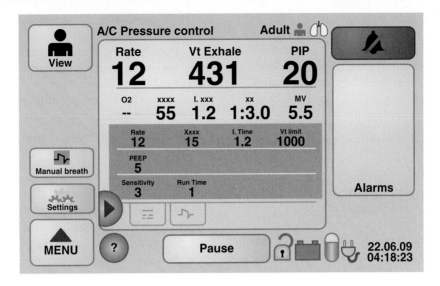

FIGURE 9-62 GE iVent 101 operator interface.

Used with permission of GE Healthcare.

TABLE 9-57
Classification of Modes for the iVent 101

Mode Name	Control Variable	Breath Sequence	Primary Breath Targeting Scheme	Secondary Breath Targeting Scheme	Tag
A/C Volume Control	volume	CMV	set-point	N/A	VC-CMVs
A/C Volume Control with Adaptive Peak Flow	volume	CMV	adaptive	N/A	VC-CMVa
SIMV Volume Control	volume	IMV	set-point	set-point	VC-IMVs,s
SIMV Volume Control with Adaptive Peak Flow	volume	IMV	adaptive	set-point	VC-IMVa,s
A/C Pressure Control	pressure	CMV	set-point	N/A	PC-CMVs
A/C Pressure Regulated Volume Control	pressure	CMV	adaptive	N/A	PC-CMVa
SIMV Pressure Control	pressure	IMV	set-point	set-point	PC-IMVs,s
Adaptive Bi-Level	pressure	IMV	set-point	set-point	PC-IMVs,s
SIMV Pressure Regulated Volume Control	pressure	IMV	adaptive	set-point	PC-IMVa,s
CPAP/Pressure Support Ventilation	pressure	CSV	set-point	N/A	PC-CSVs

Reproduced with permission from Mandu Press Ltd.

- Within-breath settings:
  - Operator-set PEEP, frequency, rise time, inspiratory time, and optional tidal volume limit
  - Ventilator-set inspiratory pressure
- *Spontaneous breaths:* Not allowed
- Between-breath targets:
  - Operator-set tidal volume

A/C Volume Control (optional Adaptive Flow and Pressure Limit)
- *Mandatory breaths:* Machine triggered (preset frequency) or patient triggered (pressure or flow sensitivity) and machine cycled (tidal volume)
  - Within-breath settings:
    - Operator-set PEEP, frequency, peak inspiratory flow or Adaptive Flow, inspiratory

time, inspiratory pressure limit, and tidal volume. The Adaptive Peak Flow algorithm will adjust peak flow so that the tidal volume is delivered in the inspiratory time determined by the Adaptive I-Time algorithm to achieve an I:E ratio of 1:2.

- *Spontaneous breaths:* Not allowed
- *Between-breath targets:* None

Adaptive BiLevel

- *Mandatory breaths:* Machine triggered (preset frequency) or patient synchronized (pressure or flow sensitivity) and machine cycled (inspiratory time) or patient cycled (percent of peak flow). Spontaneous breaths are patient triggered (pressure or flow sensitivity) and patient cycled (percent of peak flow). Spontaneous breaths suppress mandatory breaths if they occur at a frequency higher than the set frequency.
  - Within-breath settings:
    - Operator-set PEEP (called P-Low), peak inspiratory pressure (called P-High), rise time, inspiratory time, and frequency
- *Spontaneous breaths:* Patient triggered (pressure or flow sensitivity) and patient cycled (% peak inspiratory flow). Spontaneous breaths are permitted both between and during mandatory breaths.
  - Within-breath settings:
    - Operator-set inspiratory pressure, rise time, and cycle sensitivity (% peak flow)
- *Between-breath targets:* None

CPAP/PSV

- *Mandatory breaths:* Not allowed
- *Spontaneous breaths:* Patient triggered (pressure or flow sensitivity) and patient cycled (% peak inspiratory flow)
  - Within-breath settings:
    - Operator-set inspiratory pressure, rise time, and cycle sensitivity (% peak flow)
- *Between-breath targets:* None

SIMV Pressure Control

- *Mandatory breaths:* Machine triggered (preset frequency or patient synchronized using pressure or flow sensitivity) and machine cycled (inspiratory time)
  - Within-breath settings:
    - Operator-set PEEP, inspiratory pressure, frequency, rise time, and I:E ratio
- *Spontaneous breaths:* Patient triggered (pressure or flow sensitivity) and patient cycled (% peak inspiratory flow)
  - Within-breath settings:
    - Operator-set inspiratory pressure, rise time, cycle sensitivity (% peak inspiratory flow), and optional tidal volume limit
- *Between-breath targets:* None

SIMV Pressure Regulated Volume Control

- *Mandatory breaths:* Machine triggered (preset frequency) or patient triggered (pressure or flow sensitivity) and machine cycled (inspiratory time)
  - Within-breath settings:
    - Operator-set PEEP, frequency, rise time, inspiratory time, and optional tidal volume limit
    - Ventilator-set inspiratory pressure
- *Spontaneous breaths:* Patient triggered (pressure or flow sensitivity) and patient cycled (% peak inspiratory flow)
  - Within-breath settings:
    - Operator-set inspiratory pressure, rise time, and cycle sensitivity (% peak flow)
- Between-breath targets:
  - Operator-set tidal volume

SIMV Volume Control (Optional Adaptive Flow and Pressure Limit)

- *Mandatory breaths:* Machine triggered (preset frequency) or patient synchronized (pressure or flow sensitivity) and machine cycled (tidal volume)
  - Within-breath settings:
    - Operator-set PEEP, frequency, peak inspiratory flow or Adaptive Flow, inspiratory time, inspiratory pressure limit, and tidal volume. The Adaptive Peak Flow algorithm will adjust peak flow so that the tidal volume is delivered in the inspiratory time determined by the Adaptive I-Time algorithm to achieve an I:E ratio of 1:2.
- *Spontaneous breaths:* Patient triggered (pressure or flow sensitivity) and patient cycled (% peak inspiratory flow)
  - Within-breath settings:
    - Operator-set inspiratory pressure, rise time, and cycle sensitivity (% peak inspiratory flow)
- *Between-breath targets:* None

Special Features

Oxygen: The iVent 101 ventilator uses oxygen from a low pressure oxygen source such as an oxygen concentrator or a flowmeter (20 L/min maximum).

Backup ventilation: A backup mode is automatically activated when no breath has been delivered during the set apnea time interval. Ventilation will continue with an apnea rate set by the clinician with the same mandatory breath settings of the ventilation mode that is currently chosen. If the ventilation mode is CPAP/PSV at the time when apnea occurs, ventilation is delivered according to the mode chosen by the clinician or with default apnea settings. The default mode in CPAP/PSV for all patients is A/C pressure control. Modes that may be selected as backup modes are A/C Volume or Pressure Control and SIMV Volume or Pressure Control.

Gas volume compensation: All flow, volume, and pressure measurements in iVent101 are expressed at STPD conditions (standard temperature and pressure, dry) 32°F (0°C) and 101.3 kPa (760 mm mercury column).

Miscellaneous: A feature called Easy Exhale is an advanced PEEP strategy used in cases of intrinsic PEEP. Its purpose is to improve the downstream airway emptying while potentially matching the intrinsic PEEP to optimize alveolar ventilation. With this feature, the ventilator circuit is depressurized during the very early phase of expiration. The ventilator reestablishes the PEEP value as the flow begins to slow to prevent airway pressure from falling below alveolar pressure.

Nebulizer: None.

Noninvasive ventilation: The Adaptive Bi-Level mode can accommodate high leak situations, such as when using a face mask (noninvasive ventilation) or pressure support for high leak ET tube ventilation (e.g., Passy Muir and cuffless applications).

Manufacturer's Specifications

Table 9-58 lists specifications for the GE iVent 101.

Hamilton Medical Hamilton-T1

The Hamilton Medical Hamilton-T1 ventilator (**Figure 9-63**) is an electronically controlled pneumatic ventilation system with an integrated air compressing system. This ventilator is powered from an AC source with internal battery backup. It is intended to provide positive pressure ventilatory support adult and pediatric patients. This full-functioned intensive care ventilator offers a complete range of modes and a variety of monitoring capabilities. It displays monitored parameters as numbers and graphic data displayed as a combination of real-time waveforms (curves), loops, trends, and special Intelligent Panels. These Intelligent Panels include the Dynamic Lung, which shows the lung's activity, and the Vent Status, which indicates the patient's level of ventilator dependency. The Hamilton-T1 receives inputs from a disposable, proximal flow sensor (required) and other sensors within the ventilator. Based on this monitored data, the device adjusts gas delivery to the patient. This sensor lets the ventilator sense even weak patient breathing efforts. The flow sensor is highly accurate even in the presence of secretions, moisture, and nebulized medications.

TABLE 9-58
Specifications for the GE iVent 101

Setting Category	Setting	Range
Pressure	Inspiratory Pressure	5–60 cm H_2O
	Pressure Support	5–60 cm H_2O
	PEEP	0–45 cm H_2O
Volume	Tidal Volume	0.04–2.5 L
Flow	Inspiratory Flow	5–120 L/min
	Waveform	Not Specified
Time	Inspiratory Time	0.3–3.0 s
	Mandatory Breath Frequency	1–80/min
	Adjustable Rise Time	Yes
Sensitivity	Cycle Sensitivity (flow)	5–80%
Alarm Category		
Pressure	High Pressure	5–60 cm H_2O
	Low Pressure	1–55 cm H_2O
Flow	Minute Volume	0–50 L/min
Time	Respiratory Rate	1–99/min
	Apnea Time	5–60 s
Other	O_2 Sensor	Enabled/Disabled
Monitored Parameters	Exhaled Tidal Volume	
	Minute Volume Exhaled	

(continues)

TABLE 9-58
Specifications for the GE iVent 101 (*Continued*)

Setting Category	Setting	Range
	Respiratory Rate	
	Inspiratory Time	
	Peak Inspiratory Pressure	
	Peak Flow	
	PEEP	
	I:E Ratio	
	Measured Oxygen Mix (F_iO_2)	

Used with permission of GE Healthcare.

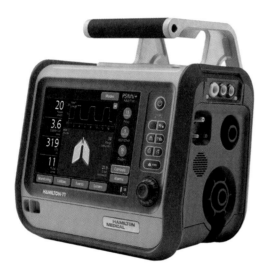

FIGURE 9-63 Hamilton Medical Hamilton-T1 ventilator.
Courtesy of Hamilton Medical.

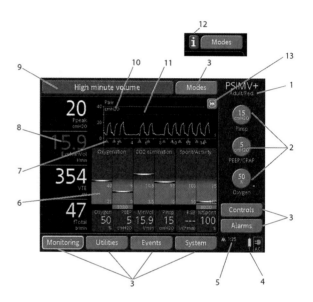

FIGURE 9-64 Hamilton Medical Hamilton-T1 operator interface. 1. Active mode and patient group. 2. Main controls. 3. Window buttons (tabs). 4. Input power. 5. Alarm silence countdown. 6. Graphic display. 7. Symbol indicating patient triggered breath. 8. Main monitoring parameters. 9. Message bar. 10. Maximum pressure indication line. 11. Pressure limitation. 12 Inactive alarm indicator. 13. Freeze button.
Courtesy of Hamilton Medical.

Operator Interface

The ventilator's operator interface (**Figure 9-64**) is based on a color touch screen, a press-and-turn knob, and keys.

Modes

Modes on the T1 are selected by mode name (e.g., PCV+, SPONT, ASV, DuoPAP, etc.) using a menu. Specific mode settings are selected using other menus. Available modes are shown in **Table 9-59**.

For the T1 ventilator, spontaneous breathing is allowed at any time in any mode.

Adaptive Support Ventilation

- *Mandatory breaths:* Machine triggered (preset frequency) and machine cycled (inspiratory time). Spontaneous breaths suppress mandatory breaths

if spontaneous minute ventilation is above target minute ventilation.
- Within-breath settings:
  - Operator-set PEEP, maximum inspiratory pressure, patient height, and percent minute ventilation to support
  - Ventilator-set inspiratory pressure
- *Spontaneous breaths:* Patient triggered (flow sensitivity) and patient cycled (% peak inspiratory flow)
  - Within-breath settings:
    - Rise time and cycle sensitivity (% peak flow)

TABLE 9-59
Classification of Modes for the Hamilton Medical Hamilton-T1 Ventilator

| Mode Name | Mode Classification | | | | |
	Control Variable	Breath Sequence	Primary Breath Targeting Scheme	Secondary Breath Targeting Scheme	Tag
Synchronized Controlled Mandatory Ventilation Plus	pressure	CMV	adaptive	N/A	PC-CMVa
Pressure Controlled Ventilation Plus	pressure	CMV	set-point	N/A	PC-CMVs
Pressure Controlled Synchronized Intermittent Mandatory Ventilation	pressure	IMV	set-point	set-point	PC-IMVs,s
Noninvasive Ventilation—Spontaneous Timed	pressure	IMV	set-point	set-point	PC-IMVs,s
Duo Positive Airway Pressure	pressure	IMV	set-point	set-point	PC-IMVs,s
Airway Pressure Release Ventilation	pressure	IMV	set-point	set-point	PC-IMVs,s
Synchronized Intermittent Mandatory Ventilation Plus	pressure	IMV	adaptive	set-point	PC-IMVa,s
Adaptive Support Ventilation	pressure	IMV	optimal/intelligent	optimal/intelligent	PC-IMVoi,oi
Spontaneous	pressure	CSV	set-point	N/A	PC-CSVs
Noninvasive Ventilation	pressure	CSV	set-point	N/A	PC-CSVs

Reproduced with permission from Mandu Press Ltd.

- Between-breath targets:
  - Ventilator-set tidal volume and minute ventilation

Airway Pressure Release Ventilation

- *Mandatory breaths:* Machine triggered (preset frequency or patient synchronized using flow trigger sensitivity) and machine cycled (inspiratory time or patient synchronized using flow cycle sensitivity).
  - Within-breath settings:
    - Operator-set PEEP (called P_{low}), peak inspiratory pressure (called P_{high}), inspiratory time (called T_{high}), and expiratory time (called T_{low})
- *Spontaneous breaths:* Patient triggered (flow sensitivity) and patient cycled (% peak inspiratory flow). Spontaneous breaths are permitted both between and during mandatory breaths.
  - Within-breath settings:
    - Operator-set inspiratory pressure (pressure support) and cycle sensitivity (% peak flow)
- *Between-breath targets:* None.

Duo Positive Airway Pressure

- *Mandatory breaths:* Machine triggered (preset frequency or patient synchronized using flow trigger sensitivity) and machine cycled (inspiratory time or patient synchronized using flow cycle sensitivity)
  - Within-breath settings:
    - Operator-set PEEP (called P_{low}), peak inspiratory pressure (called P_{high}), frequency, and inspiratory time (called T_{high})
- *Spontaneous breaths:* Patient triggered (flow sensitivity) and patient cycled (% peak inspiratory flow). Spontaneous breaths are permitted both between and during mandatory breaths.
  - Within-breath settings:
    - Inspiratory pressure (i.e., pressure support level) and cycle sensitivity (% peak flow)
- *Between-breath targets:* None.

Noninvasive Ventilation

Noninvasive ventilation (NIV) is an adaptation of the SPONT mode, whereas NIV-ST is an adaptation of the PSIMV+ mode. The primary difference is that NIV modes are designed to compensate for leaks when using a mask or other noninvasive patient interface.

- *Mandatory breaths:* Not allowed
- *Spontaneous breaths:* Patient triggered (flow sensitivity) and patient cycled (% peak inspiratory flow)
  - Within-breath settings:
    - Operator-set inspiratory pressure, cycle sensitivity (% peak inspiratory flow), and maximum inspiratory time
- *Between-breath targets:* None

Noninvasive Ventilation-Spontaneous Timed

Noninvasive ventilation (NIV) is an adaptation of the SPONT mode, whereas NIV-ST is an adaptation of the PSIMV+ mode. The primary difference is that NIV modes are designed to compensate for leaks when using a mask or other noninvasive patient interface.

- *Mandatory breaths:* Machine triggered (preset frequency or patient synchronized using flow sensitivity) and machine cycled (inspiratory time)
  - Within-breath settings:
    - Operator-set PEEP, inspiratory pressure, frequency, inspiratory time
- *Spontaneous breaths:* Patient triggered (pressure or flow sensitivity) and patient cycled (% peak inspiratory flow)
  - Within-breath settings:
    - Inspiratory pressure set for mandatory breaths applies to spontaneous breaths automatically, cycle sensitivity (% peak inspiratory flow), and maximum inspiratory time.
- *Between-breath targets:* None

Pressure Controlled Synchronized Intermittent Mandatory Ventilation

- *Mandatory breaths:* Machine triggered (preset frequency or patient synchronized using flow sensitivity) and machine cycled (inspiratory time)
  - Within-breath settings:
    - Operator-set PEEP, inspiratory pressure, frequency, and inspiratory time
- *Spontaneous breaths:* Patient triggered (flow sensitivity) and patient cycled (% peak inspiratory flow)
  - Within-breath settings:
    - Operator-set inspiratory pressure, cycle sensitivity (% peak flow), and maximum inspiratory time
- *Between-breath targets:* None

Pressure Control Ventilation Plus

- *Mandatory breaths:* Machine triggered (preset frequency) or patient triggered (flow sensitivity) and machine cycled (inspiratory time)
  - Within-breath settings:
    - Operator-set PEEP, frequency, inspiratory pressure, rise time, and inspiratory time
- *Spontaneous breaths:* Not allowed
- *Between-breath targets:* None

Spontaneous

- *Mandatory breaths:* Not allowed
- *Spontaneous breaths:* Patient triggered (flow sensitivity) and patient cycled (% peak inspiratory flow)
  - Within-breath settings:
    - Operator-set inspiratory pressure, cycle sensitivity (% peak inspiratory flow), and maximum inspiratory time
- *Between-breath targets:* None

Synchronized Controlled Mandatory Ventilation Plus

- *Mandatory breaths:* Machine triggered (preset frequency) or patient triggered (flow sensitivity) and machine cycled (inspiratory time)
  - Within-breath settings:
    - Operator-set PEEP, frequency, rise time, and inspiratory time
    - Ventilator-set inspiratory pressure
- *Spontaneous breaths:* Not allowed
- Between-breath targets:
  - Operator-set tidal volume

Synchronized Intermittent Mandatory Ventilation Plus

- *Mandatory breaths:* Machine triggered (preset frequency) or patient triggered (flow sensitivity) and machine cycled (inspiratory time).
  - Within-breath settings:
    - Operator-set PEEP, frequency, rise time, and inspiratory time
    - Ventilator-set inspiratory pressure
- *Spontaneous breaths:* Patient triggered (flow sensitivity) and patient cycled (% peak inspiratory flow)
  - Within-breath settings:
    - Operator-set inspiratory pressure, rise time, and cycle sensitivity (% peak flow)
- Between-breath targets:
  - Operator-set tidal volume

Special Features

Oxygen: The ventilator uses either high or low pressure oxygen sources. High pressure oxygen (flow ≤ 120 L/min, pressure 41 to 87 psi) can be provided by a central gas supply or a gas cylinder. Low pressure oxygen (flow ≤ 15 L/min, pressure ≤ 87 psi) can be provided by a concentrator or liquid cylinder.

Backup ventilation: Backup ventilation is activated if no breath is detected during the set apnea delay time. The backup ventilation mode is either SIMV+ or PCV+, depending on the original mode in which the apnea occurred.

Gas volume compensation: Pressure, flow, and volume measurements are based on readings from the flow sensor, and they are expressed in body temperature and pressure, saturated (BTPS).

Miscellaneous: Sigh breaths are delivered at a regular interval (every 50 breaths) at a pressure up to 10 cm H_2O higher than nonsigh breaths, as allowed by the Pressure alarm limit. Sigh breaths are available in all modes except Duo-PAP and APRV.

An optional CO_2 sensor can be connected to the ventilator, which will allow both end-tidal and volumetric exhaled CO_2 measurements and calculations.

Nebulizer: The T1's nebulization function powers a standard inline pneumatic nebulizer for delivery of

medications in the ventilator circuit. The nebulizer flow is synchronized with the inspiratory phase of each breath for 30 minutes. Nebulization can be activated in all modes of ventilation. The ventilator may also be used with an optional Aerogen Aeroneb Pro vibrating mesh nebulizer.

Noninvasive ventilation: The T1 provides two modes of noninvasive ventilation: Noninvasive Ventilation and Noninvasive Ventilation—Spontaneous Timed.

Manufacturer's Specifications

Table 9-60 lists specifications for the Hamilton Medical Hamilton-T1 ventilator.

TABLE 9-60
Specifications for the Hamilton Medical Hamilton-T1 Ventilator

Setting Category	Setting	Range
Pressure	Inspiratory Pressure	3–60 cm H_2O
	Pressure Support	0–60 cm H_2O
	PEEP	0–35 cm H_2O
Volume	Tidal Volume	0.02–2.0 L
Flow	Waveform	Square/descending ramp
	Inspiratory Time	0.1–12 s
Time	Mandatory Breath Frequency	1–80/min
	Adjustable Rise Time	Yes
Sensitivity	Trigger Sensitivity (flow)	0.1–20 L/min
	Cycle Sensitivity (flow)	5–80%
Alarm Category		
Pressure	High Pressure	20–70 cm H_2O
	Low Pressure	4–60 cm H_2O
Volume	High Tidal Volume	0.01–3.0 L
	Low Tidal Volume	0.01–3.0 L
Flow	High Expiratory Minute Volume	0.1–50 L/min
	Low Expiratory Minute Volume	0.1–50 L/min
Time	Apnea Time	15–60 s
	High Frequency	0–99/min
	Low Frequency	0–99/min
Other	High Oxygen	18–103%
	Low Oxygen	18–97%
Monitored Parameters	Airway Pressure	
	Peak Airway Pressure	
	Mean Airway Pressure	
	Inspiratory Pressure	

(continues)

TABLE 9-60
Specifications for the Hamilton-T1 Ventilator *(Continued)*

Setting Category	Setting	Range
Monitored Parameters, cont.	PEEP/CPAP	
	Tracheal Pressure	
	Plateau Pressure	
	End Inspiratory Pressure	
	Inspiratory Flow	
	Peak Inspiratory Flow	
	Peak Expiratory Flow	
	Tidal Volume	
	Expiratory Tidal Volume	
	Inspiratory Tidal Volume	
	Spontaneous Expiratory Minute Volume	
	Leakage Minute Volume	
	Leakage Percent of Airway	
	I:E Ratio	
	Total Breathing Frequency	
	Spontaneous Breathing Frequency	
	Inspiratory Time	
	Expiratory Time	
	Percentage of Spontaneous Breathing Rate	
	Static Compliance	
	AutoPEEP	
	Expiratory Time Constant	
	Inspiratory Flow Resistance	
	Rapid Shallow Breathing	
	Pressure Time Product	
	Airway Occlusion Pressure	
	F_IO_2	
	CO_2	
	Fractional End Tidal CO_2	
	End Tidal CO_2 Partial Pressure	
	Alveolar Tidal Ventilation	
	Alveolar Minute Ventilation	
	CO_2 Elimination	
	Airway Dead Space	
	Exhaled Volume of CO_2	
	Inspired Volume of CO_2	

Impact Instrumentation Uni-Vent Eagle II

Impact Instrumentation Inc. makes the Uni-Vent series of portable ventilators (**Figure 9-65**). We will describe one representative model, the model 731 series Eagle II ventilator (**Figure 9-66**). The devices in the Model 731 ventilator series are indicated for use in the management of infants (weighing 11 lb/5 kg or more) through adult patients with acute or chronic respiratory failure or during resuscitation by providing continuous positive pressure ventilation. They are appropriate for use in hospitals, outside the hospital, during transport, and in austere environments where they may be

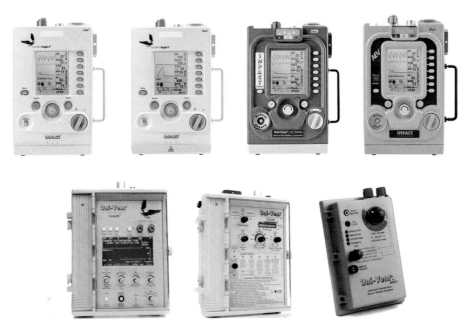

FIGURE 9-65 Impact Instrumentation Uni-Vent series of portable ventilators.
Courtesy of Impact Instrumentation.

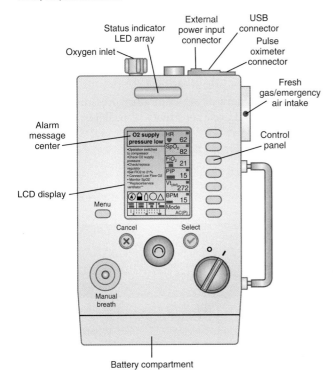

FIGURE 9-66 Impact Instrumentation Uni-Vent Model 731 Eagle II ventilator.
Courtesy of Impact Instrumentation.

exposed to rain, dust, rough handling, and extremes in temperature and humidity. With an appropriate third-party filter in place, they may be operated in environments where chemical and/or biological toxins are present. When marked with an "MRI conditional" label, they are suitable for use in an MRI environment with appropriate precautions. The unit is a volume- and pressure-targeted, time- or flow-cycled ventilator designed to use oxygen from either a 55 psig source or fresh air using its internal compressor to deliver a positive pressure breath. When the F_IO_2 is set to 21%, operators may connect a low flow oxygen source at the Fresh Gas/Emergency Air Intake using a reservoir.

Operator Interface

The Eagle II has a liquid crystal display that provides continuous display of control settings, operating conditions, power, and alarm status information. Most unit functions are controlled by pressing the PARAMETER button associated with the parameter. Pressing this button highlights the primary parameter; additional presses highlight secondary parameters moving in a clockwise direction. When the parameter of interest is highlighted, the ROTARY ENCODER is turned clockwise or counterclockwise to adjust the parameter to the desired value, and then the new value

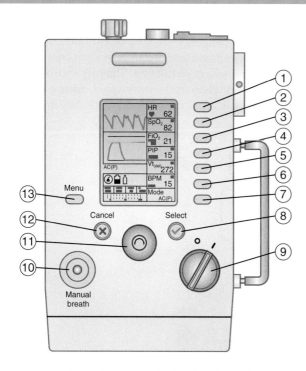

FIGURE 9-67 Impact Instrumentation Uni-Vent Model 731 Eagle II operator interface. 1. Heart rate alarm limit (active when pulse oximeter is connected). 2. SpO₂ alarm limit (active when pulse oximeter is connected). 3. F₁O₂ display and control setting. 4. Peak airway pressure (volume control modes) or inspiratory pressure setting (pressure control modes). 5. Tidal volume setting (volume control modes) or measured value (pressure control modes). 6. Breath rate setting. 7. Displays the current ventilatory mode. 8. Confirm/select a new setting. 9. Power on/off. 10. Manual breath. 11. Rotary encoder used to change a value or highlight a menu option. 12. Mute/cancel button. 13. Menu.

Courtesy of Impact Instrumentation.

is confirmed by pressing the CONFIRM/SELECT button (**Figure 9-67**).

Modes

Modes on the Eagle II are built by first selecting the breath sequence (what the manufacturer calls the mode) as either CMV (A/C), IMV (SIMV), or CSV (CPAP). Next the operator selects the control variable (what the manufacturer calls volume target or pressure target). Pressure support can also be added to spontaneous breaths. Available modes are shown in **Table 9-61**.

A/C Pressure Target
- *Mandatory breaths:* Machine triggered (preset frequency) or patient triggered (pressure sensitivity) and machine cycled (inspiratory time)
  - Within-breath settings:
    - Operator-set PEEP, frequency, inspiratory pressure, rise time, and inspiratory time or I:E
- *Spontaneous breaths:* Not allowed
- *Between-breath targets:* None

A/C Volume Target
- *Mandatory breaths:* Machine triggered (preset frequency) or patient triggered (pressure sensitivity) and machine cycled (tidal volume or pause time)
  - Within-breath settings:
    - Operator-set PEEP, frequency, inspiratory time or I:E, and tidal volume. Inspiratory flow is preset to be a square waveform.
- *Spontaneous breaths:* Not allowed
- *Between-breath targets:* None

CPAP
- *Mandatory breaths:* Not allowed
- *Spontaneous breaths:* Patient triggered (pressure sensitivity) and patient cycled (% peak inspiratory flow)
  - Within-breath settings:
    - Operator-set inspiratory pressure, rise time, and cycle sensitivity (% peak inspiratory flow)
- *Between-breath targets:* None

TABLE 9-61
Classification of Modes for the Eagle II Ventilator

Mode Name	Control Variable	Breath Sequence	Primary Breath Targeting Scheme	Secondary Breath Targeting Scheme	Tag
A/C Volume Target	volume	CMV	set-point	N/A	VC-CMVs
SIMV Volume Target	volume	IMV	set-point	set-point	VC-IMVs,s
A/C Pressure Target	pressure	CMV	set-point	N/A	PC-CMVs
SIMV Pressure Target	pressure	IMV	set-point	set-point	PC-IMVs,s
CPAP	pressure	CSV	set-point	N/A	PC-CSVs

Reproduced with permission from Mandu Press Ltd.

SIMV Pressure Target

- *Mandatory breaths:* Machine triggered (preset frequency) or patient synchronized (pressure sensitivity) and machine cycled (inspiratory time)
  - Within-breath settings:
    - Operator-set PEEP, frequency, inspiratory pressure, rise time, and inspiratory time or I:E
- *Spontaneous breaths:* Patient triggered (pressure or flow sensitivity) and patient cycled (% peak inspiratory flow)
  - Within-breath settings:
    - Operator-set inspiratory pressure, rise time, and cycle sensitivity (% peak inspiratory flow)
- *Between-breath targets:* None

SIMV Volume Target

- *Mandatory breaths:* Machine triggered (preset frequency) or patient synchronized (pressure sensitivity) and machine cycled (tidal volume or pause time)
  - Within-breath settings:
    - Operator-set PEEP, frequency, inspiratory time or I:E, and tidal volume. Inspiratory flow is preset to be a square waveform.
- *Spontaneous breaths:* Patient triggered (pressure or flow sensitivity) and patient cycled (% peak inspiratory flow)
  - Within-breath settings:
    - Operator-set inspiratory pressure, rise time, and cycle sensitivity (% peak inspiratory flow)
- *Between-breath targets:* None

Special Features

Oxygen: The unit can use oxygen from low flow sources such as flowmeters and oxygen concentrators. To do this, oxygen is entrained through the Fresh Gas/Emergency Air Intake with an Oxygen Reservoir Bag Assembly.

Backup ventilation: Depending on the preexisting conditions at the time of failure, the backup ventilator will begin operation in one of two ways:

1. If no preexisting alarm condition(s) exists: Backup operation will continue using the current settings.
2. If a preexisting alarm condition(s) exists: Backup operation will revert to the startup default settings (Mode A/C, volume target, frequency = 12, PIP = 20 cm H_2O, F_1O_2 = 21%, PEEP = 5 cm H_2O, I:E = 1:2).

Gas volume compensation: Gas volumes are displayed as atmospheric temperature and pressure, dry (ATPD).

Miscellaneous: An optional pulse oximeter probe can be connected to the ventilator.

Nebulizer: None.

Noninvasive ventilation: The Noninvasive Positive Pressure feature, when activated, provides flow during the expiratory phase to maintain the baseline pressure (CPAP) in spontaneously breathing patients with a leaking airway or face mask. The amount of leak compensation depends on the leak flow rate during the expiratory period and ranges from 0 to 15 L/min; it is automatically adjusted by the ventilator in order to maintain the CPAP target.

Manufacturer's Specifications

Table 9-62 lists specifications for the Uni-Vent Eagle II ventilator.

Philips Respironics Trilogy

The Philips Respironics Trilogy 202 ventilator (Figure 9-68) provides continuous or intermittent

---

TABLE 9-62
Specifications for the Uni-Vent Eagle II Ventilator

Setting Category	Setting	Range
Pressure	Inspiratory Pressure	10–80 cm H_2O
	Pressure Support	
	PEEP	0–25 cm H_2O
Volume	Tidal Volume	0.05–1.5 L
Flow	Inspiratory Flow	0–100 L/min
	Waveform	
Time	Inspiratory Time	0.3–3.0 s
	Mandatory Breath Frequency	1–60/min
	Adjustable Rise Time	

(continues)

TABLE 9-62
Specifications for the Uni-Vent Eagle II Ventilator (*Continued*)

Setting Category	Setting	Range
Sensitivity	Trigger Sensitivity (pressure)	–6.0 to –0.5 cm H_2O
	Trigger Sensitivity (flow)	
	Cycle Sensitivity (flow)	
Alarm Category		
Pressure	High Pressure	20–100 cm H_2O
	Low Airway Pressure	0–35 cm H_2O
Other	O_2 Sensor	Enabled/Disabled

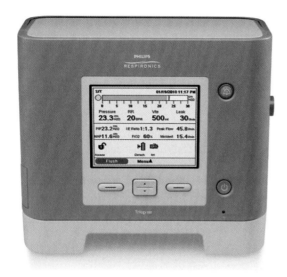

FIGURE 9-68 Philips Respironics Trilogy ventilator.
Reproduced with permission from Philips Healthcare.

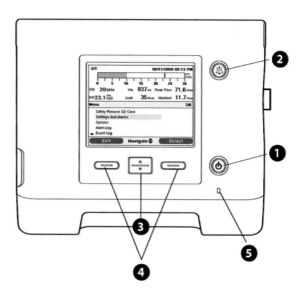

FIGURE 9-69 Philips Respironics Trilogy operator interface. 1. Start/stop button. 2. Alarm indicator and audio pause button. 3. Up/Down button for navication and settings adjustment. 4. Left/right buttons for selecting display options. 5. AC power LED. 6. Keypad backlight LEDs. 7. Red (high priority) alarm LED. 8. Yellow (medium priority) alarm LED.
Reproduced with permission from Philips Healthcare.

ventilatory support for the care of individuals who require mechanical ventilation with or without air/oxygen blending. It is intended for use in hospitals and institutions, and for portable applications such as wheelchairs and gurneys only when in an institutional setting. It may be used for both invasive and noninvasive ventilation. It is not intended to be used as a transport ventilator. The ventilator can be used with either a single-limb (passive) patient circuit or a dual-limb (active) circuit with pressurized exhalation manifold.

Operator Interface

The Trilogy uses a central screen in conjunction with up/down, left/right buttons to make parameter selections and setting adjustments (**Figure 9-69**).

Modes

Modes are selected by name (e.g., Spontaneous or Assist/Control). Average Volume Assured Pressure

Support is the name given to a feature that, when activated, allows adaptive control in several pressure control modes. Activating AVAPS actually changes the mode classification. **Table 9-63** shows the available modes.

Assist/Control

- *Mandatory breaths:* Machine triggered (preset frequency) or patient triggered (flow or Auto-Trak) and machine cycled (tidal volume or inspiratory time)
  - Within-breath settings:
    - Operator-set PEEP, frequency, flow waveform, tidal volume, inspiratory time, and sigh. (A sigh breath is 150% of set tidal volume every 100th mandatory breath.)

TABLE 9-63
Mode Classifications for the Philips Respironics Trilogy Ventilator

| Mode Name | Mode Classification | | | | Tag |
	Control Variable	Breath Sequence	Primary Breath Targeting Scheme	Secondary Breath Targeting Scheme	
Control	volume	CMV	set-point	N/A	VC-CMVs
A/C	volume	CMV	set-point	N/A	VC-CMVs
SIMV	pressure	IMV	set-point	set-point	PC-IMVs,s
Pressure Control	pressure	CMV	set-point	N/A	PC-CMVs
Pressure Control with Average Volume Assured Pressure Support	pressure	CMV	adaptive	N/A	PC-CMVs,a
Pressure Control SIMV	pressure	IMV	set-point	set-point	PC-IMVs,s
Spontaneous/Timed	pressure	IMV	set-point	set-point	PC-IMVs,s
Timed	pressure	IMV	set-point	set-point	PC-IMVs,s
Timed with Average Volume Assured Pressure Support	pressure	IMV	adaptive	set-point	PC-IMVa,s
Spontaneous/Timed with Average Volume Assured Pressure Support	pressure	IMV	adaptive	set-point	PC-IMVa,s
Spontaneous	pressure	CSV	set-point	N/A	PC-CSVs
CPAP	pressure	CSV	set-point	N/A	PC-CSVs
Spontaneous with Average Volume Assured Pressure Support	pressure	CSV	adaptive	N/A	PC-CSVa

Reproduced with permission from Mandu Press Ltd.

- *Spontaneous breaths:* Not allowed
- *Between-breath targets:* None

Control
- *Mandatory breaths:* Machine triggered (preset frequency) and machine cycled (tidal volume or inspiratory time)
  - Within-breath settings:
    - Operator-set PEEP, frequency, flow waveform, tidal volume, inspiratory time, and sigh. (A sigh breath is 150% of set tidal volume every 100th mandatory breath.)
- *Spontaneous breaths:* Not allowed
- *Between-breath targets:* None

Continuous Positive Airway Pressure
- *Mandatory breaths:* Not allowed
- *Spontaneous breaths:* Patient triggered (flow or Auto-Trak) and patient cycled (% peak flow or Auto-Trak)

- Within-breath settings:
  - Operator-set CPAP, cycle sensitivity (% peak inspiratory flow), leak compensation, ramp (the Ramp feature will reduce the pressure and then gradually increase [ramp] the pressure to the prescription pressure setting so patients can fall asleep more comfortably), leak compensation, and Bi-Flex. (The Bi-Flex attribute adjusts therapy by inserting a small amount of pressure relief during the latter stages of inspiration and during the beginning part of exhalation [Figure 9-70].)
- *Between-breath targets:* None

Pressure Control
- *Mandatory breaths:* Machine triggered (preset frequency) or patient triggered (flow or Auto-Trak) and machine cycled (inspiratory time)
  - Within-breath settings:

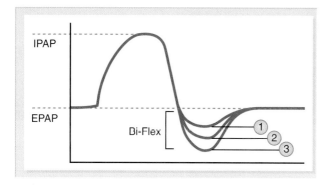

FIGURE 9-70 Pressure–time waveform showing the operation of the Bi-Flex feature. Bi-Flex level settings of 1, 2, or 3 progressively increase pressure relief during expiration. IPAP = inspiratory positive airway pressure, EPAP = expiratory positive airway pressure.

– Operator-set PEEP, frequency, inspiratory pressure, rise time, inspiratory time, ramp (the Ramp feature will reduce the pressure and then gradually increase [ramp] the pressure to the prescription pressure setting so patients can fall asleep more comfortably), and leak compensation
- *Spontaneous breaths:* Not allowed
- *Between-breath targets:* None

Pressure Control Synchronized Intermittent Mandatory Ventilation

- *Mandatory breaths:* Machine triggered (preset frequency) or patient synchronized (flow or Auto-Trak) and machine cycled (inspiratory time)
  • Within-breath settings:
    – Operator-set PEEP, frequency, inspiratory pressure, rise time, and inspiratory time
- *Spontaneous breaths:* Patient triggered (pressure, flow, or Auto-Trak) and patient cycled (% peak inspiratory flow or Auto-Trak)
  • Within-breath settings:
    – Operator-set inspiratory pressure, rise time, and cycle sensitivity (% peak inspiratory flow)
- *Between-breath targets:* None

Pressure Control with Average Volume Assured Pressure Support

- *Mandatory breaths:* Machine triggered (preset frequency) or patient triggered (flow or Auto-Trak) and machine cycled (inspiratory time)
  • Within-breath settings:
    – Operator-set PEEP, frequency, rise time, and inspiratory time
    – Ventilator-set inspiratory pressure
- *Spontaneous breaths:* Not allowed
- Between-breath targets:
  • Operator-set tidal volume

Synchronized Intermittent Mandatory Ventilation

- *Mandatory breaths:* Machine triggered (preset frequency) or patient synchronized (flow or Auto-Trak) and machine cycled (tidal volume or inspiratory time)
  • Within-breath settings:
    – Operator-set PEEP, frequency, flow waveform, tidal volume, inspiratory time, and sigh. (A sigh breath is 150% of set tidal volume every 100th mandatory breath.)
- *Spontaneous breaths:* Patient triggered (pressure or flow sensitivity) and patient cycled (% peak inspiratory flow or Flow-Trak)
  • Within-breath settings:
    – Operator-set inspiratory pressure, rise time, and cycle sensitivity (% peak inspiratory flow)
- *Between-breath targets:* None

Spontaneous

- *Mandatory breaths:* Not allowed
- *Spontaneous breaths:* Patient triggered (flow or Auto-Trak) and patient cycled (% peak flow or Auto-Trak)
  • Within-breath settings:
    – Operator-set CPAP, cycle sensitivity (% peak inspiratory flow), leak compensation, ramp (the Ramp feature will reduce the pressure and then gradually increase [ramp] the pressure to the prescription pressure setting so patients can fall asleep more comfortably), leak compensation, and Bi-Flex. (The Bi-Flex attribute adjusts therapy by inserting a small amount of pressure relief during the latter stages of inspiration and during the beginning part of exhalation.)
- *Between-breath targets:* None

Spontaneous with Average Volume Assured Pressure Support

- *Mandatory breaths:* None
- *Spontaneous breaths:* Patient triggered (flow or Auto-Trak) and patient cycled (% peak flow or Auto-Trak)
  • Within-breath settings:
    – Operator-set PEEP, rise time, and cycle sensitivity (% peak inspiratory flow)
    – Ventilator-set inspiratory pressure
- Between-breath targets:
  • Operator-set tidal volume

Spontaneous/Timed

- *Mandatory breaths:* Machine triggered (preset frequency) or patient triggered (flow or Auto-Trak) and machine cycled (inspiratory time). Spontaneous breaths suppress mandatory breaths if they occur at a frequency higher than the set mandatory rate.

- Within-breath settings:
  - Operator-set PEEP, inspiratory pressure, inspiratory time, frequency, rise time, and ramp
- *Spontaneous breaths:* Patient triggered (flow or Auto-Trak) and patient cycled (flow or Auto-Trak).
  - Within-breath settings:
    - Operator-set cycle sensitivity (% peak flow). Inspiratory pressure and rise time set for mandatory breaths apply to spontaneous breaths automatically.
- *Between-breath targets:* None.

Spontaneous/Timed with Average Volume Assured Pressure Support

- *Mandatory breaths:* Machine triggered (preset frequency) or patient triggered (flow or Auto-Trak) and machine cycled (inspiratory time). Spontaneous breaths suppress mandatory breaths if they occur at a frequency higher than the set mandatory rate.
  - Within-breath settings:
    - Operator-set PEEP, inspiratory pressure, frequency, rise time, inspiratory time, tidal volume, and ramp
- *Spontaneous breaths:* Patient triggered (flow or Auto-Trak) and patient cycled (flow or Auto-Trak).
  - Within-breath settings:
    - Operator-set cycle sensitivity (% peak flow). Inspiratory pressure and rise time set for mandatory breaths apply to spontaneous breaths automatically.
- *Between-breath targets:* None.

Timed

- *Mandatory breaths:* Machine triggered (preset frequency) or patient triggered (flow or Auto-Trak) and machine cycled (inspiratory time). Spontaneous breaths suppress mandatory breaths if they occur at a frequency higher than the set mandatory rate.
  - Within-breath settings:
    - Operator-set PEEP, inspiratory pressure, inspiratory time, frequency, rise time, and ramp
- *Spontaneous breaths:* None.
- *Between-breath targets:* None.

Timed with Average Volume Assured Pressure Support

- *Mandatory breaths:* Machine triggered (preset frequency) or patient triggered (flow or Auto-Trak) and machine cycled (inspiratory time). Spontaneous breaths suppress mandatory breaths if they occur at a frequency higher than the set mandatory rate.

- Within-breath settings:
  - Operator-set PEEP, inspiratory pressure, frequency, rise time, inspiratory time, tidal volume, and ramp
- *Spontaneous breaths:* None.
- *Between-breath targets:*
  - Operator-set tidal volume

Special Features

Backup ventilation: If the Apnea alarm is enabled, you can set the Apnea Rate from 4 to 60 breaths/min.

Gas volume compensation: All flows and volumes used in Trilogy are expressed in body temperature and pressure, saturated (BTPS).

Leak compensation: When using the Passive Circuit configuration, compensation for both intentional and unintentional leaks is included in the triggering method. When using the Active PAP Circuit configuration, leak compensation is not available. When using the Active Flow Circuit configuration, flow trigger with leak compensation may be enabled. The default setting when using the Active Flow Circuit is Leak Compensation On. The clinician has the option to turn off leak compensation; however, unintentional leaks will not be compensated.

The Passive circuit provides leak compensation. When using the Passive circuit with volume control modes, the set tidal volume is delivered to the patient above the calculated circuit and cuff (or mask) leak. This is different from traditional active circuit ventilation where the cuff (or mask) leak reduces the tidal volume delivered to the patient. Volume ventilation with the Passive circuit delivers an inspiratory tidal volume close to the device setting regardless of leak; this should be considered when transitioning a patient from an active to a passive circuit. With a Passive circuit, tidal volume is estimated based on the calculated sum of circuit and cuff (or mask) leak.

Neonatal ventilation: None.

Noninvasive ventilation: No special features other than leak compensation (discussed previously).

Manufacturer's Specifications

Table 9-64 lists specifications for the Philips Respironics Trilogy 202 ventilator.

Section 5: Neonatal Ventilators

Dräger Babylog VN500

The Dräger Babylog VN500 (Figure 9-71) is intended for the ventilation of neonatal patients from 0.88 lb (0.4 kg) up to 22 lb (10 kg) and pediatric patients from 11 lb (5 kg) up to 44 lb (20 kg) bodyweight.

TABLE 9-64
Specifications for the Philips Respironics Trilogy 202 Ventilator

Setting Category	Setting	Range
Pressure	Inspiratory Pressure	4–50 cm H_2O
	Pressure Support	0–30 cm H_2O
	PEEP	0–25 cm H_2O
Volume	Tidal Volume	0.05–2 L
Flow	Waveform	Not Specified
	Inspiratory Time	0.3–5.0 s
Time	Mandatory Breath Frequency	0–60/min
	Trigger Sensitivity (pressure)	0–25 cm H_2O
	Adjustable Rise Time	Yes
Sensitivity	Trigger Sensitivity (flow)	1–9 L/min
	Cycle Sensitivity (flow)	10–90%
Alarm Category		
Volume	High Tidal Volume	0.05–2 L
	Low Tidal Volume	0.05–2 L
Flow	High Minute Ventilation	1–99 L/min
	Low Minute Ventilation	1–99 L/min
Time	Circuit Disconnect	10–60 s
	Apnea	10–60 s
	High Respiratory Rate	4–80/min
	Low Respiratory Rate	4–80/min
Other	O_2 Sensor	Enabled/Disabled

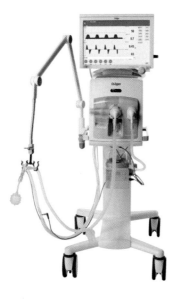

FIGURE 9-71 Dräger Babylog VN500 ventilator.

Operator Interface

The Babylog VN500 has an operator interface similar to the Dräger Infinity V500 that uses a touch screen, buttons, and a control knob (see Figure 9-26). Screen displays change according to the context of the operation, such as initial ventilator operation verification, entering ventilator settings, entering alarm settings, and reviewing monitored values including waveforms or digital values. Settings are entered by touching a virtual button on the screen to select the desired setting, turning the rotary knob to select the setting value, and then pressing the knob to finalize the setting. Other buttons provide various features related to menu navigation and alarm silencing.

The Babylog VN500 has a unique interface for monitoring the patient's pulmonary status, called Smart Pulmonary View (see Figure 9-27). This is a graphic display of the compliance and resistance as well as of the spontaneous and mandatory minute volume.

Modes

Modes on the Babylog VN500 are selected by mode name (e.g., Pressure Control A/C, Spontaneous Proportional Pressure Support, etc.) using tabs on the touch screen. When the tab is selected, the relevant ventilator setting screens are displayed. The setting screens are also tabbed, giving access to basic settings (e.g., tidal volume for volume control modes and inspiratory pressure for pressure control modes) and additional settings. The additional settings include simple things like trigger sensitivity or automatic tube compensation, as well as complicated things such as activating Volume Guarantee. There are no volume control modes available on the Babylog VN500. **Table 9-65** shows the modes available on the Babylog VN500.

Pressure Control Assist Control
- *Mandatory breaths:* Machine triggered (preset frequency) or patient triggered (flow sensitivity) and machine cycled (inspiratory time)

TABLE 9-65
Modes of Ventilation for the Dräger Babylog VN500

Mode Name	Mode Classification				Tag
	Control Variable	Breath Sequence	Primary Breath Targeting Scheme	Secondary Breath Targeting Scheme	
Pressure Control A/C	pressure	CMV	set-point	N/A	PC-CMVs
Pressure Control A/C with Automatic Tube Compensation	pressure	CMV	set-point/servo	N/A	PC-CMVsr
Pressure Control A/C with Volume Guarantee	pressure	CMV	adaptive	N/A	PC-CMVa
Pressure Control A/C with Volume Guarantee and Automatic Tube Compensation	pressure	CMV	adaptive/servo	N/A	PC-CMVar
Pressure Control Continuous Mandatory Ventilation	pressure	IMV	set-point	set-point	PC-IMVs,s
Pressure Control Continuous Mandatory Ventilation with Automatic Tube Compensation	pressure	IMV	set-point/servo	set-point/servo	PC-IMVsr,sr
Pressure Control SIMV	pressure	IMV	set-point	set-point	PC-IMVs,s
Pressure Control SIMV with Automatic Tube Compensation	pressure	IMV	set-point/servo	set-point/servo	PC-IMVsr,sr
Pressure Control Pressure Support Ventilation	pressure	IMV	set-point	set-point	PC-IMVs,s
Pressure Control Pressure Support Ventilation with Automatic Tube Compensation	pressure	IMV	set-point/servo	set-point/servo	PC-IMVsr,sr
Pressure Control Airway Pressure Release Ventilation	pressure	IMV	set-point	set-point	PC-IMVs,s
Pressure Control Airway Pressure Release Ventilation with Automatic Tube Compensation	pressure	IMV	set-point/servo	set-point/servo	PC-IMVsr,sr
Pressure Control Mandatory Minute Volume Ventilation with Volume Guarantee	pressure	IMV	adaptive	set-point	PC-IMVa,s

(continues)

TABLE 9-65
Modes of Ventilation for the Dräger Babylog VN500 *(Continued)*

| Mode Name | Mode Classification | | | | Tag |
	Control Variable	Breath Sequence	Primary Breath Targeting Scheme	Secondary Breath Targeting Scheme	
Pressure Control Continuous Mandatory Ventilation with Volume Guarantee	pressure	IMV	adaptive	set-point	PC-IMVa,s
Pressure Control Continuous Mandatory Ventilation with Volume Guarantee and Automatic Tube Compensation	pressure	IMV	adaptive/servo	set-point/servo	PC-IMVar,sr
Pressure Control SIMV with Volume Guarantee	pressure	IMV	adaptive	set-point	PC-IMVa,s
Pressure Control SIMV with Volume Guarantee and Automatic Tube Compensation	pressure	IMV	adaptive/servo	set-point/servo	PC-IMVas,sr
Pressure Control Pressure Support Ventilation with Volume Guarantee	pressure	IMV	adaptive	set-point	PC-IMVa,s
Pressure Control Pressure Support Ventilation with Volume Guarantee and Automatic Tube Compensation	pressure	IMV	adaptive/servo	set-point/servo	PC-IMVar,sr
Spontaneous CPAP/ Pressure Support	pressure	CSV	set-point	N/A	PC-CSVs
Spontaneous CPAP/ Pressure Support with Automatic Tube Compensation	pressure	CSV	set-point/servo	N/A	PC-CSVsr
Spontaneous Proportional Pressure Support	pressure	CSV	servo	N/A	PC-CSVr
Spontaneous Proportional Pressure Support with Automatic Tube Compensation	pressure	CSV	servo	N/A	PC-CSVr
Spontaneous CPAP/ Volume Support	pressure	CSV	adaptive	N/A	PC-CSVa
Spontaneous CPAP/ Volume Support wth Automatic Tube Compensation	pressure	CSV	adaptive/servo	N/A	PC-CSVar

Reproduced with permission from Mandu Press Ltd.

- Within-breath settings:
  - Operator-set PEEP, frequency, inspiratory pressure, rise time, and inspiratory time
- *Spontaneous breaths:* Permitted during mandatory breath but not between mandatory breaths
- *Between-breath targets:* None

Pressure Control Assist Control with Volume Guarantee

- *Mandatory breaths:* Machine triggered (preset frequency) or patient triggered (flow sensitivity) and machine cycled (inspiratory time)

- Within-breath settings:
  - Operator-set PEEP, frequency, rise time, and inspiratory time
  - Ventilator-set inspiratory pressure
- *Spontaneous breaths:* Permitted during mandatory breath but not between mandatory breaths
- Between-breath targets:
  - Operator-set tidal volume

Pressure Control Airway Pressure Release Ventilation

- *Mandatory breaths:* Machine triggered (preset frequency) and machine cycled (inspiratory time). Patient triggering of mandatory breaths is possible using the AutoRelease feature. This triggers inspiration once a preset expiratory flow threshold is reached. When AutoRelease is turned on, the switch from P_{high} to P_{low} is synchronized with the patient's breathing. Thus, with AutoRelease, what were formerly machine-triggered and machine-cycled (mandatory) breaths are converted to patient-triggered and patient-cycled (spontaneous) breaths.
  - Within-breath settings:
    - Operator-set PEEP (called P_{low}), peak inspiratory pressure (called P_{high}), rise time, inspiratory time (called T_{high}), and expiratory time (called T_{low}). The inspiratory trigger sensitivity may also be set (using AutoRelease) as a percentage of peak expiratory flow.
- *Spontaneous breaths:* Patient triggered (flow sensitivity) and patient cycled (% peak inspiratory flow). Spontaneous breaths are permitted both between and during mandatory breaths.
  - Within-breath settings:
    - Automatic tube compensation
- *Between-breath targets:* None.

Pressure Control Continuous Mandatory Ventilation

- *Mandatory breaths:* Machine triggered (preset frequency) and machine cycled (inspiratory time). Spontaneous breaths are permitted both between and during mandatory breaths. Because of this feature, the mode is classified as a form of intermittent mandatory ventilation, not continuous mandatory ventilation, despite the name given by Dräger.
  - Within-breath settings:
    - Operator-set PEEP, frequency, inspiratory pressure, rise time, and inspiratory time
- *Spontaneous breaths:* Patient triggered (flow sensitivity) and patient cycled (% peak inspiratory flow).
  - *Within-breath settings:* None
- *Between-breath targets:* None.

Pressure Control Continuous Mandatory Ventilation with Volume Guarantee

- *Mandatory breaths:* Machine triggered (preset frequency) and machine cycled (inspiratory time). Spontaneous breaths are permitted both between and during mandatory breaths. Because of this feature, the mode is classified as a form of intermittent mandatory ventilation, not continuous mandatory ventilation, despite the name given by Dräger.
  - Within-breath settings:
    - Operator-set PEEP, frequency, rise time, and inspiratory time
    - Ventilator-set inspiratory pressure
- *Spontaneous breaths:* Patient triggered (flow sensitivity) and patient cycled (% peak inspiratory flow).
  - *Within-breath settings:* None
- Between-breath targets:
  - Operator-set tidal volume

Pressure Control Mandatory Minute Volume Ventilation with Volume Guarantee

- *Mandatory breaths:* Machine triggered (preset frequency) or patient triggered (flow sensitivity) and machine cycled (inspiratory time). Mandatory breaths are suppressed if minute ventilation from spontaneous breaths is above preset minute ventilation target (i.e., product of tidal volume and frequency).
  - Within-breath settings:
    - Operator-set PEEP, frequency, rise time, and inspiratory time
    - Ventilator-set inspiratory pressure
- *Spontaneous breaths:* Patient triggered (flow sensitivity) and patient cycled (% peak inspiratory flow).
  - Within-breath settings:
    - Operator-set inspiratory pressure and rise time
- Between-breath targets:
  - Operator-set tidal volume.
  - The settings for tidal volume and frequency constitute a between-breath target for minimum minute ventilation. Mandatory breaths are suppressed if minute ventilation from spontaneous breaths is this target.

Pressure Control Pressure Support Ventilation

- *Mandatory breaths:* Machine triggered (preset frequency) and patient cycled (% peak inspiratory flow)
  - Within-breath settings:
    - Operator-set PEEP, frequency, inspiratory pressure, and rise time
- *Spontaneous breaths:* Patient triggered (flow sensitivity) and patient cycled (% peak inspiratory flow)
  - Within-breath settings:
    - Operator-set inspiratory pressure and rise time
- *Between-breath targets:* None

Pressure Control Pressure Support Ventilation with Volume Guarantee
- *Mandatory breaths:* Machine triggered (preset frequency) and patient cycled (% peak inspiratory flow)
  - Within-breath settings:
    - Operator-set PEEP, frequency, and rise time
    - Ventilator-set inspiratory pressure
- *Spontaneous breaths:* Patient triggered (flow sensitivity) and patient cycled (% peak inspiratory flow)
  - Within-breath settings:
    - Operator-set rise time
    - Ventilator-set inspiratory pressure
- Between-breath targets:
  - Operator-set tidal volume

Pressure Control Synchronized Intermittent Mandatory Ventilation
- *Mandatory breaths:* Machine triggered (preset frequency) or patient synchronized (flow sensitivity) and machine cycled (inspiratory time). Spontaneous breaths are permitted both between and during mandatory breaths.
  - Within-breath settings:
    - Operator-set PEEP, frequency, inspiratory pressure, rise time, and inspiratory time
- *Spontaneous breaths:* Patient triggered (flow sensitivity) and patient cycled (% peak inspiratory flow).
  - Within-breath settings:
    - Operator-set inspiratory pressure and rise time
- *Between-breath targets:* None.

Pressure Control Synchronized Intermittent Mandatory Ventilation with Volume Guarantee
- *Mandatory breaths:* Machine triggered (preset frequency) or patient triggered (flow sensitivity) and machine cycled (inspiratory time)
  - Within-breath settings:
    - Operator-set PEEP, frequency, rise time, and inspiratory time
    - Ventilator-set inspiratory pressure
- *Spontaneous breaths:* Patient triggered (flow sensitivity) and patient cycled (% peak inspiratory flow)
  - Within-breath settings:
    - Operator-set inspiratory pressure and rise time
- Between-breath targets:
  - Operator-set tidal volume

Spontaneous Continuous Positive Airway Pressure/ Pressure Support
- *Mandatory breaths:* Not allowed
- *Spontaneous breaths:* Patient triggered (flow sensitivity) and patient cycled (% peak inspiratory flow)
  - Within-breath settings:
    - Operator-set inspiratory pressure and rise time
- *Between-breath targets:* None

Spontaneous Continuous Positive Airway Pressure/ Volume Support
- *Mandatory breaths:* Not allowed
- *Spontaneous breaths:* Patient triggered (pressure or flow sensitivity) and patient cycled (% peak inspiratory flow)
  - Within-breath settings:
    - Operator-set cycle sensitivity (% peak inspiratory flow)
    - Ventilator-set inspiratory pressure
- Between-breath targets:
  - Operator-set average tidal volume

Spontaneous Proportional Pressure Support
- *Mandatory breaths:* Not allowed
- *Spontaneous breaths:* Patient triggered (pressure or flow sensitivity) and patient cycled (% peak inspiratory flow)
  - *Within-breath settings:* None
- Between-breath targets:
  - Operator-set flow assist (amount of resistance to be supported) and volume assist (amount of elastance to be supported)

Special Features

Backup ventilation: For the Babylog VN500 to be able to detect an apnea, flow measurement with the neonatal flow sensor must function and flow monitoring with the neonatal flow sensor must be activated. If apnea ventilation is activated, the Babylog VN500 starts volume-guaranteed SIMV with the preset apnea respiratory rate and tidal volume target. The inspiratory time for apnea ventilation is determined from the set apnea respiratory rate and a fixed I:E ratio of 1:2.

Gas volume compensation: Measured values for flow and volume are displayed as Body Temperature (98.6°F/37°C) and ambient Pressure Saturated (47 mm Hg) with water vapor (BTPS).

Miscellaneous: The sigh function can be activated in all ventilation modes with mandatory breaths, except for PC-APRV. When the sigh function is activated, the end-expiratory pressure PEEP increases by the set value of the intermittent PEEP. In pressure-controlled ventilation, the inspiratory pressures increase by an amount equal to the intermittent PEEP. The time between the two sigh phases can be set. The operator can also set how many respiratory cycles are covered by the sigh phase.

An optional CO_2 sensor can be connected to the ventilator, which will allow both end-tidal and volumetric exhaled CO_2 measurements and calculations.

Nebulizer: The medication nebulizer nebulizes continuously. The medication nebulizer is supplied with compressed air, oxygen, or a mixture of compressed air and oxygen by the Babylog VN500 depending on the set oxygen concentration.

Noninvasive ventilation: In the neonatal patient category, only the SPN-CPAP or PC-CMV ventilation modes may be selected. When using prongs or a mask, the neonatal flow sensor must be removed from the breathing circuit. The Babylog VN500 switches off flow monitoring with the neonatal flow sensor.

The Babylog VN500 determines the leakage flow and subtracts it from the total flow in order to determine the patient flow. Only this flow is used for the flow trigger or the inspiratory termination criterion. After a few breaths the Babylog VN500 "learns" the leakage and avoids auto-triggering. If the leakage is eliminated, the sensitivity of the flow trigger is automatically increased again. The same applies to the inspiratory termination criterion for breaths with pressure support or volume support. If leakage compensation is activated, measured volume and flow as well as the curves for flow and volume are displayed with leakage correction.

Manufacturer's Specifications

Table 9-66 lists specifications for the Dräger Babylog VN500 ventilator.

TABLE 9-66
Specifications for the Dräger Babylog VN500 Ventilator

Setting Category	Setting	Range
Pressure	Inspiratory Pressure	1–80 cm H_2O
	Pressure Support	1–80 cm H_2O
	PEEP	0–35 cm H_2O
Volume	Tidal Volume	0.002–0.3 L
Flow	Inspiratory Flow	2–30 L/min
	Waveform	Not specified
Time	Inspiratory Time	0.1–30 s
	Mandatory Breath Frequency	0.5–150/min
	Adjustable Rise Time	Yes
Sensitivity	Trigger Sensitivity (flow)	0.2–5 L/min
Alarm Category		
Pressure	Upper Airway Pressure	7–105 cm H_2O
	Upper End Expiratory CO_2 Concentration	1–98 mm Hg
	Lower End Expiratory CO_2 Concentration	0–97 mm Hg
Flow	Upper Expiratory Minute Volume	0.03–60 L/min
	Lower Expiratory Minute Volume	0.02–40 L/min
Time	Respiratory Rate	5–200/min
	Apnea Time	5–60 s
Other	O_2 Sensor	Enabled/Disabled
Monitored Parameters	Expiratory Minute Volume	
	Airway Pressure	
	Maximum Airway Pressure	
	Inspired O_2 Concentration	
	End-Expiratory CO_2 Concentration	
	Respiratory Rate	
	Volume Monitoring	
	Apnea Alarm Time	

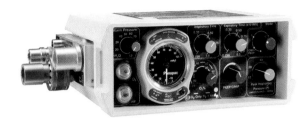

FIGURE 9-72 Smiths babyPAC 100 ventilator.
Courtesy of Smiths Medical.

Smiths Medical Pneupac babyPAC 100

The Smiths babyPAC 100 (**Figure 9-72**) is a portable gas-powered transport ventilator, suitable for use in an MRI environment up to 3 Tesla, that features a battery-powered integrated electronic pressure alarm unit. It is designed for use for ambulance, hospital, emergency, and transport ventilation of patients during respiratory distress or insufficiency. It *is not* intended for use as a critical care device. It can be used on neonates and infants up to a bodyweight of 44 lb (20 kg).

Operator Interface

The operator interface of the babyPAC 100 is composed of knobs and an aneroid pressure gauge (**Figure 9-73**).

Modes

Modes on the babyPAC 100 are selected by mode name (e.g., CMV + PEEP, CPAP, etc.). **Table 9-67** shows the modes available on the babyPAC 100.

Controlled Mandatory Ventilation + Active PEEP
- *Mandatory breaths:* Machine triggered (preset expiratory time and expiratory time) and machine cycled (preset inspiratory time). Spontaneous breaths may be drawn from the continuous flow through the patient circuit.

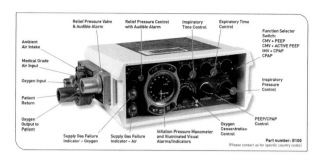

FIGURE 9-73 Smiths babyPAC 100 operator interface. 1. Controls for inspiratory and expiratory times. 2. Inspiratory pressure control. 3. Oxygen concentration control. 4. Function selector switch - used to select one of the four operating modes of the babyPAC 100 ventilator and is also used to switch off the ventilator. 5. PEEP/CPAP control. 6. Silencing and muting of electronic audible alarms. 7. Variable pressure relief valve for continuous adjustment of an independent upper patient inspiratory pressure limitation device. 8. Breath delivery indicator. 9. Low inspiratory pressure (Disconnect) alarm. 10. High inspiratory pressure / constant positive inspiratory pressure alarm. 11. Supply gas failure alarms. 12. Low battery alarm. 13. Battery. 14. Basic operating instructions. 15. Alarm information label. 16. Airway pressure gauge. 17. Gas output port. 18. Gas return port. 19. Supply gas inlet connection(s). 20. Gas intake port. 21. Patient circuit. 22. Gas supply hoses. 23. Carry sling attachment slots. 24. Mounting attachment points. 25. Audible alarm. 26. Single gas operations.
Courtesy of Smiths Medical.

- Within-breath settings:
  - Operator-set PEEP, inspiratory pressure, inspiratory and expiratory time
- Spontaneous breaths:
  - Operator-set PEEP
- *Between-breath targets:* None.

Controlled Mandatory Ventilation + PEEP
- *Mandatory breaths:* Machine triggered (preset inspiratory time and expiratory time) and machine cycled (preset inspiratory time).

TABLE 9-67
Modes of Ventilation for the babyPAC 100

| Mode Name | Mode Classification | | | | |
	Control Variable	Breath Sequence	Primary Breath Targeting Scheme	Secondary Breath Targeting Scheme	Tag
Controlled Mandatory Ventilation + PEEP	pressure	CMV	set-point	N/A	PC-CMVs
Controlled Mandatory Ventilation + Active PEEP	pressure	IMV	set-point	set-point	PC-IMVs,s
IMV + CPAP	pressure	IMV	set-point	set-point	PC-IMVs,s
CPAP	pressure	CSV	set-point	N/A	PC-CSVs

Reproduced with permission from Mandu Press Ltd.

Spontaneous breaths cannot occur because there is no continuous bias flow and inspiratory efforts are blocked by the exhalation manifold valve.
- Within-breath settings:
  - Operator-set PEEP, inspiratory pressure, inspiratory and expiratory time
- *Spontaneous breaths:* Not allowed.
- *Between-breath targets:* None.

CPAP
- *Mandatory breaths:* Not allowed.
- *Spontaneous breaths:* Patient breathes from continuous bias flow of 10 L/min.
  - Within-breath settings:
    - Operator-set CPAP
- *Between-breath targets:* None.

Intermittent Mandatory Ventilation + CPAP
- *Mandatory breaths:* Machine triggered (preset inspiratory time and expiratory time) and machine cycled (preset inspiratory time). Spontaneous breaths may be drawn from the continuous flow through the patient circuit (10 L/min).
  - Within-breath settings:
    - Operator-set CPAP, inspiratory pressure, inspiratory and expiratory time
- Spontaneous breaths:
  - Operator-set CPAP
- *Between-breath targets:* None.

Special Features

Oxygen: A unique gas mixing system enables the selection of a precise oxygen concentration by means of the calibrated rotary control. There is a double calibration in order to be able to select the concentration with the two different gas supply possibilities. If oxygen alone is available as a compressed supply gas then a range of approximately 45% to 100% oxygen concentration is possible. The air dilution is obtained by entraining atmospheric air. Because of this, the minimum oxygen concentration setting (approximately 45% on the white scale), with oxygen only as a supply, is the most economic setting in terms of gas usage. If both oxygen and air are connected as gas sources then the yellow scale becomes operative and it is possible to select from 21% to 70% oxygen concentration.

Backup ventilation: None.
Gas volume compensation: None.
Leak Compensation: None.

Manufacturer's Specifications

Table 9-68 lists specifications for Smiths babyPAC 100 ventilator.

TABLE 9-68
Specifications for the Smiths babyPAC 100 Ventilator

Setting Category	Setting	Range
Pressure	Inspiratory Pressure	
	Pressure Support	
	PEEP	0–20 cm H_2O
Volume	Tidal Volume	0–0.33 L
Flow	Inspiratory Flow	
	Waveform	Not specified
Time	Inspiratory Time	0.25–2.0 s
	Mandatory Breath Frequency	10–120/min
	Adjustable Rise Time	
Sensitivity	Trigger Sensitivity (pressure)	
	Trigger Sensitivity (flow)	
	Cycle Sensitivity (flow)	
Alarm Category		
Pressure	Pressure Relief	10–80 cm H_2O
	PEEP	> 10 cm H_2O

(continues)

TABLE 9-68
Specifications for the Smiths babyPAC 100 Ventilator *(Continued)*

Setting Category	Setting	Range
Volume	None	
Flow	None	
Time	None	
Other	None	
Monitored Parameters	I:E Ratio	
	Pressure	
	PEEP	
	Active PEEP	

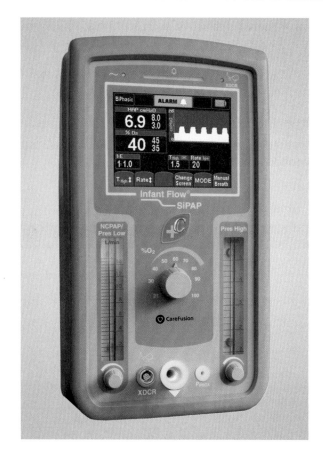

FIGURE 9-74 CareFusion Infant Flow SiPAP system.
Reproduced with permission from CareFusion.

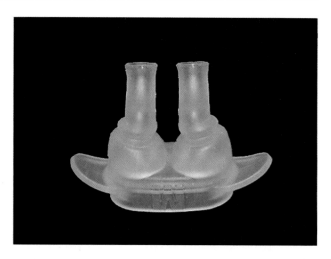

FIGURE 9-75 CareFusion Infant Flow SiPAP nasal prongs.
Reproduced with permission from CareFusion.

CareFusion Infant Flow SiPAP

CareFusion Infant Flow SiPAP (**Figure 9-74**) provides a noninvasive form of respiratory support designed for infants in hospital environments. It can also be used when transporting these patients within the hospital environment. Infant Flow SiPAP is available in a Plus or Comprehensive configuration. The Plus configuration provides nasal continuous positive airway pressure (NCPAP) and time-triggered BiPhasic modes with and without breath rate monitoring. (CareFusion defines *BiPhasic* as time-triggered, time-cycled pressure assists at two separate pressure levels. Using the ventilator mode taxonomy described in this text, the name *BiPhasic* is classified as pressure control intermittent mandatory ventilation.) The Comprehensive configuration offers these features plus a patient-triggered BiPhasic mode with apnea backup breaths. The Infant Flow SiPAP system is designed for noninvasive ventilation of infants using either nasal prongs (**Figure 9-75**) or a nasal mask (**Figure 9-76**).

Operator Interface

The operator interface of the Infant Flow SiPAP (**Figure 9-77**) consists of an LCD touch screen display with keypad, separate flowmeter controls for adjustment of NCPAP and inspiratory pressure above CPAP, and an oxygen blender control. Patient circuit connections are located along the bottom panel. LEDs along

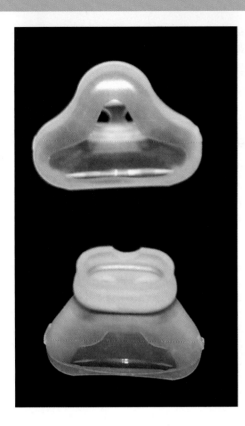

FIGURE 9-76 CareFusion Infant Flow SiPAP nasal mask.
Reproduced with permission from CareFusion.

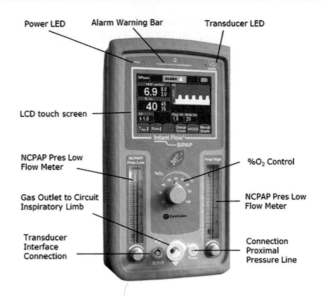

FIGURE 9-77 CareFusion Infant Flow SiPAP operator interface.
Reproduced with permission from CareFusion.

the top of the front panel indicate power on, connection to wall AC, active alarms, and Transducer Interface connection to the driver. An ambient light sensor is located under the front panel to adjust the backlight of the screen display in high and low light environments.

Modes

Modes on the Infant Flow SiPAP are selected by name (i.e., Nasal CPAP, BiPhasic, and BiPhasic tr). The available modes are shown in Table 9-69.

BiPhasic

■ *Mandatory breaths:* Machine triggered (preset frequency) and machine cycled (inspiratory time). Spontaneous breaths are permitted both between and during mandatory breaths.

- Within-breath settings:
  - Operator-set PEEP (set indirectly by adjusting the Pres Low flowmeter), frequency, inspiratory pressure (set indirectly by adjusting the Pres High flowmeter), and inspiratory time (called T_{High}).
■ *Spontaneous breaths:* Patient breathes from continuous bias flow.
  - *Within-breath settings:* None
■ *Between-breath targets:* None.

BiPhasic tr

This mode is currently not available in the United States. It requires the use of an abdominal sensor for the trigger signal.

■ *Mandatory breaths:* Patient triggered (pressure signal from abdominal movement sensor) and machine cycled (inspiratory time). Spontaneous breaths are permitted both between and during mandatory breaths.

TABLE 9-69
Modes for the Infant Flow SiPAP

Mode Name	Control Variable	Breath Sequence	Mode Classification		Tag
			Primary Breath Targeting Scheme	Secondary Breath Targeting Scheme	
BiPhasic	pressure	IMV	set-point	set-point	PC-IMVs,s
BiPhasic tr	pressure	IMV	set-point	set-point	PC-IMVs,s
Nasal CPAP	pressure	CSV	set-point	N/A	PC-CSVs

Reproduced with permission from Mandu Press Ltd.

- Within-breath settings:
  - Operator-set PEEP (set indirectly by adjusting the Pres Low flowmeter), inspiratory pressure (set indirectly by adjusting the Pres High flowmeter), and inspiratory time (called T_{High})
  - *Spontaneous breaths:* Patient breathes from continuous bias flow.
    - *Within-breath settings:* None
  - *Between-breath targets:* None.

CPAP

- *Mandatory breaths:* Not allowed
- Spontaneous breaths:
  - Within-breath settings:
    - Operator-set CPAP (set indirectly by adjusting the Pres Low flowmeter)
- *Between-breath targets:* None

Special Features

Backup ventilation: None, but there is an apnea or low breath rate alarm.

Gas volume compensation: None.
Nebulizer: None.

Manufacturer's Specifications

Table 9-70 lists specifications for the CareFusion SiPAP system.

Section 6: High Frequency Ventilators

High frequency ventilators[37] are designed to provide the lowest possible tidal volume by ventilating at frequencies much higher than conventional ventilators. The idea behind this design is to minimize the risk of volutrauma. Unfortunately, after more than 30 years of clinical research, the evidence for the attainment of this goal remains controversial. In the United States, conventional ventilators are limited to a maximum frequency of 150 breaths/minute, but they are rarely used clinically above about a fourth (adults) to a half (neonates) of that limit. In contrast, high frequency ventilators are approved for operation at many hundreds of cycles per minute (up to 15 Hz for the CareFusion 3100 high frequency oscillator). Many different models of

TABLE 9-70
Specifications for the CareFusion SiPAP System

Setting Category	Setting	Range
Pressure	Inspiratory Pressure	
	Pressure Support	
	PEEP	
Volume	Tidal Volume	
Flow	Low Pressure Inspiratory Flow	0–15 L/min
	High Pressure Inspiratory Flow	0–5 L/min
Time	Inspiratory Time	0.1–3.0 s
	Mandatory Breath Frequency	1–120/min
Alarm Category		
Pressure	High Airway Pressure	Automatic
	Low Airway Pressure	Automatic
Time	Apnea Interval	10–30 s
Other	O_2 Sensor	Enabled/Disabled
Monitored Parameters	nCPAP	
	Mean Airway Pressure	
	Peak Inspiratory Pressure	
	PEEP	
	Oxygen	

high frequency ventilator have come and gone over the last three decades and they continue to evolve outside the United States. Within the United States, there are only two basic designs for delivering low tidal volumes at high frequencies. One design is called a jet ventilator. A jet is a stream of gas forced out of a small-diameter opening (e.g., 2 mm) into a relatively larger diameter tube (e.g., an endotracheal tube at 8 mm). This pneumatic configuration leads to what is called *jet entrainment*, whereby the faster moving gas molecules in the jet stream drag along slower moving molecules in the surrounding gas. The result is that the total gas flow delivered to the endotracheal tube is higher than the flow from the jet orifice itself. This device becomes a ventilator when the jet orifice is supplied with timed pulses of driving pressure such that the operator can control frequency and duty cycle of the jet pulses. In simple jet ventilators, the pressure, volume, and flow delivered to the patient for any given ventilator settings are dependent on the impedance of the patient's respiratory system. The key concept of jet ventilation is that the ventilator forces gas into the lungs but it depends on the passive recoil of the respiratory system to "exhale" that gas. Such a mode of ventilation is classified as **time control** because pressure, volume, and flow are uncontrolled, leaving only the timing of the pulses as preset values (see Figure 9-10 earlier in the chapter). Jet ventilation is considered a form of intermittent mandatory ventilation because spontaneous breathing is uninhibited and because the patient's inspiratory efforts do not affect the frequency of mandatory breaths set on the ventilator as with simple IMV on conventional ventilators. The flow pulsations are superimposed on the patient's spontaneous breaths (if any). In more sophisticated devices (e.g., the Bunnell LifePulse ventilator) the airway pressure is adjusted by an automatic feedback control mechanism, allowing the ventilator to deliver a mode classified as pressure control intermittent mandatory ventilation with set-point targeting. The Percussionaire VDR-4 ventilator is also a jet ventilator but uses a much more complex jet mechanism composed of a "sliding venture." In the case of the VDR-4, airway pressure is not feedback controlled, so the mode the device delivers is time control, intermittent mandatory ventilation with set-point targeting.

The other design of high frequency ventilator available in the United States is known as a high frequency oscillator. An oscillator is something like a piston or a diaphragm that forces gas *both* into and out of the airway, in contrast to a jet ventilator that just forces gas into the airway and relies on passive recoil of the respiratory system to force gas out. As with simple jets, simple oscillators (e.g., the CareFusion 3100 high frequency oscillatory ventilator) do not use feedback control to maintain a consistent airway pressure waveform. Pressure, volume, and flow oscillations for a given ventilator setting are all dependent on the

impedance of the respiratory system. Spontaneous breathing is generally unimpeded and, hence, the mode is classified as time control intermittent mandatory ventilation with set-point targeting.

Bunnell Life Pulse High-Frequency Ventilator

The Bunnell Life Pulse High-Frequency Ventilator (**Figure 9-78**) is indicated for use in ventilating critically ill infants with pulmonary interstitial emphysema (PIE). Infants studied ranged in birth weight from 1.65 to 7.8 pounds (750 to 3,529 grams) and in gestation age from 24 to 41 weeks. The Bunnell Life Pulse High-Frequency Ventilator (HFV) is also indicated for use in ventilating critically ill infants with respiratory distress syndrome (RDS) complicated by pulmonary air leaks that are, in the opinion of their physicians, failing on conventional ventilation. Infants of this description studied ranged in birth weight from 1.32 to 8 pounds (600 to 3,660 grams) and in gestational age from 24 to 38 weeks. The Bunnell Life Pulse High-Frequency Ventilator is a microprocessor-controlled infant ventilating system capable of delivering and monitoring between 240 and 660 humidified high frequency "breaths" per minute. All hardware elements in the system, from the initial gas input connection to the integral humidifier to the LifePort adapter, have been specifically designed to convey information back to the controlling software elements. Together, these elements form a fully integrated, self-regulating unit that maximizes both machine efficiency and patient safety (**Figure 9-79**).

Operator Interface

The operator interface of the Bunnell Life Pulse consists of LED displays and membrane switches (up and down arrows) for adjusting settings (**Figure 9-80**).

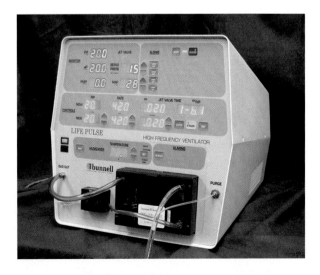

FIGURE 9-78 Bunnell Life Pulse High-Frequency Ventilator.
Courtesy of Bunnell Incorporated.

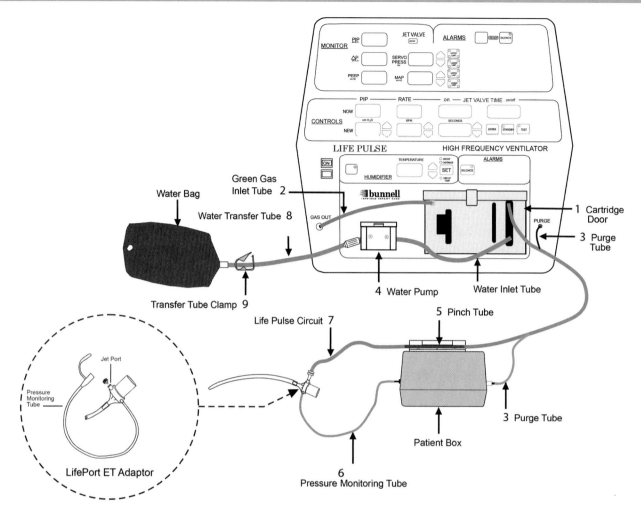

Water Bag

Green Gas Inlet Tube 2

Water Transfer Tube 8

GAS OUT

1 Cartridge Door

3 Purge Tube

Transfer Tube Clamp 9

4 Water Pump

Water Inlet Tube

PURGE

Life Pulse Circuit 7

Jet Port

Pressure Monitoring Tube

LifePort ET Adaptor

5 Pinch Tube

3 Purge Tube

Patient Box

6 Pressure Monitoring Tube

FIGURE 9-79 Unique elements of the Bunnell Life Pulse ventilator.
Courtesy of Bunnell Incorporated.

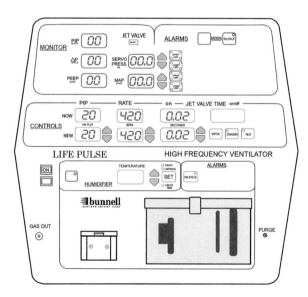

FIGURE 9-80 Bunnell Life Pulse operator interface.
Courtesy of Bunnell Incorporated.

Modes

The Life Pulse is unique among ventilators in that it is designed to be used with a conventional infant ventilator at all times (i.e., the ventilator must provide PC-IMV with time-triggered, time-cycled mandatory breaths, PEEP/CPAP, and continuous bias flow from a separate heated humidifier). The Life Pulse produces pulses (jets) of flow that create breaths that are provided in tandem with PC-IMV of the conventional ventilator. The Life Pulse allows the operator to set the peak inspiratory pressure, the breath rate (frequency), and the jet valve on time or inspiratory time (essentially controlling the duty cycle of the jet pulse). The conventional ventilator is essential for providing gas for the patient's spontaneous breathing, PEEP, and periodic normally sized breaths (background intermittent mandatory ventilation). The Life Pulse monitors the pressures in the patient's airway by using a pressure transducer located in the Patient Box. It is recommended that the Life Pulse be connected to the patient

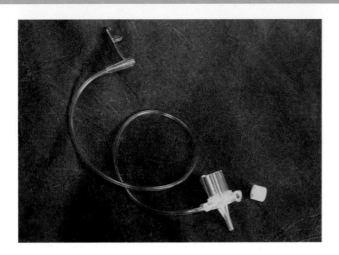

FIGURE 9-81 Bunnell LifePort endotracheal tube adapter.
Courtesy of Bunnell Incorporated.

and the PIP, PEEP, and mean airway pressure (MAP) values produced by the conventional ventilator be monitored using the pressure monitoring capability of the Life Pulse.

Special Features

The Life Pulse is designed to be used with a special endotracheal tube adapter (the LifePort, **Figure 9-81**) and a standard endotracheal tube.

Unlike most conventional ventilators, the Life Pulse has been programmed to automatically establish high and low alarm limits around servo pressure, mean airway pressure, and peak inspiratory pressure, and to automatically check for other alarm conditions.

Manufacturer's Specifications

Table 9-71 lists specifications for the Bunnell Life Pulse high frequency ventilator.

CareFusion 3100B High Frequency Oscillatory Ventilator

The CareFusion 3100B is a high frequency oscillator ventilator (**Figure 9-82**). An earlier version of this device (the 3100A HFOV) has approval for treatment of respiratory failure in infants and children. This version of the device, the 3100B HFOV, has increased power capability and other modifications to allow treatment of adults.

Operator Interface

The operator interface of the 3100B is composed of LED displays and knobs (**Figure 9-83**).

Modes

The 3100B high frequency oscillatory ventilator is essentially a high-flow CPAP system with superimposed pressure oscillations created by an electrically driven diaphragm, similar to an audio loudspeaker cone. The oscillation frequency, duty cycle, mean pressure, and oscillatory pressure amplitude are operator preset. The frequency can be set between 3 and 15 Hz

TABLE 9-71
Specifications for the Bunnell Life Pulse High Frequency Ventilator

Setting Category	Setting	Range
Pressure	Inspiratory Pressure	8–50 cm H_2O
Time	Jet Valve on Time	0.020–0.034 s
	Jet Pulse Frequency	240–660/min
Alarm Category		
	Automatic Adjustment of Peak, Mean and Servo Pressure Alarms	
Monitored Parameters	Peak Inspiratory Pressure	
	ΔP	
	PEEP	
	Mean Airway Pressure	
	Servo Pressure	
	I:E Ratio	

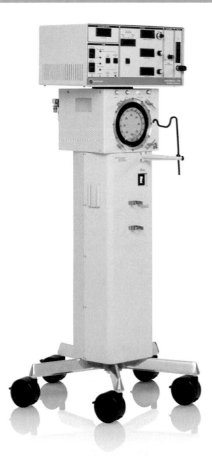

FIGURE 9-82 CareFusion 3100B high frequency oscillatory ventilator.

Reproduced with permission from CareFusion.

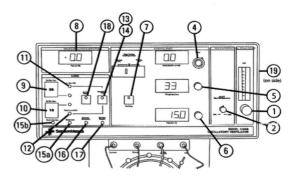

FIGURE 9-83 CareFusion 3100B operator interface. 1. Bias flow control. 2. Mean airway pressure control. 3. Not used. 4. Power driving the oscillator piston, an indirect control of oscillatory pressure amplitude. 5. Percent inspiratory time control. 6. Frequency control. 7. Start/stop. 8. Mean airway pressure display. 9. Set maximum mean airway pressure. 10. Set minimum mean airway pressure. 11. Mean airway pressure > 60 cm H_2O. 12. Mean airway pressure < 5 cm H_2O. 13. Power failure. 14. Alarm reset. 15a. Low battery indicator. 15b. Low source gas indicator. 16. Oscillator overheated. 17. Oscillator stopped. 18. Audible alarm silence. 19. Patient circuit calibration.

Reproduced with permission from CareFusion.

(cycles per second). The mean airway pressure can be set from 5 to 55 cm H_2O and the bias flow (generating the CPAP) can be set from 0 to 60 L/min. The duty cycle can be set from 30% to 50%. Mean airway pressure is adjusted with a control that varies the resistance of the exhalation manifold; however, mean airway pressure is not feedback controlled, so it varies with changes in bias flow, duty cycle, and oscillatory pressure amplitude (the "power" setting). Oscillatory pressure amplitude is not feedback controlled and is adjusted indirectly by adjusting the "power" setting that determines the power driving the oscillator piston. The actual pressure amplitude will vary with the impedance of the patient's respiratory system and artificial airway. The maximum airway pressure oscillatory amplitude is about 140 cm H_2O. Corresponding pressure swings in the trachea would be in the range of 10% of this value because of attenuation due to airway resistance. The maximum tidal volume will be approximately 250 mL depending on the ventilator settings, tracheal tube size, and patient's respiratory system mechanics. Typical tidal volumes (although not measured) are considerably

less than this maximum value and may be as small as the patient's anatomic dead space.

Special Features

The 3100B is intended to be used with a specially designed patient circuit and a conventional heated humidifier.

Manufacturer's Specifications

Table 9-72 lists specifications for the CareFusion 3100B oscillatory ventilator.

Percussionaire VDR-4

The Percussionaire Volumetric Diffusive Respirator (VDR-4), shown in **Figure 9-84**, is a pneumatically powered and pneumatically controlled high frequency ventilator suitable for use with neonates through adults. It is the most sophisticated in a line of interpulmonary percussive ventilators, called percussionators (**Figure 9-85**). The VDR-4 is operated with a separate electronic airway pressure monitor called the Monitron II Waveform Analyzer (see Figure 9-84). This device also provides a basic airway pressure alarm capability.

Operator Interface

The operator interface of the VDR-4 consists of dials for adjusting the various parameters of the high frequency airway pressure waveform (**Figure 9-86**).

Modes

The VDR-4 generates a high frequency airway pressure waveform that the manufacturer calls interpulmonary percussive ventilation (IPV); it is sometimes referred to

TABLE 9-72
Specifications for the CareFusion 3100B Oscillatory Ventilator

Setting Category	Setting	Range
Pressure	Inspiratory Pressure	3–55 cm H_2O
Flow	Inspiratory Flow	0–60 L/min
	Waveform	Not specified
Time	Inspiratory Time	30–50%
	Mandatory Breath Frequency	
Alarm Category		
Pressure	Maximum Airway Pressure	0–59 cm H_2O
	Minimum Airway Pressure	0–59 cm H_2O
Monitored Parameters	Bias Flow	
	Mean Pressure	
	Frequency	
	Airway Pressure	

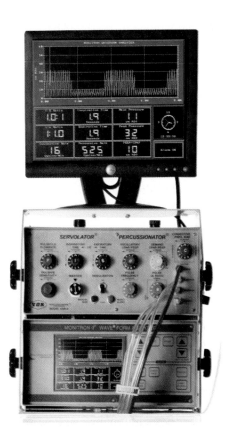

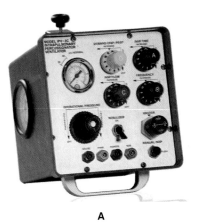

A

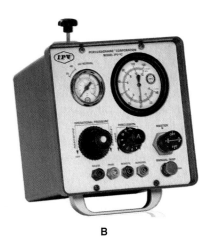

B

FIGURE 9-84 Percussionaire VDR-4 ventilator.

Courtesy of Percussionaire® Corporation.

FIGURE 9-85 Percussionaire family of IPV percussionators.

Photos courtesy of Percussionaire® Corporation.

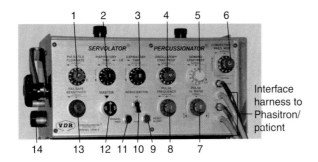

FIGURE 9-86 Percussionaire VDR-4 operator interface. 1. Pulsatile flow: Determines the amplitude or peak inspiratory pressure (PIP) delivered to the patient during inspiratory time. 2. Inspiratory time: Selects the time interval (programmable from 0.5 seconds to 5 seconds) that high frequency volumes are delivered to which the amplitude or PIP is determined by the Pulsatile Flowrate control. 3. Expiratory time: Selects the interval (programmable from 0.5 seconds to 5 seconds) that high frequency volumes are not being delivered. Expiratory time can be programmed for Oscillatory/Demand CPAP/PEEP or a static baseline. 4. Oscillatory CPAP/PEEP: Provides for a high frequency baseline pressure during the expiratory phase. 5. Demand CPAP/PEEP: Provides for the establishment of "static PEEP" that automatically increases flow to the patient as the inspiratory demand warrants. 6. Convective Pressure Rise: Programmed to occur 1 second into the inspiratory phase when activated and controls the pressure rise above that programmed with the Pulsatile Flowrate. To be used with caution and when low compliance requires very high delivery pressures. 7. Pulse i/e Ratio: Controls the i/e ratio of the high frequency volumes delivered. 8. Pulse Frequency: Controls the rate of the high frequency volumes delivered. 9. Alarm reset. 10. Nebulization: Controls the flow of gas to the aerosol circuit. 11. Manual Inspiration button. 12. Master: Activates unit when placed into the on position. When master switch is in off position Manual Inspiration, Nebulization, Demand CPAP/Peep are still functional for weaning purposes. 13. Failsafe Sensitivity: Limits a maximum sustained pressure over a programmed time. 14. Alarm Body.

Courtesy of Percussionaire® Corporation.

in the literature as high frequency percussive ventilation. IPV is a form of high frequency jet ventilation, relying on a jet orifice and entrainment as discussed previously. However, IPV is delivered with a specially designed sliding venturi that allows for enhanced flow delivery (compared to simple jet orifices) to patients ranging from neonates to large adults (**Figure 9-87**). The venturi is inside a housing called the Phasitron, which provides a means for connecting the high pressure source gas from the ventilator to the venturi, a port for air entrainment, a port for monitoring airway pressure, and a port for connection to the artificial airway. IPV is defined by the manufacturer as follows:

> A cyclic method of controlled percussive intrapulmonary (sub tidal) breath stacking, increasing the existing Functional Residual Capacity of the pulmonary structures to a selected level (pulsatile equilibrium) at which

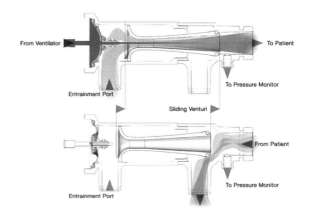

FIGURE 9-87 Phasitron section of the VDR-4 ventilator containing the sliding venturi. Top: Jet pulse from ventilator is on, forcing the sliding venturi to the right, closing the exhalation port and increasing airway pressure and delivering flow to the patient. Bottom: Jet pulse is off, allowing the venturi to slide to the left, opening the exhalation port, and depressurizing the lungs.

Courtesy of Percussionaire® Corporation.

point repetitive sub tidal volume delivery does not further increase lung volumes. Each percussive inspiratory interval (timed in seconds) is associated with percussive, diffuse intrapulmonary gas mixing concomitant with aerosol delivery; followed by passive exhalation of a Gross Tidal Volume to a selected baseline.

The manufacturer defines volumetric diffusive ventilation as follows:

> A cyclic method of precisely controlling the intrapulmonary delivery of successive (aggregate) sub tidal volumes to a selected equilibrium (increase in lung volume) ultimately reaching an Oscillatory Apneustic Plateau (Oscillatory Equilibrium), followed by the passive exhalation of a gross tidal volume down to a programmed static and/or pulsatile baseline.

The airway pressure waveform created by the VDR-4 is shown in **Figure 9-88**. As can be seen from inspection of Figure 9-88, the airway pressure waveform produced by the VDR-4 looks like a high frequency oscillation superimposed on a low frequency PC-IMV waveform (spontaneous breathing is unrestricted at all times). However, the actual pressures, volumes, and flows delivered to the patient are determined by the mechanical load of the respiratory system (once the ventilator parameters are preset by the operator).[38] Thus, examination of Figure 9-10 indicates that the mode of ventilation delivered by the VDR-4 is a form of time control (because neither pressure, volume, or flow are preset so it cannot be a form of pressure control or volume control). A brief description of high frequency percussive ventilation is given in a recent paper on treatment

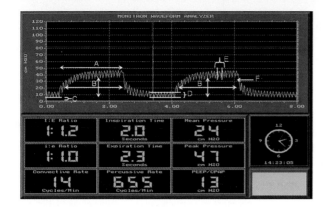

FIGURE 9-88 Example airway pressure waveform produced by VDR-4 ventilator. A. Pulsatile flow during inspiration at 655 cycles/min. B. Convective pressure-limited breath with low frequency cycle. C. Demand CPAP. D. Oscillatory CPAP. E. Single percussive breath. F. Periodic programmed interruptions signifying end of inspiration and onset of exhalation.

Courtesy of Felix Khusid.

options for severe hypoxemic respiratory failure.[39] A list of references for high frequency percussive ventilation is available in a recent letter to the editor of *Respiratory Care Journal*.[40]

Operator's Manuals Used for Reference

Intensive Care Ventilators

- Avea, CareFusion, July 2011, Revision M
- Vela, CareFusion, May 2012, Revision H
- Newport Medical e360-T, Covidien, December 2010, Revision B
- Puritan Bennett 840, Covidien, August 2005, Revision F
- EvitaXL, Dräger Medical, July 2004, 1st edition, Software 6.n
- Evita Infinity V500, Dräger Medical, June 2009, 1st edition, Software 2.n
- Engström Carestation, GE Healthcare, Software Revision 7.X
- VersaMed iVent 201, GE Medical, December 2006, Revision 11
- C3, Hamilton Medical, 2012, Software Version 1.0
- Galileo, Hamilton Medical, 2006
- G5, Hamilton Medical, 2012, Software Version 2.2X
- Servo-i, Maquet, Version 3.1
- V60, Philips Respironics, 2009–2010, Revision D
- V200, Philips Respironics, 2009, Revision A

Portable Ventilators

- pNeuton Model A, Airon Corporation, August 2011, Revision F
- Crossvent-4+, Bio-Med Devices, 2005, Revision 071012

- EnVe, CareFusion, Revision EVA 2034
- ReVel, CareFusion, September 2011, Revision A
- Carina, Dräger, August 2012, 1st Edition, Software 3.2n
- Oxylog 3000 plus, Dräger Medical, September 2011, 5th Edition, Software 1.n
- Puritan Bennett 540, Covidien, 2009, Revision C
- Newport Medical HT70 Plus, Covidien, November 2011, Revision B
- VersaMed iVent 101, GE Medical, March 2010, Revision 2
- T1, Hamilton Medical, 2011, Software Version 1.1.x
- Uni-Vent Eagle Model 754, Impact Instrumentation, September 2006, Revision 1.85J
- Trilogy, Philips Respironics, 2009, REF 1067236

Neonatal Ventilators

- Babylog VN500, Dräger Medical, August 2010, 4th Edition, Software 2.n
- Pneupac babyPAC 100, Smiths Medical, April 2005, Issue 1
- Infant Flow SiPAP, CareFusion, March 2013, Revision N

High Frequency Ventilators

- Life Pulse, Bunnell, GBC–01289-27.30
- 3100B, CareFusion, July 2011, Revision R
- VDR-4, Percussionaire, 2009, Document ID: F-032309 DCO 10282 06-22-10

References

1. Mushin WW, Rendell-Baker L, Thompson PW, et al. *Automatic ventilation of the lungs.* Philadelphia: FA Davis; 1980.
2. McPherson SP, Spearman CB. *Respiratory therapy equipment.* 1st ed. St. Louis: CV Mosby; 1977.
3. Chatburn RL, Mireles-Cabodevila E. Basic principles of ventilator design and operation. In: Tobin MJ, ed. *Principles and practice of mechanical ventilation.* 3rd ed. New York: McGraw-Hill; 2012:65-97.
4. Sanborn WG. Microprocessor-based mechanical ventilation. *Respir Care.* 1993;38(1):72-109.
5. Morch ET. History of mechanical ventilation. In: Kerby RR, Smith RA, Desautels DA, eds. *Mechanical ventilation.* New York: Churchill Livingstone; 1985:158.
6. Russell IF, Ross DG, Manson HJ. Fluidic cycling devices for inspiratory and expiratory timing in automatic ventilators. *J Biomed Eng.* 1983;5(3):227-234.
7. Chatburn RL. Classification of mechanical ventilators. In: Branson RD, Hess DR, Chatburn RL, eds. *Respiratory care equipment.* Philadelphia: Lippincott Williams & Wilkins; 1999:359-393.
8. MacIntyre NR, Branson RD. *Mechanical ventilation.* 2nd ed. St. Louis: Saunders Elsevier; 2009:153-156.
9. de Wit M. Monitoring of patient-ventilator interaction at the bedside. *Respir Care.* 2011;56(1):61-72.
10. Henderson WR, Sheel AW. Pulmonary mechanics during mechanical ventilation. *Respir Physiol Neurobiol.* 2012; 180(2-3):162-172.
11. Sassoon CSH. Triggering of the ventilator in patient-ventilator interactions. *Respir Care.* 2011;56(1):39-48.

12. Grooms DA, Sibole SH, Tomlinson JR, Marik PE, Chatburn RL. Customization of an open-lung ventilation strategy to treat a case of life-threatening acute respiratory distress syndrome. *Respir Care*. 2011;56(4):514-519.

13. Cairo JM, Pilbeam SP. *Mosby's respiratory care equipment*. 8th ed. St. Louis: Mosby; 2010.

14. Chatburn RL, Khatib ME, Mireles-Cabodevila E. A taxonomy for mechanical ventilation: 10 fundamental maxims. *Respir Care*. 2014;59(11):1747-1763.

15. Chatburn RL, Carlo WA. A taxonomy for mechanical ventilation. In: Berhardt LV, ed., *Advances in biology and medicine*, vol. 78. Hauppauge, NY: Nova Science Publishers; 2014.

16. Cairo JM. *Pilbeam's mechanical ventilation. Physiological and clinical applications*. 5th ed. St. Louis: Mosby; 2012.

17. Fedor K. Mechanical ventilators. In: Walsh BK, Czervinske MP, DiBlasi RM, eds. *Perinatal and pediatric respiratory care*. 3rd ed. St. Louis: Saunders; 2010:267-304.

18. Hess DR, Kacmarek RM. *Essentials of mechanical ventilation*. 3rd ed. New York: McGraw-Hill; 2014.

19. Chatburn RL, Volsko TA, Hazy J, Harris LN, Sanders S. Determining the basis for a taxonomy of mechanical ventilation. *Respir Care*. 2012;57(4):514-524.

20. Chatburn RL, Daoud EG. Ventilation. In: Kacmarek RM, Stoller JK, Heuer AH, eds. *Egan's fundamentals of respiratory care*. 10th ed. St. Louis: Mosby Elsevier; 2012:225-249.

21. Sassoon CSH. Triggering of the ventilator in patient-ventilator interactions. *Respir Care*. 2011;56(1):39-48.

22. Rodarte JR, Rehder K. Dynamics of respiration. In: Fishman AP, Macklem PT, Mead J, Geiger SR, eds. *Handbook of Physiology. The Respiratory System*. Volume III, Mechanics of breathing, Part 1. Bethesda, MD: American Physiological Society; 1986:131-144.

23. Chatburn RL, Volsko TA. Documentation issues for mechanical ventilation in pressure-control modes. *Respir Care*. 2011;55(12):1705-1716.

24. Marini JJ, Crooke PS III, Truwit JD. Determinants and limits of pressure-preset ventilation: A mathematical model of pressure control. *J Appl Physiol*. 1989;67:1081-1092.

25. Babic MD, Chatburn RL, Stoller JK. Laboratory evaluation of the Vortran Automatic Resuscitator Model RTM. *Respir Care*. 2007;52(12):1718-1727.

26. Chatburn RL, Mireles-Cabodevila E. Basic principles of ventilator design and operation. In: Tobin MJ, ed. *Principles and practice of mechanical ventilation*. 3rd ed. New York: McGraw-Hill; 2012:65-97.

27. Chatburn RL, Mireles-Cabodevila E. Closed-loop control of mechanical ventilation: Description and classification of targeting schemes. *Respir Care*. 2011;56(1):85-102.

28. Amato MB, Barbas CS, Bonassa J, Saldiva PH, Zin WA, de Carvalho CR. Volume-assured pressure support ventilation (VAPSV). A new approach for reducing muscle workload during acute respiratory failure. *Chest*. 1992;102(4):1225-1234.

29. Volsko TA, Hoffman J, Conger A, Chatburn RL. The effect of targeting scheme on tidal volume delivery during volume control mechanical ventilation. *Respir Care*. 2012;57(8):1297-1304.

30. Mutch WA, Harms S, Ruth GM, et al. Biologically variable or naturally noisy mechanical ventilation recruits atelectatic lung. *Am J Respir Crit Care Med*. 2000;162:319-323.

31. Spieth PM, Güldner A, Beda A, et al. Comparative effects of proportional assist and variable pressure support ventilation on lung function and damage in experimental lung injury. *Crit Care Med*. 2012;40(9):2654-2661.

32. Chatburn RL, Volsko TA. Mechanical ventilators. In: Kacmarek RM, Stoller JK, Heuer AH, eds. *Egan's fundamentals of respiratory care*. 10th ed. St. Louis: Mosby Elsevier; 2012:1006-1040.

33. Chatburn RL, Volsko TA. Mechanical ventilators: Classification and principles of operation. In: Hess DR, MacIntyre NR, Mishoe SC, Galvin WF, Adams AB, Saposnick AB, eds. *Respiratory care: Principles and practice*. 2nd ed. Philadelphia: W.B. Saunders; 2012:444-461.

34. Chatburn RL. Classification of mechanical ventilators and modes of ventilation. In: Tobin MJ, ed. *Principles and practice of mechanical ventilation*. 3rd ed. New York: McGraw-Hill; 2012:45-64.

35. Mireles-Cabodevila E, Chatburn RL. A rational basis for comparing modes of mechanical ventilation. *Respir Care*. 2013;58(2):348-366.

36. Covidien. *840 Ventilator system operator's and technical reference manual*. Rev. M, August 2010.

37. Froese AB, Ferguson ND. High-frequency ventilation. In: Tobin MJ, ed. *Principles and practice of mechanical ventilation*. 3rd ed. New York: McGraw-Hill Medical; 2013:495-515.

38. Lucangelo U, Antonaglia V, Zin WA, et al. Effects of mechanical load on flow, volume, and pressure delivered by high-frequency percussive ventilation. *Respir Physiol Neurobiol*. 2004;142(1):81-91.

39. Esan A, Hess DR, Raoof S, George L, Sessler CN. Severe hypoxemic respiratory failure: Part 1—ventilatory strategies. *Chest*. 2010;137(5):1203-1216.

40. Short K, Bougatef A, Khusid F, Kenny BD, Miller K. High-frequency percussive ventilation. *Resp Care*. 2010;55(12):1762-1764.

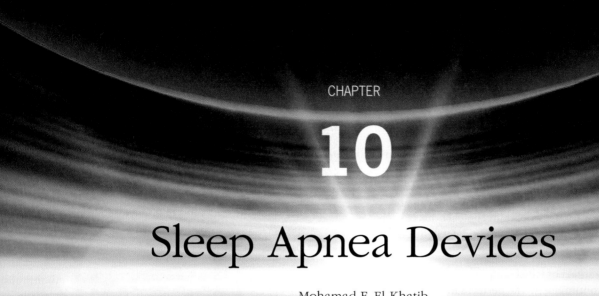

CHAPTER

10

Sleep Apnea Devices

Mohamad F. El-Khatib

CHAPTER OBJECTIVES

1. Describe the classification of devices used for sleep apnea patients.
2. Understand the principle of operation of CPAP devices.
3. Understand the principle of operation of BiPAP devices.
4. Recognize the different types of patient interfaces used with sleep apnea devices.
5. Compare and contrast technical specifications of currently available CPAP and BiPAP devices.

KEY TERMS

Autotitration
Bilevel positive airway pressure (BiPAP)
Continuous positive airway pressure (CPAP)

Expiratory release
Interface
Masks
Obstructive sleep apnea (OSA)

Introduction

Obstructive sleep apnea (OSA) is a relatively common disorder in the United States and worldwide. In 2005, a poll conducted by the National Sleep Foundation indicated that as many as one in four American adults are at high risk of OSA.[1] The defining characteristic of OSA is a partial or complete obstruction of the airway while sleeping; it is usually indicated by loud snoring and frequent, sudden, and severe snorting. During the day, OSA is reflected by an increased daytime somnolence and tiredness as well as other severe comorbidities (arterial hypertension, stroke, arrhythmias, and all-cause mortality).[2] The main therapy for OSA is the application of some form of positive airway pressure during sleep with the aim

of increasing luminal pressure that will oppose the collapsing pressure, thereby splinting the airway open and functioning as a pneumatic stent.[2]

Classification of Devices

Devices that are based on the application of positive airway pressure for the treatment of obstructive sleep apnea are in the form of either **continuous positive airway pressure (CPAP)** or **bilevel positive airway pressure (BiPAP)**. When used properly and consistently, CPAP and BiPAP result in improved sleep patterns and quality of life due to decreased daytime somnolence.[3]

- *CPAP:* CPAP devices are, in essence, blowers that are capable of generating high flows. When the device is connected through special **interfaces** to either the patient's nose, mouth, or both, a fixed level of continuous positive pressure is transmitted to the upper airways to keep them open. CPAP devices are not true ventilators because they do not actively assist inspiration. They require a spontaneously breathing patient and are unable to support ventilation in the case of apnea.[4] **Autotitration** allows for varying the applied positive airway pressure. With autotitration, the level of positive airway pressure is not fixed during the CPAP therapy and varies according to the patient's needs.[5]
- *BiPAP:* Similar to CPAP devices, BiPAP devices are also blowers and flow generators; however, they have the capability of creating two levels of pressures rather than one. The BiPAP devices

are able to alternate between these two levels of pressures. In that sense, BiPAP devices are considered true ventilators and are the most widely used devices for noninvasive mechanical ventilation. Although patients are required to be spontaneously breathing with BiPAP, most modern BiPAP devices incorporate a backup mode that delivers positive pressure ventilation in the event of apnea.[6] As with CPAP, autotitration can be applied with BiPAP devices to meet the patient's requirements by varying the high and low pressures as per certain clinical criteria such as airflow resistance, targeted tidal volume, or minute ventilation.[5,6]

New generations of CPAP and BiPAP devices are popping up continuously. The performance, features, monitoring capability, shape, and weight are being updated to allow patients to more easily control their sleep apnea and at the same time meet the clinician's requirements for superior and more efficient therapies. This has made sleep therapy more user friendly and has significantly improved the patient's compliance with the therapy and subsequently the patient's outcome. Later in the chapter we will present the specifications for currently available CPAP and BiPAP devices.

CPAP Devices

CPAP devices (**Figure 10-1**) provide an increase in the baseline pressure, from atmospheric pressure as with spontaneous breathing up to a clinician-specified fixed level of pressure (**Figure 10-2**). Meanwhile, the patient breathes as he or she does during spontaneous breathing with full control of tidal volume and minute ventilation. As mentioned previously, CPAP is not a true ventilator because it does not actively assist inspiration. It requires a spontaneously breathing patient and is unable to support ventilation in the case of apnea. A single hose is used either through a direct connection to the patient's airway interface or via an integrated humidifier. Patient interfaces such as nasal **masks**, full face masks, nasal pillows, and helmets can be used with CPAP devices, as long as they incorporate or provide an exhalation port. Most CPAP devices can function on AC and DC power supplies for more flexibility.

Principles of Operation

By delivering constant pressure during both inspiration and expiration (Figure 10-2, middle), CPAP acts as a pneumatic splint that counteracts collapsible pressures on the airways and prevents upper airway collapse during sleep in patients with obstructive sleep apnea syndrome. Also, CPAP increases functional residual capacity (FRC), which is the main oxygen store; recruits underventilated and/or collapsed alveoli; and ultimately improves oxygenation

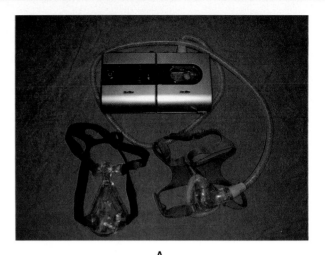

A

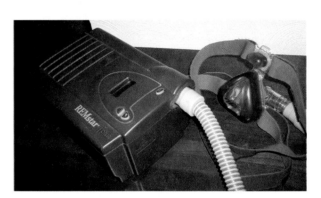

B

FIGURE 10-1 CPAP devices.

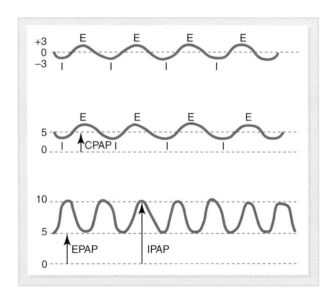

FIGURE 10-2 A spontaneous breathing pattern (top), with a CPAP of 5 cm H_2O (middle), and with a BiPAP of 10 and 5 cm H_2O (bottom).

and creates a safety net against episodes of desaturation usually associated with obstructive sleep apnea syndrome.[7] The increase in FRC may also increase lung compliance and decrease the work of breathing. With acute cardiogenic pulmonary edema, the use of CPAP lowers left ventricular transmural pressure and thus reduces afterload, increases cardiac output, and helps in resolving acute pulmonary edema. In chronic obstructive pulmonary disease (COPD), the tonic increase in baseline pressure with CPAP counterbalances the inspiratory threshold load imposed by auto-positive end-expiratory pressure (auto-PEEP). However, BiPAP devices remain the more suitable form of positive pressure support in COPD patients (see the following section).[8]

Autotitration

Many patients refuse to use or cannot comply with CPAP or BiPAP therapy during sleep, particularly when the therapy is applied at high levels of pressure.[9] In addition, several studies have shown that the degree of airway obstruction and subsequent airflow resistance are not uniform throughout sleep in patients with obstructive sleep apnea.[10,11] These important facts have fueled the development of a number of technological solutions. The most common solution that allows for variations in the applied positive airway pressure is autotitration. Fixed CPAP provides continuous fixed therapeutic pressure during the entire sleep period. In contrast, with autotitration, the delivered pressure varies depending on changes in airflow resistance. The level of CPAP is continuously adjusted (increased and decreased) to achieve the minimal pressure that will relieve the obstruction and as such eliminate the need for high and unnecessary pressure levels. Varying the applied pressure would promote an improvement in breathing synchrony with the CPAP device and therefore could optimize patient comfort and thus enhance compliance with the therapy. A 2009 Cochrane review comparing autotitrating CPAP with fixed CPAP concluded that autotitrating CPAP was superior to fixed CPAP in increasing patient comfort and compliance.[12]

Expiratory Release Features

A typical complaint of sleep apnea patients using CPAP is the discomfort or even difficulty in exhaling against the continuous positive airway pressure level, particularly when high CPAP levels of greater than 10 cm H_2O are prescribed to patients.[13] Different algorithms by different manufactures of CPAP devices have been implemented on newer CPAP devices to increase the patient's comfort and improve patient compliance and outcomes. The general feature of all **expiratory release** algorithms involves reducing pressure at the beginning

of exhalation and then returning to therapeutic pressure just before inhalation.

- *Respironics algorithm:* The algorithm for Respironics machines involves tracking the patient's breathing pattern to lower the amount of pressure delivered at the beginning of exhalation and then increasing the pressure at the end of exhalation to prevent airway collapse during the respiratory phase transition to inhalation. Usually there is more than one pressure relief level that is user selected. The amount of pressure relief is based on the patient's expiratory flow and the pressure relief setting level (**Figure 10-3**). At the heart of this concept is the use of a Digital Auto-Trak and Sensitivity algorithm. Digital Auto-Trak is a highly sensitive algorithm that tracks each breath and detects the onset of

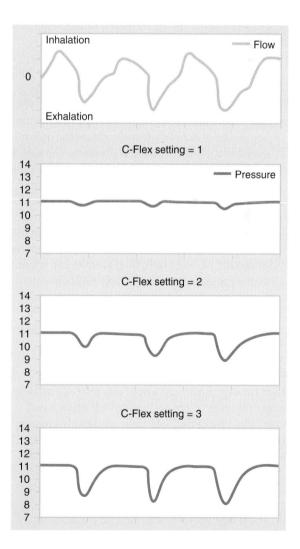

FIGURE 10-3 Changes in CPAP level as per the expiratory release feature (C-Flex) with Respironics sleep apnea devices.

Reproduced with permission from Philips Healthcare.

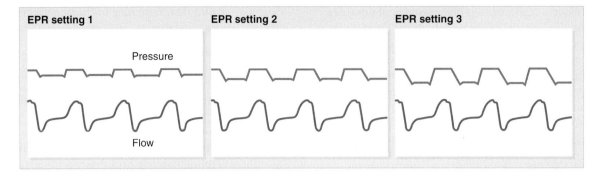

FIGURE 10-4 The pressure and flow during three different settings of expiratory pressure relief (EPR) with the ResMed CPAP devices.
© ResMed 2007. Used with permission.

inspiration and expiration—even in the presence mask leak. It automatically adjusts the variable trigger and cycle thresholds to ensure optimum system response with every breath.[14,15]

- *ResMed algorithm:* New models of ResMed CPAP devices (S9 Series) feature the Enhanced Easy-Breathe waveform that allows variable expiratory pressure relief (EPR). The Easy-Breathe EPR waveform provides a gentler pressure during exhalation for more comfortable breathing. With Easy-Breathe EPR, the CPAP device detects the beginning of exhalation and reduces the motor speed to drop the treatment pressure. The patient or clinician can select one of three comfort levels for the detection of exhalation: Setting 1 = mild comfort (1 cm H_2O); Setting 2 = medium comfort (2 cm H_2O); and Setting 3 = maximum comfort (3 cm H_2O) (**Figure 10-4**). EPR has an automatic time-out feature in which the CPAP device determines the baseline breathing average and whenever a patient's breathing drops 75% below the baseline for 10 seconds or more, pressure relief is suspended. After the event is over, EPR will start again.[16]

Memory/Information Storage

Patient management is an important part of any sleep therapy regimen to ensure patient adherence and results. Most modern CPAP devices include memory cards for storage of data over a long period of time (3–12 months). Commonly stored data, which can be presented in either numerical or graphical forms, include patient's compliance data, time spent at a certain therapeutic pressure, apnea/hypopnea index, leak, and usage pattern. The data on these memory cards can be downloaded for the clinician's review and influence future recommendations for the therapy plan.

Cleaning and Maintenance

Patients must ensure that their CPAP devices are well maintained and always clean. All CPAP devices come with clear instructions for the cleaning procedure and the maintenance program. Upon purchasing the devices, patients should familiarize themselves with these topics. In general, cleaning involves surface cleaning of the device when it is not used and is unplugged from the electrical supply. Usually a cloth dampened with water and a mild detergent is used for surface cleaning of the device. During the cleaning process, fluid should not penetrate the enclosure, inlet filter, or any other opening. If the device is used with multiple people, all inlet bacterial and dust filters should be removed and discarded each time the device is used on a different person. As for the cleaning agents, it is highly recommended to coordinate with the institutional infection control program to create a short list of cleaning agents that can ensure full disinfection of the device and yet do not cause any damage to the device. CPAP devices should be maintained as per the manufacturer's recommended periodic maintenance.

Currently Available Devices

In the last decade, a plethora of CPAP devices have come onto the market for sleep apnea patients. Devices with superior performance, complex features, comprehensive monitoring capability, and different sizes and shapes are released to meet the needs and requirements of both patients and clinicians. The general specifications of different currently available CPAP devices in the U.S. market are presented in **Table 10-1**.

BiPAP Devices

Similar to CPAP devices, bilevel positive airway pressure (BiPAP) devices are also flow generators; however, in contrast to CPAP devices, BiPAP devices are capable of delivering and toggling between two levels of positive airway pressures: inspiratory positive airway pressure (IPAP) and expiratory positive airway pressure (EPAP) (Figure 10-2, bottom). Because of its capability for generating two pressure levels, BiPAP devices can provide a wider range of modality for ventilatory support than can CPAP devices. BiPAP devices are the main devices for providing noninvasive ventilation for patients with chronic obstructive lung diseases, acute lung injury and acute respiratory distress syndrome, and immunocompromised patients, and for end-of-life support of terminal patients.[17-19] However, they can also be used for patients with obstructive sleep apnea syndrome, particularly for patients with severe obstructions that necessitate the use of high positive airway pressures for the relief of obstructions.[20,21] The rest of this chapter describes BiPAP devices and evaluates their capacity as a therapy for obstructive sleep apnea syndrome rather than as a noninvasive ventilator.

BiPAP devices can look exactly like CPAP devices, and most of the time can function as CPAP devices (**Figure 10-5**); however, CPAP devices cannot function as BiPAP devices. Similar to CPAP devices, BiPAP devices use a hose to connect the device either directly or via an inline humidifier (whether directly integrated or added) to the patient's interface, which can be a nasal or full face mask, nasal pillows, a lip-seal mouthpiece, or a helmet. BiPAP devices can function on either AC or DC power.

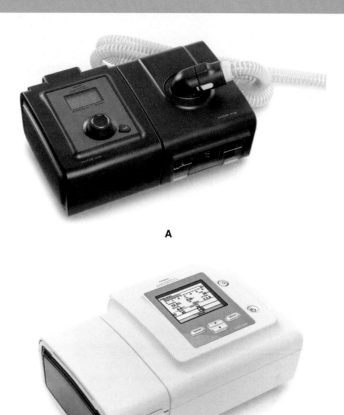

A

B

FIGURE 10-5 BiPAP devices.
Photos courtesy of Philips Healthcare.

Principles of Operation

As described previously, BiPAP devices provide two levels of pressure. In other words, BiPAP is just another name for a pressure control mode of ventilation, often similar or identical to the mode called Pressure Support found on standard mechanical ventilators. On top of the increase in baseline pressure seen with CPAP, there is an additional phasic increase in airway pressure that is usually triggered by a patient breathing effort. During BiPAP therapy, the clinician needs to set two levels of pressures: IPAP and EPAP (Figure 10-2, bottom). By using two levels of positive airway pressure, the clinician can influence the delivered tidal volume and minute ventilation as well as the functional residual capacity. Widening or narrowing the gradient between IPAP and EPAP will directly impact the delivered tidal volume and minute ventilation. An increased gradient results in increases of tidal volume and minute ventilation and vice versa. Selecting an appropriate EPAP is equivalent to selecting a CPAP or PEEP level and has the physiological effect of increasing the functional residual lung capacity or end-expiratory lung volume and subsequently improving oxygenation. At the same time, both IPAP and EPAP prevent airway collapse and

serve as a variable pneumatic stent for maintaining the patency of the upper airway in obstructive sleep apnea patients.[20,21] Usually BiPAP machines can function as CPAP machines whenever IPAP and EPAP are set equally; however, the opposite is not true. These devices deliver a low CPAP in expiration (EPAP), which cycles with a higher pressure that assists inspiration (IPAP).

In general, when used to treat obstructive sleep apnea, most BiPAP devices operate in three different modes:

1. *Spontaneous mode:* In this mode the device triggers IPAP when the flow sensors detect spontaneous inspiratory efforts and then the device cycles back to EPAP. This would be classified as PC-CSV.
2. *Timed mode:* In this mode the IPAP/EPAP cycling is purely device triggered at a set rate, typically expressed in breaths per minute (BPM). This would be classified as PC-CMV.

TABLE 10-1
Specifications of Currently Available CPAP Devices for Patient with Obstructive Sleep Apnea Syndrome

Manufacturer	CareFusion	CareFusion	DeVilbiss Healthcare, Inc.	DeVilbiss Healthcare, Inc.	DeVilbiss Healthcare, Inc.	evo Medical Solutions	evo Medical Solutions	evo Medical Solutions	evo Medical Solutions	Fisher & Paykel Healthcare, Inc.	Fisher & Paykel Healthcare, Inc.	Fisher & Paykel Healthcare, Inc.	Fisher & Paykel Healthcare, Inc.
Model	PureSom	PureSom CPAP Plus	IntelliPAP Standard	IntelliPAP Standard Plus	IntelliPAP AutoAdjust	RemRest 901	RemRest 903	Comfort CPAP 803	ComfortPAP Auto 804	SleepStyle 200 HC231	SleepStyle 200 HC232	SleepStyle 200 HC233	SleepStyle 200 HC234
Modes	CPAP	CPAP	CPAP	CPAP	CPAP, AutoAdjust	CPAP	CPAP	CPAP	CPAP, Auto	CPAP	CPAP	CPAP	CPAP
Controls													
Pressure, cm H$_2$O	4–18	4–18	3–20	3–20	3–20	3.5–20	3.5–20	4–20	4–20	4–20	4–20	4–20	4–20
Pressure increments, cm H$_2$O	1	0.5	0.5	0.5	0.5	Not specified	Not specified	Not specified	Not specified	Not specified	Not specified	Not specified	Not specified
Pressure accuracy, cm H$_2$O	± 2	± 0.5	Not specified	Not specified	Not specified	Not specified	Not specified	Not specified	Not specified	Not specified	Not specified	Not specified	Not specified
Ramp time (min)	0–45 min (5 min increment)	0–45 min (5 min increment)	Not specified	Not specified	Not specified	Not specified	Not specified	0–45	0–45	Not specified	Not specified	Not specified	Not specified
Ramp starting pressure (cm H$_2$O)	4	3	Not specified	Not specified	Not specified	Not specified	Not specified	3	3–19	Not specified	Not specified	Not specified	Not specified
Leak compensation	NA	Not specified	Not specified	Not specified	Not specified	Not specified	Not specified	Not specified	Not specified	Not specified	Not specified	Not specified	Not specified
Panel lock	Yes	Yes	Yes	Yes	Yes	Yes	Yes	Yes	Yes	Yes	Yes	Yes	Yes
Expiratory release	NA	NA	NA	NA	NA	No	No	No	No	Not specified	Not specified	Not specified	Not specified
Monitored Parameters													
Apnea/ hypopnea index	No	Not specified	Not specified	Not specified	Not specified	No	No	No	No	Not specified	Not specified	Not specified	Not specified
Pressure	Yes	Yes	Yes	Yes	Yes	Yes	Yes	Yes	Yes	Yes	Yes	Yes	Yes
Leak %	No	Yes	No	Yes	Yes	Not specified	Yes	Yes	Yes	No	No	No	No
Patient compliance	Yes	Yes	Yes	Yes	Yes	No	Direct download to PC	Yes	Yes	Not specified	Not specified	Not specified	Not specified
Running time	Yes	Yes	Yes	Yes	Yes	No	Yes	Not specified	Not specified	Not specified	Not specified	Not specified	Not specified
Equipment Alarms													
Power failure	Yes	Yes	No	No	No	Yes	Yes	Yes	Yes	No	No	No	No
Fault	No	No	Visual	Visual	Visual	Yes	Yes	Yes	Yes	Yes	Yes	Yes	Yes
Mask alarm	No	No	No	Visual	Visual	No	Yes	Yes	Yes	No	No	No	No
Waveforms displayed	No	No	Through DeVilbiss software	Through DeVilbiss software	Through DeVilbiss software	Not specified	Not specified	Not specified	Not specified	No	No	No	No

	Fisher & Paykel Healthcare, Inc.	Fisher & Paykel Healthcare, Inc.	Fisher & Paykel Healthcare, Inc.	Fisher & Paykel Healthcare, Inc.	Philips Respironics, Inc.	Philips Respironics, Inc.	Philips Respironics, Inc.	ResMed	ResMed	ResMed	ResMed	ResMed	ResMed	ResMed
	SleepStyle 200 HC236	SleepStyle 200 HC238	SleepStyle 600 HC604	SleepStyle 600 HC608	System One REMstar Plus	System One REMstar Pro	System One REMstar Auto	S8 Escape II	S8 Escape II Auto	S8 AutoSet Spirit II	S9 Escape	S9 Escape Auto	S9 Elite	S9 AutoSet
	CPAP	CPAP	CPAP	CPAP	CPAP	CPAP	CPAP, Auto	CPAP	CPAP, Auto	CPAP, Auto	CPAP	CPAP, Auto	CPAP	CPAP, Auto
	4–20	4–20	4–20	4–20	4–20	4–20	4–20	4–20	4–20	4–20	4–20	4–20	4–20	4–20
	Not specified	Not specified	Not specified	Not specified	Not specified	Not specified	Not specified	Not specified	Not specified	Not specified	Not specified	Not specified	Not specified	Not specified
	Not specified	Not specified	Not specified	Not specified	Not specified	Not specified	Not specified	Not specified	Not specified	Not specified	Not specified	Not specified	Not specified	Not specified
	Not specified	Not specified	Not specified	Not specified	0–45	0–45	0–45	0–45	0–45	0–45	0–45	0–45	0–45	0–45
	Not specified	Not specified	Not specified	Not specified	4	4	4	Not specified	Not specified	Not specified	Not specified	Not specified	Not specified	Not specified
	Not specified	Not specified	Not specified	Not specified	Yes	Yes	Yes	Automatic	No	Automatic	Automatic	Automatic	Automatic	Automatic
	Yes	Yes	Yes	Yes	Yes	Yes	Yes	Yes	Yes	Yes	Yes	Yes	Yes	Yes
	Not specified	Not specified	Not specified	Not specified	Yes	Yes	Yes	Yes	Yes	Yes	Yes	Yes	Yes	Yes
	Not specified	Not specified	Not specified	Not specified	Yes	Yes	Yes	Yes	Yes	Yes	No	No	Yes	Yes
	Yes	Yes	Yes	Yes	Yes	Yes	Yes	Yes	Yes	Yes	Yes	Yes	Yes	Yes
	No	No	No	No	Yes	Yes	Yes	No	No	Yes	No	No	Yes	Yes
	Not specified	Not specified	Not specified	Not specified	Yes	Yes	Yes	Yes	Yes	Yes	No	No	Yes	Yes
	Not specified	Not specified	Not specified	Not specified	Yes	Yes	Yes	No	No	Yes	No	No	Yes	Yes
	No	No	No	No	Not specified	Not specified	Not specified	Not specified	Not specified	Not specified	Not specified	Not specified	Not specified	Not specified
	Yes	Yes	Yes	Yes	Not specified	Not specified	Not specified	Not specified	Not specified	Not specified	Not specified	Not specified	Not specified	Not specified
	No	No	No	No	Yes	Yes	Yes	Yes	Yes	Yes	Yes	Yes	Yes	Yes
	No	No	No	No	Yes, on software	Yes, on software	Yes, on software	Yes, on software	Yes, on software	Yes, on software	Yes, on software	Yes, on software	Yes, on software	Yes, on software

(continues)

TABLE 10-1
Specifications of Currently Available CPAP Devices for Patient with Obstructive Sleep Apnea Syndrome (*Continued*)

Manufacturer	CareFusion	CareFusion	DeVilbiss Healthcare, Inc.	DeVilbiss Healthcare, Inc.	DeVilbiss Healthcare, Inc.	evo Medical Solutions	evo Medical Solutions	evo Medical Solutions	evo Medical Solutions	Fisher & Paykel Healthcare, Inc.	Fisher & Paykel Healthcare, Inc.	Fisher & Paykel Healthcare, Inc.	Fisher & Paykel Healthcare, Inc.
Model	PureSom	PureSom CPAP Plus	IntelliPAP Standard	IntelliPAP Standard Plus	IntelliPAP AutoAdjust	RemRest 901	RemRest 903	Comfort CPAP 803	ComfortPAP Auto 804	SleepStyle 200 HC231	SleepStyle 200 HC232	SleepStyle 200 HC233	SleepStyle 200 HC234
Display type	LCD	LCD	LCD	LCD	LCD	Not specified	LCD	LCD	LCD	LCD, LED	LCD, LED	LCD, LED	LCD, LED
Noise level, dBA	< 30	< 30	26 at 10 cm H_2O	26 at 10 cm H_2O	26 at 10 cm H_2O	< 30	< 30	< 30	< 30	≤ 30	≤ 30	≤ 30	≤ 30
Air filter	Yes	Yes	Yes	Yes	Yes	Yes	Yes	Yes	Yes	Yes	Yes	Yes	Yes
Altitude adjustment	Not specified	Not specified	Automatic	Automatic	Automatic	No	Automatic	Automatic	Automatic	Not specified	Not specified	Not specified	Not specified
PC compatible	No	No	Yes	Yes	Yes	Not specified	Yes	Not specified	Not specified	Yes	Yes	Yes	Yes
Data storage (hrs)	9999.9	9999.9	Not specified	Not specified	Not specified	No	Time since last reset	No	Yes	Not specified	Not specified	Not specified	Not specified
Software	NA	NA	Yes	Yes	Yes	No	Yes	No	No	Windows 95 or later	Windows 95 or later	Windows 95 or later	Windows 95 or later

Accessories

Humidifier	Optional	Optional	Optional	Optional	Optional	Optional	Optional	Optional	Optional	Conversion kit	Conversion kit	Integrated	Integrated
Power requirements, VAC	100V–240V, 50/60 Hz	100V–240V, 50/60 Hz	100–240, 50/60 Hz	100–240, 50/60 Hz	100–240, 50/60 Hz	100–240, 50–60 Hz	100–240, 50–60 Hz	100–240, 50–60 Hz	100–240, 50–60 Hz	110–115, 220–240	110–115, 220–240	110–115, 220–240	110–115, 220–240
DC input	NA	NA	12 VDC	12 VDC	12 VDC	12 VDC	12 VDC	12 VDC	12 VDC	Yes	Yes	Yes	Yes

Battery

Type	None	None	None	None	None	None	None	None	None	None	None	None	None
Operating time, hr	NA	NA	NA	NA	NA	NA	NA	NA	NA	NA	NA	NA	NA
Rechargeable	NA	NA	NA	NA	NA	NA	NA	NA	NA	NA	NA	NA	NA
Recharge time, hr	NA	NA	NA	NA	NA	NA	NA	NA	NA	NA	NA	NA	NA
H × W × D, in	3.9 × 5.8 × 5	3.9 × 5.8 × 5	6.4 × 6.5 × 8.4	6.4 × 6.5 × 8.4	6.4 × 6.5 × 8.4	4.7 × 8.6 × 9.4	4.7 × 8.6 × 9.4	5.7 × 5.1 × 3.9	5.8 × 5 × 3.9	5.3 × 6.5 × 11.6	5.3 × 6.5 × 11.6	5.3 × 6.5 × 11.6	5.3 × 6.5 × 11.6
Weight, lb	1.76	1.76	4.45 with humidifier	4.45 with humidifier	4.45 with humidifier	< 5 lb	< 5 lb	3.63	2.13	5	5	5	5
Operating conditions	41°F to 95°F; 15% to 95% relative humidity	41°F to 95°F; 15% to 95% relative humidity	Not specified	Not specified	Not specified	Not specified	Not specified	Not specified	Not specified	Not specified	Not specified	Not specified	Not specified
Green features	None specified	None specified	None specified	None specified	None specified	None specified	None specified	None specified	None specified	None specified	None specified	None specified	None specified

NA: Not Applicable

Fisher & Paykel Healthcare, Inc.	Fisher & Paykel Healthcare, Inc.	Fisher & Paykel Healthcare, Inc.	Fisher & Paykel Healthcare, Inc.	Philips Respironics, Inc.	Philips Respironics, Inc.	Philips Respironics, Inc.	ResMed	ResMed	ResMed	ResMed	ResMed	ResMed	ResMed
SleepStyle 200 HC236	SleepStyle 200 HC238	SleepStyle 600 HC604	SleepStyle 600 HC608	System One REMstar Plus	System One REMstar Pro	System One REMstar Auto	S8 Escape II	S8 Escape II Auto	S8 AutoSet Spirit II	S9 Escape	S9 Escape Auto	S9 Elite	S9 AutoSet
LCD, LED	LCD, LED	LCD, LED	LCD, LED	LCD	LCD	LCD	LCD	LCD	LCD	LCD	LCD	LCD	LCD
≤ 30	≤ 30	≤ 30	≤ 30	< 30	< 30	< 30	26	26	24	24	24	24	24
Yes	Yes	Yes	Yes	Yes	Yes	Yes	Yes	Yes	Yes	Yes	Yes	Yes	Yes
Not specified	Not specified	Not specified	Not specified	Manual	Automatic	Automatic	Automatic	Automatic	Automatic	Automatic	Automatic	Automatic	Automatic
Yes	Yes	Yes	Yes	Yes, with SD card	Yes, with SD card	Yes, with SD card	Yes	Yes	Yes	Yes	Yes	Yes	Yes
Not specified	Not specified	Not specified	Not specified	> 8760 with SD card	> 8760 with SD card	> 8760 with SD card	SD card	SD card	SD card	SD card	SD card	SD card	SD card
Windows 95 or later	Windows 95 or later	Windows 95 or later	Windows 95 or later	Yes	Yes	Yes	Yes	Yes	Yes	Yes	Yes	Yes	Yes
Conversion kit	Integrated	Integrated	Integrated	Optional	Optional	Optional	Integrated	Integrated	Integrated	Integrated	Integrated	Integrated	Integrated
110–115, 220–240	110–115, 220–240	110–115, 220–240	110–115, 220–240	100–240, 50/60 Hz	100–240, 50/60 Hz	100–240, 50/60 Hz	100–240, 50/60 Hz	100–240, 50/60 Hz	100–240, 50/60 Hz	100–240, 50/60 Hz	100–240, 50/60 Hz	100–240, 50/60 Hz	100–240, 50/60 Hz
Yes	Yes	Yes	Yes	Yes	Yes	Yes	Yes	No	Yes	Yes	Yes	Yes	Yes
None	None	None	None	Optional	Optional	Optional	Not specified	Not specified	Not specified	30W or 90W power supply unit	30W or 90W power supply unit	30W or 90W power supply unit	30W or 90W power supply unit
NA	NA	NA	NA	Not specified	Not specified	Not specified	Not specified	Not specified	Not specified	Not specified	Not specified	Not specified	Not specified
NA	NA	NA	NA	Not specified	Not specified	Not specified	Not specified	Not specified	Not specified	Not specified	Not specified	Not specified	Not specified
NA	NA	NA	NA	Not specified	Not specified	Not specified	Not specified	Not specified	Not specified	Not specified	Not specified	Not specified	Not specified
5.3 × 6.5 × 11.6	5.3 × 6.5 × 11.6	10.7 × 6.7 × 6.9	10.7 × 6.7 × 6.9	4 × 5.5 × 7	4 × 5.5 × 7	4 × 5.5 × 7	4.5 × 6.6 × 5.8	4.6 × 6.5 × 5.7	4.5 × 6.6 × 5.8	3.4 × 5.6 × 6.1	3.4 × 5.6 × 6.1	3.4 × 5.6 × 6.1	3.4 × 5.6 × 6.1
	5	3.4	3.4	3	3	3	2.9	2.9	3.1	1.8	1.8	1.8	1.8
Not specified	Not specified	Not specified	Not specified	Not specified	Not specified	Not specified	41°F to 95°F; 10% to 95% relative humidity	41°F to 95°F; 10% to 95% relative humidity	41°F to 97°F; 10% to 95% relative humidity	41°F to 95°F; 10% to 95% relative humidity	41°F to 95°F; 10% to 95% relative humidity	41°F to 95°F; 10% to 95% relative humidity	41°F to 95°F; 10% to 95% relative humidity
None specified	None specified	None specified	None specified	None specified	None specified	None specified	None specified	None specified	None specified	None specified	None specified	None specified	None specified

3. *Spontaneous/timed mode:* In this mode, the patient receives the therapy as if he or she is in the spontaneous mode and the device triggers to IPAP on the patient's inspiratory effort. However, in spontaneous/timed mode a "backup" rate is also set to ensure that the patient still receives a minimum number of breaths per minute if he or she fails to breathe spontaneously. This would be classified as PC-IMV.

One of the major complains of OSA patients is the difficulty in falling asleep when using BiPAP, particularly at high therapeutic prescribed pressure levels. Therefore, most BiPAP devices are equipped with a Ramp feature for a gradual increase to the prescribed pressure if the patient does not immediately fall asleep. The pressure gradually rises to the prescribed level over a period of time that can be adjusted by the clinician and/or patient.

Autotitration

Patients who have difficulty complying with traditional sleep therapy that uses fixed levels of pressure during CPAP or BiPAP can benefit from a special feature that autotitrates the prescribed pressure levels and applies the most appropriate levels for a well-tolerated, comfortable yet efficient treatment. This is usually accomplished with a proactive, multilevel algorithm that analyzes several parameters to monitor and respond to a patient's breathing pattern. With autotitration and with detection of flow limitation or hypopnea, the device slowly increases or decreases IPAP while monitoring for limitations or improvements in the flow signals. This will ensure that effective therapy is maintained at the minimal pressure and yet maximum therapeutic levels are obtained.[22,23] Furthermore, when snoring or apneas are detected, EPAP will be quickly but smoothly increased to eliminate the event. Finally, with the presence of elevated leak, the IPAP level is lowered improve mask seal and decrease the leak.

Memory/Information Storage

Similar to CPAP devices, BiPAP devices are equipped with memory/information storage capability for analysis and interpretation by the clinician. With the use of appropriate software, data that are usually stored on memory cards can be downloaded to allow the clinician to verify treatment effectiveness. The comprehensive statistical analysis of all relevant variables will help the clinician to optimize the patient's compliance and response to the therapy.

Cleaning and Maintenance

BiPAP devices can be cleaned and maintained similar to CPAP devices. See the previous section on cleaning and maintenance of CPAP devices.

Currently Available Devices

BiPAP devices are considered the main devices for providing noninvasive ventilator support; however, they can be used for patients with obstructive sleep apnea syndrome and might provide some advantages in terms of increased comfort and patient's compliance whenever high pressure levels are needed.[21,24] **Table 10-2** shows the currently available BiPAP devices in the U.S. market that are intended for primary use on OSA patients, along with their technical specifications.

Patient Interface Devices

The selection of an interface device is a very crucial component for the success of positive airway pressure therapy in OSA patients.[25–27] Once the pressure level is selected, the attention should be directed to selecting the appropriate interface that will optimize the therapy and increase the chance of success by minimizing leaks and loss of pressure as well as side effects (e.g., claustrophobia, nasal and facial skin breakdowns and ulcerations). The more comfortable the patient is with his or her interface, the higher the chance for increased therapy compliance and successful outcome.[25–27]

In general there is no ideal interface for all patients; every patient should be fitted separately for his or her own interface. However, five important criteria should be considered when searching for a specific patient's ideal interface: amount of air leakage, pressures from cushion and headgear, range of sleep positions, skin irritation, and noise. The clinicians and the patient have to try an array of interfaces that fall under three major categories: nasal masks, oral–nasal masks, and full face masks. A fourth, recent development has been the use of a helmet.

> *Nasal masks:* Nasal masks are the simplest interfaces. They cover the patient's nose, with major contact points at the patient's forehead or nasal bridge (**Figure 10-6**). These masks might not be suitable for patients who are mouth-breathers or patients with severe nasal congestion because significant leaks will occur through the mouth that will prevent the implementation of adequate pressure to the airways. Historically, chin straps that ensure adequate mouth closure were used with nasal masks. A wide range of nasal masks are provided by each manufacturer to meet the requirements of a variety of patients. The currently available nasal masks along with their specifications are presented in **Table 10-3**.
>
> *Oral–nasal masks:* Oral–nasal masks cover the patient's mouth and nose (**Figure 10-7**). These interfaces are more suitable for patients who are unable to keep their mouth closed during sleep or for patients who are prescribed a high level of pressure for their obstructive sleep apnea syndrome. The currently available nasal masks along with their specifications are presented in **Table 10-4**.

TABLE 10-2
Specifications of Currently Available BiPAP Devices for Patients with Obstructive Sleep Apnea Syndrome

Manufacturer	DeVilbiss Healthcare, Inc.	DeVilbiss Healthcare, Inc.	Philips Respironics, Inc.	Philips Respironics, Inc.	ResMed
Model	IntelliPAP Bilevel S	IntelliPAP AutoBilevel	System One BiPAP Auto	System One BiPAP autoSV Advanced	AutoSet CS-A
Modes	BiPAP	BiPAP, Auto	BiPAP	BiPAP	BiPAP, Auto
Controls					
Inspiratory					
Time, sec	NA	NA	Not specified	0.5–3	Not specified
Pressure, cm H$_2$O	3–25 (0.5 increments)	3–25 (0.5 increments)	4–25	4–25	4–30
Trigger sensitivity	1–10, increments of 1	1–10, increments of 1	Automatic	Automatic	Automatic
Expiratory					
Pressure, cm H$_2$O	3–25	3–25	4–IPAP	4–25	4–30
Trigger Sensitivity	1–10, increments of 1	1–10, increments of 1	Automatic	Automatic	Automatic
Rate, bpm	NA	NA	Not specified	4–30	Automatic
Ramp Time (min)	Not specified	Not specified	0–45 (5 min increments)	0–45 (5 min increments)	0–45
Starting Ramp Pressure	Not specified	Not specified	4 to EPAP	4 to EPAP	Not specified
Trigger Sensitivity	Yes	Yes	Yes	Yes	Yes
Leak Sensitivity	NA	NA	Not specified	Not specified	Not specified
Leak Compensation	Automatic	Automatic	Yes	Yes	Yes
Panel Lock	Yes	Yes	Yes	Yes	Yes
Monitored Parameters					
Respiratory rate	Not specified	Not specified	Yes	Yes	Yes
Inspiratory pressure	Yes	Yes	Yes	Yes	Yes
Expiratory pressure	Yes	Yes	Yes	Yes	Yes
Leak %	Not specified	Not specified	Yes	Yes	Yes
Patient's compliance	Not specified	Not specified	Yes	Yes	Yes

(continues)

TABLE 10-2
Specifications of Currently Available BiPAP Devices for Patients with Obstructive Sleep Apnea Syndrome *(Continued)*

Manufacturer	DeVilbiss Healthcare, Inc.	DeVilbiss Healthcare, Inc.	Philips Respironics, Inc.	Philips Respironics, Inc.	ResMed
Equipment Alarms					
Power failure	No	No	Not specified	Not specified	Yes
Fault	Visual	Visual	Yes	Yes	Yes
Mask alarm	Visual	Visual	Yes	Yes	Yes
Other alarms	None	None	None specified	None specified	High leak, low minute ventilation
Waveforms displayed	Through SmartLink DeVilbiss software	Through SmartLink DeVilbiss software	Yes, on software	Yes, on software	Yes
Display type	Backlit LCD	Backlit LCD	LCD	LCD	Color screen
Noise level, dBA	26 at 10 cm H_2O	26 at 10 cm H_2O	< 30	< 30	26
Air filter	Yes	Yes	Yes	Yes	Yes
Data storage	Not specified	Not specified	Yes (SD card)	Yes (SD card)	Yes
PC compatible	Yes	Yes	Yes, with SD card	Yes	Yes
Software	SmartCode and SmartLink Therapy Management software, DeVilbiss software	SmartCode and SmartLink Therapy Management software, DeVilbiss software	Encore Pro/Encore Basic	Encore Pro/Encore Basic	ResScan
Accessories					
Humidifier	Optional, integrated	Optional, integrated	Optional, integrated	Optional, integrated	Optional, integrated
Altitude adjustment	Automatic	Automatic	Automatic	Automatic	Automatic
Power requirements, VAC	100–240, 50/60 Hz	100–240, 50/60 Hz	100–240, 50/60 Hz	100–240, 50/60 Hz	110–240, 50/60 Hz
Battery	12 VDC capable	12 VDC capable	12 VDC capable	12 VDC capable	12 VDC capable
H × W × L, in	6.4 × 6.5 × 8.4	6.4 × 6.5 × 8.4	4 × 5.5 × 7	4 × 5.5 × 7	3.5 × 6.9 × 6.1
Weight, lb	4.45 (with humidifier)	4.45 (with humidifier)	3 without humidifier	3 without humidifier	4.6
Green features	None specified	None specified	None specified	None specified	None specified
Compliance with Federal Aviation Administration	Not specified	Not specified	Not specified	Not specified	Yes

NA: Not Applicable

TABLE 10-3
Specifications of Currently Available Nasal Masks Used with Sleep Apnea Devices

Manufacturer	Forehead Support	Adjustable Fitting	Rotational Connection with Circuit	Integrated Venting Port	Integrated Oxygen Port	Headgear Clips	Swivel	Cushion	Replaceable Cushion	Latex Free
AG Industries										
Sopora	Yes	No	Yes	Yes	Yes	Yes	Yes	Silicone	Yes	Yes
CareFusion										
Advantage Series Nasal Mask	Yes	Not specified	Yes	Yes	Yes	No	Yes	Silicone	Not specified	Yes
IQ	No	Yes	Yes	Not specified	Not specified	No	Yes	Gel	No	Yes
MiniMe	No	Yes	Yes	Not specified	Not specified	No	Yes	Gel	No	Yes
Phantom	No	Yes	No	Yes	Yes	No	Yes	Gel	No	Yes
Circadiance										
SleepWeaver	No	No	No	Yes	No	No	Yes	Soft Cloth	No	Yes
DeVilbiss Healthcare										
EasyFit	Yes	Yes	Yes	Yes	Not specified	Yes	Yes	Silicone	Yes	Yes
EasyFit SilkGel	Yes	Yes	Yes	Yes	Not specified	Yes	Yes	Gel	Yes	Yes
FlexSet	Yes	Yes	Yes	Yes	Not specified	Yes	Yes	Silicone & Gel	Yes	Yes
Innova	No	Yes	Yes	Yes	Not specified	Yes	Yes	Gel	No	Yes
Serenity	Yes	Yes	Yes	Yes	Not specified	Yes	Yes	Silicone & Gel	Yes	Yes
SomnoPlus	Yes	Yes	Yes	Yes	Yes	Yes	Yes	Silicone	Yes	Yes
evo Medical Solutions										
ComfortFit Nasal Deluxe+	Yes	No	Yes	Yes	Yes	Yes	No	Silicone	Not specified	Yes
ComfortFit Nasal Deluxe+ EZ	Yes	No	Yes	Yes	Yes	Yes	No	Silicone	Not specified	Yes

(continues)

TABLE 10-3
Specifications of Currently Available Nasal Masks Used with Sleep Apnea Devices (Continued)

Manufacturer	Forehead Support	Adjustable Fitting	Rotational Connection with Circuit	Integrated Venting Port	Integrated Oxygen Port	Headgear Clips	Swivel	Cushion	Replaceable Cushion	Latex Free
Fisher & Paykel Healthcare										
Acclaim 2	Yes	Yes	No	Yes	Not specified	Yes	Not specified	Silicone	Not specified	Yes
Eson	No	Yes	Yes	Yes	No	Yes	Yes	Silicone	Not specified	Yes
FlexiFit 405/406/407	No	No	Yes	Yes	No	Yes	Yes	Silicone	Not specified	Yes
FreeMotion	Yes	No	Yes	Not specified	Not specified	Yes	Yes	Silicone	Not specified	Yes
LadyZest Q	Yes	No	Yes	Yes	No	Yes	Yes	Foam/Silicone	Yes	Yes
Zest	Yes	No	Yes	Yes	No	Yes	Yes	Foam/Silicone	Yes	Yes
Zest Q	Yes	No	Yes	Yes	No	Yes	Yes	Foam/Silicone	Yes	Yes
GE Health Products, Inc.										
John Bunn CPAP Mask	Yes	No	Yes	Yes	Yes	No	No	Silicone	No	Yes
Philips Respironics										
ComfortClassic	Yes	No	Yes	Yes	Yes	Yes	Yes	Silicone	No	Yes
ComfortFusion	Yes	Yes	Yes	Yes	Yes	Yes	Yes	Silicone	Yes	Yes
ComfortGel	Yes	Yes	Yes	Yes	Yes	Yes	Yes	Gel	Yes	Yes
EasyLife	Yes	Yes	Yes	Yes	Not specified	Yes	Yes	Silicone	Yes	Yes
ProfileLite	Yes	No	Yes	Yes	Yes	Yes	Yes	Gel	No	Yes
TrueBlue	Yes	No	Yes	Yes	Not specified	Yes	No	Gel	Yes	Yes
Wisp	No	No	Yes	Yes	Not specified	Yes	No	Silicone	Yes	Yes

TABLE 10-3
Specifications of Currently Available Nasal Masks Used with Sleep Apnea Devices (*Continued*)

Manufacturer	Forehead Support	Adjustable Fitting	Rotational Connection with Circuit	Integrated Venting Port	Integrated Oxygen Port	Headgear Clips	Swivel	Cushion	Replaceable Cushion	Latex Free
Pediatric										
Profile Life Youth	Yes	No	Yes	Yes	Yes	Yes	Yes	Gel	No	Yes
Small Child Contour	Yes	No	Yes	Yes	Yes	Yes	No	Silicone	No	Yes
Small Child Profile Lite	Yes	No	Yes	Yes	Yes	Yes	Yes	Gel	No	Yes
ResMed										
Mirage Activa	Yes	Yes	Yes	Yes	Yes	Yes	Yes	Silicone	Yes	Yes
Mirage Activa LT	Yes	Yes	Yes	Yes	Yes	Yes	Yes	Silicone	Yes	Yes
Mirage FX	Yes	No	Yes	Yes	Yes	No	No	Silicone	No	Yes
Mirage FX for Her	Yes	No	Yes	Yes	Yes	No	No	Silicone	No	Yes
Mirage Micro	Yes	Yes	Yes	Yes	Yes	Yes	Yes	Silicone	Yes	Yes
Mirage SoftGel	Yes	Yes	Yes	Yes	Yes	Yes	Yes	Silicone/Gel	Yes	Yes
Mirage Vista	No	NA	Yes	Yes	Yes	Yes	Yes	Silicone	Yes	Yes
Pediatric										
Mirage Kidsta	Yes	Yes	Yes	Yes	Yes	Yes	Yes	Silicone	Yes	Yes
Pixi	No	NA	Yes	Yes	Not specified	No	No	Silicone	Not specified	Yes

NA: Not Applicable

TABLE 10-4
Specifications of Currently Available Oral–Nasal Masks Used with Sleep Apnea Devices

Manufacturer	Forehead Support	Adjustable Fitting	Rotational Connection with Circuit	Integrated Venting Port	Integrated Oxygen Port	Headgear Clips	Swivel	Cushion	Replaceable Cushion	Latex Free
AG Industries										
Miran	Yes	No	Yes	Yes	Yes	Yes	Yes	Silicone	Yes	Yes
CareFusion										
Advantage Series Oronasal Masks	Yes	Yes	Yes	Yes	Yes	No	Yes	Silicone	Not specified	Yes
Mojo	Yes	Yes	Yes	Yes	Yes	Yes	Yes	Silicone	Not specified	Yes
DeVilbiss Healthcare										
EasyFit	Yes	Yes	Yes	Yes	Not specified	Yes	Yes	Silicone	Yes	Yes
EasyFit SilkGel	Yes	Yes	Yes	Yes	Not specified	Yes	Yes	Gel	Yes	Yes
V2	No	No	Yes	Yes	Not specified	Yes	Yes	Silicone	No	Yes
evo Medical Solutions										
ComfortFitFull Face	No	NA	Yes	Yes	Yes	Yes	No	Silicone	Not specified	Yes
ComfortFitFull Face Deluxe	No	NA	Yes	Yes	Yes	Yes	No	Silicone	Not specified	Yes
ComfortFitFull Face Deluxe+	Yes	No	Yes	Yes	Yes	Yes	No	Silicone	Not specified	Yes
ComfortFitFull Face Deluxe EZ	No	NA	Yes	Yes	Yes	Yes	No	Silicone	Not specified	Yes
Fisher & Paykel Healthcare										
FlexiFit 431/432	Yes	No	Yes	Yes	Not specified	Yes	Yes	Silicone	Yes	Yes
Forma	Yes	No	Yes	Yes	Not specified	Yes	Yes	Foam/Silicone	Not specified	Yes
FreeMotion	Yes	No	Yes	Yes	Yes	Yes	Yes	Silicone	Yes	Yes

TABLE 10-4
Specifications of Currently Available Oral–Nasal Masks Used with Sleep Apnea Devices (*Continued*)

Manufacturer	Forehead Support	Adjustable Fitting	Rotational Connection with Circuit	Integrated Venting Port	Integrated Oxygen Port	Headgear Clips	Swivel	Cushion	Replaceable Cushion	Latex Free
Hans Rudolph, Inc.										
V2 Mask	No	No	Yes	Yes	Yes	Yes	Yes	Silicone	No	Yes
Philips Respironics										
Amara	Yes	Yes	Yes	Yes	No	Yes	Yes	Silicone	Yes	Yes
ComfortFull 2	Yes	Yes	Yes	Yes	Yes	Yes	Yes	Silicone	No	Yes
ComfortGel Full	Yes	Yes	Yes	Yes	Yes	Yes	Yes	Gel	Yes	Yes
FullLife	No	NA	Yes	Yes	Not specified	Yes	Yes	Silicone	Yes	Yes
ResMed										
Mirage Liberty	No	NA	Yes	Yes	Yes	Yes	Yes	Silicone	Yes	Yes
Mirage Quattro	Yes	Yes	Yes	Yes	Yes	Yes	Yes	Silicone	Yes	Yes
Quattro Fx	No	NA	Yes	Yes	Yes	Yes	Yes	Silicone	Yes	Yes
InnoMed Tec/Respcare										
Hybrid	No	NA	Yes	Yes	Yes	Yes	Yes	Silicone	Not specified	Yes
Silent	Yes	Yes	Yes	Yes	Yes	No	Yes	Silicone	Not specified	Yes

NA: Not Applicable

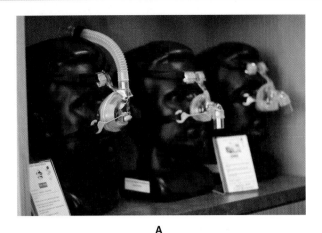

A

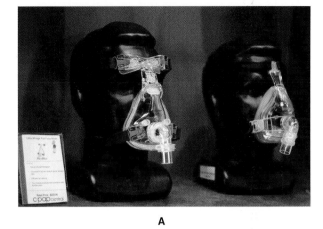

A

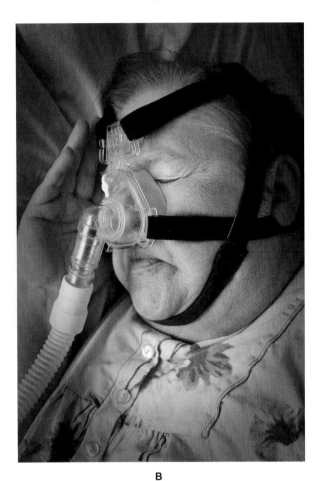

B

FIGURE 10-6 Types of nasal masks for CPAP and BiPAP devices.

Photo A courtesy of Rachel Tayse. Licensed under Creative Commons Attribution 2.0 Generic via Flickr https://www.flickr.com/photos/11921146@N03/6835826092. Photo B © Jonny Kristoffersson /iStockphoto.

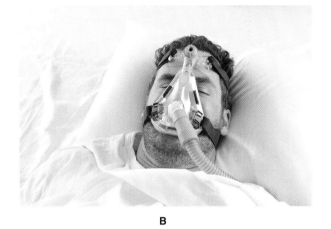

B

FIGURE 10-7 Types of oral–nasal masks for CPAP and BiPAP devices.

Photo A courtesy of Rachel Tayse. Licensed under Creative Commons Attribution 2.0 Generic via Flickr https://www.flickr.com/photos/11921146@N03/6981942677. Photo B © stockmachine/iStockphoto.

Full face masks: Full face masks are usually confused with oral–nasal masks; however, in addition to covering the patient's mouth and nose, these masks usually also cover the patient's eyes (**Figure 10-8**). The main purpose of a full face mask is to reduce the contact pressure exerted by nasal and oral–nasal masks at the patient's nasal bridge, thus eliminating the nasal bridge ulceration frequently seen with nasal and oral–nasal masks.[26] With full face masks, gentler pressure is spread over the patient's forehead with minimal risk for ulceration. On the down side, the full face mask is bulkier and may limit the patient's range of sleep positions. The currently available full face masks along with their specifications are presented in **Table 10-5**.

Helmet: A helmet is a patient interface device that covers the patient's head while making a seal at the neck level with the fixations below the armpits (**Figure 10-9**). This interface is mainly intended for use with positive airway pressure therapy (e.g., CPAP or BiPAP devices) in patients with cardiogenic pulmonary edema, COPD exacerbation, asthma, or acute respiratory distress syndrome. There is no evidence in the literature for the helmet to play a role in helping patients with obstructive sleep apnea devices. The technical specifications of this interface are indicated in Table 10-5.

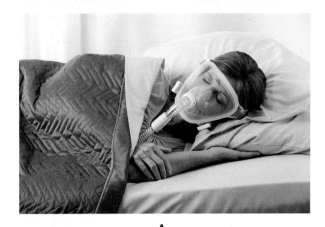

A

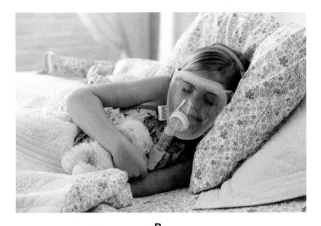

B

FIGURE 10-8 Types of full face masks for CPAP and BiPAP devices.
Photos courtesy of Philips Healthcare.

Almost all of these interfaces usually include an exhalation port and an adaptation for supplemental oxygen whenever needed. These interfaces are intended for a single patient's use, but reusable interfaces are available. Reusable interfaces should be well maintained and cleaned and/or disinfected as per the manufacturer's instructions because these devices tend to lose their efficiency with repetitive cleaning and disinfection.

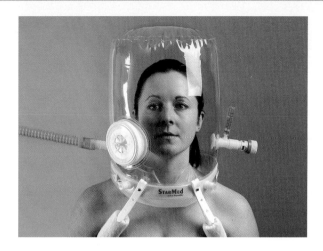

FIGURE 10-9 Helmet for CPAP and BiPAP devices.
Courtesy of Intersurgical Spa.

Also, it is advisable to involve the institutional infection control program in the process of cleaning and disinfection of the reusable interfaces.

Criteria for Selecting the Appropriate Device

With the availability of a wide range of sleep apnea devices and patient interfaces, it is becoming confusing and difficult for clinicians as well as patients to select the appropriate device. Several important issues should be considered. The technical performance of the device along with whether its clinical features meet the patient's therapeutic objectives and goals are paramount in deciding on a specific device. However, other factors are also important to consider for the final decision (see **Table 10-6**).

Humidification Issues

Not all patients will need some form of humidification during sleep therapy; however, sleep apnea devices should be capable of providing humidification during

TABLE 10-5
Specifications of Currently Available Full Face Masks and Helmet Used with Sleep Apnea Devices

Manufacturer	Forehead Support	Adjustable Fitting	Rotational Connection with Circuit	Integrated Venting Port	Integrated Oxygen Port	Headgear Clips	Swivel	Cushion	Replaceable Cushion	Latex Free
Philips Respironics										
FitLife	NA	NA	Yes	Yes	Yes	Yes	Yes	Silicone	No	Yes
Total Face Mask	NA	NA	Yes	Yes	Yes	Yes	Yes	Silicone	No	Yes
StarMed										
Starcase Helmet	NA	NA	No	Yes	Yes	NA	No	Plastic	NA	No

NA: Not applicable

TABLE 10-6
Criteria for Selecting the Appropriate Sleep Apnea Device

- Technical and clinical features
- Manufacturer's/supplier's support
- Range of compatible masks
- Flexibility for buying/rental
- Warranty
- Price
- Exchange possibility
- Support for humidification

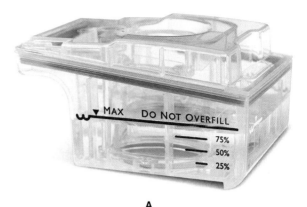

A

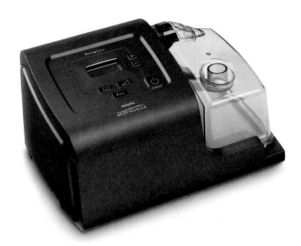

B

FIGURE 10-10 Stand-alone pass-over humidification devices (top) and CPAP/BiPAP devices equipped with integrated humidifiers (bottom).

Photos courtesy of Philips Healthcare.

therapy should the need arise. Usually this is indicated by a dry mouth, nose, or throat on the morning following the therapy.[28,29] Humidification during CPAP or BiPAP therapy is usually provided by a pass-over humidifier that can be heated or not. Most modern CPAP and BiPAP have the capability to integrate an active humidifier; otherwise, a stand-alone and simple pass-over humidifier can be used (**Figure 10-10**).

Instructions for Proper Use of CPAP/BiPAP Devices

Sleep apnea therapy and the use of sleep apnea devices start with adequate education and training of the patient and/or family members. Putting in the time and effort early on with sufficient training and interaction with patients will prevent future problems. The patient should be adequately and clearly instructed on all aspects of the therapy: how to operate the device, how to wear the interface, how to clean and maintain the device and interface, and how to troubleshoot and solve common simple problems that might arise as the patient is receiving the therapy.

Common Problems

Sleep apnea therapy is associated with problems that are usually simple and common. A list of these problems along with potential solutions is presented in **Table 10-7**.

References

1. Hiestand DM, Britz P, Goldman M, Phillips B. Prevalence of symptoms and risk of sleep apnea in the US population: Results from the National Sleep Foundation Sleep in America 2005 poll. *Chest.* 2006;130:780-786.
2. Simon S, Collop N. Latest advances in sleep medicine: Obstructive sleep apnea. *Chest.* 2012;142(6):1645-1651. doi: 10.1378/chest.12-2391.
3. Piper AJ, Stewart DA. An overview of nasal CPAP therapy in the management of obstructive sleep apnea. *Ear Nose Throat J.* 1999;78(10):776-778, 781-782, 784-790.
4. International Consensus Conferences in Intensive Care Medicine: Noninvasive positive pressure ventilation in acute respiratory failure. *Am J Respir Crit Care Med.* 2001;163:283-291.
5. Anstead M, Phillips B, Buch K. Tolerance and intolerance to continuous positive airway pressure. *Curr Opin Pulm Med.* 1998;4(6):351-354.
6. Calzia E, Bein T. Breath by breath, spontaneously or mechanically supported: Lessons from biphasic positive airway pressure (BIPAP). *Intensive Care Med.* 2004;30(5):744-745.
7. Mehta S, Hill NS. Noninvasive ventilation. *Am J Respir Crit Care Med.* 2001;163:540-577.
8. Kolodziej MA, Jensen L, Rowe B, Sin D. Systematic review of noninvasive positive pressure ventilation in severe stable COPD. *Eur Respir J.* 2007;30(2):293-306.
9. Veasey SC, Guilleminault C, Strohl KP, Sanders MH, Ballard RD, Magalang UJ. Medical therapy for obstructive sleep apnea: A review by the Medical Therapy for Obstructive Sleep Apnea Task Force of the Standards of Practice Committee of the American Academy of Sleep Medicine. *Sleep.* 2006;29:1036-1044.
10. Simon S, Collop N. Latest advances in sleep medicine: Obstructive sleep apnea. *Chest.* 2012;142(6):1645-1651.
11. Mannarino MR, Di Filippo F, Pirro M. Obstructive sleep apnea syndrome. *Eur J Intern Med.* 2012;23(7):586-593.

TABLE 10-7
Common Problems Seen with CPAP/BiPAP Sleep Therapy

Problems	Solutions
Wrong size or style of mask	Appropriate fitting and selection of mask
Trouble getting used to wearing the mask	Adequate demonstration and training
Difficulty breathing with forced high flow	Adequate training on use of ramp feature
Dry and stuffy nose	Use of humidifier
Claustrophobia	Appropriate selection of mask
Leaky masks	Adequate fixation of mask
Skin irritation or pressure sores	Using minimal pressure for adequate seal
Difficulty falling asleep while on therapy	Adequate training on use of ramp feature
Dry mouth	Use of humidifier
Eye irritation	Appropriate selection of mask or adequate seal at the nasal bridge
Unintentional removal of mask during sleep	Adequate fixation of interface
Annoyance by the device noise and mask	Appropriate selection of device; time and patience

12. Smith I, Lasserson TJ. Pressure modification for improving usage of continuous positive airway pressure machines in adultswith obstructive sleep apnoea. *Cochrane Database Syst Rev.*2009;4:CD003531. Update of *Cochrane Database Syst Rev.* 2004;(4):CD003531.

13. Massie Clifford A, McArdle N, Hart RW, Schmidt-Nowara WW, Lankford A, et al. Comparison between automatic and fixed positive airway pressure therapy in the home. *Am J Resp Crit Care Med.* 2003;167:20-23.

14. Aloia MS, Stanchina M, Arnedt JT, Malhorta A, Millman RP. Treatment adherence and outcomes in flexible vs standard continuous positive airway pressure therapy. *Chest.* 2005;127(6): 2085-2093.

15. Dolan DC, Okonkwo R, Gfullner F, Hansbrough JR, Strobel RJ, Rosenthal L. Longitudinal comparison study of pressure relief (C-flex) vs CPAP in OSA patients. *Sleep Breath.* 2009;13(1): 73-77.

16. Pepin JL, Muir JF, Gentina T, Dauvilliers Y, Tamisier R, Sapene M, et al. Pressure reduction during exhalation in sleep apnea patients treated by continuous positive airway pressure. *Chest.* 2009;136(2):490-497.

17. McCurdy BR. Noninvasive positive pressure ventilation for acute respiratory failure patients with chronic obstructive pulmonary disease (COPD): An evidence-based analysis. *Ont Health Technol Assess Ser.* 2012;12(8):1-102.

18. Charlesworth M, Elliott MW, Holmes JD. Noninvasive positive pressure ventilation for acute respiratory failure in delirious patients: Understudied, underreported, or underappreciated? A systematic review and meta-analysis. *Lung.* 2012;190(6):597-603.

19. Boldrini R, Fasano L, Nava S. Noninvasive mechanical ventilation. *Curr Opin Crit Care.* 2012;18(1):48-53.

20. Blau A, Minx M, Peter JG, Glos M, Penzel T, Baumann G, et al. Auto bi-level pressure relief-PAP is as effective as CPAP in OSA patients—a pilot study. *Sleep Breath.* 2012;16(3):773-779.

21. Randerath WJ, Nothofer G, Priegnitz C, Anduleit N, Treml M, Kehl V, et al. Long-term auto-servoventilation or constant positive pressure in heart failure and coexisting central with obstructive sleep apnea. *Chest.* 2012;142(2):440-447.

22. Allam JS, Olson EJ, Gay PC, Morgenthaler TI. Efficacy of adaptive servoventilation in treatment of complex and central sleep apnea syndromes. *Chest.* 2007;132(6):1839-1846.

23. Morgenthaler TI, Gay PC, Gordon N, Brown LK. Adaptive servoventilation versus noninvasive positive pressure ventilation for central, mixed, and complex sleep apnea syndromes. *Sleep.* 2007;30(4):468-475.

24. Gali B, Whalen FX Jr, Gay PC, Olson EJ, Schroeder DR, Plevak DJ, et al. Management plan to reduce risks in perioperative care of patients with presumed obstructive sleep apnea syndrome. *J Clin Sleep Med.* 2007;3(6):582-588.

25. Borel JC, Gakwaya S, Masse JF, Melo-Silva CA, Sériès F. Impact of CPAP interface and mandibular advancement device on upper airway mechanical properties assessed with phrenic nerve stimulation in sleep apnea patients. *Respir Physiol Neurobiol.* 2012;183(2):170-176.

26. Bachour A, Vitikainen P, Virkkula P, Maasilta P. CPAP interface: Satisfaction and side effects. *Sleep Breath.* 2013;17(2):667-672.

27. Parthasarathy S. Mask interface and CPAP adherence. *J Clin Sleep Med.* 2008;4(5):511-512.

28. Koutsourelakis I, Vagiakis E, Perraki E, Karatza M, Magkou C, Kopaka M, et al. Nasal inflammation in sleep apnoea patients using CPAP and effect of heated humidification. *Eur Respir J.* 2011;37(3):587-594.

29. Ruhle KH, Franke KJ, Domanski U, Nilius G. Quality of life, compliance, sleep and nasopharyngeal side effects during CPAP therapy with and without controlled heated humidification. *Sleep Breath.* 2011;15(3):479-485.

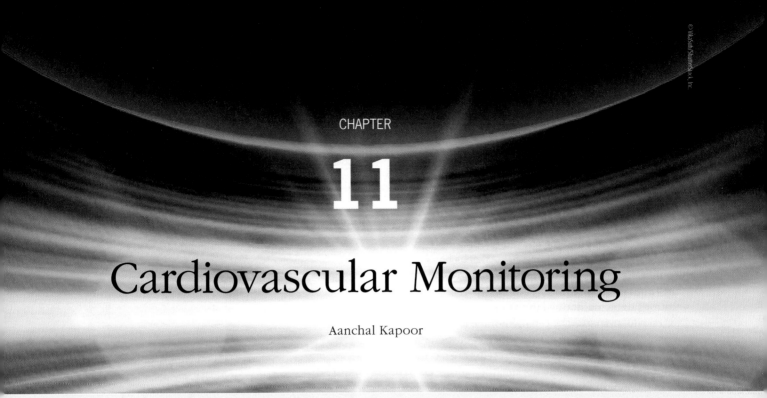

CHAPTER

11

Cardiovascular Monitoring

Aanchal Kapoor

CHAPTER OBJECTIVES

1. Explain the importance of cardiovascular monitoring in respiratory care.
2. Demonstrate the proper placement of ECG electrodes.
3. Describe the components of a vascular pressure monitoring system.
4. Describe the proper insertion and pressure readings obtained from a pulmonary artery catheter.
5. Describe the measurement of cardiac output.

KEY TERMS

Atrioventricular (AV) node
Cardiac output
Damping
Electrocardiogram (ECG)
Electrode
Frequency response

Pulmonary artery catheter (PAC)
Pulmonary artery wedge pressure (PAWP)
Flush test
Zeroing

Introduction

In the intensive care unit, the monitoring and assessment of cardiovascular function is essential. The technology used for cardiovascular monitoring ranges from recording the **electrocardiogram (ECG)** to measuring intravascular pressures and **cardiac output**. Hemodynamic monitoring becomes crucial in mechanically ventilated patients. Respiratory care practitioners should be familiar with the operation and troubleshooting of devices used for cardiorespiratory assessment. This chapter discusses the equipment and techniques commonly used for cardiovascular monitoring.

ECG Monitoring

An ECG is the graphic representation of electrical voltage generated by the muscular contraction and

relaxation of the heart examined by 11 leads, which allows capturing of heart rhythm in three dimensions. Einthoven's invention of the string galvanometer in 1901 provided a direct method for registering electrical activity of the heart. By 1910, use of the string galvanometer had emerged from the research laboratory into the clinic. Subsequently, the ECG became the first and most common bioelectric signal to be computer-processed and the most commonly used cardiac diagnostic tests.

Recent advances have extended the importance of the ECG. It is a vital test for determining the presence and severity of acute myocardial ischemia, localizing sites of origin and pathways of tachyarrhythmias, assessing therapeutic options for patients with heart failure, and identifying and evaluating patients with genetic diseases who are prone to arrhythmias.

Cardiac Conduction System

Electric activity in the heart is accomplished by a conduction system (**Figure 11-1**). Depolarization of the sinoatrial (SA) node, which is called the pacemaker of the heart, initiates the heartbeat. The wave of excitation spreads throughout the left and right atria and moves towards the **atrioventricular (AV) node**. Movement of impulse between the SA and AV nodes occurs through internodal conduction pathways. As the impulse travels through the AV node a delay of approximately 100 milliseconds occurs, which allows the atria to fully depolarize and contract before the ventricular excitation begins, thus allowing atrial emptying. From the AV node, the impulse spreads to the ventricular musculature via a high speed conduction system that starts at the bundle of His and then splits into right and left bundle branches, which further divide into a complex network of conducting fibers called Purkinje fibers. Excitation of ventricular muscles occurs from the inner endocardial surface and travels outward toward epicardial surfaces. Repolarization has the opposite polarity.

The Electrocardiograph

The electrical activity of the heart is monitored with a device called an electrocardiograph, which produces a graphical output, the electrocardiogram (ECG). The ECG is the final outcome of a complex series of physiologic and technologic processes. All cells have a cell membrane that separates the interior and exterior of the cell. The cell membrane allows different ion concentrations to be maintained in the intracellular space and extracellular space. The cell membrane is composed of a phospholipid bilayer, within which cholesterol molecules and proteins are found. Proteins are a critical component of the cell membrane; they allow selective movement of different ions at different times in the cardiac cycle. For the cardiac cells, voltage difference between the inside and outside of the cell is generated by sequential opening and closing of different ion channels. These currents are synchronized by cardiac activation and recovery sequences to generate a cardiac electrical field in and around the heart that varies with time during the cardiac cycle. This electrical field passes through numerous other structures, including the lungs, blood, and skeletal muscle, that perturb the cardiac electrical field. The currents reaching the skin are then detected by **electrodes** placed in specific locations on the extremities and torso that transduce ionic potentials into electrical impulses. The outputs of these leads are amplified, filtered, and displayed by a variety of devices to produce an electrocardiographic recording.

Continuous ECG Monitoring

The ECG is monitored in two basic ways: continuously and intermittently. Continuous monitoring is most often used in telemetry and intensive care units (**Figure 11-2**). This type of ECG monitoring requires only three electrodes—one negative polarity, one positive polarity, and one ground. The ECG is traced on a standardized grid. The individual boxes created by grids are 1 millimeter (mm) by 1 mm and one box (darker lines) is 5 mm by 5 mm. The horizontal axis on the paper depicts the time based on the graph display speed, which is commonly 25 mm/sec. At this speed, each 1-mm box represents 0.04 seconds and each 5-mm box represents 0.2 seconds. So, five of the 5-mm boxes are equivalent to 1 second. The vertical axis represents the signal amplitude and is measured in millivolts (mV). Standard ECG recordings use 10 mm (10 small or 2 large boxes) to represent 1 mV. The determination of

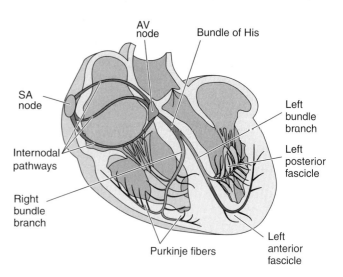

FIGURE 11-1 Electrical conduction system of the heart. The electrical signal normally starts at the sinus node, which causes the right and left atria to contract. The atrioventricular (AV) node is triggered next. The AV node sends a signal through the His/Purkinje system conduction pathways. The conduction pathways then signal the right and left ventricles to contract.

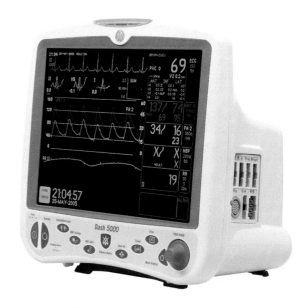

FIGURE 11-2 GE Dash 5000 patient monitor.
Used with permission of GE Healthcare.

time and voltage is important for detecting abnormalities in heart rate and rhythm.

Intermittent monitoring for diagnostic purposes uses more than three electrodes. The specific placement of the electrodes on the patient's chest are called *leads*. Lead I provides information about the left lateral wall of the heart (**Figure 11-3**). Leads II and III provide information about the inferior wall of the heart (**Figure 11-4** and **Figure 11-5**). The lead called the modified chest lead provides information about the anterior wall of the heart (**Figure 11-6**).

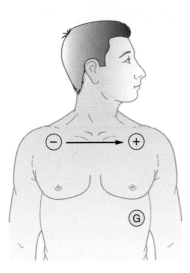

FIGURE 11-3 Location of chest electrodes for ECG lead I (G = ground).
Adapted from Aehlert B. *ACLS Quick Review Study Guide*. Mosby; 1994.

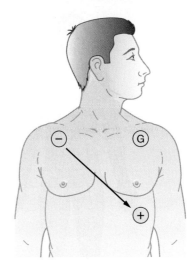

FIGURE 11-4 Location of chest electrodes for ECG lead II (G = ground).
Adapted from Aehlert B. *ACLS Quick Review Study Guide*. Mosby; 1994.

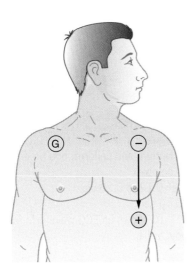

FIGURE 11-5 Location of chest electrodes for ECG lead III (G = ground).
Adapted from Aehlert B. *ACLS Quick Review Study Guide*. Mosby; 1994.

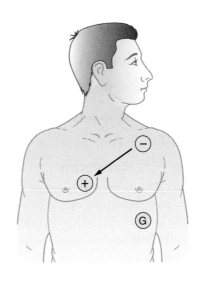

FIGURE 11-6 Location of chest electrodes for modified chest lead (G = ground).
Adapted from Aehlert B. *ACLS Quick Review Study Guide*. Mosby; 1994.

Intermittent ECG Monitoring

A more detailed view of cardiac electrical activity is often obtained using more electrodes and a portable electrocardiograph (**Figure 11-7**). Such devices are often seen in physician offices but are also used in emergency rooms as well as acute and intensive care settings.

Ten electrodes are used to generate a 12-lead ECG. Four electrodes are placed on the extremities (wrists and ankles) and six are placed on the chest (**Figure 11-8**). The 12 leads are divided into two groups: Six limb leads are called leads I, II, III, aV_R, aV_L, and aV_F. Six additional chest or precordial leads are called V_1, V_2, V_3, V_4, V_5, and V_6. Once the electrodes are placed, the ECG machine is activated. Modern ECG machines are fully automated

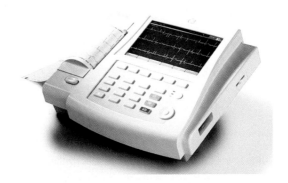

FIGURE 11-7 GE Mac 800 portable ECG machine.
Used with permission of GE Healthcare.

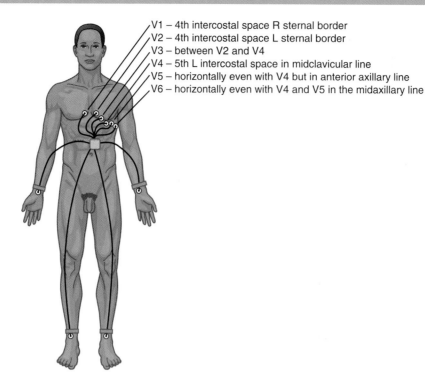

V1 – 4th intercostal space R sternal border
V2 – 4th intercostal space L sternal border
V3 – between V2 and V4
V4 – 5th L intercostal space in midclavicular line
V5 – horizontally even with V4 but in anterior axillary line
V6 – horizontally even with V4 and V5 in the midaxillary line

FIGURE 11-8 Placement of electrodes for 12-lead ECG.

and provide computer-interpreted analysis of adult and pediatric patients.

Interpreting ECG Waveforms

The following ECG patterns are the most important ones that respiratory therapists should be able to recognize at the bedside. The following information was adapted from Sing.[1]

Normal Sinus Rhythm

Rate: 60 to 100 beats/min
Rhythm: Regular
P waves: Upright and uniform, one preceding each QRS complex
PR interval: 0.12 to 0.20 sec
QRS: < 0.10 sec
Figure 11-9 shows a normal sinus rhythm.

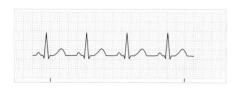

FIGURE 11-9 ECG waveform for normal sinus rhythm.
Reproduced from *Arrhythmia Recognition: The Art of Interpretation*, courtesy of Tomas B. Garcia, MD.

Sinus Bradycardia

Rate: < 60 beats/min
Rhythm: Regular
P waves: Upright and uniform, one preceding each QRS complex
PR interval: 0.12 to 0.20 sec
QRS: < 0.10 sec
Figure 11-10 shows an ECG waveform for sinus bradycardia.

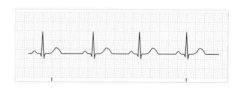

FIGURE 11-10 ECG waveform for sinus bradycardia.
Reproduced from *Arrhythmia Recognition: The Art of Interpretation*, courtesy of Tomas B. Garcia, MD.

Sinus Tachycardia

Rate: 100 to 160 beats/min
Rhythm: Regular
P waves: Upright and uniform, one preceding each QRS complex
PR interval: 0.12 to 0.20 sec
QRS: < 0.10 sec

Figure 11-11 shows an ECG waveform for sinus tachycardia.

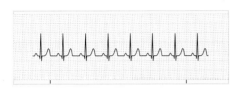

FIGURE 11-11 ECG waveform for sinus tachycardia.

Premature Atrial Complexes (PACs)

Rate: < 60 beats/min
Rhythm: Regular
P waves: Upright and uniform, one preceding each QRS complex
PR interval: 0.12 to 0.20 sec
QRS: < 0.10 sec
Figure 11-12 shows premature atrial complexes (PACs).

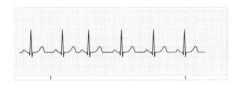

FIGURE 11-12 ECG waveform for premature atrial complexes (PACs).

Atrial Flutter

Rate: Atrial rate 250–350 beats/min, ventricular rate variable
Rhythm: Atrial rhythm regular, ventricular rhythm usually regular
P waves: Sawtooth flutter waves
PR interval: Not measurable
QRS: Usually < 0.10 sec but may be wider
Figure 11-13 shows atrial flutter.

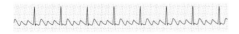

FIGURE 11-13 Atrial flutter.

Atrial Fibrillation

Rate: Atrial rate usually > 400 beats/min, ventricular rate variable
Rhythm: Atrial and ventricular rhythm very irregular

P waves: None identifiable
PR interval: None
QRS: Usually < 0.10 sec
Figure 11-14 shows atrial fibrillation.

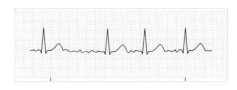

FIGURE 11-14 Atrial fibrillation.

Premature Ventricular Contractions

Rate: Atrial and ventricular rate depend on the underlying rhythm
Rhythm: Irregular
P waves: None identifiable
PR interval: None
QRS: > 0.12 sec, wide, T wave frequently in the opposite direction of QRS complex
Figure 11-15 shows premature ventricular contractions.

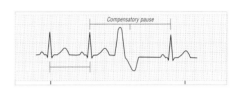

FIGURE 11-15 Premature ventricular contractions.

Ventricular Tachycardia

Rate: Atrial not discernable; ventricular 100–250 beats/min
Rhythm: Atrial not discernable; ventricular regular
P waves: If present, not related to QRS complexes
PR interval: None
QRS: > 0.12 sec
Figure 11-16 shows ventricular tachycardia.

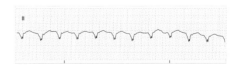

FIGURE 11-16 Ventricular tachycardia.

Ventricular Fibrillation

Rate: Cannot be determined
Rhythm: Rapid with no pattern
P waves: Not discernable
PR interval: Not discernable
QRS: Not discernable
Figure 11-17 shows ventricular fibrillation.

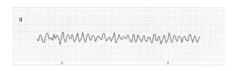

FIGURE 11-17 Ventricular fibrillation.
Reproduced from *Arrhythmia Recognition: The Art of Interpretation*, courtesy of Tomas B. Garcia, MD.

First Degree AV Block

Rate: Atrial and ventricular rates the same and within
    normal limits
Rhythm: Regular
P waves: Normal
PR interval: > 0.20 sec but constant
QRS: < 0.10 sec
Figure 11-18 shows first degree AV block.

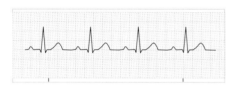

FIGURE 11-18 First degree AV block.
Reproduced from *Arrhythmia Recognition: The Art of Interpretation*, courtesy of Tomas B. Garcia, MD.

Second Degree AV Block

Rate: Atrial rate greater than ventricular but both within
    normal limits
Rhythm: Atrial regular, ventricular irregular
P waves: Normal, some P waves not followed by QRS
    complexes
PR interval: Lengthens with each cycle until P wave
    appears without QRS
QRS: < 0.10 sec but dropped periodically
Figure 11-19 shows second degree AV block.

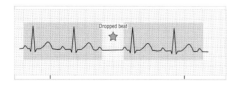

FIGURE 11-19 Second degree AV block.
Reproduced from *Arrhythmia Recognition: The Art of Interpretation*, courtesy of Tomas B. Garcia, MD.

Third Degree AV Block

Rate: Atrial rate greater than ventricular
Rhythm: Atrial regular, ventricular regular
P waves: Normal, some P waves not followed by QRS
    complexes
PR interval: None—the atria and ventricles beat
    independently
QRS: Narrow: junctional pacemaker; wide: ventricular
    pacemaker
Figure 11-20 shows third degree AV block.

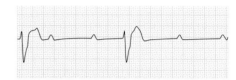

FIGURE 11-20 Third degree AV block.
Reproduced from *Arrhythmia Recognition: The Art of Interpretation*, courtesy of Tomas B. Garcia, MD.

Hemodynamic Monitoring

Hemodynamic monitoring includes invasive and non-invasive means for measuring vascular pressures and cardiac output. Indwelling monitoring catheters are used when continuous monitoring of blood pressure and cardiac output is required in intensive care settings or when frequent blood sampling is required, especially arterial blood gases. Blood pressure can be measured noninvasively.

Vascular Pressure Monitoring

Arterial blood pressure, when considered alone, is at best a crude indicator of a patient's hemodynamic state. The cardiac output, systemic vascular resistance, aortic impedance, and diastolic arterial blood volume all interact to determine arterial blood pressure. In addition, the sympathetic tone of blood vessels, which is regulated by the autonomic nervous system, adjusts for changes in body position, blood volume, and cardiac output. Pressure waveforms from the vascular monitoring system are helpful in diagnosing problems and provide information in the same fashion as the ECG or ventilator graphics. Continuous arterial blood pressure monitoring is indicated when rapid fluctuations of blood pressure are expected; when abrupt shifts in antihypertensives, vasodilators, or vasopressor therapy are anticipated; and in order to monitor response to therapy.

Noninvasive Arterial Pressure Monitoring

Several methods are used to measure blood pressure noninvasively, but two are most common to respiratory therapists. The auscultatory or Korotkoff method

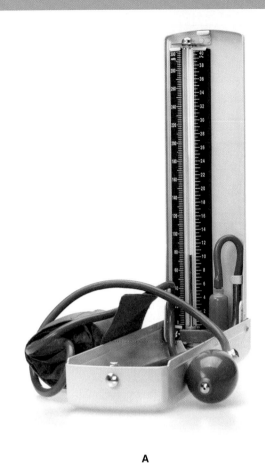

A

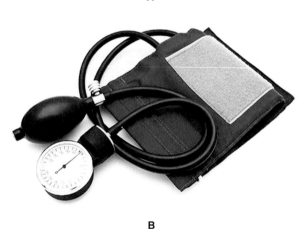

B

FIGURE 11-21 A. Mercury sphygmomanometer. B. Aneroid sphygmomanometer.

Photo A © iStock/Thinkstock. Photo B © Sergej Razvodovskij/Shutterstock

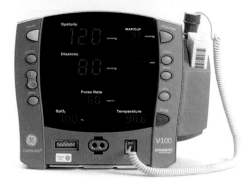

FIGURE 11-22 Automatic sphygmomanometer built into a device for taking vital signs.

Courtesy of General Electric Healthcare.

the stethoscope. The pressure in the cuff at this time is approximately the systolic blood pressure. As the cuff pressure continues to fall, the pulse sounds gradually diminish and finally disappear. The pressure in the cuff at the moment the sounds stop is considered the diastolic blood pressure. The device that comprises the cuff and the pressure gauge is called a sphygmomanometer (**Figure 11-21**).

Automated sphygmomanometers are often used on nursing floors when taking patients' vital signs (**Figure 11-22**). These devices automatically inflate and deflate the cuff (**Figure 11-23**) and use the oscillometric technique for measuring blood pressure. The method is based on the observation that oscillations of pressure in the sphygmomanometer cuff begin above the systolic pressure and continue to below the diastolic pressure. Computer algorithms (different for each manufacturer) interpret the oscillations and calculate the systolic, mean, and diastolic blood pressures (**Figure 11-24**). Advantages of this method include that it does not require a stethoscope, cuff placement is not as critical, and it is less susceptible to external noise.

The sphygmomanometer cuff should have a bladder length that is 80% of the arm circumference and a width at least 40% of the arm circumference (length to width ratio of 2:1). **Table 11-1** shows recommended sizes for different types of patients.

Invasive Arterial Pressure Monitoring

Invasive arterial pressure measurement is required for continuous monitoring of critically ill patients. These measurements are made by a small diameter catheter (18–20 gauge) that is placed into the radial, femoral, axillary, dorsalis pedis, or brachial artery. The cannula is connected with small-bore, high pressure tubing to a pressurized (usually 300 mm Hg) bag of plain or

has been the standard technique for the past 100 years. Blood flow through the brachial artery is occluded by a cuff placed around the upper arm and inflated to a pressure above the systolic blood pressure. A stethoscope is placed over the artery below the cuff. The cuff is gradually deflated and as the pressure falls to the systolic blood pressure, pulsatile blood flow is heard with

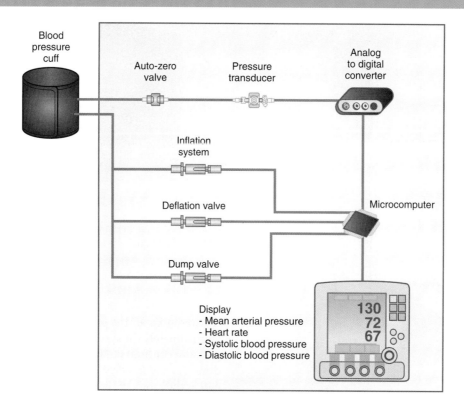

FIGURE 11-23 Simplified schematic of an automated sphygmomanometer.

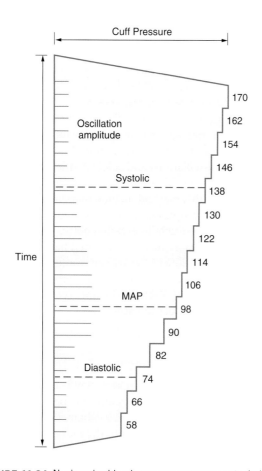

FIGURE 11-24 Noninvasive blood pressure measurements derived from analysis of cuff pressure oscillations during cuff deflation.

Modified from materials courtesy of Critikon LLC, Tampa, Fla. (GE Healthcare Monitoring Solutions)

TABLE 11-1
Recommended Dimensions for Blood Pressure Cuff Bladders

Age Range	Width (cm)	Length (cm)	Maximum Arm Circumference (cm)*
Newborn	4	8	10
Infant	6	12	15
Child	9	18	22
Small adult	10	24	26
Adult	13	30	34
Large adult	16	38	44
Thigh	20	42	52

* Calculated so that the largest arm would still allow bladder to encircle arm by at least 80%.

Reproduced from *The Fourth Report on Diagnosis, Evaluation, and Treatment of High Blood Pressure in Children and Adolescents.* NIH Publication No. 05-5267. National Institutes of Health and National Heart, Lung, and Blood Institute. May 2005.

heparinized 0.9% saline. A slow infusion rate (e.g., 2–4 mL/hr) helps prevent occlusion of the cannula by thrombus. The fluid in the tubing is in contact with an electronic pressure transducer, which provides the signal for the display of pressure and calculated values on a monitor. The transducer must be kept level with the patient, usually in line with the right atrium. Raising or lowering

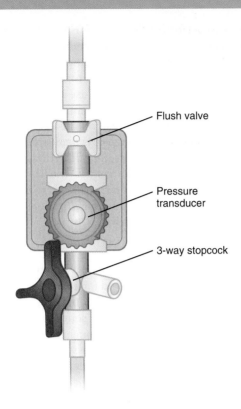

FIGURE 11-25 Three-way stopcock and flush valve.

the transducer relative to the patient will introduce a bias in the reading. For example, a 10-cm change in height corresponds to a pressure change of 10 cm H_2O, which is reflected in a change in the blood pressure reading of about 7.5 mm Hg.

The tubing also has a three-way stopcock for obtaining blood samples and a flush valve (**Figure 11-25**). The flush valve allows for rapid flushing of the system (e.g., after drawing a blood sample) and also makes possible the flush test to assure adequate frequency response of

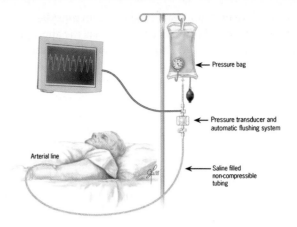

FIGURE 11-26 Arterial blood pressure monitoring system.

Reproduced with permission, Cleveland Clinic Center for Medical Art & Photography © 2012. All Rights Reserved.

the system (discussed later in this section). The measurement system is shown in **Figure 11-26**.

Arterial pressure reflects both cardiac output and systemic vascular resistance. The typical pressure waveform is shown in **Figure 11-27**. The waveform shows the peak (systolic) pressure corresponding to cardiac contraction and the nadir (diastolic) pressure corresponding to cardiac relaxation. The waveform also shows a dicrotic notch, which corresponds to the closure of the aortic valve.

If invasive hemodynamic monitoring is used, it is essential that it is accurate; otherwise, the patient will be subjected to the risks associated with this type of monitoring. Hemodynamic readings are often used to titrate therapy, and inaccuracies in measurement can lead to inappropriate treatment strategies and potential harm to the patient. The errors in the shape of pressure waveforms during vascular pressure monitoring are usually related to problems in the tubing set. To maintain

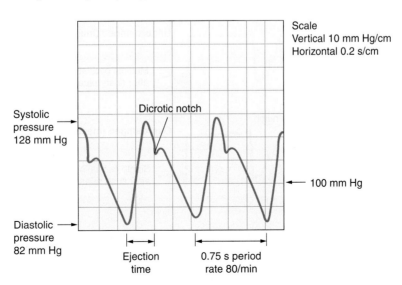

FIGURE 11-27 Arterial blood pressure waveform.

Courtesy of Dr. Dean Hess.

an accurate pressure reading, the system must be **zeroed** and checked to assure that it has the appropriate **frequency response**. Zeroing the monitor eliminates the effect of atmospheric pressure on the pressure readings. Zeroing is accomplished by opening the transducer to atmospheric pressure and adjusting the output reading to zero.

Frequency response refers to the relation between the input and output of a measurement system as a function of frequency. As the frequency of the signal increases, the output amplitude will generally start to increase (introducing error) and reach a peak value at the resonant frequency of the system (also called the natural frequency). After that, the output amplitude starts to decrease with frequency (called **damping**, also causing error). Thus, an accurate system has a resonant frequency high enough to avoid distortion of the pressure waveform (typically above 30 Hz for blood pressure measurement). The system must also be optimally damped, avoiding underdamping (causing loss of signal information) and overdamping (causing noise in the signal). Damping can also be caused by air bubbles or kinks in the tubing. A simple way to evaluate both of these characteristics (also called the dynamic response) of a blood pressure

system is to perform a **flush test** (also called a snap test or square wave test). The procedure is to open the flush valve in the infusion tubing, exposing the pressure transducer to a constant high pressure from the bag, and then quickly close it, causing the pressure to drop immediately and creating a rectangular pressure waveform on the display.

The ideal flush test waveform is depicted in **Figure 11-28**. The initial sharp upstroke is produced by activation of the fast flush system. The flat line is produced for the duration of activation of the fast flush system, and reflects the high pressure present in the flush bag. The sharp down stroke represents release of the fast flush device.

The square wave should return quickly to baseline after a few rapid sharp waves called oscillations. If the oscillations are sluggish and far apart, the system is referred to as *overdamped*. Think of the way sound carries in a soundproofed room; it sounds muffled and flat. The sound waves in such a room are dampened. An overdamped system muffles pressure waves, and will underestimate systolic pressures and overestimate diastolic pressures as a result.

Formal analysis of the resultant waveform (Figure 11-28) gives estimates of the resonant frequency

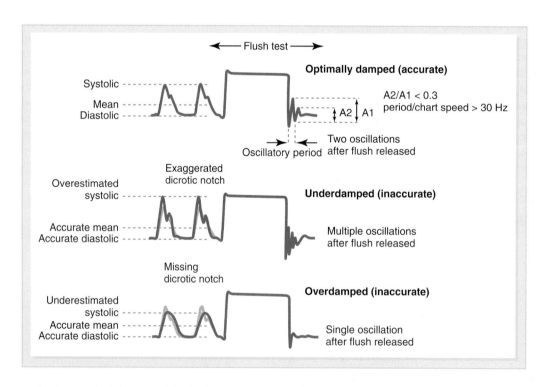

FIGURE 11-28 Waveform analysis for determining the frequency response of a blood pressure system. The resonant frequency is estimated from the period between two successive oscillation waveforms. The resonant frequency is the display (chart) speed divided by the period. For example, if the period is 1.7 mm and the display speed is 25 mm/sec, then the resonant frequency is 25/1.7 = 15 Hz. The system should have a resonant frequency greater than 30 Hz. The system is optimally damped if the amplitude ration (A2/A1) is less than 0.3.

and the degree of damping. Frequency response is evaluated from the amplitudes and period of the oscillatory waveforms that happen as the pressure drops suddenly after releasing the flush valve. The system has an adequate frequency response if the resonant frequency is greater than 30 Hz and if the amplitude ratio (A2/A1) is less than 0.3.[2]

Overdamping is a common cause of errors in blood pressure systems. It reduces the waveform magnitude and causes the loss of some waveform components. This leads to a falsely low systolic pressure and a falsely high diastolic pressure reading.

Potential sources of overdamping include:

- *Distensible tubing:* Use only the semi-rigid tubing that comes with the transducer setup.
- *Overly long extension tubing:* Extension tubing should never exceed 3–4 feet in length.
- *Air bubbles in the circuit:* Check stopcocks and connections with meticulous care, because air bubbles tend to cling to these components.
- *Catheter diameter, length, and stiffness:* Small diameter catheters, long catheters, and soft, compliant catheters can all cause overdamping.

Perhaps even more common is an underdamped system, in which the square wave is followed by multiple large oscillations. Underdamping will cause a false high systolic pressure reading and a false low diastolic pressure reading, resulting in an inaccurate assessment of the patient's hemodynamic status. Underdamping occurs when the natural frequency of the system is identical to one frequency of the pressure waves being transmitted by the patient. When this happens the tubing vibrates more intensely, producing overshoot and undershoot spikes. The end result is falsely high systolic pressures and falsely low diastolic pressures. These discrepancies are often referred to as artifact or whip. At times, artifact may be so pronounced that accurate waveform interpretation is impossible.

The arterial pulse waveform shows variations in amplitude due to the breathing pattern. For normal, unassisted breathing, blood pressure decreases on inspiration, a phenomenon called *pulsus paradoxus.* However, during assisted ventilation, a reverse phenomenon is observed due to a complex interaction of intrapleural pressure and cardiac responses.[3] In this situation, systolic blood pressure and pulse pressure (PP, which equals systolic pressure minus diastolic pressure) are maximum and end inspiration and minimum blood pressure and PP occur a few heartbeats later (**Figure 11-29**). This phenomenon has been used to assess whether giving fluids will improve cardiac output. One index of pulse pressure variation (PPV) is calculated as follows:

$$PPV\ (\%) = 100\% \times (PP_{max} - PP_{min})/PP_{mean}$$

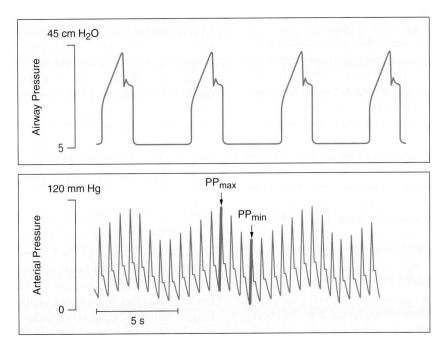

FIGURE 11-29 Blood pressure variation during mechanical ventilation.

Reproduced with permission from BioMed Central. Michard F, Teboul J. Using heart-lung interactions to assess fluid responsiveness during mechanical ventilation. *Crit Care.* 2000;4:282-289.

where PP_{max} and PP_{min} indicate the mean value of four maximum or minimum pulse pressures of the previous 30 seconds of monitoring, respectively. PP_{mean} is the mean value of pulse pressure over the same time interval. This is one of the indices available on the PiCCO-plus monitor (Pulsion Medical Systems AG, Munich, Germany). Huang et al. have shown that a threshold value for the baseline PPV greater than 11.8% predicted a significant positive response to subsequent volume expansion therapy by an increase of cardiac index ≥ 15% with a sensitivity of 68% and a specificity of 100%.[4]

Central Venous Catheters

Central venous pressure (CVP) is measured in the superior vena cava and reflects the filling pressure of the right atrium (**Figure 11-30**). CVP can be elevated in different disease states, and an increase in CVP may be interpreted as a positive response to fluid challenge.[5] Causes of low CVP include fluid loss through hemorrhage (e.g., trauma or surgery), excessive diuresis, and poor venous return (e.g., cardiogenic shock).[6] In some patients (those with sepsis and congestive heart failure without pulmonary hypertension), a CVP target of 8 mm Hg for volume repletion may optimally balance perfusion and respiratory function.[7]

Catheters for adults are about 2.3 mm in diameter (7 French), are about 16 to 20 cm long, and may have several ports. CVP catheters are connected to flush lines similar to those used for arterial lines. One major difference, however, is that the pressure transducer in the flush line must be leveled as well as zeroed. Modern disposable transducers facilitate these two procedures by placing a three-way stopcock near the transducer and making the transducer small enough that it can be attached to the patient's body. As with the arterial line, zeroing means to close the stopcock to the patient and open it to the atmosphere while pressing the appropriate button on the monitor to zero it, meaning to display a value of zero for the CVP pressure. Next, the transducer must be leveled, meaning that it must be at the same distance above the floor as the tip of the CVP catheter. If the tip and the transducer are at different levels, the liquid in the tubing will generate a hydrostatic pressure that will cause an error in the reading of CVP. A difference of only 3 cm (a little over an inch) will cause an error of about 2 mm Hg. Because the normal CVP is only 2–6 mm Hg, this is a huge error. In the supine patient, the transducer is leveled by placing it (sometimes taping it to the chest) at the mid-chest position (fourth intercostal space) in the mid-axillary line (sometimes called the phlebostatic axis). This site is easy to estimate by eye and

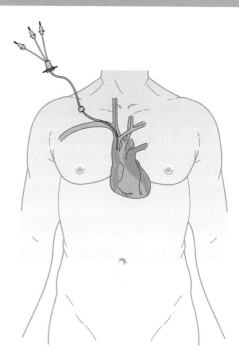

FIGURE 11-30 Placement of central venous catheter.

Adapted from Taylor, C., et al. *Fundamentals of Nursing*. 5th ed. (Figure 16-10). Lippincott Williams & Wilkins; 2005.

provides a reasonable approximation for the location of the CVP catheter tip.

The CVP waveform shows several permutations that correspond to the ECG,[8] as shown in **Figure 11-31**. The *a wave* is produced by right atrial (RA) contraction (systole) and occurs between 80 and 100 ms after the P wave on the ECG. The *x descent* is the fall in pressure corresponding to RA relaxation. The *c wave* is caused by closure of the tricuspid valve and follows the QRS complex on the ECG. The *v wave* reflects the rise in RA pressure as it fills against a closed tricuspid valve in late ventricular systole. It follows the T wave on the ECG. The *y descent* shows the fall in RA pressure as the tricuspid valve opens and blood from the RA empties into the right ventricle during diastole.

Pulmonary Artery Catheters

The most well-known method of invasive hemodynamic monitoring is the **pulmonary artery catheter (PAC)**, also known as the Swan-Ganz Catheter, referring to the inventors Drs. Jeremy Swan and William Ganz at Cedars-Sinai in California. This flow-directed balloon-tipped pulmonary artery catheter has been in clinical use for more than 30 years (**Figure 11-32**). Initially developed for the management of acute myocardial

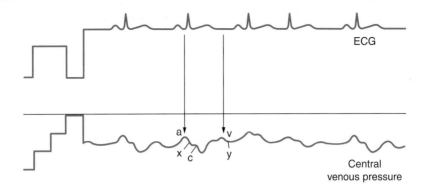

FIGURE 11-31 CVP waveform.

Courtesy of Dr. Dean Hess.

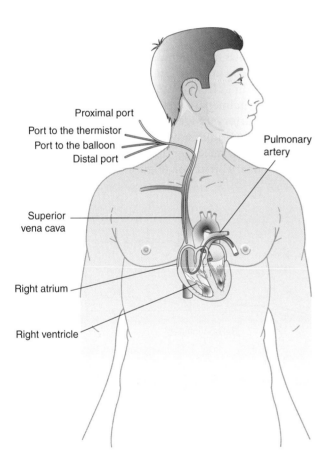

FIGURE 11-32 Pulmonary artery catheter.

Adapted from Schulte am Esch J. *Atlas of Anaesthesia*. 3rd ed. Thieme Medical Publishers; 2006.

catheters, the larger lumen terminates at the distal tip of the catheter and is used to monitor pulmonary artery and wedge pressures. The smaller lumen permits balloon inflation and deflation. Triple-lumen monitoring catheters have the same capabilities as double-lumen catheters with the additional (proximal) lumen for central venous pressure monitoring.

Despite widespread use of the PAC for more than three decades, no validated indications exist for its general use.[9] Some publications present only authors' suggestions for indications and contraindications for the use of the PAC. Various association and subspecialty guidelines exist as consensus statements. Pulmonary artery catheterization is necessary for the diagnosis of pulmonary hypertension. **Table 11-2** gives general guidelines for clinical use of the PAC.

The PAC is a 7.5-French, multilumen catheter that is 110 cm long with extra connecting tubes for attachment to the pressure transducer. At the tip is the PA lumen, or distal lumen. A 1.5-cc balloon is located just proximal to the tip. Approximately 4 cm proximal to the balloon is the thermistor, which is used to measure temperature changes for calculation of cardiac output. Two additional lumens are present at 19 cm and 30 cm from the tip. Depending on the degree of right heart enlargement and the position of the catheter (i.e., distance advanced into the patient), these lumens reside within the right ventricle (RV), right atrium (RA), or superior vena cava (SVC). Some catheters are coated with heparin to reduce thrombogenicity and have connections for temporary ventricular pacing. The former is important to remember in case the patient develops heparin-induced thrombocytopenia, because only a small amount of heparin is necessary to sustain this process.

During placement of the catheter, the balloon at the tip is inflated once the waveform indicates the location of the right atrium. The inflated balloon enhances the

infarction, it gained widespread use in the management of a variety of critical illnesses and surgical procedures. PAC provides a rapid and effective method for monitoring right heart pressures, sampling mixed venous blood, and infusing solutions. In double-lumen

TABLE 11-2
General Guidelines for Clinical Use of a Pulmonary Artery Catheter

Diagnostic
• Diagnosis of shock states
• Differentiation of high- versus low-pressure pulmonary edema
• Diagnosis of idiopathic pulmonary hypertension
• Diagnosis of valvular disease, intracardiac shunts, cardiac tamponade, and pulmonary embolus (PE)
• Monitoring and management of complicated AMI
• Assessing hemodynamic response to therapies
• Management of multiorgan system failure and/or severe burns
• Management of hemodynamic instability after cardiac surgery
• Assessment of response to treatment in patients with idiopathic pulmonary hypertension

Therapeutic
• Aspiration of air emboli

effect of blood flow in directing the catheter through the heart (**Figure 11-33**). The physician advances the PAC following the path of the blood flow through the right ventricle and finally "wedging" it in the pulmonary artery (PA), as evidenced by the waveform. The PAC is attached to a flush and transducer system similar to the CVP system. The transducer must be zeroed and leveled as described for the CVP transducer. The frequency response of the PAC should be checked with a flush test as described in the section on invasive arterial pressure monitoring.

Pulmonary artery catheters have several ports for making pressure measurements, injecting ice water for thermal dilution determination of cardiac output, medication infusion, and blood sampling. Some catheters have a sensor for measuring mixed venous oxygen saturation. CVP measurements are made from the proximal port of the PAC. The pulmonary circulation, having no valves, allows for obtaining left atrium pressures with the balloon inflated. The inflated balloon blocks pressure readings from the pulmonary artery. This is called the pulmonary artery occlusion pressure or **pulmonary artery wedge pressure (PAWP)**. The PAWP is measured intermittently by inflating the balloon with 1.5 mL of air for no longer than 10–15 seconds to prevent pulmonary infarction (**Figure 11-34**). PAWP can

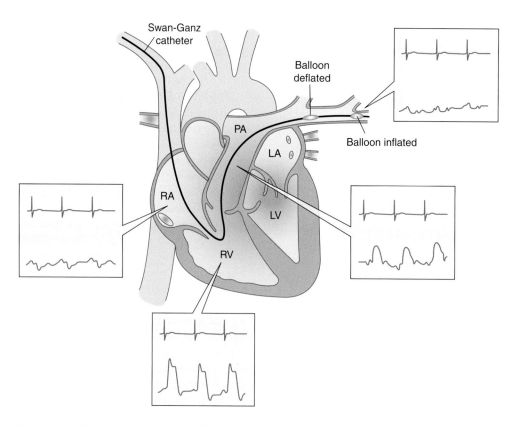

FIGURE 11-33 Pressure waveforms correlated with the ECG as the pulmonary artery catheter passes through the heart.

Modified from Longnecker D, Brown D, Newman M, Zapol, W. 2007. *Anesthesiology.* McGraw-Hill, New York. (© The McGraw-Hill Companies, Inc.)

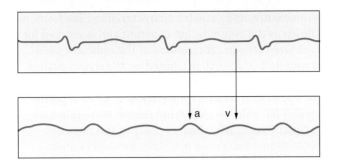

FIGURE 11-34 Pulmonary artery wedge pressure waveform.
Courtesy of Dr. Dean Hess.

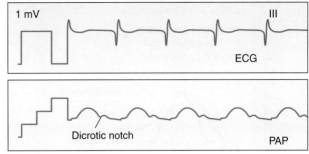

FIGURE 11-35 Pulmonary artery pressure waveform.
Courtesy of Dr. Dean Hess.

be used to identify the presence of a hydrostatic component to pulmonary edema and to assess pulmonary vascular resistance. The central venous pressure and the pulmonary artery pressure (**Figure 11-35**) are measured continuously.

Other important information provided by a PAC includes the cardiac output, mixed venous oxygen saturation ($S\bar{v}O_2$), and oxygen saturations in the right heart chambers to assess for the presence of an intracardiac shunt. Using these measurements, other variables can be derived including pulmonary or systemic vascular

resistance and the difference between arterial and venous oxygen content. Obtaining CO and PCWP measurements is the primary reason for inserting most PACs; therefore, understanding how they are obtained and what factors alter their values are of prime importance. **Table 11-3** shows the normal range of pressures for some hemodynamic parameters.

Cardiac Output Monitoring

There are many ways to measure cardiac output, but only three have evolved to be implemented on

TABLE 11-3
Normal Values for Standard Hemodynamic Parameters

MAP	70–110 mm Hg
$SVR = \dfrac{MAP - CVP}{CO} \times 80$	900–1,600 dynes·sec/cm^5
$CO = \dfrac{\dot{V}O_2}{(CaO_2 - C\bar{v}O_2) \times 10}$	4–8 L/min
$SV = \dfrac{CO \times 1,000}{HR}$	60–130 mL/beat
$PVR = \dfrac{MPAP - PAWP}{CO}$	< 160 dynes·sec/cm^5
$VO_2 = (CaO_2 - C\bar{v}O_2) \times CO \times 10$	200–250 mL/min
$DO_2 = CaO_2 \times CO \times 10$	950–1,150 mL/min
$CaO_2 = (Hb \times 1.34 \times SaO_2) + 0.0031 \times PaO_2$	20 mL/dL blood (for Hb in g/dL)
$C\bar{v}O_2 = (Hb \times 1.34 \times S\bar{v}O_2) + 0.0031 \times P\bar{v}O_2$	15 mL/dL blood (for Hb in g/dL)

MAP = mean arterial pressure, SVR = systemic vascular resistance, PVR = pulmonary vascular resistance, CO = cardiac output, DO_2 = oxygen delivery, $\dot{V}O_2$ = oxygen consumption, CaO_2 = arterial oxygen content, $C\bar{v}O_2$ = mixed venous oxygen content.

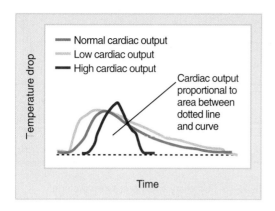

FIGURE 11-36 Thermodilution curves.

commercially available devices commonly used in intensive care units.[10]

Thermodilution

Measuring cardiac output by the thermodilution method was first described by Fegler in the 1950s. It became a standard practice to measure cardiac output during the 1970s when Doctors Swan and Ganz demonstrated the reliability of this method using the Swan-Ganz catheter. The thermodilution method relies on measuring a change in temperature caused by the injection of a solution cooler than blood, typically iced saline at 35.6°F–41°F (2°C–5°C), although the development of catheters with multiple thermistors makes this unnecessary. A specific quantity of the iced saline (generally 10 mL) is injected in a rapid and smooth manner into the proximal injectate port of the PAC. The fluid is dispelled into the right atrium and then passes to the right ventricle and subsequently the pulmonary artery, where the temperature of the mixed blood is recorded by the thermistor at the distal tip of the PAC. The cooler solution cools the surrounding blood. The monitor calculates the CO based on the temperature change and the time it takes the injected volume of solution to pass the thermistor. The temperature change is graphically displayed on the monitor as a function of time. A normal curve will have a sharp upstroke representing rapid injection of the fluid and rapid cooling of the blood, followed by a smooth curve and a prolonged downslope representing change in temperature back to normal (**Figure 11-36**). The area under the curve is inversely proportional to cardiac output.

Most monitors can automatically calculate the cardiac index (CI) as long as the height and weight information have been entered. For the purpose of calculation, it is required to know the volume of the indicator, temperature of the indicator, blood temperature, and catheter characteristics. The latter is known as the computation constant and is entered for each size catheter. The volume of the indicator used is usually 2.5, 5, or 10 mL based on the size of patient and the catheter. Earlier consensus recommended the use of iced saline as the standard. More recently studies have shown that room temperature injectate is equally accurate, which is cheaper and does not require the clinician to maintain the iced containers. The injection times should be less than 4 seconds and ideally should be approximately 2 seconds. The thermodilution cardiac output is measured three times and the average of three readings within 10% of each of each other are recorded. The advantages of this technique are its reliability, easy bedside performance, and ease of getting serial cardiac outputs. Errors in the measurement of cardiac output can be introduced in conditions such as malposition of the catheter, intracardiac shunts, mitral valve regurgitation, contamination of the catheter, thermistor breakage, inappropriate computation constant entered on the computer, and a difference between the actual and measured injectate temperatures.

Note that there are two common forms of thermodilution: (1) right heart thermodilution and (2) transpulmonary thermodilution. Right heart thermodilution uses a right heart pulmonary artery catheter (Swan-Ganz). Transpulmonary thermodilution uses both a central line and a special femoral artery catheter with an embedded thermistor.

Pulse Contour Analysis

The FloTrac/Vigileo (Edwards Lifesciences LLC, United States), LiDCO Plus (LiDCO Ltd, London, England), and PulsioFlex (Pulsion Medical Systems, Munich, Germany) systems provide real-time continuous monitoring through pulse contour analysis and (with the exception of FloTrac) allow for intermittent thermodilution measurement via the transpulmonary thermodilution (TPTD) method (**Figure 11-37**).[11] These devices estimate cardiac output using a radial or femoral arterial catheter connected to an external disposable pressure sensor. The PulsioFlex requires a femoral arterial catheter with an embedded thermistor for the TPTD measurement. The PulsioFlex system or the LiDCO Plus system require calibration by either transpulmonary thermodilution or lithium dilution and therefore depend on a central venous catheter. The solution for thermodilution is injected through the central venous catheter. This thermal signal reaches the arterial thermister, which detects the temperature difference, and a dissipation curve is generated (as explained in the section on thermodilution) and cardiac output is calculated.[12] Pulse contour analysis gives consistent and reproducible results because the readings are not

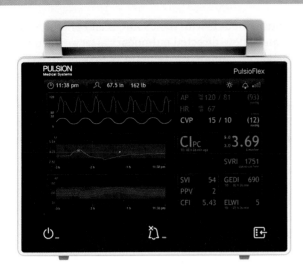

FIGURE 11-37 PulsioFlex device.
Courtesy of PULSION Medical Systems SE.

affected by ventilator or unassisted breathing cycles. Several studies support that cardiac output measurements obtained using the PulsioFlex method are comparable to those obtained using traditional Swan-Ganz thermodilution.[13] FloTrac/Vigileo uses a self-calibrated system in which vascular tone (a function of vascular resistance and compliance) is assessed by a calculation within its algorithm, which is then used to calculate stroke volume.

Pulse contour analysis uses the arterial pressure waveform as an input for a mathematical model that relates pressure and flow for the systemic circulation. The model allows prediction of flow from pressure. The model parameters (resistance, compliance, and characteristic impedance) are related to the patient's sex and age. Initial estimates for model parameters are refined following a calibration using the thermodilution technique.

The FloTrac/Vigileo system (**Figure 11-38**) does not require calibration, and therefore is very easy to use. The system, consisting of the Vigileo monitor and the FloTrac sensor, uses a clinically validated algorithm to provide continuous cardiac output, stroke volume, and stroke volume variation in real time. The FloTrac algorithm utilizes arterial pressure, age, gender, and body surface area to calculate SV. The patient-specific SV is then multiplied by pulse rate to get cardiac output. Patient-specific stroke volume is updated as fast as every 20 seconds.

Fick Equation

This equation was proposed by Adolf Fick in the 1870s for calculating cardiac output, with the assumption that normal oxygen consumption is 250 mL/min. The principle behind this equation is that blood flow through the lungs can be calculated from the amount of oxygen absorbed by every 100 mL of blood during its passage through the lungs and the total oxygen uptake per minute. The blood flow through the lungs is equal to the output of the left ventricle. The difference between arterial and mixed venous oxygen content is measured by sampling arterial and venous blood. Oxygen consumption can be calculated from the inspired minus expired oxygen content and ventilation rate (see Table 11-3 earlier in the chapter).[14]

The Philips NM3 system (formerly the NICO) is a noninvasive device for determining cardiac output based on a modified version of the Fick equation using carbon dioxide instead of oxygen (**Figure 11-39**). Carbon dioxide is generated by intermittent partial rebreathing through a disposable rebreathing loop. The NM3 monitor is the first commercially available

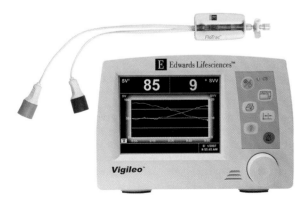

FIGURE 11-38 FlowTrack/Vigileo.
Courtesy of Edwards Lifesciences LLC, Irvine, CA.

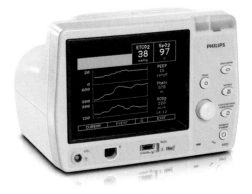

FIGURE 11-39 Philips NM3 device.
Courtesy of Philips Healthcare

cardiac output system making use of the partial rebreathing of CO_2 and can provide real-time and continuous cardiac output monitoring.

The monitor consists of a carbon dioxide sensor (infrared light absorption), a disposable airflow sensor (differential pressure pneumotachometer), and a pulse oximeter. Cardiac output (CO) is calculated from minute ventilation and its CO_2 content. Arterial CO_2 content ($CaCO_2$) is estimated from end-tidal CO_2 ($etCO_2$). The partial rebreathing maneuver reduces CO_2 elimination and hence increases $etCO_2$. The Fick equation for carbon dioxide elimination is:

$$CO = \frac{\dot{V}CO_2}{CvCO_2 - CaCO_2}$$

Assuming that cardiac output remains unchanged under normal (N) and rebreathing (R) conditions

$$CO = \frac{\dot{V}CO_2 N}{CvCO_2 N - CaCO_2 N} = \frac{\dot{V}CO_2 R}{CvCO_2 R - CaCO_2 R}$$

By subtracting the normal and rebreathing ratios, the following differential Fick equation is obtained:

$$CO = \frac{\dot{V}CO_2 N - \dot{V}CO_2 R}{(CvCO_2 N - CaCO_2 N) - (CvCO_2 R - CaCO_2 R)}$$

Because carbon dioxide diffuses quickly in blood (22 times faster than oxygen), one can assume that $CvCO_2$ does not differ between normal and rebreathing conditions. Therefore, the venous contents disappear from the equation.

$$CO = \frac{\Delta \dot{V}CO_2}{\Delta CaCO_2}$$

The delta in $CaCO_2$ can be approximated by the delta in $etCO_2$ multiplied by the slope (S) of the carbon dioxide dissociation curve. This curve represents the relation between carbon dioxide volumes (used to calculate carbon dioxide content) and partial pressure of carbon dioxide. This relation can be considered linear between 15 and 70 mm Hg of partial pressure of carbon dioxide.

$$CO = \frac{\Delta \dot{V}CO_2}{S \times \Delta etCO_2}$$

Mixed Venous Oxygen Saturation Monitoring

The technology to measure mixed venous oxygen saturation continuously through oximetry became available in the early 1980s. This system uses a microprocessor, an optical module with light sources and photo-detectors, and a flow-directed pulmonary artery catheter. By using fiber optics, wavelengths of light between 650 and 1000 nanometers (nm) are pulsed into the pulmonary artery. The light reflected off the red blood cells in the pulmonary artery is returned to the optic module through another fiber-optic bundle. The mixed venous oxygen saturation ($S\overline{v}O_2$) is calculated as the ratio of transmitted and reflected light. Before insertion, the system is calibrated using an in-vitro calibration standard. Calibration can be updated periodically by in-vivo calibration using an $S\overline{v}O_2$ determined by a laboratory oximeter. Factors affecting the measurement of $S\overline{v}O_2$ using this method include temperature, pH, blood flow velocity, hematocrit, and occlusion of the catheter tip.

Three systems are commercially available to measure $S\overline{v}O_2$ by oximetry. Each of these uses different methods to deal with interference and drift:

Edwards Sat-One Catheter: This system uses two reference wavelengths and one detecting fiber-optic filament and allows the user to periodically update the hematocrit, which will control the effects of hematocrit on $S\overline{v}O_2$ measurements.

Oxymetrix Opticath Catheter: This system uses three reference wavelengths and one detecting filament to improve the accuracy of the system in the presence of physiological changes such as hematocrit.

Spectramed Spectracath Catheter: This system uses two reference wavelengths and two detecting filaments. The second detecting filament improves the accuracy of the system when hematocrit changes.

Most studies have found three-wavelength systems to correlate better with oximeter $S\overline{v}O_2$ than two-wavelength systems. Drift is less with three-wavelength systems.

References

1. Sing J. Cardiac assessment. In Hess DR, MacIntyre NR, Mishoe SC, Galvin WF, Adams AB, eds. *Respiratory care: Principles and practice.* 2nd ed. Sudbury, MA: Jones & Bartlett Learning; 2012:101-125.
2. Gardner RM. Direct blood pressure measurement: Dynamic response requirements. *Anesthesiology.* 1981;54:227-236.
3. Michard F. Changes in arterial pressure during mechanical ventilation. *Anesthesiology.* 2005;103(2):419-428.
4. Huang CC, Fu JY, Hu HC, Kao KC, Chen NH, Hsieh MJ, et al. Prediction of fluid responsiveness in acute respiratory distress syndrome patients ventilated with low tidal volume and high positive end-expiratory pressure. *Crit Care Med.* 2008;36(10): 2810-2816.
5. Pinsky MR, Didier P. Functional hemodynamic monitoring. *Critical Care.* 2005;9(6):556-572.

6. Woodrow P. Central venous catheters and central venous pressure. *Nurs Stand.* 2002;16(26):45-51.

7. Manoach S, Weingart SD, Charchaflieh J. The evolution and current use of invasive hemodynamic monitoring for predicting volume responsiveness during resuscitation, perioperative, and critical care. *J Clin Anesth.* 2012;24:242-250.

8. Burchell PL, Powers KA. Focus on central venous pressure monitoring in an acute care setting. *Nursing.* 2011;41(12):38-43.

9. Harvey S, Young D, Brampton W, et al. Pulmonary artery catheters for adult patients in intensive care. *Cochrane Database Syst Rev.* 2006;3:CD003408.

10. Berton C, Cholley B. Equipment review: New techniques for cardiac output measurement—oesophageal Doppler, Fick principle using carbon dioxide, and pulse contour analysis. *Crit Care.* 2002;6(3):216-221.

11. Cottis R, Magee N, Higgins DJ. Haemodynamic monitoring with pulse-induced contour cardiac output (PiCCO) in critical care. *Intensive Crit Care Nurs.* 2003;19(5):301-307.

12. Salukhe TV, Wyncoll DLA. Volumetric haemodynamic monitoring and continuous pulse contour analysis—an untapped resource for coronary and high dependency care units? *Br J Cardiol (Acute Intervent Cardiol).* 2002;9:20-25.

13. Goedje O, Hoke K, Goetz AE, et al. Reliability of a new algorithm for continuous cardiac output determination by pulse-contour analysis during hemodynamic instability. *Crit Care Med.* 2002;30(1):52-58.

14. Kendrick AH, West J, Papouchado M, Rozkovec A. Direct Fick cardiac output: Are assumed values of oxygen consumption acceptable? *Eur Heart J.* 1988;9:337-342.

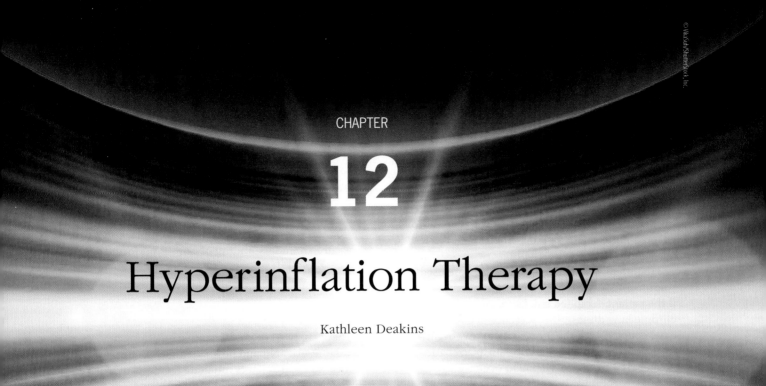

CHAPTER

12

Hyperinflation Therapy

Kathleen Deakins

CHAPTER OBJECTIVES

1. Define hyperinflation therapy.
2. Describe the types of therapies used to perform hyperinflation therapy.
3. Explain the differences in operation between flow-oriented and volume-oriented incentive spirometers.
4. Compare techniques for IPPB using mechanical ventilators and stand-alone devices.
5. List the common problems that may occur when performing IPPB.
6. Discuss how IPV devices operate.
7. Explain how IPV can be used to accomplish hyperinflation therapy.
8. Discuss the principles of operation for positive airway pressure adjuncts including CPAP and devices that accomplish positive expiratory pressure maneuvers.

KEY TERMS

Continuous positive airway pressure (CPAP)
Incentive spirometer
Intermittent positive pressure breathing (IPPB)

Intrapulmonary percussive ventilation IPV
Positive airway pressure (PAP) devices
Positive expiratory pressure (PEP)

Introduction

Hyperinflation therapy (HT), also referred to as lung expansion maneuvers, encompasses subjecting the lungs to volumes greater than normal to reinflate the collapsed areas of the lung and improve gas exchange.[1] HT may be utilized for the treatment or prevention of atelectasis by improving lung mechanics and oxygenation.[1,2] Atelectasis, or loss of lung volume resulting in the collapse of alveolar spaces, can result in respiratory compromise and other complications.

Atelectasis is classified by its origin: airway obstruction (resorption), abdominal distention (compression), hypoventilation (passive), or increased surface tension (adhesive).[3] The treatment of atelectasis is dependent on its underlying origin and pathophysiology. Passive and adhesive atelectasis may benefit from hyperinflation therapy using positive pressure on inspiration or expiration.[3] Incentive spirometers, intermittent positive pressure breathing devices, and positive airway pressure devices including positive expiratory pressure devices are used to accomplish hyperinflation therapy goals.

Incentive Spirometer

Incentive spirometry (IS) is a low-level resistance breathing exercise that incorporates an inspiratory technique called sustained maximal inspiration (SMI), the equivalent of a deep breath or sigh that is routinely generated by a spontaneous yawn.[4] **Incentive spirometers** are goal-oriented devices that use visual aids such as raising a lightweight ball or indicator when breathing in at a specific flow or volume.[5] During an SMI, when a deep breath is generated, the transpulmonary pressure and inspiratory volume rise when achieving the specific flow or volume target.[5] Clinical outcomes associated with the use of incentive spirometers are based on repetition of deep breaths that results in airway patency and in turn treats the underlying cause of the atelectasis.[5] Evidence of lung expansion including observation of chest rise and confirmation of lung volume achieved is greater using a volume-oriented compared to a flow-oriented incentive spirometer.[6]

Application

Incentive spirometers are used as adjuncts for deep breathing in both inpatient and outpatient settings. Depending on the type of spirometer selected (flow or volume oriented), the correct use of these devices can be easily achieved when basic instruction is provided. In the majority of cases, a simple inspiratory breath-holding for at least 3 to 10 seconds followed by passive exhalation will meet the primary goal of therapy.[4] Incentive spirometers can be used with a mouthpiece or adapted for use with a permanent artificial airway (tracheostomy), if needed.

Historically, incentive spirometers were used just prior to and following thoracic and abdominal surgery if the patient exhibited risk factors associated with chronic lung disease. The presence of chronic lung disease, coupled with the propensity for hypoventilation from anesthetic agents and/or pain, place patients at greater risk for the development of atelectasis, mucostasis, and infection.[4,5] Incentive spirometry is also indicated for patients with mild underlying restrictive diseases affected by abnormal diaphragm function.[5] The primary and evidence-based indication for incentive spirometry is in the management of atelectasis in sickle cell disease patients to prevent pulmonary complications associated with acute chest syndrome.[7]

Patients who are not conscious, do not have the cognitive ability to understand or cooperate with instructions, or are unable to reproduce the maneuver because of significant reduction in pulmonary mechanics (vital capacity less than 10 mL/kg or inspiratory capacity less than one-third predicted normal) should not use incentive spirometry.[5] Incentive spirometers are still used routinely for the purpose of preventing or treating postoperative complications following cardiac or abdominal surgery, but evidence has not demonstrated its benefit in this situation and therefore there is not an absolute indication for this reason.[4,8–10]

This form of hyperinflation therapy is not completely benign; risks are associated with its use. Incentive spirometry is not intended to be the sole treatment for atelectasis or lung consolidation. Hyperventilation may be induced by a high respiratory rate or volume.[4] Patients may experience hypoxia if supplemental oxygen therapy is interrupted while the patient performs the maneuver. However, some devices such as the Coach 2 (Smith's Medical) incorporate a port through which low flow oxygen may be titrated, to facilitate oxygen delivery and minimize the risk of hypoxemia during therapy. Patients may experience weakness or fatigue from the physical work associated with taking a deep breath. Patients may also experience discomfort related to incisional or procedural pain. Patients at risk for air leak or those who present with underlying obstructive lung disease may be at risk for bronchospasm (asthma) or barotrauma (emphysema). Patients with underlying obstructive lung disease may have air-trapping and hyperinflation and may experience adverse effects from the additional lung volume. Repeating SMI maneuvers without adequate rest periods between sets of deep breathing may impose an additional load on the deconditioned muscles of patients with moderate to severe lung disease. In this instance, performing incentive spirometry may mimic the effect this patient population feels during persistent exercise, which may slow expiratory flows and extend dynamic hyperinflation.[11] Care should be taken to monitor patients and assure an understanding of how to perform the technique properly.[5]

Principles of Operation

There are two types of incentive breathing devices, volume-oriented and flow-oriented. Volume-oriented incentive spirometers integrate concepts of true volume displacement during inspiration. During a deep inspiration, the device's indicator rises concomitantly with the change in volume. Once the target maximum volume is achieved for a given breath, the patient is instructed to perform an inspiratory hold of 5 to 10 seconds.[4] During a passive exhalation, gravity returns the indicator (i.e., ball or plastic bellows) to its initial starting position. The literature reports diaphragmatic motion is increased when using a volume-oriented spirometer compared to its flow-oriented counterpart.[12] Volume-oriented incentive spirometers are also recommended for larger (adolescent or adult) patients, although pediatric devices are commercially available.[12]

Flow-oriented incentive spirometers directly measure flow. Because volume is a function of flow and time, the volume of air inspired during an SMI maneuver can be calculated. During inhalation, the patient's inspiratory flow is directed to a column containing a lightweight ball.[13] The ball rises in proportion to the flow generated as the patient inspires. There are different manufacturer designs to this type of incentive breathing device. The specific design will determine the action flow will have on the ball enclosed within the column. For example, as flow is generated the higher the ball rises within the column, the longer the ball is held at the desired level, or the greater the number of balls that rise within their respective columns. When flow ceases, the ball or indicator drops. This occurs during an inspiratory hold or with exhalation. Flow is measured in mL/sec and operational ranges vary among devices. Incentive spirometers containing more than one ball require higher flows to raise each ball consecutively.[13] A rise in flow is an indirect indicator that the tidal volume has increased. Tidal volume can also be directly measured independently by connecting a measuring device to the spirometer.[5,13] The beneficial effects of therapy are directly related to the patient's ability to perform an SMI.

The more compliant the patient is with performing a slow deep breath, the better the chest expansion and the greater the diaphragmatic motion and subsequent volume delivery that will occur.[4,14] Equipment malfunction and/or problems with patient technique can occur during treatment. A list of common problems and a troubleshooting guide are found in Table 12-1.

Currently Available Devices

There are several different types of incentive spirometers on the market. These devices can be divided into volume-based and flow-based on their operating principles. A few of the commercially available devices are described below.

Volume-Oriented Incentive Spirometers

The Voldyne Exerciser and Coach 2 are examples of two incentive breathing devices that integrate concepts of true volume displacement during inspiration.

Voldyne Exercisers

The Voldyne Volumetric Exerciser is a volume-oriented incentive spirometer that utilizes plastic bellows contained within a plastic column (Figure 12-1). An indicator is located on the side of the column, which can be adjusted by the clinician to mark the patient's inspiratory target. A short piece of corrugated tubing attaches the patient mouthpiece to the incentive breathing device. As the patient inhales, the bellows rise.[4] This

TABLE 12-1

Troubleshooting Guide for Patient and Equipment Problems Commonly Associated with Incentive Spirometers

| Problem | Possible Causes | | Suggested Solutions |
	Patient	Equipment	
No volume or flow indicated on the device		Leak in the system	Assess the device. Ensure all components are connected and connections are tight.
	Poor inspiratory effort		Instruct patient in proper technique. Coach patient during the sustained inspiratory maneuver.
	Patient exhaling into the device		Instruct patient to exhale through the nose and then take a slow deep breath in through the mouthpiece. Coach patient during the maneuver.
Patient unable to achieve the operator-set volume or flow target not achieved		Leak in the system	Assess the device. Ensure all components are connected and connections are tight.
	Improper patient technique		Assess the patient's technique. Ensure the patient's mouth is sealed around the mouthpiece and that the patient is mouth breathing throughout inspiration. Evaluate the need for nose clips.
	Poor patient effort		Instruct patient in proper technique. Coach patient during the sustained inspiratory maneuver. Evaluate patient's level of pain and coordinate administration of prescribed pain medications with therapy.
		Volume or flow target set too high	Adjust (lower) volume and flow target. Evaluate patient's performance of the technique to ensure patient is able to perform maneuver and operate device correctly.
Patient exceeds the operator-set volume or flow target		Volume or flow target set too low	Adjust (increase) volume and flow target. Evaluate patient's performance of the technique to ensure patient is able to perform maneuver and operate device correctly.
		Supplemental oxygen flow is affecting device performance.	Adjust (increase) volume and flow target to ensure patient is able to perform maneuver and operate device correctly.
	The patient is able to adequately deep breathe. Therapeutic goals met.		Evaluate patient for discontinuation of therapy.

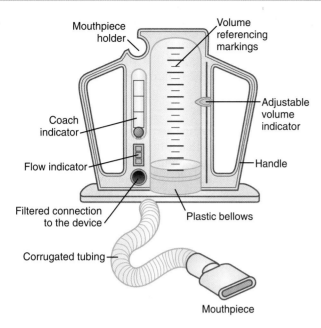

FIGURE 12-1 Schematic of the Voldyne Volume-Dependent Incentive Spirometer.

device also has a flow indicator, a lightweight plastic ball that also rises with inspiration. The flow indicator or float provides visual feedback to the patient in order to promote a slow, steady, and deep inspiratory maneuver. During the inspiratory hold, the flow indicator will drop to baseline, but the volume indicator will not return to its resting position until exhalation occurs. This particular design is available in three sizes: the Voldyne 5000, Voldyne 2500, and Voldyne Pediatric; volume measurement of the former is up to 5.0 L, and 2.5 L for the latter two devices (**Figure 12-2**).

The Coach 2

The Coach 2 (Smiths Medical) is a volume-oriented incentive spirometer that also incorporates a plastic bellows for volume displacement and a feedback device to gauge patient adherence to performing a slow inspiration. Rather than use words to describe how well the patient is performing a slow inspiratory maneuver, this device uses pictures in the form of happy and sad faces. A one-way valve is located between the

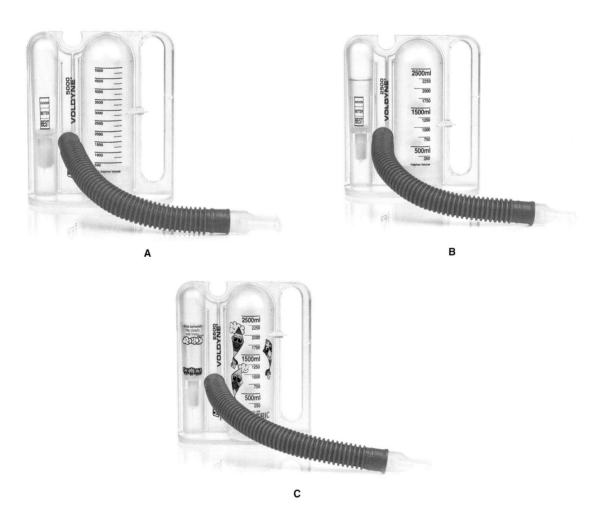

FIGURE 12-2 Sizing variations commercially available for the Voldyne Volume-Dependent Incentive Spirometer. A. The Voldyne 5000. B. The Voldyne 2500. C. The Pediatric Voldyne.

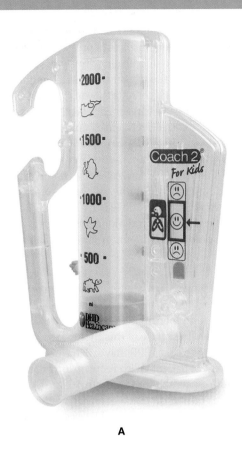

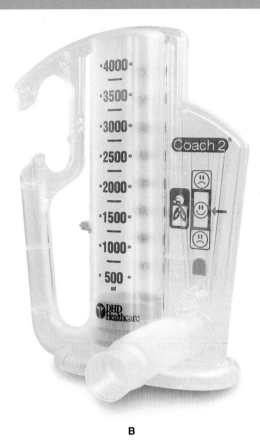

A

B

FIGURE 12-3 The Coach Volume-Dependent Incentive Spirometer. A. The pediatric model with maximum volume displacement of 2.0 L. B. The adult model with maximum volume displacement of 4.0 L.

Photos courtesy of Smiths Medical.

corrugated tubing and the device to prevent the patient from exhaling into the device and performing the maneuver incorrectly. The patient handle is notched to allow the device to be secured to the patient's bedrail (**Figure 12-3**). This brand of volume-dependent incentive spirometer is available in two models: an adult and pediatric model with volume measurement of up to 4.0 L and 2.0 L, respectively.

Flow-Oriented Incentive Spirometers

The Clini-Flow and the Hudson RCI LVE are examples of incentive spirometers that directly measure flow. The volume of air inspired during an SMI maneuver with these devices is a function of flow and time, and can be calculated.

Clini-Flow

Clini-Flow (**Figure 12-4**) is a flow-based incentive spirometer designed for patients with weak respiratory muscles such as those with neuromuscular disease, or those with low flow rates (geriatric or pediatric patients). As the patient inspires, the yellow plastic disc, enclosed in the device, will rise. A happy face is imprinted on the column containing the flow indicator. The happy face

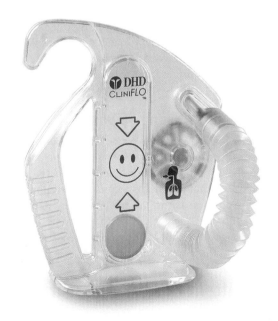

FIGURE 12-4 The CliniFlow (Smiths Medical) is an example of a flow-oriented incentive spirometer. The flow setting is adjustable, from 100 to 600 mL/sec, enabling this device to be used across a spectrum of patient populations.

Courtesy of Smiths Medical.

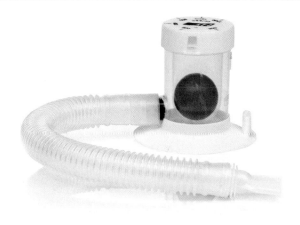

FIGURE 12-5 The Hudson RCI LVE lung volume exerciser (Teleflex Medical) is a flow-oriented incentive spirometer with operational flow ranges of 200–1200 cc/sec.

Courtesy of Teleflex.

provides a target for the correct technique as well as visual feedback for patient effort. If the patient performs the technique properly, the yellow indicator will be centered or hover around the happy face. Patients are instructed to continue inhaling, keeping the yellow indicator centered on the happy face for approximately 5 seconds. Arrows are located above and below the happy face to guide patients to slow down their flow (downward arrow), or inspire more deeply (upward pointing arrow). A dial at the rear of the spirometer facilitates adjustment of inspiratory flow. Flow rates can be adjusted by 100 mL/sec increments in a range from 100 to 600 mL/sec. Supplemental oxygen may also be provided by attaching supply tubing to a port on the back of the spirometer, if needed. The addition of supplemental oxygen will augment the patient's inspiratory flow; the manufacturer recommendations specify increasing the flow rate setting in this instance.

Hudson RCI LVE Lung Volume Exerciser

The Hudson RCI LVE (**Figure 12-5**) lung volume exerciser accomplishes lung expansion as the patient inhales slowly through a mouthpiece connected to a dual chamber that maintains a constant resistance during inspiration as the ball rises.[4] The resistance is equivalent to the selected inspiratory flow setting.[4] Higher flow rates result in greater chest rise and thoracic motion than lower flow rates.[4]

Intermittent Positive Pressure Breathing

Intermittent positive pressure breathing (IPPB) is a modality that utilizes a mechanical positive pressure device that provides lung expansion by delivering a controlled flow of air into the lungs at a predetermined pressure above atmospheric when triggered by a spontaneously breathing patient's effort.[15] IPPB can be flow,

pressure, or time cycled.[15] Breaths are pressure triggered, meaning as the patient inspires, a pressure drop below baseline is needed to initiate a positive pressure breath. With most devices, the trigger threshold is adjustable. Once the breath is triggered, a flow of gas is provided until a preset pressure is reached; flow then ceases, pressure is released to the lungs, and then the patient passively exhales to a baseline pressure.[15] Clinical studies in the early to mid-1960s demonstrated positive patient outcomes in terms of an increase in vital and inspiratory capacity, improved quality of breath sounds, and improved expiratory flow rates (FEV_1 or peak flow).[16,17] IPPB is delivered by a stand-alone positive pressure device or through an invasive or noninvasive ventilator.

Application

The lack of evidence in the literature supporting positive patient outcomes and the emergence of newer, low cost devices for hyperinflation therapy have contributed to the decline in use of this therapy over the past 20 years. Despite this, IPPB may still have a role in the management of patients with reduced lung volumes. The American Association for Respiratory Care (AARC) recognized this limitation in its recommendations regarding the use of IPPB in its Clinical Practice Guidelines. According to the AARC's Clinical Practice Guidelines, IPPB is not the therapeutic modality of choice for improving hyperinflation therapy or delivering medicated aerosols. As a result, this form of therapy is recommended only either when other less expensive hyperinflation therapies are not suitable or when the clinical objectives have not been met after other lower technology therapies have been used.[15] Currently available devices still make it possible for IPPB to be administered across the continuum of care. The use of electrically and pneumatically powered machines facilitate use in the inpatient, outpatient, and in-home settings as part of the patient's hyperinflation therapy regime. Treatment may be applied with a variety of patient interfaces, including mouthpiece, mask mouth shield, or connected directly to an artificial airway (tracheostomy or endotracheal tube). Treatment length is usually brief; studies recommend therapy should usually last about 20 minutes, and should not exceed 1 hour.[18] If possible, patients should be seated in semi-Fowler's position to achieve an even distribution of ventilation.[19] To avoid increased work of breathing the trigger threshold should be set at lower levels, to reduce the patient's inspiratory work but minimize the risk of auto-triggering. The literature supports the use of volume-oriented IPPB. Initially the pressure used to deliver a positive pressure is set relatively low, typically between 10 and 15 cm H_2O with an inspiratory to expiratory (I:E) ratio of about 1:3. Inspiratory pressure is then slowly increased until a minimum delivered volume of at least one-third of the patient's inspiratory capacity is achieved.[15,20]

IPPB is indicated for patients with low lung volumes who are at risk for or require treatment for atelectasis in the postoperative period.[21] For postoperative patients, incisional pain, residual effects of anesthesia, or analgesics may inhibit proper performance of other hyperinflation techniques, such as incentive spirometry or breathing exercises, for example. In these instances, patients may benefit from a device that can assist with lung expansion.[22] This form of therapy may also be indicated when treatment of atelectasis is refractory to other therapies. IPPB may be beneficial in patients whose cognitive impairment limits their ability to cooperate with other forms of hyperinflation therapy or when obstructive, restrictive diseases[23,24] or chest wall deformities[25] inhibit patients from maximizing the benefits of other forms of hyperinflation therapies. Volume-oriented IPPB has been shown to improve peak cough flows by means of hyperinflation and enhancing secretion clearance as a result of improving cough.[23] Patient assessment is essential; it should occur initially when determining if the therapy is appropriate and then on a continual basis to ensure goals of therapy are met, complications are identified and treated, and end-points are determined.

An absolute contraindication for IPPB is an untreated tension pneumothorax.[15] Relative contraindications to IPPB include intracranial pressure greater than 15 mm Hg; hemodynamic instability; active hemoptysis; radiographic evidence of air leak including blebs; recent facial, oral, skull, or esophageal surgeries; tracheoesophageal fistula; active tuberculosis; and nausea.[15]

Some hazards and complications of performing IPPB treatments include gastric distention, nosocomial infection, hypoxemia, hypocarbia, hemoptysis, hyperoxia, decreased venous return, increased ventilation perfusion mismatch, air trapping, intrinsic positive end-expiratory pressure (PEEP), or barotrauma including pneumothorax.[18,26] Precautions should be taken to consider stopping enteral feedings or waiting a specified period of time after a meal when patients are receiving IPPB treatments. As with any respiratory equipment, device malfunction and/or problems with patient technique can occur. These factors can interfere with achieving maximum benefits of the treatment. A list of common problems that may occur and a troubleshooting guide are found in **Table 12-2**.

Principles of Operation

IPPB can be accomplished through the use of any mechanical ventilator with a noninvasive option. Therapy can be accomplished by setting a peak inspiratory pressure (PIP) on an invasive or noninvasive pressure control (PC) mode with or without PEEP. Typically, the patient interface is a mask. Positive pressure breaths are initiated when either a change in bias flow (flow triggered) or a pressure drop from baseline (pressure triggered) occurs when the patient makes a spontaneous breathing effort. PIP or P_{high} is the amount of pressure delivered on inspiration. Because the ventilator is in pressure control mode, the flow delivered to the patient will vary and is dependent upon patient demand. The trigger level (pressure or flow) should be preset to assure that the breath can be generated easily, without permitting auto-triggering to occur.

Pressure support ventilation can also be used to deliver IPPB therapy. The operator would adjust the pressure support level to achieve the desired inspired volumes. Flow will vary and is dependent upon patient need. Inspiratory time is also variable and is dependent upon the time needed to reach the pressure support level, in addition to the operator-set criteria for the termination of the breath or manufacturer preset maximum inspiratory time (T_{supp}) limit. Most modern ventilators allow the clinician to make adjustments in the cycle criteria and terminate the breath early. The manner in which this is accomplished is manufacturer specific. The ventilator-provided application for IPPB is an expensive method for employing hyperinflation therapy and is not meant to be a permanent means of providing mechanical ventilatory support.

Pneumatically or electrically powered devices also can be used to deliver IPPB therapy. Generally these devices are pressure triggered. Depending on the device, inspiration is flow, pressure, or time cycled. Only a few types of devices are currently available on the market.

Hybrid flow devices are commercially available to provide IPPB therapy. These devices are small and lightweight, and connect to a compressed gas source by means of a standard flowmeter. This type of device has a port that allows attachment to a pressure manometer to measure inspiratory and expiratory pressures. Hybrid flow devices do not require special instructions to perform the maneuver and can be used with a mouthpiece or mask to provide hyperinflation therapy to patients with normal breathing patterns. Because of their relative ease of use and low cost, hybrid devices may function as an alternative to use of mechanical ventilators or devices used to deliver IPPB therapy.

Currently Available Devices
Puritan Bennett AP-5

The Puritan Bennett AP-5 is an electronically powered, pressure-triggered, pressure-targeted, and flow-cycled device. Its primary use is in settings where high pressure compressed gas is not available. Therefore, it is most commonly used in the home or an extended care facility, but it may also be used in outpatient offices and clinics. Gas is provided by an electrically powered compressor. When a positive pressure breath is triggered, gas flow is directed through a filter to either a nebulizer or a pressure control. A safety mechanism in the form of a pressure pop-off is incorporated into the unit at the filter outlet. The pressure control knob actually adjusts the tension of a simple spring disk pressure relief valve. Turning the knob clockwise increases the spring tension on the disk and permits the flow of gas at a variety of pressure settings, ranging from 0 to 30 cm H_2O. A pressure gauge is located on the front panel of the device, which allows the clinician to monitor pressures delivered to the patient during

TABLE 12-2
Troubleshooting Guide for Patient and Equipment Problems Commonly Associated with IPPB

Problem	Possible Causes Patient	Possible Causes Equipment	Suggested Solutions
Machine does not trigger		Leak in the system	Assess the device. Ensure all components are connected and connections are tight.
		Trigger threshold not set correctly.	Adjust the sensitivity setting to lower the trigger threshold and reduce the amount of patient effort needed to initiate a positive pressure breath.
		Power source not connected.	Connect pneumatically operated devices to a 50-psi gas source. Ensure pneumatically operated devices are not connected to the flowmeter of a high pressure compressed gas source (e.g., flowmeter connected to a piped-in gas system, flowmeter connected to a high pressure tank) or a low pressure gas source (e.g., stationary liquid oxygen container).
			Connect electrically powered devices to a wall outlet.
Machine auto-triggers		Trigger threshold not set correctly	Adjust the sensitivity setting to raise the trigger threshold and increase the amount of patient effort needed to initiate a positive pressure breath.
Machine does not cycle		Leak in the system	Assess the device. Ensure all components are connected and connections are tight.
	Patient technique causes leak in the system		Assess the patient's technique. Ensure the patient's mouth is sealed around the mouthpiece and that the patient is mouth breathing throughout inspiration and expiration. Evaluate the need for nose clips.
		Pressure set too high	Lower the set-inspiratory pressure. Evaluate the patient after pressure adjustments. Monitor patient for proper technique. Coach patient during maneuver. Monitor volumes delivered to patient and compare to targets.
		Flow is set too low	Increase the set flow rate. Evaluate the patient after flow adjustments. Monitor the patient for proper technique and ease of breathing during therapy.
Very short inspiratory time		Flow is set too high	Decrease the set flow rate. Evaluate the patient after flow adjustments. Monitor for proper technique and ease of breathing during therapy.
		Pressure set too low	Raise the set-inspiratory pressure. Evaluate the patient after pressure adjustments. Monitor patient for proper technique. Coach patient during maneuver if needed. Monitor volumes delivered to patient and compare to targets.
Very long inspiratory time		Leak in the system	Assess the device. Ensure all components are connected and connections are tight.
	Patient technique causes leak in the system		Assess the patient's technique. Ensure the patient's mouth is sealed around the mouthpiece and that the patient is mouth breathing throughout inspiration and expiration. Evaluate the need for nose clips.
		Pressure set too high	Lower the set-inspiratory pressure. Evaluate the patient after pressure adjustments. Monitor patient for proper technique. Coach patient during maneuver. Monitor volumes delivered to patient and compare to targets.
		Flow is set too low	Increase the set flow rate. Evaluate the patient after flow adjustments. Monitor the patient for proper technique and ease of breathing during therapy.
Tidal volume delivery is less than the patient target		Leak in the system	Assess the device for small leaks due to loose connections. Ensure all components are connected and connections are tight.
	Patient technique causes leak in the system		Assess the patient's technique. Ensure the patient's mouth is sealed around the mouthpiece and that the patient is mouth breathing throughout inspiration and expiration. Evaluate the need for nose clips.
		Flow is set too low	Increase the set flow rate. Evaluate the patient after flow adjustments. Monitor the patient for proper technique and ease of breathing during therapy.
		Pressure set too low	Raise the set-inspiratory pressure. Evaluate the patient after pressure adjustments. Monitor patient for proper technique. Coach patient during maneuver if needed. Monitor volumes delivered to patient and compare to targets.

inspiration. Gas exits the pressure relief valve and enters a hollow cylinder that is closed at either end with two rectangular openings on opposite sides, also known as the Bennett valve. A counterweight is contained within the cylinder and a drum vane attached to its external surface. During exhalation, the counterweight keeps the drum rotated in a counterclockwise position. While the drum is in this downward position, gas flowing from the pressure relief valve is blocked and gas is directed to the atmosphere through a dump port (**Figure 12-6**). During inspiration the drum moves clockwise to an upward or open position, allowing flow to enter the patient.[16] A separate nebulizer control incorporates a needle valve that receives gas from the compressor and increases or decreases gas that supplies the nebulizer.[27]

Bird Mark 7

The Bird Mark 7 (**Figure 12-7**) is one of the Bird Mark Series ventilators that was designed in the late 1950s

and 1960s by Forrest M. Bird and is still used today. This pressure controller is capable of delivering inspiratory pressures in the range of 10–60 cm H_2O.[27] A high pressure compressed gas source is used to both power and control this device. Inspiration may be triggered in one of three ways: by time, pressure, or manually pushing the hand timer rod. Positive pressure breaths are pressure or time cycled. Both breath phases incorporate a change in pressure and depend on an attraction of a metal clutch plate to a magnet to trigger or initiate a positive pressure breath or to cycle the breath off. **Figure 12-8** shows a conceptual diagram of the Bird Mark 7. This schematic displays a diaphragm, located in the center of the unit, that separates the central core into two chambers that communicate with ambient pressure. A metal plate is attached to both sides of the diaphragm and is positioned adjacent to a magnet in each compartment. When the pressure of both chambers is equal (Figure 12-8A) there is equal magnetic attraction on both sides of the diaphragm, so the diaphragm remains centered and does not move. When the patient makes an inspiratory effort, pressure on the patient or right side of the diaphragm drops, shifting the plate toward the magnet (Figure 12-8B). When the plate touches the magnet the pressure must increase to greater than ambient in the patient chamber to overcome the magnetic attraction. As pressure builds in the right chamber the plate and magnet shift to the left, increasing the pressure on the patient side (Figure 12-8C). During exhalation, a switch attached to the metal plate moves toward the ambient chamber (left), or the ambient magnet touches the plate. This action prevents positive pressure from entering the patient or circuit, completing the breath cycle. The pressure limit adjusts the proximity of the pressure magnet to the plate.

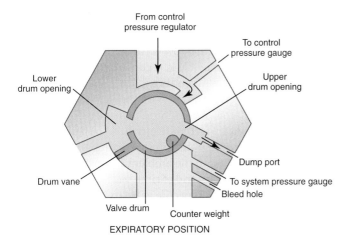

EXPIRATORY POSITION

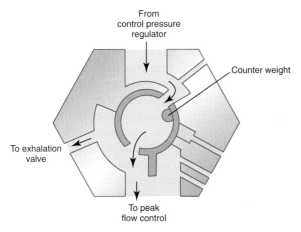

INSPIRATORY POSITION

FIGURE 12-6 The Bennett valve controls the flow of gas during inspiration and expiration. During inspiration, the vane drum rotates clockwise or upward into an open position to let gas flow from the pressure control regulator to the nebulizer. The vane drum with the Bennett valve rotates counterclockwise during expiration, directing the flow of gas from the pressure regulator to the dump port.

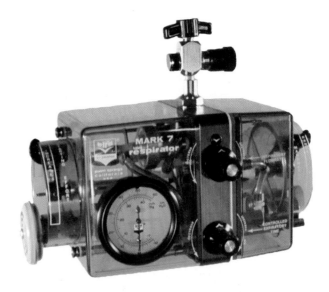

FIGURE 12-7 The Bird Mark 7. The first of several generations of Bird IPPB units that were commercially available from the early 1950s.

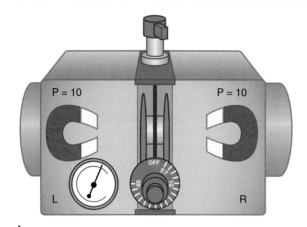

A

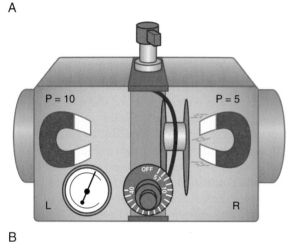

B

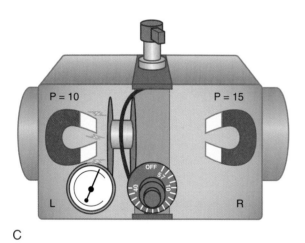

C

FIGURE 12-8 The use of pressure gradients and magnetism with the Bird series of devices used for IPPB. A. The pressure of both chambers is equal. B. The pressure on the patient side of the chamber drops as a result of an inspiratory effort. C. The clutch plate and magnet shift to the left as pressure on the right side, or patient side, increases during inspiration.

In addition to the movement of the plate toward the magnet, a ceramic switch moves to the right and allows gas flow to enter the flow control valve and an opening in the ceramic switch to the patient. Flow is then directed to the (air/mix) control. The air mixture valve is a plunger

mechanism that controls F_IO_2 by allowing flow to go in and out of a venturi jet entrainment device. The venturi entrains gas from the ambient part of the chamber, lowering the concentration of oxygen delivered to the patient. If the plunger is pushed in, O rings block the pathway to the venturi. The air/O_2 mix knob is closed and the concentration of oxygen remains at 100%. When there is no air entrainment, gas flows to the nebulizer output. When the air/O_2 mix plunger is pulled out or is in the open position, gas enters from the nebulizer output and the venturi. Air from the ambient portion of the chamber is entrained, lowering the F_IO_2. Because the device relies on pressure to entrain ambient air, the concentration of oxygen delivered to the patient during the ventilator cycle varies.[27] A spring-loaded valve is located at the outlet to the venturi. This valve functions as a gate that prevents gas from inadvertently entering the pressure compartment from the ambient compartment during inspiration. A pressure of 2 cm H_2O is needed to open this gate and allow gas to enter the pressure chamber.

In addition to affecting the F_IO_2, the air-mix controller affects the shape of the pressure waveform. When in mix position, the pressure waveform uses the Venturi and creates a descending flow waveform. In the closed position the flow waveform is rectangular while the pressure waveform is ascending.[27]

When manual inspiration is desired, a hand timer rod moves a ceramic switch into the inspiratory position. On a patient-triggered inspiration, spontaneous effort causes pressure in the pressure compartment to fall below pressure in the ambient compartment. An expiratory timer cartridge time triggers breaths by diverting gas to an open needle valve in the pressure compartment. On exhalation, pressure drops in the cartridge and gas exits through the needle valve to a bleed hole, pushing the spring and diaphragm to the right in preparation for the next inhalation. The velocity that gas travels through the needle valve determines the length of expiratory time in seconds.

The trigger threshold on the Bird Mark 7 is controlled by the sensitivity arm. Changes in the arm position alter the proximity of the magnet to the ambient clutch plate. The closer the plate is to the magnet, the more effort the patient must exert to overcome the magnetic pull of the magnet on the plate, making it more difficult to initiate a positive pressure breath. Conversely, the farther away the plate is from the magnet, the less effort the patient must exert to overcome the magnetic pull.

Vortran IPPB

The Vortran IPPB is a small device that uses a single-patient-use manifold to provide medicated aerosol therapy in conjunction with intermittent positive pressure ventilation. This device requires no maintenance, and the disposable patient manifold may be used by the same patient for several therapies.

Therefore, the relative cost for operating and maintaining this type of device is relatively low. The device can be operated by connecting it to a 50-psi gas source or a standard medical grade flowmeter. The device operates from a continuous flow of gas. A high inspiratory flow, up to 40 L/min, can be achieved when the unit is connected to a 50-psi source. When connected to a standard flowmeter, flow rates of 15 to 40 L/min can be generated. Breaths are pressure triggered and are time or pressure cycled. A spring-loaded pressure modulator and a nebulizer are the main components of this device (**Figure 12-9**). The modulator is an adjustable spring-loaded valve that is capable of providing inspiratory pressures from 20 to 50 cm H_2O and baseline pressures of PEEP from 2 to 5 cm H_2O. A pressure manometer is incorporated into the manifold to monitor inspiratory pressures delivered to the patient. The aerosol generator operates from a demand valve. This air entrainment valve allows the patient to access fresh gas, which

is drawn in through the nebulizer, if needed. Air entrainment affects and dilutes F_IO_2. The F_IO_2 will vary proportionally with the amount of air entrained. The more air the patient entrains, the lower the F_IO_2 will be. The nebulizer reservoir can hold up to 20 mL of an aqueous solution. Inspiratory time and breath rate are adjustable from 0.5 to 3.0 seconds and 8 to 20 breaths per minute, respectively. Tidal volume is a product of inspiratory time and flow. It can be estimated by first converting the units of measure for flow from L/min to mL/sec, and then multiplying flow (L/sec) by inspiratory time (sec). The following provides an example:

Flow = 20 L/min
Inspiratory time = 0.5 sec

Equation needed to determine V_T:

$$V_T = \text{Flow (mL/sec)} \times \text{Inspiratory time (seconds)}$$

1. Convert flow from mL/min to mL/sec:

20 L/min/60 sec = 0.333 L/sec
0.333 L/sec × 1,000 mL/L = 333 mL/sec

2. Multiply flow (mL/sec) by inspiratory time (sec):

333 mL/sec × 0.5 sec = 167 mL

However, the manufacturer provides a quick reference chart for clinicians in the device operator's guide (**Table 12-3**). Turning the rate dial clockwise decreases trigger sensitivity and counterclockwise increases trigger sensitivity. The Voltran IPPB is not equipped with a redundant safety pop-off valve. Therefore, it is not recommended for use with patients requiring tracheal airways (endotracheal tubes or tracheostomy tubes) and should be used cautiously when administering therapy by mask.

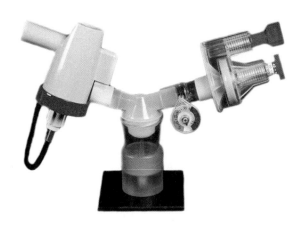

FIGURE 12-9 The Vortran IPPB, a disposable, single-patient-use device.

Courtesy of VORTRAN® Medical Technology1, Inc., Sacramento, CA.

TABLE 12-3
The Vortran IPPB Quick Reference Chart for Estimating Tidal Volume Delivery (mL) at Different Inspiratory Time and Flow Combinations

Flow (L/min)	Inspiratory Time (seconds)					
	0.5	1	1.5	2	2.5	3
15	125	250	375	500	625	750
20	167	333	500	667	833	1,000
25	208	417	625	833	1,042	1,250
30	250	500	750	1,000	1,250	1,500
35	282	583	875	1,167	1,458	1,750
40	333	667	1,000	1,333	1,667	2,000

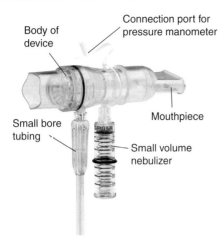

FIGURE 12-10 Parts of the EzPAP (Smiths Medical) illustrating the use of a small volume nebulizer in-line with the device to provide medicated aerosol therapy in tandem with hyperinflation therapy.
Courtesy of Smiths Medical.

Hybrid IPPB/PEP Device

EzPAP

The EzPAP device uses flow from a compressed gas source (air or oxygen) to generate positive airway pressure on inspiration. The device also incorporates a fixed orifice threshold resistor to impede exhaled flow and generate positive expiratory pressure (PEP). Medicated aerosol therapy can be delivered in conjunction with this device by attaching a nebulizer between the patient mouthpiece and the device (**Figure 12-10**). The application of PEP enhances collateral ventilation in the airways by creating a back pressure that stents conducting airways open and positive pressure throughout exhalation to open up collapsed or partially collapsed alveoli. Snyder and colleagues tested the effect that the addition of a small volume nebulizer as well as the effect increasing compressed gas flow rates had on positive inspiratory and expiratory pressures on healthy volunteers. The researchers demonstrated that the addition of a nebulizer had little effect on the airway pressures generated.[28] Their data verified that airway pressure was a function of the flow set on the flowmeter and that the device maintained controllable, clinically useful airway pressures throughout the respiratory cycle with the inspiratory pressure averaging 45% of the expiratory pressure.[28]

Principles of Operation

Oxygen supply tubing is connected to a compressed gas source on one end and to the gas inlet port on the other and flow is set at 5–15 L/min (Figure 12-10). A pressure gauge attaches to the pressure port for monitoring.[17] The patient inspires through the device with little effort at a preset flow, and then exhales against a flow or resistance that generates an expiratory pressure.[17] The greater the inspiratory flow, the lower the pressure

delivered to the airway. As the patient's expiratory flow increases, the expiratory pressure generated is higher. A nebulizer can be placed in line with EzPAP for medication delivery because it has minimal effect on the delivered airway pressure.[17]

Intrapulmonary Percussive Ventilation (IPV)

Intrapulmonary percussive ventilation (IPV) is a therapy that combines hyperinflation therapy with airway clearance therapy. The delivery of positive pressure during inspiration eases some of the work of the patient's respiratory muscles and augments inspired volumes in order to improve gas exchange.[29] The application of high frequency pulses of flow (100–300/minute) superimposed on the patient's spontaneous breathing pattern provides changes in transrespiratory pressure and facilitates the cephalad movement of secretions during passive exhalation.[30,31] Convective flow, molecular diffusion, Taylor dispersion, and step-by-step inflation are integrated into IPV and promote alveolar gas mixing, augment gas exchange, and enhance airway clearance.[30–32] IPV has been shown to stabilize mean airway pressure while increasing lung volume at a preset pressure, to deliver aerosolized medications, and to facilitate the mobilization of airway secretions.[33]

Application

IPV was invented by Dr. Forrest Bird and first described in the literature in the mid-1980s as a method of delivering aerosolized bronchodilators to patients with chronic obstructive lung disease (COPD).[34] This therapy can be administered manually or automatically using applications for both inpatient and outpatient settings to expand collapsed alveoli or facilitate the mobilization of secretions due to impaired airway clearance mechanisms including for patients who do not respond to or cannot tolerate unassisted forms of hyperinflation therapy (i.e., incentive spirometry, thoracic expansion exercises), standard chest physical therapy, or other forms of airway clearance. The literature reports the use of IPV in the treatment of atelectasis[33] and as a method to facilitate secretion removal in patients with neurodegenerative diseases,[35] COPD,[32] and cystic fibrosis.[30,31] IPV is applied noninvasively via a mouthpiece, mask, or mouth guard, or invasively in-line with a ventilator circuit during continuous mechanical ventilation. IPV may be used in conjunction with a stand-alone PEEP valve or by adjusting a setting on the respective device or mechanical unit. The patient circuit is designed to enable the delivery of aerosolized medication in conjunction with positive inspiratory pressure and percussive breaths.

The definitive and relative contraindications for IPV are similar to those for IPPB. The only absolute contraindication to therapy is an untreated tension pneumothorax. Relative contraindications include increased intracranial pressure; tracheoesophageal fistula; hemodynamic instability; active hemoptysis; recent postoperative esophageal, facial, oral, or cranial surgery; active and untreated tuberculosis; and nausea.[29]

Because a positive pressure is applied on inspiration and expiration, gastric insufflation, hyperventilation, hemodynamic compromise, air leak, pneumothorax or barotraumas, air trapping, and alveolar overdistention remain potential hazards of this form of therapy.[29] Care should be taken to assess the patient prior to, during, and after the treatment. Close monitoring of the patient's vital signs, breath sounds, and oxygen saturation may minimize hazards and reduce complications of therapy by promoting identification and applying the appropriate intervention. To minimize the occurrence of vomiting and risk of aspiration, precautions should be taken to coordinate a patient's meals or feeding schedule with therapy. It is advisable to schedule treatments at least 1 hour after eating or to temporarily discontinue feedings during treatment when a patient is receiving intermittent or continuous enteral nutrition via artificial means using gastrostomy or nasogastric tube.

Currently Available Devices

Percussionator IPV-1C

The Percussionator (Percussionaire, Sandpoint, ID) is a pneumatically powered device that disperses aerosolized medications simultaneously with positive pressure percussive breaths to the lungs. The Percussionator creates high frequency bursts (100 to 300 bursts per minute) of flow through activation of the venturi system within a flow interrupter called a Phasitron. High frequency percussive breaths, superimposed on a positive pressure breath, can be triggered manually by the patient or automatically by a triggering mechanism. A 50-psi compressed gas source is needed to operate this device.

The Percussionator IPV-1C has only four operator controls (**Figure 12-11**). Gas enters the device at 50 psi from a high pressure compressed source. Gas is directed through a pressure regulator. The operational pressure control makes adjustments to the device's working pressure (20–50 psig). The front panel contains an aneroid gauge, which displays the operational pressure. The On/Off switch will open up or prevent the flow of gas from the compressed gas source into the pressure regulator. In the Off position, the unit may remain connected to the high pressure gas source but does not consume gas, rendering the unit nonfunctional.

Gas exits the IPV-1C through sockets on the front panel of the device. The sockets direct gas flow to the nebulizer, phasitron, and remote outputs in the

patient circuit as well as to a pressure manometer. The percussion control determines the number of flow bursts that occur during the breathing cycle. The percussion frequency affects the pressure amplitude delivered. Percussion frequency is adjustable from 1 to 11 Hz. Percussion frequency and pressure amplitude are inversely related. As the frequency is increased pressure amplitude decreases, and vice versa. A fixed inspiratory to expiratory (I:E) ratio of 1:2 to 1:2.5 is used.[31,34] A button is available on the front panel to allow inspiration to be manually triggered. The unit will remain in the inspiratory phase as long as this button is depressed. Manual releasing of this button will allow for passive exhalation.

During IPV, therapeutic delivery of gas through the phasitron or sliding venturi (**Figure 12-12**) adjusts inspiratory flow and results in a pressure that varies to some degree in response to the patient's lung compliance and resistance. Gas diverted through the nebulizer orifice flows to the nebulizer jet and an orifice sleeve that covers the jet. Negative pressure between the jet and sleeve draws medication up through the sleeve from holes located at the bottom of the sleeve.

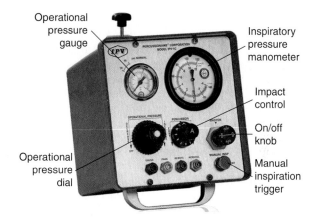

FIGURE 12-11 The Percussionator IPV-1C with labeled controls.
Courtesy of Percussionaire® Corporation.

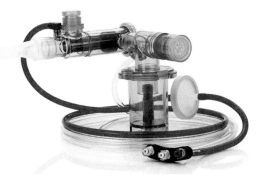

FIGURE 12-12 The Phasitron portion of the IPV breathing circuit incorporating the sliding venturi and the small volume nebulizer.
Courtesy of Percussionaire® Corporation.

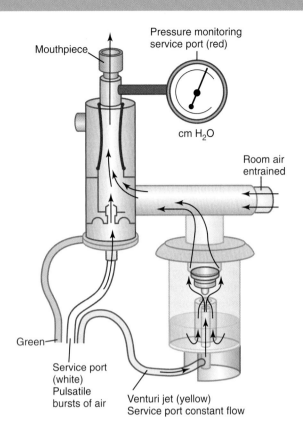

FIGURE 12-13 A cross-sectional view of the IPV breathing circuit that shows the flow of gas and medicated aerosol to the patient. The service ports are color coded on the device, as well as the circuit. Ambient air, entrained through the venturi, mixes with the gas exiting the nebulizer socket to aerosolize medication in the nebulizer. This drawing shows a mouthpiece as the patient interface.

Medication scatters at the top of the sleeve when particles reach a diffractor. Medication combines with gas entrained from room air through the entrainment port and enters the phasitron (**Figure 12-13**). As gas proceeds through the phasitron tubing attached to a sliding venturi, aerosolized particles from the nebulizer enter the phasitron. As the venturi moves back and forth it creates the percussion, further directing the flow from the venturi to the patient connection. The sliding venturi moves over the exhalation port, creating some loss of inspiratory gas and reduction in F_IO_2 (**Figure 12-14**). Patient or peak pressure is monitored at the distal portion of the phasitron assembly and displayed on the manometer on the face of the machine. The patient continues to breathe spontaneously through the entire cycle, independent of the percussion interval (treatment) that is controlled by the patient or caregiver.

Percussive Neb IPPV

Percussive Neb (Vortran Medical Technology, Sacramento, CA) is a disposable IPV device approved for single-patient use (**Figure 12-15**). The Percussive Neb incorporates a pneumatic flow interrupter to

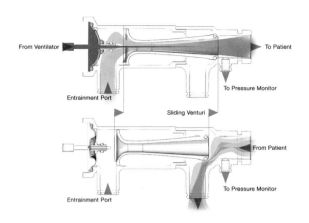

FIGURE 12-14 A cross-section of the phasitron showing the flow of gas. A. Inspiratory phase. B. Expiratory phase.
Courtesy of Percussionaire® Corporation.

generate small bursts of gas at high flows to a mouthpiece at frequencies of 11 to 30 Hz. Oxygen or compressed air from a standard flowmeter set at 15–16 L/min is used to power this device. Pressures of 20 to 40 cm H_2O may be delivered and adjusted by rotating the amplitude dial. The amplitude dial does not have reference marks, rather, it is visually displayed on the pressure manometer incorporated into the unit. I:E ratios of 1:2 to 1:3 are delivered and vary depending on the oscillation frequency. The higher the frequency, the lower the I:E. This device is also capable of delivering medicated aerosol therapy in addition to positive pressure required for lung expansion. The nebulizer output is approximately 1 mL/min. The single-patient-use manifold device cannot be used with a mechanical ventilator.

MetaNeb

The MetaNeb (HillRom Respiratory Care, St. Paul, MN) is a device that can deliver IPV or continuous positive expiratory pressure (CPEP). This device requires a 50-psi compressed gas source for operation. Gas first passes through the internal circuitry of the controller to power it and then is directed to the patient as therapy gas. As it passes through the controller it may be sent through an internal chopper valve, which chops the linear flow into pulses for continuous high frequency oscillation, or through a series of internal circuits that allow it to be controlled and delivered as CPEP. The high frequency pulses are calibrated to deliver I:E ratios of approximately 1:2. A portion of the supply gas is used to power the nebulizer. The front panel contains a pressure manometer, a tri-connector for the patient circuit, and three control knobs (**Figure 12-16**). The mode selector knob allows the operator to choose which form of therapy to provide to the patient. Choices include continuous high frequency oscillation (CHFO), continuous positive expiratory pressure (CPEP), or just

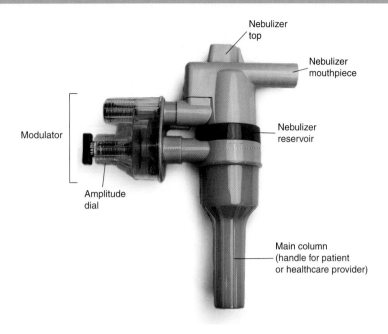

FIGURE 12-15 The Percussive Neb is a disposable single-patient-use IPV device.

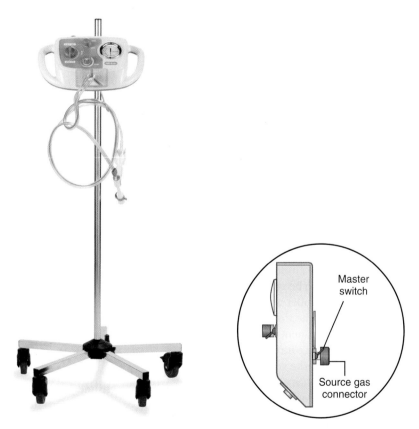

FIGURE 12-16 The MetaNeb.

the nebulizer (Aerosol Only). If CHFO is selected, a second control switch allows for pressure adjustment of the pulsatile breath rate and pulse amplitude. Clinicians have two choices—Higher or Lower—which will cause simultaneous directional changes in both pressure and

breath rate. The third control knob allows the inspiratory flow to be set and is functional in the CPEP mode.

The patient circuit (**Figure 12-17**) is connected to the controller by means of a tri-connector located just below the mode selector. A single connector is located

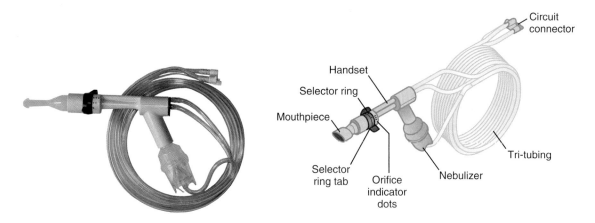

FIGURE 12-17 MetaNeb circuit with labeling.

on the distal end of the patient circuit, which attaches to the controller and is secured in place with two locking mechanisms. Proximal to the tri-connector are three tubes connected to one another, and a handset. One tube transports therapy gas from the controller to the back of the handset. A second tube supplies flow to the nebulizer. A third tube transmits pressure from the handset directly to the manometer. The handset is made up of a patient opening, selector ring, venturi, proximal pressure tube, jet, entrainment ports, nebulizer port, and nebulizer. The patient opening can be connected to a mouthpiece, a cushion mask, or a tracheostomy tube or placed in-line with a ventilator (**Figure 12-18B**). The selector ring enables expiratory resistance to be adjusted to one of three settings. Rotating the ring will change the size of the expiratory orifices underneath the selector ring. The ring is shown in **Figure 12-18A**. An occlusion ring is included with the circuit to replace the selector ring for use in-line with a ventilator. The venturi serves as a safety mechanism and regulates flow to the patient. The proximal pressure tube links the patient connection end of the handset to the pressure tubing of the circuit, which in turn allows the proximal pressures to be read at the manometer on the front of the controller. A jet in the rear of the handset funnels gas into the throat of the venturi and is surrounded by entrainment ports. The entrainment ports serve not only as a source of ingress for ambient gas, which is drawn into the venturi, but also of egress, allowing them to serve as a safety pop-off of sorts in the event of excessive back pressure. Aerosolized medication is produced by the nebulizer and entrained into the venturi via the nebulizer port.

Positive Airway Pressure Devices

Positive airway pressure (PAP) devices are used to treat atelectasis and reduce the work of breathing by increasing intraluminal bronchial pressure, which maintains airway patency, reduces airway resistance,

and minimizes airway obstruction.[36] Positive expiratory pressure (PEP), and continuous positive airway pressure (CPAP) are PAP approaches that are used for bronchial hygiene or lung expansion therapy.[37]

Positive Expiratory Pressure

During **positive expiratory pressure (PEP)** therapy, positive expiratory pressure is applied to the airways as the patient exhales against a resistance. A back pressure is created during the expiratory maneuver, which stents the airways open and improves airway patency. This may be beneficial in reducing premature airway closure in patients with alterations in bronchial smooth muscle tone, such as patients with bronchoconstriction or bronchomalasia (i.e., bronchiectasis). An active, not forced, exhalation produces expiratory pressures up to 20 cm H_2O with most commercially available devices, with 10–20 cm H_2O cited as the therapeutic range. This maneuver mimics the physiological effects of pursed lip breathing, often performed by individuals with chronic obstructive pulmonary diseases.

Continuous Positive Airway Pressure

Continuous positive airway pressure (CPAP) is a constant airway pressure maintained during both the inspiratory and expiratory phases. CPAP elevates intrathoracic pressure and alveolar pressure, which in turn increases functional residual capacity (FRC) and improves collateral ventilation by improving the distribution of ventilation.[38] The application of positive pressure for patients with bronchoconstriction or bronchospasm decreases the work of breathing by reducing the respiratory effort required to initiate a spontaneous breath in the face of intrinsic PEEP.[39] Expiratory positive airway pressure (EPAP) increases intraluminal airway pressure, stents the airway open, and stabilizes end expiratory lung volume.[39] CPAP may provide additional benefit by enhancing the mechanism of secretion

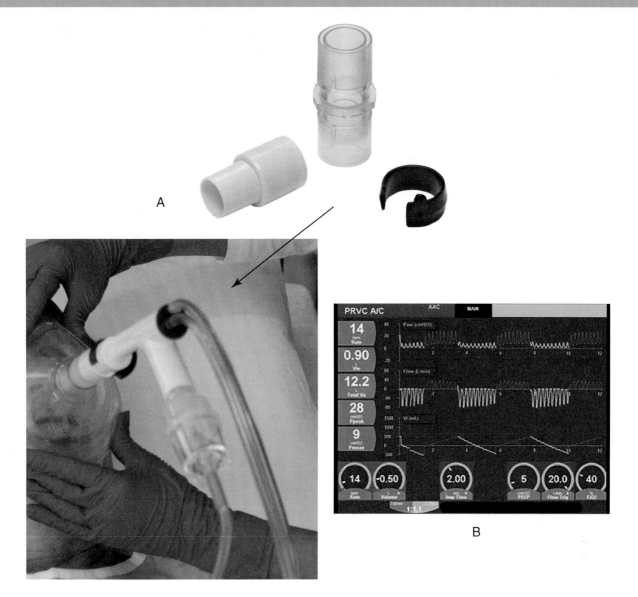

FIGURE 12-18 The MetaNeb inline with a ventilator circuit. A. A view of the adaptors necessary to incorporate the handset into the ventilator circuit. B. Waveform display of high frequency oscillations when the MetaNeb is used inline with a ventilator.

removal. CPAP can be applied intermittently or continuously through a valved mask, but there is no consensus on one mask preference over another.[40] Threshold resistors and flow resistors are two types of expiratory pressure valve systems that can be used to provide CPAP.

CPAP may also be administered invasively through a tracheal tube (endotracheal tube or tracheostomy tube) or noninvasively (nasal mask, oronasal mask, full face mask, etc.) by a mechanical ventilator. If a mechanical ventilator is used, the patient is placed in the continuous spontaneous mode of ventilation. Infant ventilators will use a continuous flow or demand flow system. During inspiration, the flow of gas from the ventilator to the patient must be maintained above the patient's inspiratory flow to maintain the operator-set CPAP. During spontaneous breathing the CPAP level will vary with changes in the breathing cycle, decreasing during inspiration and increasing with exhalation. Changes in baseline pressure of up to 2 cm H_2O are associated with a normal work of breathing.[38] Some infant ventilators do not provide a constant fresh flow of gas through the ventilator circuit during inspiration and expiration. Flow during exhalation is reduced to minimize the resistive work of breathing associated with breathing against a fixed flow of gas. The patient is able to access more flow by opening a demand valve. Ventilators that use demand flow have been shown to decrease the work of breathing by fulfilling flow demands required by the patient.[36]

Threshold Resistors

During intermittent PAP therapy, using a threshold resistor, patients breathe from a pressurized circuit against a fixed resistance (i.e., resistance is constant with varying flow). There are different types of threshold resistors. Some devices use a water-column, weighted-ball, or spring-loaded device to maintain a consistent airway pressure, typically from 5 to 20 cm H_2O. Depending on the device, this airway pressure may be constant only during the expiratory phase, such as with positive expiratory pressure (PEP) devices, or throughout the entire respiratory cycle, as with CPAP devices. Threshold resistors create pressure that does not require the patient's flow rate to remain constant and impose minimal resistance above opening pressure to achieve the desired pressure.[41] When placed in the expiratory limb of a breathing circuit, a threshold resistor slows or stops exhalation while maintaining a preset pressure higher than ambient.

Gravity-dependent threshold resistors require a specific position that severely restricts movement and are typically inconvenient to use. The disadvantage of these devices is any change in its position may result in changes in the expiratory pressure. An example of a gravity-dependent threshold resistor is the weighted-ball principle incorporated within a PEEP valve.

Non–gravity-dependent threshold resistor devices are most popular. Upon selection of a specific level of PEEP, spring-loaded valves maintain pressure as a coil is compressed, resulting in positive pressure being maintained on the other side of the spring (PEEP valve added to a ventilator exhalation valve). The amount of positive pressure maintained is proportional to the tension on the spring. Valved diaphragms maintain positive pressure that is dependent on the position of the valve and where it is seated. Balloon-type devices establish PEEP by maintaining a force in the balloon that must be exceeded in order for exhalation to occur (ventilator with exhalation diaphragm in the circuit) (**Figure 12-19**).

Flow-Dependent Resistors

Flow resistor–type devices produce expiratory positive pressure that varies with the patient's expiratory flow. Generally, commercially available devices that use this principle of operation allow the clinician to adjust the expiratory pressure by changing the size of the orifice. Expiratory positive pressure varies inversely with the orifice size, assuming the expiratory flow rate is constant. As the orifice size decreases, resistance to expiratory flow increases.

Figure 12-19C illustrates a screw-clamp variable orifice. As the clamp tightens, the orifice becomes smaller. The smaller the orifice, the greater the expiratory resistance and pressure will be. Expiratory flow has a direct proportional effect on the pressure generated by this type of device (**Figure 12-20**). Expiratory flow is depicted in Figure 12-20A. As expiratory flow decreases, pressure decreases as well, as shown in Figures 12-20B and 12-20C.

Uses

CPAP delivered by mask or prongs with devices that utilize threshold resistors may help decrease the work of breathing and reduce air trapping in patients with obstructive diseases such as asthma and chronic obstructive pulmonary disease.[42, 43] CPAP may also help facilitate the cephalad mobilization of retained secretions (in certain chronic conditions such as cystic fibrosis and chronic bronchitis) as well as prevent or reverse atelectasis.[42] CPAP may help by providing positive pressure to upper airway structures during the expiratory phase and has been used extensively in the treatment of obstructive sleep apnea.[44] Bronchodilator delivery may be optimized in patients who are receiving bronchial hygiene therapy and positive airway pressure combined.[26] As with CPAP, PAP may also be used as an intermittent treatment option for secretion removal and treatment and/or prevention of atelectasis.

Types

Underwater Seal (Bubble CPAP) Water Column

Water column threshold resistors are gravity dependent and achieve CPAP using the force exerted by a column of water.[45] Adjusting the water level of the column will

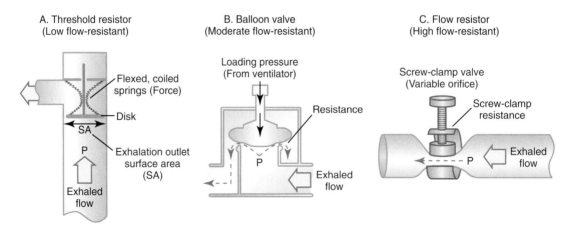

FIGURE 12-19 A. Threshold resistor valve. B. Balloon valve. C. Flow resistor.

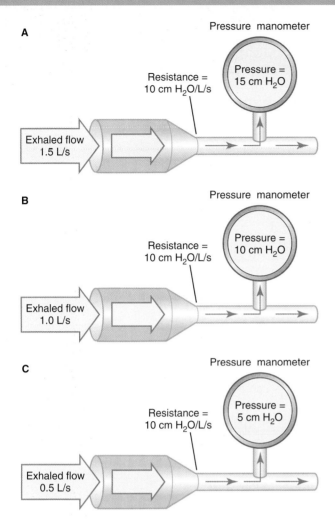

FIGURE 12-20 A schematic drawing of the effect expiratory flow has on PEP. A. For a fixed resistance (R = 10 cm H_2O/L/sec), the greater the flow, the higher the pressure generated during exhalation is. B. and C. As flow is reduced, expiratory pressure decreases concomitantly.

change the expiratory pressure. CPAP can be achieved by applying the positive pressure to a mask, nasal prongs, or an endotracheal tube.[45]

Bubble CPAP is an inexpensive method of providing PAP that is typically used in neonates with respiratory distress to provide a form of lung recruitment.[45–47] Bubble CPAP devices may be used instead of a mechanical ventilator for infants who present with atelectasis related to surfactant-deficient lungs. Studies have demonstrated that bubble CPAP is cost efficient and as effective as CPAP provided through a mechanical ventilator in reducing the infant's work of breathing and improving gas exchange.[48,49]

Portable commercially available devices exist for short- or long-term use.

Principles of Operation

Bubble CPAP uses a continuous flow source gas at a specified F_1O_2. The expiratory limb of the patient circuit is submersed a specific depth underwater that correlates with the level of desired CPAP (i.e., 5 cm depth produces 5 cm H_2O CPAP). **Figure 12-21** shows a schematic of bubble CPAP designed for manual ventilation. The expiratory tubing bubbles and generates positive pressure on exhalation.[45,47] Oscillations from the bubbling have been reported to transmit back into the airway and produce vibrations that in turn enhance gas exchange.[45]

Examples of Current Equipment Using This Technology

The following are examples of current equipment that use this technology:

> *Infant Nasal CPAP Assembly (INCA):* The Infant Nasal CPAP Assembly (**Figure 12-22**) is a commercially available bubble CPAP device used for therapeutic (rather than resuscitation) purposes. INCA uses a

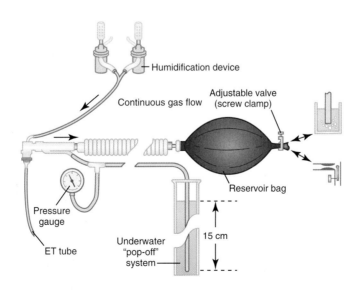

FIGURE 12-21 Basic CPAP setup.

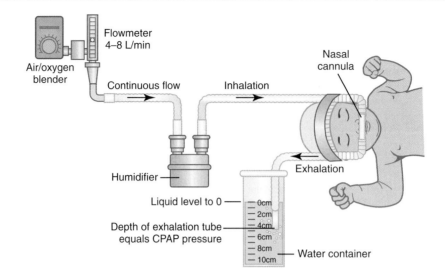

FIGURE 12-22 The INCA Bubble CPAP.
Image provided by CooperSurgical, Inc.

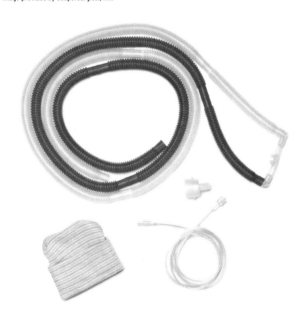

FIGURE 12-23 Hudson Infant Nasal CPAP cannula system.
Courtesy of Teleflex.

CPAP cannula attached to flex tubing that can be used with a standardized bubble/water column. A pressure line is attached to a manometer while the tubing adapter connects to standard size tubing that is submersed in a water column downstream. A source gas is attached to blended oxygen and creates the flow within the system. The CPAP is dependent on how far the tubing is submersed below the surface. This setup is available in 7.5 to 15 French interfaces, which generally meet the size requirements of most infants.

Hudson RCI: The Hudson RCI infant nasal prong CPAP cannula system (Teleflex Medical) (**Figure 12-23**) is compatible with a water seal or spring-loaded valve or can be used with any standard mechanical ventilator circuit. On one side of the cannula, the source gas tubing attaches to a flow source of blended gas that is supplied to the infant. On the opposing side of the cannula, an adapter is attached to the cannula and a T-piece adapter is connected to a pressure manometer. The expiratory tubing is submersed underwater to create CPAP.

Commercially Available Devices That Use Threshold Resistors

Weighted Ball Devices

Weighted ball threshold resistors are gravity dependent and generate PEP as the weight of the ball exerts force over a precise calibrated exhalation orifice. These devices have preset values that generate pressures from 2.5 to 15 cm H_2O. The heavier the ball, the greater the force it exerts and the greater the PEP generated.

Weighted ball threshold resistors utilize the dead-weight measurement principle, which consists of a precision ball of known size and density that restricts the gas flow through a calibrated orifice until a threshold back pressure is achieved. As the ball floats off the orifice inside the resistor the system is opened to pressure. These systems require a minimal flow rate to maintain a constant pressure over time.

Examples of current equipment using this technology include the following:

Boehringer Laboratories PEEP valves: Boehringer Laboratories PEEP valves (**Figure 12-24**) are threshold resistors that use a weighted ball to provide resistance to exhaled gas flow and positive expiratory pressure. Valves are individually calibrated from 2.5 to 15 cm H_2O and are changed with each level of PEP or PEEP, if used in-line with a mechanical ventilator. These valves are considered to have consistent measured PEEP or PEP, exhibiting stable pressure in most applications.

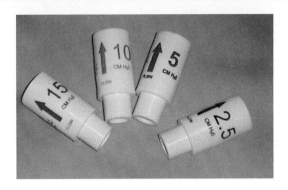

FIGURE 12-24 Boehringer valves use a weighted ball technology to provide positive expiratory pressure for PEP therapy, or continuous positive expiratory pressure (PEEP) if placed inline with a ventilator circuit.

Courtesy of Boehringer Laboratories.

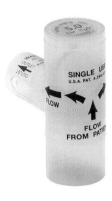

FIGURE 12-25 AccuPEEP valve.

Reproduced with permission from CareFusion.

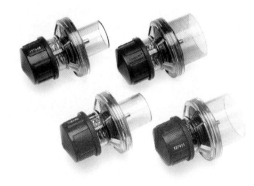

FIGURE 12-26 Spring-loaded PEEP valve.

Courtesy of Ambu Medical.

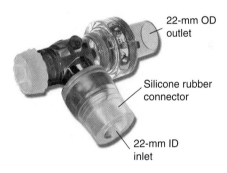

FIGURE 12-27 Magnetic PEEP valve.

Courtesy of Instrumentation Industries.

Accu PEEP valve: Accu PEEP valves (Vital Signs GE, Totowa, NJ), shown in **Figure 12-25**, are used for invasive ventilation when attached to a mechanical ventilator circuit or anesthesia circuit. The fixed orifice valves are available in 2.5, 5, 7.5, 10, 12.5, 15, and 20 cm H_2O settings. These valves can also be used noninvasively to provide PAP therapy when attached to a mask's lower expiratory port.[38] The upper port of the mask receives flow to the circuit from a gas source while the lower port with PEEP valve maintains and controls expiratory gas flow.[38]

Spring-Loaded Valve

Spring-loaded valves create positive expiratory pressure as coiled springs exert force against a plastic disk. The greater the force exerted on the disk across the valve surface area, the higher the pressure. PEEP valves are available in individual preset spring tensions of 2.5 to 20 cm H_2O or are adjustable to different PEEP settings, usually from 5 to 20 cm H_2O.

AMBU PEEP valves (AMBU Medical, Glen Burnie, MD), shown in **Figure 12-26**, are spring-loaded valves

that have been designed to provide PEEP through a manual resuscitator, anesthesia ventilator, or other breathing circuits requiring PEEP. Upon exhalation, the patient's expiratory flow encounters the resistance relative to the set expiratory pressure. The expiratory pressure is determined by the amount of tension placed on the spring and is adjustable from 0 to 20 cm H_2O for reusable valves and 1.5 to 20 cm H_2O for single-patient-use valves. Valves that are designed for multipatient use may be autoclaved at temperatures of 273°F (134°C).

Magnetic Valve

A magnetic valve threshold resistor uses a coil of wire, or solenoid, that produces an electromagnetic force when an electric current passes through it. This current is applied over the surface of a diaphragm. The expiratory pressure delivered is proportional to the amount of electric current supplied to the solenoid. The control knob on a ventilator regulates the amount of CPAP delivered to the patient.

The BE142 Magnetic PEEP valve (Instrumentation Laboratories, Bethel Park, PA), shown in **Figure 12-27**,

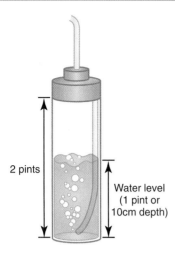

FIGURE 12-28 Basic design of a PEP bottle.

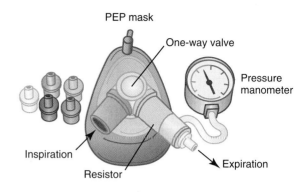

FIGURE 12-29 Schematic of a commercially available PEP mask setup.

maintains expiratory pressure at the end of exhalation through the use of a magnet that is set at an adjustable distance from a check valve. The valve remains closed until the check valve pressure overcomes the force of the magnetic field, allowing the valve to open. The pressure drops at end expiration, causing the valve to close and maintain a constant PEEP at the operator-desired level. PEEP is adjustable from 3 to 30 cm H_2O. The magnetic PEEP valve is designed to be used with mechanical ventilators, as an adjunct to resuscitator devices, and for anesthesia ventilators.

Devices Used to Provide PEP Therapy
PEP Bottle

A PEP bottle (**Figure 12-28**) uses a bottle partially filled with water to provide resistance to expiratory flow.[50] This device is also known as a blow bottle or bubble PEP. A gas source provides flow to the system through a tube or a piece of small-bore tubing. The distal tip of the tube conducting the gas is submersed in the water column at a desired level that is proportional to the amount of expiratory pressure delivered. As the patient exhales through the tube, pressure increases until it overcomes the weight of the water column.

PEP Mask

The PEP mask (**Figure 12-29**) is a plastic mask applied to the face for intermittent therapy to achieve positive expiratory pressure treatments. A variable orifice resistor is connected to the mask and delivers a flow-dependent expiratory pressure. The patient inhales flow through an inspiratory valve and then exhales into the PEP mask through one of the orifices. The patient is instructed to exhale at a constant flow and at a rate that generates the dyesired pressure as monitored on an attached pressure gauge.

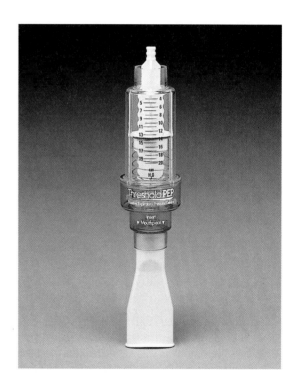

FIGURE 12-30 Threshold PEP.
Courtesy of Philips Healthcare.

Adjustable Orifice

PEP is delivered through an adjustable orifice device by passing expiratory flow through a preset resistance. As the caregiver tightens the adjustable expiratory resistor, the flow through the device slows and creates a positive pressure on exhalation.

The following are examples of adjustable orifice devices:

Respironics Threshold PEP: Threshold PEP (Philips Respironics, Andover, MA), shown in **Figure 12-30**, incorporates a one-way valve to maintain constant pressure despite the amount of

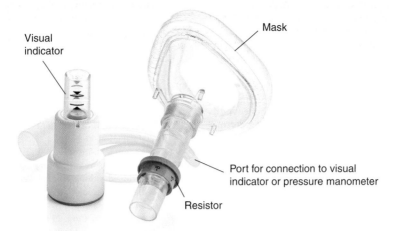

Visual indicator

Mask

Port for connection to visual indicator or pressure manometer

Resistor

FIGURE 12-31 TheraPEP.
Courtesy of Smiths Medical.

exhaled flow passing through the device. PEP pressures are adjustable in 1–2 cm H_2O increments by adjusting the tension on the spring-loaded valve.

TheraPEP: TheraPEP (Smiths Medical, Watford, UK), shown in **Figure 12-31**, is a flow resistor. Gas is drawn in on inspiration through a mouthpiece and one-way valve. On exhalation the gas flows through a fixed orifice. As the number on the device increases, a lower resistance or larger orifice is encountered. Higher flow will generate more pressure if the resistance setting is kept constant. The resistance setting is adjusted to enable the patient to produce expiratory pressures within the therapeutic range of 10–20 cm H_2O. This device also incorporates a visual pressure indicator to provide feedback to the patient as the therapy is performed.

Summary

Hyperinflation therapy is used for the prevention or treatment of atelectasis. The effects of lung underinflation or atelectrauma are underestimated. Defining and treating the specific type of atelectasis is important to meeting a patient's long-term goals. Hyperinflation therapy modalities available today are primarily noninvasive in nature. Technological advances have enhanced the function, reduced the size, and increased the portability of available devices. The underlying principles of operation of each modality should be considered when choosing the device for a patient with a specific need. There is no substitute for techniques or modalities that are supported by clinically based evidence and accompanying practice guidelines. With the increased focus on utilization and resources, it is imperative that the clinician choose the precise modality that fits the clinical condition while providing the greatest benefit and preventing untoward complications.

References

1. Malbouisson LMS, Szeles TF, Barbalho L, Massoco CO, Carmona MJC, Carvalho CRR, et al. Lung hyperinflation stimulates the release of inflammatory mediators in spontaneously breathing subjects. *Braz J Med Bio Res.* 2010;43:201-205.
2. Denehy L. The use of manual hyperinflation in airway clearance. *Eur Respir J.* 1999;14(4):958-965.
3. Schindler MB. Treatment of atelectasis: Where's the evidence? *Crit Care Forum.* 2005;9(4):341-342.
4. Agostini P, Singh S. Incentive spirometry following thoracic surgery: What should we be doing? *Physiotherapy.* 2009;95:76-82.
5. American Association for Respiratory Care. AARC clinical practice guideline for incentive spirometry. *Respir Care.* 1991; 36(12):1402-1405.
6. Rafea A, Wagih K, Amin H, El-Sabagh R, Yousef S. Flow oriented versus volume oriented incentive spirometers training on pulmonary ventilation after upper abdominal surgery. *Egypt J Bronchol.* 2009;3(2);110-118.
7. Crabtree EA, Mariscalo M, Hesselgrave J, Iniguez SF, Hilliard TJ, Katkin JP, et al. Improving care for children with sickle cell disease/acute chest syndrome. *Pediatrics.* 2011;127(2):e480-e488.
8. Bartlett RH, Gazzaniga AB, Geraghty TR. Respiratory maneuvers to prevent postoperative pulmonary complications. *JAMA.* 1973;224:1017-1021.
9. Craven JL, Evans GA, Davenport PJ, Williams RH. The evaluation of the incentive spirometer in the management of postoperative pulmonary complications. *Br J Surg.* 1974;61:793-797.
10. Overend TJ, Anderson CM, Lucy DS, Bhatia C, Jonsson BI, Timmermans C. The effect of incentive spirometry on postoperative complications. *Chest.* 2001;120:971-978.
11. Gibson GJ. Editors: Brusasco V, Fitting JW. Pulmonary hyperinflation: Clinical overview. *Eur Respir J.* 1996;9:2640-2649.
12. Yamaguti WP, Sakamoto ET, Panazzolo D, Peixoto Cda C, Cerri GG, Albuquerque AL. Diaphragmatic mobility in healthy subjects during incentive spirometry with a flow-oriented device and with a volume-oriented device. *J Braz Pneumol.* 2010;3(6):738-745.
13. Verma PK. Incentive spirometry. In: *Principles and practice of critical care.* New Delhi, India: BI Publications; 2006:19-21.
14. Parriera V, Tomich GM, Britto RR, Sampaio RF. Assessment of tidal volume and thoraco-abdominal motion using flow and volume oriented incentive spirometers in healthy subjects. *Braz J Med Bio Res.* 2003;38:1105-1112.

15. American Association for Respiratory Care. AARC clinical practice guideline: Intermittent positive pressure breathing—2003 revision and update. *Respir Care.* 2003;48(5):540-546.
16. Emmanuel G, Smith W, Briscoe W. The effect of intermittent positive pressure breathing and voluntary hyperventilation upon the distribution of ventilation and pulmonary blood flow to the lung in chronic obstructive pulmonary disease. *J Clin Invest.* 1966;45:1221-1223.
17. Torres G, Lyons H, Emerson P. The effects of intermittent positive pressure breathing on the interpulmonary distribution of inspired air. *Am J Med.* 1960;29:946-954.
18. Schilling JP, Kasik JE. Intermittent positive pressure breathing: A continuing controversy. *J Iowa Med Soc.* 1980;70(3):99-100, 102-103.
19. Stiller K, Simionato R, Rice K, Hall B. The effect of intermittent positive pressure breathing on lung volumes in acute quadriparesis. *Paraplegia.* 1992;30(2):121-126.
20. Shelledy DC, Mikles SP. Patient assessment and respiratory care plan development. In: Mishoe SC, Welch MA Jr, eds. *Critical thinking in respiratory care.* New York: McGraw-Hill; 2002:181-285.
21. Hall JC, Tarala RA, Tapper J, Hall JL. Prevention of respiratory complications after abdominal surgery: A randomised clinical trial. *BMJ.* 1996;312:148-152.
22. Jenkins S, Soutar S, Loukota J, Johnson L, Moxhham J. A comparison of breathing exercises, incentive spirometry and mobilisation after coronary artery surgery. *Physiother Theory Pract.* 1990;6:117-126.
23. Ledsome J, Sharp J. Pulmonary function in acute spinal cord injury. *Am Rev Respir Dis.* 1981;124:41-44.
24. Estenne M, Gevenois P, Kinnear W, Soudon P, Heilporn A, De Troyer A. Lung volume restriction in patients with chronic respiratory muscle weakness: The role of microatelectasis. *Thorax.* 1993;48:698-701.
25. Sinha R, Bergofsky E. Prolonged alteration of lung mechanics in kyphoscoliosis by positive pressure hyperinflation. *Am Rev Respir Dis.* 1972;106:47-57.
26. Mancebo J, Isabey D, Lorino H, Lofaso F, Lemaire F, Brochard L. Comparative effects of pressure support ventilation and intermittent positive pressure breathing (IPPB) in non-intubated healthy subjects. *Eur Respir J.* 1995;8(11):1901-1909.
27. Hess DR, Branson RD. Chest physiotherapy, incentive spirometers, intermittent positive pressure breathing, secretion clearance, and inspiratory muscle training. In: Branson RD, Hess DR, Chatburn RC, eds. *Respiratory care equipment.* Philadelphia: Lippincott; 1995:258-259.
28. Snyder RJ, Slaughter SL, Chatburn RL. Pressure and flow characteristics of the EzPAP positive airway pressure therapy system [Abstract]. *Resp Care.* 2001;46(10):1089.
29. Reardon CC, Christiansen D, Barnett ED, Cabral HJ. Intrapulmonary percussive ventilation vs incentive spirometry for children with neuromuscular disease. *Arch Pediatr Adolesc Med.* 2005;159:526-531.
30. Seferian EG, Henry NK, Wylam ME. High-frequency oscillatory ventilation in an infant with cystic fibrosis and bronchiolitis. *Respir Med.* 2006;100:1466-1469.
31. Dmello D, Nayak RD, Matuschak GM. High frequency percussive ventilation for airway clearance in CF; a brief report. *Lung.* 2010;188(6):9252-9255.
32. Antonaglaa V, Lucangdo V, Zin WA, Peratonei A, DeSimoni L, Capitano G, et al. Intrapulmonary percussive ventilation improves the outcomes of patients with acute exacerbation of COPD using a helmet. *Crit Care Med.* 2006;34(12):2940-2945.
33. Deakins K, Chatburn RL. A comparison of intrapulmonary percussive ventilation and conventional chest physiotherapy for the treatment of atelectasis in the pediatric patient. *Respir Care.* 2002;47:1162-1167.
34. McInturff SL, Shaw LI, Hodgkin JE, Rumble L, Bird FM. Intrapulmonary percussive ventilation (IPV) in the treatment of COPD [Abstract]. *Respir Care.* 1985;30(10):885.
35. Toussaint M, DeWin H, Steens M, Sandon P. Effects of intrapulmonary percussive ventilation on mucus clearance in Duchenne's muscular dystrophy patients: A preliminary report. *Respir Care.* 2003;48(10):940-947.
36. Martin JG, Shore S, Engel LA. Effect of continuous positive airway pressure on respiratory mechanics and pattern of breathing in induced asthma. *Am Rev Respir Dis.*1982;126:812-817.
37. American Association for Respiratory Care. Clinical practice guideline: Use of positive pressure adjuncts to bronchial hygiene therapy. *Respir Care.* 1993;38(5):516-521.
38. Antonescu-Turcu A, Parthasarathy S. CPAP and bi-level PAP therapy: New and established roles. *Respir Care.* 2010;55(9):1216-1229.
39. Miro AM, Pinsky MR, Rogers PL. Effects of the components of positive airway pressure on work of breathing during bronchospasm. *Crit Care.* 2004;2:R72-R81.
40. Archbold KH, Parthasarathy S. Adherence to positive pressure airway therapy in adults and children. *Current Opin Pulm Med.* 2009, Aug 26 [Epub].
41. Walterspacher S, Walker DJ, Kabitz HJ, Windisch W, Dreher M. The effect of continuous positive airway pressure on stair-climbing performance in severe COPD patients. *COPD.* 2013;10(2):193-199.
42. Donoghue FJ, Catcheside PG, Jordan AS, Berstein AD, McEvoy RD. Effect of CPAP on intrinsic PEEP, inspiratory effort and lung volume in severe stable COPD. *Thorax.* 2002;57:533-539.
43. Thille AW, Bertholon JF, Becquemin MH, Roy M, Lyazidi A, Lellouche F, et al. Aerosol delivery and humidification with the Boussignac continuous positive airway pressure (CPAP) device. *Respir Care.* 2011;56(10):1526-1532.
44. Pronzato C. Chronic obstructive pulmonary disease and obstructive sleep apnea. Association, consequences and treatment. *Monaldi Arch Chest Dis.* 2010;73(4):155-161.
45. Lee KS, Dunn MS, Fenwick M, Shennan AT. A comparison of underwater bubble continuous positive airway pressure with ventilator-derived continuous positive airway pressure in premature neonates ready for extubation. *Biol Neonate.* 1998;73(2):69-75.
46. Tagare A, Kadam S, Vaidya U, Pandit A, Patole S. Bubble CPAP versus ventilator CPAP in preterm neonates with early onset respiratory distress: A randomized controlled trial. *J Trop Pediatr.* 2013;59(2):113-119.
47. Chan KM, Chan HB. The use of bubble CPAP in premature infants: A local experience. *Hong Kong J Paediatr.* 2007;12:86-92.
48. Courtney SE, Kahn DJ, Singh R, Habib RH. Bubble and ventilator-derived nasal continuous positive airway pressure in premature infants: Work of breathing and gas exchange. *J Perinatol.* 2011;31(1):44-50.
49. Tagare A, Kadam S, Vaidya U, Pandit A, Patole S. A pilot study of comparison of BCPAP vs. VCPAP in preterm infants with early onset respiratory distress. *J Trop Pediatr.* 2010;56(3):191-194.
50. Sehlin M, Ohberg F, Johansson G, Winso O. Physiological responses to positive pressure breathing: A comparison of PEP bottle and PEP mask. *Respir Care.* 2007;52(8):1000-1005.

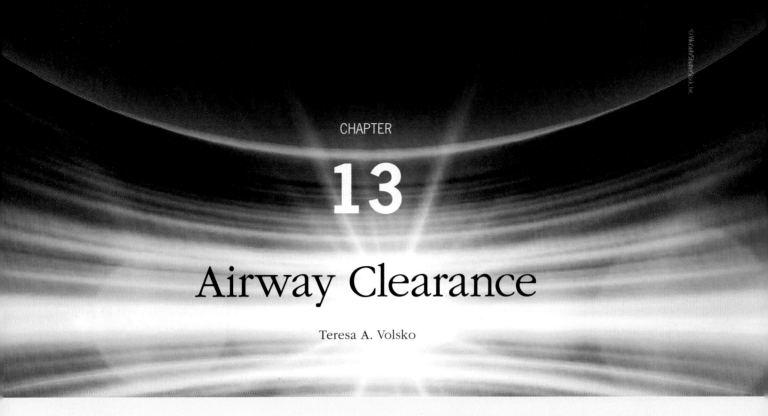

CHAPTER

13

Airway Clearance

Teresa A. Volsko

CHAPTER OBJECTIVES

1. List the indications and contraindications of oscillatory positive expiratory pressure devices.
2. Differentiate between high frequency chest wall compression and high frequency chest wall oscillation devices.
3. Describe the devices that can be used for airway clearance and lung hyperinflation therapy.
4. Explain the clinical application for mechanical insufflation-exsufflation.

KEY TERMS

Airway clearance therapy (ACT)
High frequency chest wall compression (HFCWC)
High frequency chest wall oscillation (HFCWO)
Intrapulmonary percussive ventilation
Mechanical insufflation-exsufflation
Oscillatory positive expiratory pressure (OPEP)

Introduction

The mucociliary escalator and cough reflex maintain optimal function of the respiratory system by facilitating secretion clearance and preventing airway obstruction. In healthy people, 10–100 mL[1] of airway secretions are continuously produced and cleared by the movement of the mucociliary escalator and with the aid of transient increases in expiratory airflow.[2] A variety of factors can interfere with the body's natural defense mechanism, making it difficult to mobilize and evacuate airway secretions. The aging process, tobacco use, and environmental exposures reduce the efficacy of ciliary structure and function.[3–5] Disease processes such as progressive neurodegenerative conditions inhibit the normal cough reflex.[6,7] Chronic obstructive

pulmonary disorders such as cystic fibrosis and bronchiectasis alter the production and composition of mucus, and mucociliary clearance disorders, such as primary ciliary dyskinesia, reduce the efficacy of ciliary structure and function.[8–10]

Airway obstruction and structural damage to the airways and lung parenchyma result from recurring infection, inflammatory changes, and secretion retention. As a result, clinicians employ airway therapy to aid in mucus mobilization and expectoration. **Airway clearance therapy (ACT)** utilizes physical or mechanical means to manipulate airflow, aid in the mobilization of tracheal bronchial phlegm cephalad, and facilitate evacuation by coughing. Breathing maneuvers, gravity-assisted drainage, manual techniques, and/or mechanical devices can be used to alter airflow and/or produce a cough or cough-like effect. This chapter will focus on the mechanical devices used to clear airway secretions. Mechanical devices can be divided into two distinct categories: (1) those that assist with the cephalad mobilization of secretions in the airways, and (2) those that assist with expectoration. It is important to note that devices that assist with the cephalad mobilization of secretions require the patient to perform a cough maneuver (e.g., huff cough) to facilitate expectoration.

Some devices described in this chapter subject the lungs to volumes greater than normal and are able to reinflate the collapsed areas of the lung, as well as generate expiratory flow rates that can move airway secretions cephalad. Therefore, they provide the dual function of hyperinflation and secretion removal to maintain or improve gas exchange.

515

Mechanical Devices Used for Hyperinflation Therapy and Secretion Clearance

Intrapulmonary Percussive Ventilation

Intrapulmonary percussive ventilation (IPV) is a special form of high frequency jet ventilation that can be used as a breathing treatment with spontaneously breathing patients.[11] IPV devices are pneumatically powered, using 50 psi, and deliver small bursts of high-flow gas at 100–300 cycles/min. Airflow bursts result in airway pressure changes of 5–35 cm H_2O and vibrations that facilitate secretion removal from the airway walls and aid in their mobilization toward the central airways.[12]

Application

IPV is administered manually or automatically using applications for both inpatient and outpatient settings.[13] IPV is applied noninvasively via a mouthpiece, mask, or mouth guard, or invasively in-line with a ventilator circuit during continuous mechanical ventilation.

Indications

IPV is indicated in disease states that impair the body's ability to mobilize and remove airway secretions. The literature shows IPV improves airway secretion clearance in patients with bronchiectasis,[12] cystic fibrosis,[14,15] neuromuscular disease,[16] and chronic obstructive pulmonary disease (COPD) during an acute exacerbation,[17,18] and with tracheostomized patients with poor expiratory flows.[19] There is also utility with airway burns[20] and inhalation injury[21] to mobilize the extensive sloughing of airway epithelial cells, reduce cast formation, and treat or prevent severe airway obstruction, atelectasis, and pneumonia.[22] The mechanism by which IPV may promote pulmonary secretion clearance is twofold: (1) shear forces loosen secretions from the walls of the airways, and (2) an asymmetrical flow pattern augments the movement of secretions cephalad. During inspiration, the turbulent gas stream flows over a mucus layer, creating shear forces that loosen secretions from the airway wall and propelling them in one of two directions, either deeper into the lung periphery or toward the central airways.[23] During therapy, expiratory flow exceeds inspiratory flow, which moves secretions in the central airways cephalad, where they can be coughed out or removed by mechanical means, such as suctioning.[24]

Contraindications

An untreated tension pneumothorax is the only definitive contraindication for IPV. There are several relative contraindications, which include increased intracranial pressure; tracheoesophageal fistula; hemodynamic instability; active hemoptysis; recent postoperative esophageal, facial, oral, or cranial surgery; active and untreated tuberculosis; and nausea.[25]

Hazards

Improper application of IPV may result in gastric insufflation, hyperventilation, hemodynamic compromise, air leak, pneumothorax or barotrauma, air trapping, alveolar overdistention, or inadvertent positive end-expiratory pressure (PEEP). Because there is a risk of gastric insufflation, precautions should be taken to avoid the risk for aspiration. Clinician's should wait at least 1 hour after meals to administer therapy to patients able to eat by mouth. Patients receiving intermittent or continuous enteral nutrition through a gastrostomy or nasogastric tube should have feedings temporarily discontinued during IPV therapy.

Currently Available Devices

The Percussionator IPV-1C, Percussive Neb IPPV-IPPB, and MetaNeb are examples of devices that can provide IPV therapy.

Oscillatory Positive Expiratory Pressure Devices

Oscillatory positive expiratory pressure (OPEP) therapy was first developed as an adjunct or supplement to chest physiotherapy and/or breathing techniques such as autogenic drainage and active cycle of breathing.[26] OPEP, also known as vibratory PEP, combines positive pressure during exhalation with airway vibrations or oscillations. The same theoretical benefits of airflow oscillations, described in the section on IPV therapy, are applicable with devices in this category. During exhalation, the gas flow or velocity of the airflow oscillations increases and becomes more turbulent, which has a shearing effect on the secretions adhering to the walls of the conducting airways. The shear forces that peel away the mucus layer from the airway wall also decrease the viscoelastic properties of mucus, which makes it easier to mobilize.[27] Expectoration can occur with a spontaneous or assisted cough, or with suctioning.

Application

OPEP devices are typically used with a mouthpiece; however, some of these devices can be adapted for use with a tracheostomy tube or resuscitation mask. Some devices have a standard 15-mm interior diameter and 22-mm outer diameter connection that allows the device to be directly connected to other interfaces should the patient be unable to perform the therapy with a mouthpiece. Some OPEP devices can easily adapt to a tracheostomy tube; however, when directly attached to the tracheostomy tube, the OPEP device may not be a comfortable fit for children or adults with a wide, short neck. A flex connector (e.g., Airlife OmniFlex, Carefusion, San Diego, CA) can provide an additional length of tubing to connect the patient's tracheostomy tube to the device. This allows for enhanced patient comfort by moving the device away from the neck and reducing the torque on the tracheostomy tube. Flex connectors typically expand from 5 cm to 6.5 cm and have 15-mm inner diameter and 22-mm outer diameter connections.

For small children or patients who are unable to use a mouthpiece, many OPEP devices can attach to a resuscitation mask. The mask can be held against the face to facilitate the OPEP maneuver.

Indications

OPEP is a form of ACT that utilizes a mechanical means to manipulate airflow and aid in the mobilization of tracheal bronchial phlegm. It is used as a primary form of therapy or in conjunction with other airway clearance therapies to relieve airway obstruction in pulmonary disorders such as cystic fibrosis, chronic obstructive pulmonary disease, and bronchiectasis in which the production and composition of mucus are altered, as well as in mucociliary clearance disorders such as primary ciliary dyskinesia, in which the efficacy of ciliary structure and function are reduced.[28,29]

The literature reports OPEP devices significantly enhanced mucus displacement,[30] ciliary movements, and respiratory system resonance and have clinical utility with patients receiving pulmonary rehabilitation.[31]

Contraindications

OPEP device contraindications mirror those of any positive airway adjunct to bronchial hygiene therapy, and can be found in **Table 13-1**.[32]

Hazards

An active exhalation is required to perform an OPEP maneuver correctly. Performing this positive expiratory pressure procedure properly may impose an increased work of breathing that can lead to hypoventilation and hypercarbia, or contribute to cardiovascular compromise, pulmonary barotrauma, and/or increased intracranial pressure.[32] If a mask is used as an interface there is a risk for claustrophobia, facial discomfort, and skin irritation and/or breakdown. The potential for gastric insufflation is minimal, but does exist. Therefore, patients should be monitored for the increased likelihood of vomiting and the potential for aspiration of gastric contents.

Currently Available Devices

Currently available OPEP devices include the Flutter, Acapella, Quake, and RC-Cornet.

TABLE 13-1
Contraindications to OPEP by Body System

System	Contraindication
Gastrointestinal	Esophageal surgery
	Nausea
Maxial/Facial	Known or suspected tympanic membrane rupture or middle ear pathology
	Acute sinusitis
	Epistaxis
	Recent face, mouth, or skull surgery
Cardiopulmonary	Untreated pneumothorax
	Hemodynamic instability
	Inability to tolerate the increased work of breathing the device may impose
	Active or gross hemoptysis
	Subcutaneous emphysema
Cerebral	Intracranial pressures greater than 20 mm Hg

The Flutter

The Flutter (Scandipharm, Birmingham, AL) is a handheld device shaped like a pipe, which contains a high-density stainless steel ball that sits in a circular cone inside the bowl of the pipe (**Figure 13-1**). The bowl's cover has perforations that allow expiratory airflow to pass through the device. During an active exhalation, airflow passes through the housing and mobilizes the steel ball. The weight of the steel ball against expiratory flow produces expiratory pressure, while the rise and fall of the steel ball generate airflow oscillations. Positive expiratory pressure of between 5 cm H_2O and 35 cm H_2O and airflow oscillations of 2–32 Hz were reported.[33] The characteristics of the waveform, oscillatory frequency, and PEP are dependent upon the position of the ball within the housing and the amount of flow through the device. Although the device can be tilted slightly upward or downward to change the resistance of the steel ball against expiratory flow, it is important to note that the bowl of the device must be pointed upward for maximum efficiency and proper function.[34] Tilting the device will alter the PEP and vibration frequency. **Figure 13-2** shows the position of the Flutter in a patient's mouth.

The Acapella

The Acapella (Smiths Medical, St Paul, MN) combines the principles of high frequency oscillation and PEP by employing a counterweighted lever and magnet. Exhaled gas passes through a cone, which is

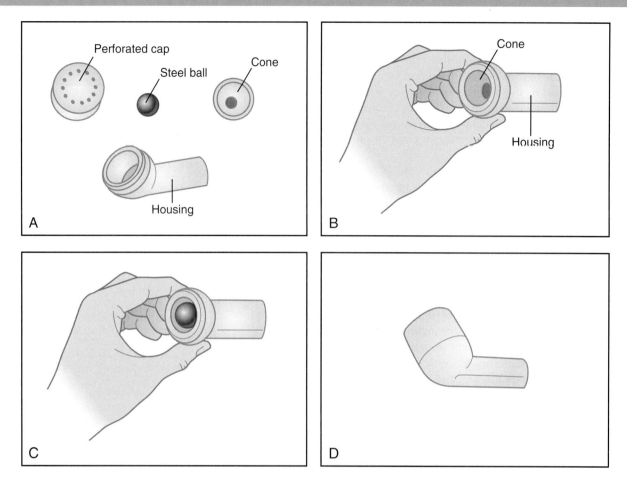

FIGURE 13-1 The Flutter airway clearance device. A. The device is dismantled to display the four components of the device. B. and C. The cone seats within the housing to form a base for the steel ball. D. The perforated cap is attached, and the device is ready for use.

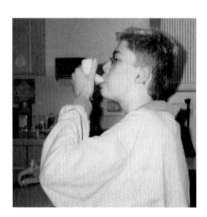

FIGURE 13-2 The position of the Flutter in the patient's mouth. Note that the patient has the Flutter tilted slightly upward.

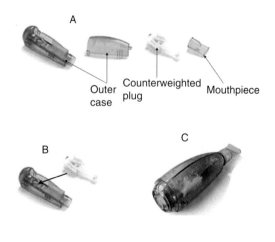

FIGURE 13-3 The Acapella Choice. A. The parts are dismantled and displayed. B. The counterweighted plug fits into the lower portion of the housing. C. An assembled device.

intermittently occluded by a plug attached to the lever, producing airflow oscillations (**Figure 13-3**). A knob located at the distal end of the device adjusts the proximity of the magnet and counterweighted plug, thereby adjusting the frequency (**Figure 13-4**).

This device comes in a variety of models. The blue and green Acapella devices were the first designs available. The initial designs cannot be disassembled to be cleaned and have flow limitations. The blue Acapella was designed for expiratory flows less than 15 L/min

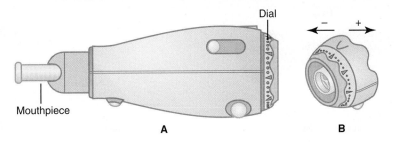

FIGURE 13-4 The Acapella's positive expiratory pressure (PEP) level is adjusted with a dial on the distal end of the device (B).

Courtesy of Smiths Medical.

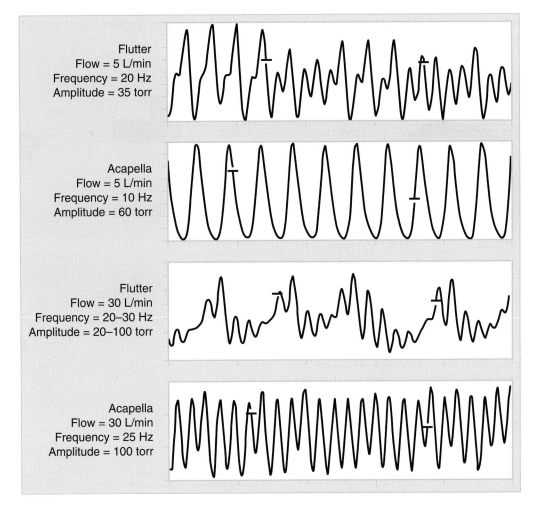

FIGURE 13-5 Representative pressure waveforms for Flutter and Acapella at the medium flows (10 and 25 L/min). The waveforms are comparable for amplitude and frequency.

Adapted from Volsko TA, DiFiore J, Chatburn RL. Performance comparison of two oscillating positive expiratory pressure devices: Acapella versus Flutter. *Respir Care*. 2003;48(2):124-130.

and the green for flows greater than 15 L/min. The Acapella Choice incorporates the range of all flows, and minimizes the need to switch devices when expiratory flows either improve or decline. This model can be disassembled and cleaned by autoclave or boiling and is dishwasher safe.

In a laboratory investigation comparing the performance characteristics of the Acapella and the Flutter, Volsko et al. reported similar PEP and pressure amplitudes between the devices (**Figure 13-5**).[35] However, at the extreme higher and lower flows, the Flutter produced a much lower amplitude and a less stable waveform.[35]

The Quake

The Quake (Thayer Medical, Tucson, AZ) is a manually operated OPEP device that uses a hand crank to direct expiratory flow through vanes housed in the casing of

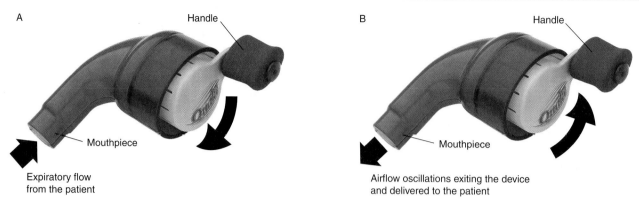

FIGURE 13-6 The Quake airway clearance device. A. As the handle rotates, expiratory flow is directed through vanes, creating expiratory pressure and airflow oscillations. B. The airflow oscillations exit the device and are transmitted to the patient through the mouthpiece.
Photos courtesy of Thayer Medical.

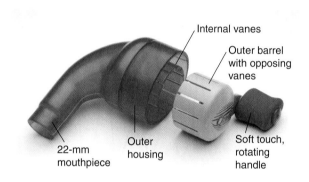

FIGURE 13-7 The dissembled components of the Quake.
Courtesy of Thayer Medical.

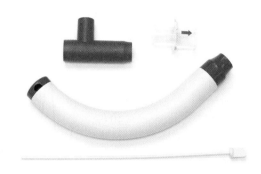

FIGURE 13-8 The RC-Cornet device.

the device, creating airflow oscillations (**Figure 13-6**). Rotating the handle slowly creates lower frequency oscillations and higher PEP. Conversely, rotating the hand crake at a higher speed creates a higher frequency of airflow oscillations and lower PEP.[30] This device can be disassembled for cleaning (**Figure 13-7**) with soap and water, by boiling in water, or in the dishwasher and can also be put in a Medela Quick-Clean Micro Steam bag and steam cleaned in the microwave. Medela Quick-Clean Micro Steam bags can be found at discount stores and retail pharmacies.

The RC-Cornet

The RC-Cornet (Curaplex Medical, Dublin, OH) has been available in Europe since the 1970s but is not Food and Drug Administration (FDA) approved for use in the United States. This device consists of a mouthpiece connected to a curved tube housing that encases a hose and a sound damper (**Figure 13-8**). The mouthpiece can be rotated to one of five settings, which changes the size of the expiratory resistor (**Figure 13-9**). The higher the setting (i.e., 4 or 5), the more expiratory pressure and pressure amplitude are generated.

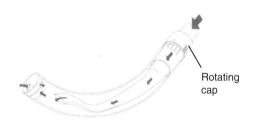

FIGURE 13-9 Diagram showing expiratory flow through the device. The cap can be rotated to provide varying levels of PEP.
Courtesy of R. Cegla GmbH & CO. KG

High Frequency Chest Wall Compression Devices

High frequency chest wall compression (HFCWC) devices depend on changes in transrespiratory pressure to generate sufficient expiratory flow behind the airway secretions to move the secretions to the larger airways, where they can be removed by cough and expectoration or suctioning.[36] This type of airway clearance device generates intermittent negative transrespiratory pressure pulses (i.e., causing short expiratory flow bursts) through the use of a garment to encase the chest and externally compress the chest wall with short, rapid expiratory flow pulses. The elastic recoil of the chest wall allows the lung volume to return to functional residual capacity.

Application

The vest and wrap are the two inflatable garment options used to encase the chest. The vest encases the chest from the shoulders to the end of the rib cage (**Figure 13-10A**). The wrap encases the center portion of the chest, with the upper border resting just under the axilla (**Figure 13-10B**). Manufacturers of HFCWC devices have reusable and disposable or single-patient-use versions of these garments.

The wrap or vest is attached to a high-output compressor, which rapidly inflates and deflates the encasing device. On inflation, pressure is exerted on the body surface, which forces the chest wall to compress and generates short bursts of expiratory flow. Inflation pressure may range from 5 to 20 cm H_2O and is dependent upon the size of the patient and comfort of fit. The garment should fit snugly against the chest wall when inflated, without being restrictive. Patient feedback regarding comfort of fit is essential. Pressure pulses are superimposed on a small (about 12 cm H_2O) positive pressure baseline. The frequency with which the chest wall compression is applied varies and can generate volume changes from 17 to 57 mL and flows up to 1.6 L/sec. Lower frequencies are used to loosen secretions from the walls of the conducting airways. Mid-level frequencies are used to mobilize the secretions in cephalad direction toward the central airways.

A typical treatment may last from 15 to 30 minutes with huff coughing performed in between each differing frequency session. **Table 13-2** compares HFCWC prescriptions common to the three HFCWC devices

currently on the market.[37] Upon completion of therapy, the garment is deflated and the chest wall recoils to its resting position.

Indications

High frequency chest wall oscillation uses an air compressor attached to an external garment—vest or wrap—to compress the chest and apply short bursts of expiratory flows. These short expiratory flow bursts create "mini coughs" that mobilize secretions without requiring the patient to actively participate in the therapy. Similar to other airway clearance devices previously described in this chapter, this form of therapy is used to relieve airway obstruction in pulmonary disorders such as cystic fibrosis,[38] chronic obstructive pulmonary disease, and bronchiectasis.[39] Because mobilization of secretions is not dependent on patient effort, HFCWC also has utility in neuromuscular diseases, which weaken respiratory muscles, in addition to conditions that result in neurological impairment, which increase the risk for secretion retention and bronchiectasis formation.[40,41] The literature also reports the use of HFCWC, in conjunction with adequate pain control, is a safe, well-tolerated airway clearance modality following thoracic surgery.[42]

Contraindications

Contraindications for HFCWC devices include an untreated pneumothorax, hemoptysis, hemodynamic instability, intracranial pressures greater than 20 mm Hg, chest or spinal trauma, surgical wound or healing tissue, recent skin grafts or flaps on the thorax and/or spine, as well as the inability to tolerate the increased work of breathing the device may impose.[32] Adequate pain control after thoracic surgery is essential.[42]

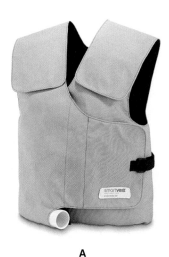

A

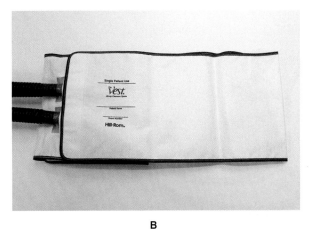

B

FIGURE 13-10 An example of the two types of garments used to encase the chest to administer high frequency chest wall compression therapy. A. The SmartVest. B. The wrap.

Photo A courtesy of Electromed, Inc.

TABLE 13-2
Manufacturer Recommended Protocols or Prescriptions Used for HFCWC Therapy, Adapted From Reference

Device Type	Frequency (Hz)	Garment Inflation Pressure (cm H₂O)	Time (min)	Comments
Vest	6, 8, 10	10	5	5 minutes at each frequency. Pause the machine, cough three times, and then resume the session.
	16, 18, 20	6	5	5 minutes at each frequency. Pause the machine, cough three times, and then resume the session.
SmartVest	10	—	10	Huff cough and move to next session.
	12	—	10	Huff cough and move to next session.
	14	—	10	Huff cough.
InCourage	—	—	30	Push the Quick start button to initiate preprogrammed 30-minute automatic ramping session. The Pause button may be pushed at any time. Push the Run button to resume therapy. Pressure can be increased or decreased during a therapy session.

Hazards

Performing this procedure properly may impose an increased work of breathing that can lead to hypoventilation and hypercarbia, or contribute to cardiovascular compromise, pulmonary barotrauma, and/or increased intracranial pressure.[32] Minor skin irritation or discomfort to indwelling central lines, such as surgically implanted medication ports, may be more likely to occur with the vest garment than the wrap.

Currently Available Devices

There are three commercially available devices on the market: The Vest (Hill-Rom, St. Paul, MN), InCourage System (RespirTech, St. Paul, MN), and SmartVest (ElectroMed, New Prague, MN). All three are shown in **Figure 13-11**. The operating principles, volume, and flow changes for each system are outlined in **Table 13-3**. In a randomized, double-blind, cross-over study, Kempainen et al. found no differences in sputum production (mean sputum wet and dry weight

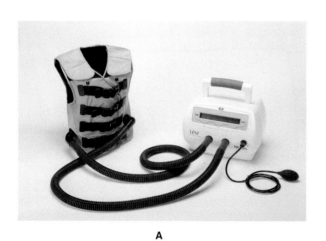

A

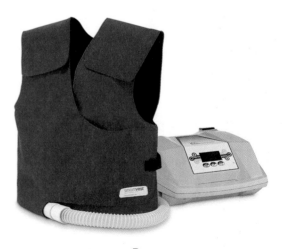

B

FIGURE 13-11 High frequency chest wall compression devices. A. The Vest. B. SmartVest.

TABLE 13-3
The Operating Principles, Volume, and Flow Changes for Each of the HFCWC Systems

Device	Manufacturer	Waveform	Frequency Range (Hz)	Pause Feature	Weight (lb)	Hose Configurations
The Vest	Hill-Rom St. Paul, MN	Sine	2–25	Yes	17	Double hoses Nonlocking connectors
InCourage System	RespirTech St.Paul, MN	Triangular	5–30	Yes	17	Double hoses Locking connectors
SmartVest	ElectroMed New Prague, MN	Sine	5–30	Yes	23	Single hose Nonlocking connector

produced) or patient comfort rating between the Vest and InCourage systems.[43]

High Frequency Chest Wall Oscillation Devices

High frequency chest wall oscillation (HFCWO) devices generate positive and negative pressures to the chest wall to achieve changes in transrespiratory pressure in order to generate enough expiratory flow behind the airway secretions to move the secretions to the larger airways, where they can be removed by cough and expectoration or suctioning.[36] Rather than the wrap or vest-like garment used by HFCWC devices, the HFCWO device uses a rigid external enclosure or chest cuirass connected to a compressor that can deliver biphasic pressures to the chest wall. The negative pressure generated by the external enclosure causes the chest wall to expand and inspiration to occur. Expiratory pressure may be atmospheric, allowing for the normal elastic recoil of the chest to return the patient's functional residual capacity (FRC) to normal, negative or positive. Positive pressure applied to the chest wall may be used to produce a forceful exhalation. The device also allows for control of inspiration to expiration (I:E) ratios. In addition to being used for airway clearance,[44] the literature reports the use of HFCWO for noninvasive ventilatory support.[45]

Indications

Indications for the use of HFCWO mirror those of HFCWC. The airway clearance regimens recommended by the manufacturers is found in **Table 13-4**.[46]

Contraindications

Contraindications for HFCWO mirror those for HFCWC.

Hazards

Hazards for HFCWO mirror those of HFCWC.

Currently Available Device

The Hayek SCS is an easy-to-use airway clearance device that has 12 sizes of cuirass, enabling treatment of both adult and pediatric patients. The Hayek SCS is

TABLE 13-4
Manufacturer Recommended Protocol Used for HFCWO Therapy

Mode	Mode Purpose	Device Settings				
		Inspiratory Pressure (cm H$_2$O)	Expiratory Pressure (cm H$_2$O)	I:E Ratio	Frequency (cpm)	Cycle Time (minutes)
Vibration	Loosen and mobilizes secretions	−8	8	1:1	800*	3–4
Cough	Expel airway secretions	−25	15	4:1	50	3

* Decrease the frequency for more tenacious secretions.

Manufacturer notes that the expiratory pressures in vibration mode are defaulted to the same as inspiratory pressures. Higher pressures such as +15 cm H$_2$O have been well tolerated.

Typical session lasts 30–60 minutes, allowing for rest periods between repeating cycle sessions.

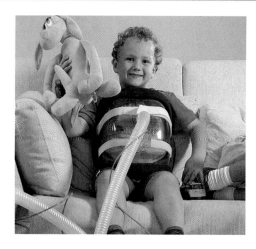

FIGURE 13-12 The Hayek SCS high frequency chest wall oscillator with assist cough functions via a cuirass shell.

Courtesy of United Hayek Medical, UK. www.hayekmedical.com.

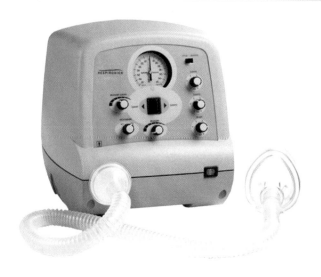

FIGURE 13-13 CoughAssist mechanical insufflator-exsufflator.

Courtesy of Philips Healthcare.

an electrically powered, fully computerized oscillator with assist cough functions (**Figure 13-12**). It is the only device currently available on the market approved to deliver HFCWO. The Hayek SCS operates at frequencies from 240 to 1200 cycles per minute, with I:E ratios of 1:6 to 6:1. Inspiratory and expiratory pressures are adjustable from 50 cm H_2O to −50 cm H_2O. The Hayek SCS delivers two modes. The first mode is called the Vibration Mode. The Vibration Mode generates a true HFCWO via the cuirass shell. The second mode is called the Cough Mode. The Cough Mode mimics a huff cough to force up secretions using an inverse I:E ratio with an extended inspiration and sharp expiration via the cuirass shell. The Hayek SCS facilitates mobilization and removal of pulmonary secretions.

Mechanical Cough Assist Devices

The cough is an essential phase of secretion clearance. A cough can be broken down into four phases: irritation, inspiration, glottis closure, and expulsion. The thoracic and abdominal muscles are instrumental in allowing for a deep inspiration and an explosive release of gas during the expiration.[47] During a normal cough, abdominal and thoracic muscles can generate pressures of greater than 80 mm Hg just before the expulsion phase. Some cough maneuvers, such as a huff cough or forced expiratory maneuver, rely on thoracic and abdominal muscle strength to forcefully move air and excretions out of the lungs after a deep inspiration. During this type of maneuver the glottis remains open throughout the respiratory cycle.

The key factor with the cough techniques just described is the muscle strength needed to expand the lungs and then forcefully exhale. Disease processes such as motor neuron defects, spinal trauma, and neuromuscular diseases can weaken muscles and inhibit an effective cough. The presence of a tracheostomy tube

also can impair a patient's ability to generate sufficient peak cough flows.[48] Peak cough flows of less than 270 L/min are associated with respiratory distress, oxygen desaturation, and hospitalizations.[49] Absence of peak cough flow is associated with increased mortality.[50] **Mechanical insufflation-exsufflation** devices deliver positive and negative pressure to the airway to produce airflow changes, simulate a cough, and propel secretions toward the oropharynx for removal by expectoration or suctioning.

Application

This type of therapy can be administered by a variety of interfaces including an oronasal mask, a mouthpiece, or a connection to an artificial airway (endotracheal tube or tracheostomy tube). The interface is connected to the device by a breathing circuit (large-bore tubing and a bacterial/viral filter).

Indications

Mechanical cough assistance is indicated in patients with an ineffective cough due to disease condition or trauma, including muscular dystrophy, myasthenia gravis, poliomyelitis, and/or neurologic disorders with some paralysis of the respiratory muscles, such as spinal cord injury.[51–53]

Contraindications

Contraindications are similar to the other airway clearance devices discussed in this chapter and include untreated pneumothorax, hemodynamic instability, intracranial pressures greater than 20 mm Hg, recent maxillofacial and/or skull surgery or trauma, active or gross hemoptysis, and known or suspected tympanic membrane rupture or middle ear pathology.[32]

Hazards

Careful consideration should be used before administering therapy to patients with a history of bullous emphysema, known susceptibility to pneumothorax or pnuemomediastinum, or recent barotrauma or those prone to airway closure (i.e., COPD).[54]

Currently Available Device

The CoughAssist (Phillips Healthcare, Andover, MA), a mechanical insufflator-exsufflator, is the only device that is commercially available to augment a cough (**Figure 13-13**). It is an electrically powered blower device that can produce inspiratory and expiratory flows up to 3.3 and 10 L/sec, respectively. Positive inspiratory pressures and negative expiratory pressures are adjustable from 60 to −60 cm H_2O. Timing of inspiratory and expiratory phases may be manually set or automatically set on the device. This device allows for pauses lasting from 0 to 5 seconds between inspiration and expiration. The pause can be programmed into the machine or manually activated.

The breathing circuit and interface are single patient use. The exterior surfaces of the device may be washed with a mild detergent and water, or with a bactericidal cleaning solution such as 70% isopropyl alcohol.

Summary

A variety of factors can impair the body's ability to mobilize and remove airway secretions. Airway clearance devices provide options to patients and caregivers; however, evidence in the literature has not demonstrated that any one type of device is superior to another. Therefore, the respiratory therapist must have an innate knowledge of the device's operational characteristics and limitations as well as information about the patient's disease state, cognitive ability, and preferences in order to match the airway clearance device(s) to the therapeutic goals.

References

1. Rubin BK. Physiology of airway mucus clearance. *Respir Care.* 2002;47(7):761–768.
2. Warwick WJ. Mechanisms of mucous transport. *Eur J Respir Dis Suppl.* 1983;127:162–167.
3. Foster WM. Mucociliary transport and cough in humans. *Pulm Pharmacol Ther.* 2002;15(3):277–282.
4. Zaugg M, Lucchinetti E. Respiratory function in the elderly. *Anesthesiol Clin N Am.* 2000;18(1):47–58.
5. Hernandez ML, Harris B, Lay JC, Bromberg PA, Diaz-Sanchez D, Devlin RB, et al. Comparative airway inflammatory response of normal volunteers to ozone and lipopolysaccharide challenge. *Inhal Toxicol.* 2010;22(8):648–656.
6. Chaudri MB, Liu C, Hubbard R, Jefferson D, Kinnear WJ. Relationship between supermaximal flow during cough and mortality in motor neuron disease. *Eur Respir J.* 2002;19(3):434–438.
7. Hadjikoutis S, Wiles CM. Respiratory complications related to bulbar dysfunction in motor neuron disease. *Acta Neurol Scand.* 2001;103(4):207–213.
8. Van der Schans CP. Bronchial mucus transport. *Respir Care.* 2007;52(9):1150–1158.
9. Voynow JA, Rubin BK. Mucins, mucus, and sputum. *Chest.* 2009;135(2):505–512.
10. Rubin BK. Mucus, phlegm, and sputum in cystic fibrosis. *Respir Care.* 2009;54(6):726–732; discussion 732.
11. Riffard G, Toussaint M. Indications for intrapulmonary percussive ventilation (IPV): A review of the literature. *Rev Mal Respir.* 2012;29(2):178–190.
12. Paneroni M, Clini E, Simonelli C, Bianchi L, Degli Antoni F, Vitacca M. Safety and efficacy of short-term intrapulmonary percussive ventilation in patients with bronchiectasis. *Respir Care.* 2011;56(7):984–988.
13. Reardon CC, Christiansen D, Barnett ED, Cabral HJ. Intrapulmonary percussive ventilation vs incentive spirometry for children with neuromuscular disease. *Arch Pediatr Adolesc Med.* 2005;159(6):526–531.
14. Van Ginderdeuren F, Verbanck S, Van Cauwelaert K, Vanlaethem S, Schuermans D, Vincken W, et al. Chest physiotherapy in cystic fibrosis: Short-term effects of autogenic drainage preceded by wet inhalation of saline versus autogenic drainage preceded by intrapulmonary percussive ventilation with saline. *Respiration.* 2008;76(2):175–180.
15. Varekojis SM, Douce FH, Flucke RL, Filbrun DA, Tice JS, McCoy KS, et al. A comparison of the therapeutic effectiveness of and preference for postural drainage and percussion, intrapulmonary percussive ventilation, and high-frequency chest wall compression in hospitalized cystic fibrosis patients. *Respir Care.* 2003;48(1):24–28.
16. Toussaint M, De Win H, Steens M, Soudon P. Effect of intrapulmonary percussive ventilation on mucus clearance in Duchenne muscular dystrophy patients; a preliminary report. *Respir Care.* 2003;48(10):940–947.
17. Vargas F, Bui HN, Boyer A, Salmi LR, Gbikpi-Benissan G, Guenard H, et al. Intrapulmonary percussive ventilation in acute exacerbation of COPD patients with mild respiratory acidosis: A randomized controlled trial. *Crit Care.* 2005;9(4):382–389.
18. Antonaglia V, Lucangelo U, Zin WA, Peratoner A, De Simoni L, Capitanio G, et al. Intrapulmonary percussive ventilation in tracheostomized patients with acute exacerbation of chronic obstructive disease using a helmet. *Crit Care Med.* 2006;34(12):2940–2945.
19. Clini EM, Antoni FD, Vitacca M, Crisafulli E, Paneroni M, Chezzi-Silva S, et al. Intrapulmonary percussive ventilation in tracheostomized patients: A randomized controlled study. *Intensive Care Med.* 2006;32(12):1994–2001.
20. Ortiz-Pujols S, Boschini LA, Klatt-Cromwell C, Short KA, Hwang J, Cairns BA, et al. Chest high-frequency oscillatory treatment for severe atelectasis in a patient with toxic epidermal necrolysis. *J Burn Care Res.* 2013;34(2):e112–e115.
21. Lentz CW, Peterson HD. Smoke inhalation is a multilevel insult to the pulmonary system. *Curr Opin Pulm Med.* 1997;3(3):221–226.
22. Reper P, van Looy K. Chest physiotherapy using intrapulmonary percussive ventilation to treat persistent atelectasis in hypoxic patients after smoke inhalation. *Burns.* 2013;39(1):192–193.
23. Toussaint M, DeWin H, Steens M, Soudon P. Effect of intrapulmonary percussive ventilation on mucus clearance in Duchenne muscular dystrophy patients: A preliminary report. *Respir Care.* 2003;48(10):940–947.
24. Freitag L, Long WM, Kim CS, Wanner A. Removal of excessive bronchial secretions by asymmetric high-frequency oscillations. *J Appl Physiol.* 1989;67(2):614–619.
25. Reardon CC, Christiansen D, Barnett ED, Cabral HJ. Intrapulmonary percussive ventilation vs incentive spirometry for children with neuromuscular disease. *Arch Pediatr Adolesc Med.* 2005;159:526–531.
26. Pryor JA. Physiotherapy for airway clearance in adults. *Eur Respir J.* 1999;14(6):1418–1424.

27. Kim CS, Rodriguez CR, Eldridge MA, Sackner MA. Criteria for mucus transport in the airways by two-phase gas liquid flow mechanism. *J Appl Phsyiol.* 1986;60(3):901–907.

28. Van der Schans CP. Bronchial mucus transport. *Respir Care.* 2007;52(9):1150–1158.

29. Voynow JA, Rubin BK. Mucins, mucus, and sputum. *Chest.* 2009; 135(2):505–512.

30. Ragavan AJ. Comparing performance of three oscillating positive expiratory pressure devices at similar amplitude and frequencies of oscillations on displacement of mucus inside trachea during cough. *Respir Care.* 2012 Mar 13 [Epub ahead of print].

31. Alves CE, Nunes LQ, Melo PL. Mechanical analysis of an oscillatory positive expiratory pressure device used in respiratory rehabilitation. *Conf Proc IEEE Eng Med Biol Soc.* 2010: 2477–2480.

32. AARC clinical practice guideline: Use of positive airway pressure adjuncts to bronchial hygiene therapy. *Respir Care.* 1993;38(5): 516–521.

33. Myers TR. Positive expiratory pressure and oscillatory positive expiratory pressure therapies. *Respir Care.* 2007;52(10): 1308–1326.

34. Alves LA, Pitta F, Brunetto AF. Performance analysis of the Flutter VRP1 under different flows and angles. *Respir Care.* 2008;53(3):316–323.

35. Volsko TA, DiFiore J, Chatburn RL. Performance comparison of two oscillating positive expiratory pressure devices: Acapella versus Flutter. *Respir Care.* 2003;48(2):124–130.

36. Chatburn RL. High-frequency assisted airway clearance. *Respir Care.* 2007;52(9):1224–1235.

37. Lester MK, Flume PA. Airway-clearance therapy guidelines and implementation. *Respir Care.* 2009;54(6):733–750.

38. Warwick WJ, Hansen LG. The long-term effect of high-frequency chest compression therapy on pulmonary complication of cystic fibrosis. *Pediatr Pulmonol.* 1991;11(3):265–271.

39. Stafler P, Carr SB. Non-cystic fibrosis bronchiectasis: Its diagnosis and management. *Arch Dis Child Educ Pract Ed.* 2010;95(3):73–82.

40. Lange DJ, Lechtzin N, Davey C, David W, Heiman-Patterson T, Gelinas D, et al. High-frequency chest wall oscillation in ALS: An exploratory randomized, controlled trial. *Neurology.* 2006;67(6):991–997.

41. Piccione JC, McPhail GL, Fenchel MC, Brody AS, Boesch RP. Bronchiectasis in chronic pulmonary aspiration: Risk factors and clinical implications. *Pediatr Pulmonol.* 2012;47(5):447–452.

42. Allan JS, Garrity JM, Donahue DM. High-frequency chest-wall compression during the 48 hours following thoracic surgery. *Respir Care.* 2009;54(3):340–343.

43. Kempainen RR, Williams CB, Hazelwood A, Rubin BK, Milla CE. Comparison of high-frequency chest wall oscillation with differing waveforms for airway clearance in cystic fibrosis. *Chest.* 2007;132(4):1227–1232.

44. Scherer T, Barandun J, Martinez E, Wanner A, Rubin EM. Effect of high frequency oral airway and chest wall oscillation and conventional chest physical therapy on expectoration in patients with stable cystic fibrosis. *Chest.* 1998;113(4):1019–1027.

45. Kameyama Y, Wagatsuma T, Nakamura M, Kurosawa S, Saito K, Hoshi K. A case of congenital central hypoventilation syndrome. *J Anesth.* 2012;26(6):922–924.

46. United Hayek Medical. Secretion clearance. Available at: http://www.unitedhayek.com/clinicians#clearance. Accessed June 29, 2012.

47. Naire S. Dynamics of voluntary cough maneuvers: A theoretical model. *J Biomech Eng.* 2009;131(1):011010.

48. McKim DA, Hendin A, LeBlanc C, King J, Brown CR, Woolnough A. Tracheostomy decannulation and cough peak flows in patients with neuromuscular weakness. *Am J Phys Med Rehabil.* 2012;91(8):666–670.

49. Tzeng AC, Bach JR. Prevention of pulmonary morbidity for patients with neuromuscular disease. *Chest.* 2000;118(5):1390–1396.

50. Chaudri MB, Liu C, Hubbard R, Jefferson D, Kinnear WJ. Relationship between supramaximal flow during cough and mortality in motor neuron disease. *Eur Respir J.* 2002;19(3):434–438.

51. Finder JD, Birnkrant D, Carl J, Farber HJ, Gozal D, Iannaccone ST, et al., American Thoracic Society. Respiratory care of the patient with Duchenne muscular dystrophy: ATS consensus statement. *Am J Respir Crit Care Med.* 2004;170(4):456–465.

52. Chatwin M, Ross E, Hart N, Nickol AH, Polkey MI, Simonds AK. Cough augmentation with mechanical insufflation/exsufflation in patients with neuromuscular weakness. *Eur Respir J.* 2003; 21:502–508.

53. McCool DF, Rosen MJ. Nonpharmocologic airway clearance therapies: AACP evidence-based clinical practice guidelines. *Chest.* 2006;129:250–259.

54. Winck JC, Goncalves MR, Lourenco C, Viana P, Almeida J, Bach JR. Effects of mechanical insufflation-exsufflation on respiratory parameters for patients with chronic airway secretion encumbrance. *Chest.* 2004;126:774–780.

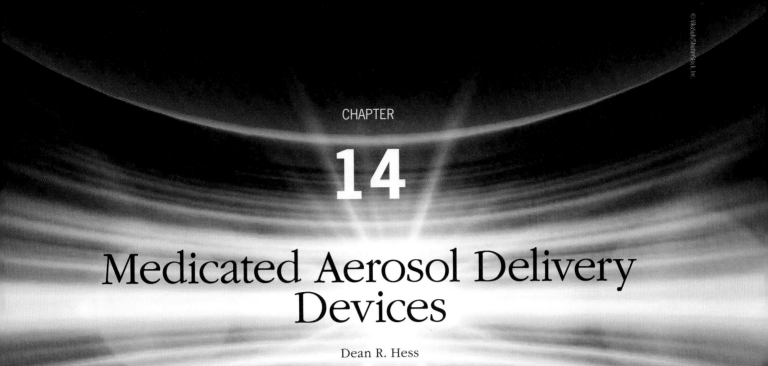

14

Medicated Aerosol Delivery Devices

Dean R. Hess

CHAPTER OBJECTIVES

1. Define mass median aerodynamic diameter and geometric standard deviation.
2. Describe the effects of inertial impaction, gravitational sedimentation, and diffusion on aerosol deposition in the lungs.
3. List the advantages of various aerosol delivery devices.
4. Compare jet nebulizers, mesh nebulizers, ultrasonic nebulizers, pressurized metered dose inhalers, and dry powder inhalers for aerosol drug administration.
5. Distinguish between spacers and valved holding chambers.
6. Discuss issues involved in the selection of a device for aerosol delivery.
7. Discuss issues pertinent to aerosol drug delivery during mechanical ventilation.

KEY TERMS

Aerosol	Mesh nebulizer
Dry powder inhaler (DPI)	Nebulizer
Geometric standard deviation (GSD)	Pressurized metered dose inhaler (pMDI)
Jet nebulizer	Spacer
Large-volume nebulizer	Ultrasonic nebulizer (USN)
Mass median aerodynamic diameter (MMAD)	Valved holding chamber

Introduction

An **aerosol** is composed of solid or liquid particles suspended in air. Common aerosol-generating devices include **nebulizers, pressurized metered dose inhalers (pMDIs)**, and **dry powder inhalers (DPIs)**.[1-7] For some of these, such as bronchodilators and steroids, the intent is to maximize airway effects and minimize systemic side effects. For others, such as pulmonary vasodilators, the intent is delivery across the alveolar–capillary membrane but with localized effects in the pulmonary circulation. For others, such as mucokinetic agents, the drug is only effective if delivered directly into the lungs. Drugs that can be administered by aerosol are shown in **Table 14-1**.

The geometric size of the particles is commonly expressed as the **mass median aerodynamic diameter (MMAD)**. By definition, half the mass of particles in an aerosol is less than the MMAD and the other half is greater (**Figure 14-1**). Relatively few particles larger than the median particle diameter comprise the mass above the MMAD, with a much greater number of particles less than the median required to reach comparable mass. Most clinical aerosol generators produce particles with an MMAD of 1 to 5 micrometers (μm). **Geometric standard deviation (GSD)** is a measure of how spread out the particles are in relation to their size. It is calculated as the ratio of particle size below which 84% of the particles occur to the particle size below which 50% occur, in a lognormal distribution. A monodisperse aerosol has a GSD under 1.2, whereas a heterodisperse aerosol has a GSD more than 1.2. Most therapeutic aerosols are heterodisperse.

The time that particles can remain suspended is related to the their size, density, and forward velocity. Inertia is the tendency of an object with mass, once it is in motion, to travel in a straight line. Inertia is determined by mass and velocity. Inertial impaction is the primary mechanism of deposition of aerosol particles ≥ 5 μm and an important mechanism

TABLE 14-1
Drugs Administered as Inhaled Aerosols

Category	Examples
Bronchodilators	Beta agonists Anticholinergics
Secretion modifiers	Dornase alfa Hypertonic saline
Antimicrobials	Antibiotics Ribavirin Pentamadine
Vasodilators	Prostacylins
Diagnostics	Methacholine Mannitol
Others	Insulin Vaccines Opioids Antirejection immunosuppressants

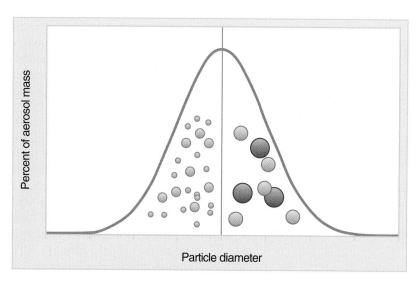

FIGURE 14-1 Illustration of a mass median aerodynamic diameter (MMAD). Half the mass of particles in an aerosol is less than the MMAD and the other half is greater.

for particles as small as 2 µm. A higher inspiratory flow increases the tendency of smaller particles to deposit at branch points in the airway. Sedimentation occurs when aerosol particles settle out of suspension because of gravity. Very small particles (those less than 0.5 µm in diameter) tend not to settle. An end-inspiratory breath hold lengthens the residence time, or the time that aerosol particles remain in the lungs, specifically in the last six generations of the airway. Diffusion, or Brownian movement, is the primary mechanism of deposition of particles less than 3 µm. Aerosol droplets in the respirable range (1 to 5 µm MMAD) are more likely to deposit in the lower respiratory tract than are larger or smaller particles. For particles ≥ 0.5 µm, the depth of penetration into

the lungs is inversely proportional to the particle size. Particles between 0.1 and 1 µm are so small a significant proportion of those that enter the lungs may be exhaled. Particles greater than 5 µm deposit in the upper airway.

The amount of delivered drug is also affected by disease severity, which affects airway lumen and breathing pattern. Humidity influences the delivery of aerosol medications, particularly during mechanical ventilation.[8-10] Droplets of solution evaporate or grow, depending on the water content and temperature of the gas, and powder can clump or aggregate in high humidity. Penetration and deposition of aerosol are also affected by inspired gas density, such as a helium–oxygen gas mixture (heliox).[11,12]

Jet Nebulizers

Jet nebulizers use the Bernoulli principle to drive a high pressure gas through a restricted orifice across the top of a capillary tube, with the bottom of the tube immersed in the solution (**Figures 14-2** and **14-3**).[10,13-17] An aerosol is formed when the jet stream shears fluid from the capillary tube and drives the particles against a solid or liquid surface that acts as a baffle. Impaction against a baffle removes larger particles from suspension and allows them to return to the reservoir, whereas smaller particles remain suspended in the gas and travel from the nebulizer. An effective small-volume pneumatic nebulizer should deliver more than 50% of its fill volume as aerosol in the respirable range (1 to 5 µm MMAD) in ≤ 10 minutes of nebulization time. A number of studies have reported large differences in performance among commercially available nebulizers.[18-20]

A gas source, usually air or oxygen, powers the nebulizer. The nebulizer is attached to a delivery system, which includes the patient interface.[13] The nebulizer and delivery system act as the reservoir for the generated aerosol. There may be additional volume that serves as aerosol storage (e.g., a reservoir bag or reservoir tubing). The delivery system also communicates with a reservoir to accommodate the patient's inspiratory flow when it exceeds the source gas flow. The inspiratory flow reservoir may be a part of the delivery system (e.g., a reservoir bag) or may simply be a communication to the atmosphere. As little as 1% of the prescribed drug placed in the nebulizer may be deposited in the patient's respiratory tract, although deposition in the range of 10–20% may be more common. Loss of drug delivery can occur at several stages, as shown in **Figure 14-4**.[13]

Nebulizer output varies with initial charge (fill volume), flow, gas density, and nebulizer model.[20] One reason that output varies is that not all of the solution is nebulized. Some of the solution remains as droplets on the reservoir walls and some simply cannot be sucked up into the capillary tube due to the shape of the reservoir. The retained charge (residual

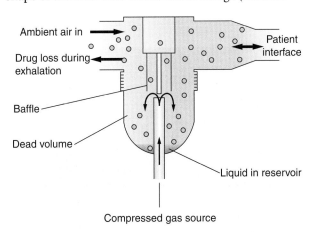

FIGURE 14-2 Illustration of a small-volume jet nebulizer.

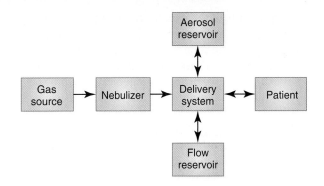

FIGURE 14-3 Schematic of a typical nebulizer system.

Reproduced from Chatburn RL, McPeck M. A new system for understanding nebulizer performance. *Respir Care*. 2007;52(8):1037-1050.

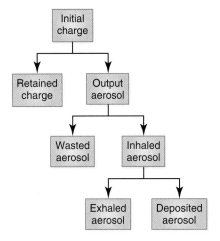

FIGURE 14-4 Stages at which drug can be lost in a nebulizer system. Initial charge: The amount of drug initially placed in the nebulizer. Retained charge: The amount of initial charge remaining in the reservoir that is not nebulized. Output aerosol: The difference between the initial charge and the retained charge. Wasted aerosol: The portion of the initial charge that is aerosolized but lost to the atmosphere or deposited on the device walls. Inhaled aerosol: Any aerosol that enters the patient's airway opening. Exhaled aerosol: Aerosol composed of particles so small that they are not retained in the lung and are subsequently exhaled. Deposited aerosol: Aerosol composed of particles large enough (i.e., in the respirable range) to be retained in the lung.

Reproduced from Chatburn RL, McPeck M. A new system for understanding nebulizer performance. *Respir Care*. 2007;52(8):1037-1050.

volume or dead volume) is the volume of solution that remains in commercial small-volume nebulizers, which varies from 0.5 to 1.5 mL, depending on the specific device. Once the solution has been nebulized down to the residual volume, the nebulizer starts to make a sputtering sound, and nebulizer output is drastically reduced. Therefore, increasing the fill volume allows a greater proportion of the medication to be nebulized. That is why a drug's volume is increased by using a dilutant before adding it to the nebulizer reservoir. An example of this would be adding 0.5 mL albuterol to 2.5 mL normal saline solution to increase the volume of solution well beyond the residual volume. Within the design limits of the nebulizer, the higher the flow to the nebulizer, the smaller the particle size generated and the shorter the time required to nebulize the full dose. Clinicians and patients commonly tap a nebulizer periodically to shake droplets of medication from the walls of the nebulizer into the reservoir. However, continuing the treatment past the point of initial jet nebulizer sputter is ineffective.

Unless labeled otherwise, small volume nebulizers perform best when they are powered with a flow of air or oxygen at 6 to 8 L/min. In the hospital setting, the nebulizer is attached to a flowmeter connected to a 50-psig gas source. In the home or ambulatory setting, however, a portable compressor is often used. Nebulizer/compressor combinations are often marketed together for home use.[18,19,21-23] In one recent study of compressor performance, the flows from five commercially available compressors ranged from about 3.1 L/min to 5.5 L/min.[18] With a lower flow, nebulizer output decreases, particle size increases, and treatment time is longer.

Humidity and temperature affect the particle size and concentration of drug remaining in the nebulizer.[8] Evaporation of water and adiabatic expansion of gas reduce the temperature of the aerosol more than 41°F (5°C) below the ambient temperature. When the inspiratory flow reservoir is dry ambient air, aerosol particles may decrease in size. An inspiratory reservoir bag can be used when it is important to control the inspired gas concentration, such as with heliox therapy (**Figure 14-5**).

Gas density affects both aerosol generation in the nebulizer and delivery of aerosol to the lungs.[12,24-26] A carrier gas of lower density (e.g., heliox) produces less turbulent flow, reducing aerosol impaction losses during inspiration and improving delivery of aerosol to the lungs. However, when heliox is used to drive a jet nebulizer, aerosol output is reduced, requiring a twofold increase in flow to produce a comparable respirable aerosol output per minute.[12] Consequently, heliox may increase the percentage of aerosol available to the lungs but impairs the production of the aerosol by the jet nebulizer.

Breathing pattern affects aerosol delivery with a nebulizer.[13,27] Commonly used nebulizers are continuous; that is, they operate throughout the patient's respiratory cycle. This wastes aerosol produced during the expiratory phase. A typical inspiration to expiration ratio of 1:3 results in 75% of the aerosol emitted from the nebulizer being lost to the atmosphere. If 50% of the nominal dose is emitted, 50% is in the respirable range, and 25% of that is inhaled, then only 12.5% of the nominal dose is inhaled and 20% of that is exhaled. This correlates with the 10% deposition observed with in vivo measurements.

A reservoir on the expiratory limb of the nebulizer conserves drug by collecting some of the nebulizer output that otherwise would be wasted to the atmosphere. A reservoir can be created by placing 15 cm of tubing on the expiratory side of the nebulizer (**Figure 14-6**). As an

alternative, commercial devices such as bag reservoirs provide a greater volume reservoir in which the smaller aerosol particles remain in suspension for inhalation and larger particles rain out (**Figure 14-7**).

Vented nebulizer systems (**Figure 14-8**) allow the patient to inhale additional air through the nebulizer,

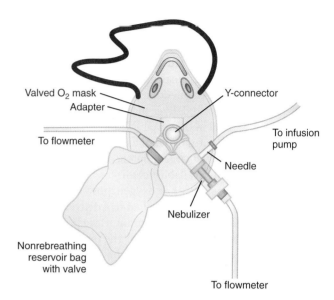

FIGURE 14-5 An inspiratory reservoir bag can be used when it is important to control the inspired gas concentration, such as with heliox therapy.

Modified from Moler FW, et al. Continuous versus intermittent nebulized terbutaline: Plasma levels and effects. *Am J Respir Crit Care Med.* 1995;151:602-606.

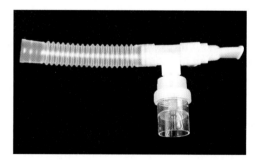

FIGURE 14-6 Small volume jet nebulizer with reservoir tubing.
Courtesy of Dr. Dean Hess.

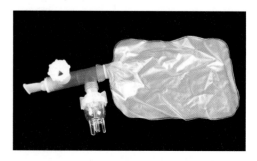

FIGURE 14-7 Nebulizer with reservoir bag to capture aerosol during the expiratory phase.
Courtesy of Dr. Dean Hess.

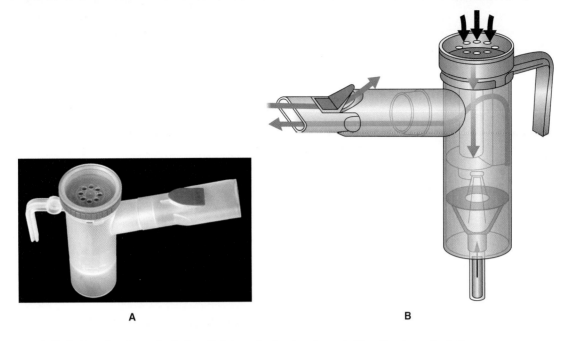

FIGURE 14-8 A. Vented breath-enhanced nebulizer. B. Schematic drawing of a vented breath-enhanced nebulizer.

Photo courtesy of Dr. Dean Hess.

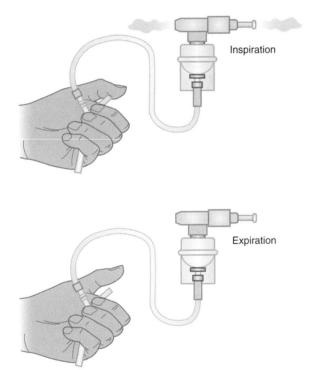

FIGURE 14-9 Schematic illustration of the function of a manual breath-actuated jet nebulizer.

Reproduced from Fink JB. Humidity and aerosol therapy. In: Cairo JM, Pilbeam SP (eds.), *Mosby's Respiratory Care Equipment*. St. Louis, MO: Mosby-Elsevier; 2010:91-140.

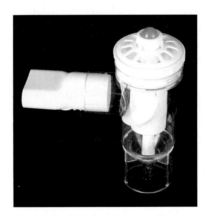

FIGURE 14-10 The Monaghan AeroEclipse, an example of a breath-actuated nebulizer.

Courtesy of Dr. Dean Hess.

increasing drug delivery on inspiration. The inlet vent closes on exhalation, and aerosol exits via a one-way valve in the mouthpiece. Because this design boosts aerosol output during inspiration, these are sometime called breath-enhanced nebulizers. This design reduces

aerosol waste and increases the inhaled dose by as much as 50% without increasing the treatment time.

A breath-actuated nebulizer synchronizes aerosol generation with inspiration, increasing the amount of inhaled aerosol.[28] Inspiratory phase nebulization can be accomplished with a thumb control port that allows the patient to manually direct gas to the nebulizer only on inspiration, but this requires good hand–breath coordination (**Figure 14-9**). More effective systems do not require hand–breath coordination and operate by synchronization of aerosol production to the patient's inspiratory phase. The Monaghan AeroEclipse (**Figure 14-10**) is a pneumatically controlled breath-actuated nebulizer.

Some nebulizers are valved and have expiratory filters (**Figure 14-11**); these are designed specifically for

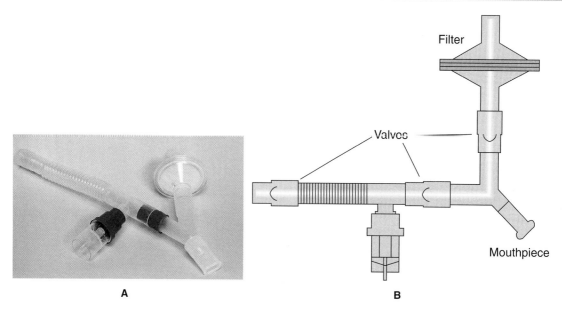

FIGURE 14-11 A. Respirgard nebulizer for pentamidine administration. B. Schematic drawing of Respirgard nebulizer.

the delivery of pentamidine. The filter minimizes ambient contamination with the aerosol and the patient's exhaled gases. These nebulizers also produce very small particles to enhance parenchymal deposition.

For patients who cannot use a mouthpiece, the nebulizer can be fitted to an appropriate mask. Clinical response has been reported to be similar with a mouthpiece compared with a close-fitting mask. Therefore, patient adherence and preference should guide selection of the device. If a mask is used, care should be taken to avoid aerosol delivery in the eyes.[29-31] Crying is a long exhalation preceded by a short and rapid inhalation; this reduces lower airway deposition of an aerosol. Blow-by, in which the practitioner directs the aerosol from the nebulizer toward the patient's nose and mouth, is not supported by available evidence.[32,33] Aerosols can be delivered by high-flow nasal cannula, which may be a reasonable alternative to a face mask for continuous aerosol delivery.[34,35] Technique for use of a jet nebulizer is given in **Table 14-2**.

The small particle aerosol generator (SPAG) is a jet nebulizer used to administer ribavirin (**Figure 14-12**). The SPAG reduces the inlet pressure of 50 psig to 26 psi, which is connected to flowmeters that control flow to the nebulizer (7 L/min) and the drying chamber (8 L/min). The aerosol generated in the medication reservoir enters the long cylindrical drying chamber, where additional flow of dry gas reduces the size of the aerosol particles through evaporation to 1.2 µm with a GSD of 1.4. The administration of ribavirin has highlighted concerns about secondhand exposure. To protect healthcare workers, ribavirin administration should be limited to a negative-pressure, single-patient room with six air exchanges per hour. Procedures used to reduce the release of ribavirin into the environment include containment of the aerosol with a canopy over the

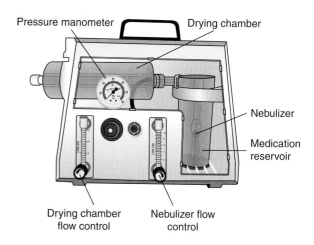

FIGURE 14-12 A schematic drawing of the small particle aerosol generator (SPAG) for ribavirin administration.

TABLE 14-2
Technique for Use of a Jet Nebulizer

1. Assemble tubing, nebulizer cup, and mouthpiece (or mask).
2. Place medicine into the nebulizer cup; use fill volume of 4–5 mL.
3. The patient should be seated in an upright position.
4. Connect to power source; set a flow of 6–8 L/min or compressor.
5. Breathe normally with occasional deep breaths until sputter or no more aerosol produced.
6. Keep nebulizer vertical during treatment.
7. Rinse nebulizer with sterile or distilled water and allow to air dry.

delivery device, use of a scavenging system, and filtering of the expiratory limb of the circuit of a mechanically ventilated patient.

If patient symptoms with an exacerbation of asthma are not relieved with standard bronchodilator dosing,

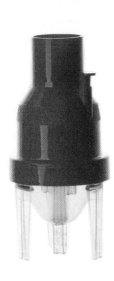

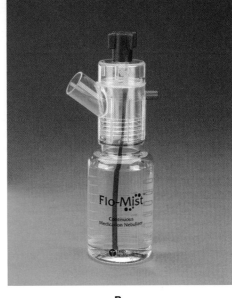

A   B

FIGURE 14-13 Commercially available nebulizers for continuous aerosol administration. A. A small volume nebulizer that can be adapted for continuous use. The port allows for tubing attachment to an intravenous (IV) pump, which feeds the medication mixture to the small volume nebulizer. B. The Flo-Mist Nebulizer (Smiths Medical) has a 200-mL reservoir to allow for up to 8 hours of nebulized medication delivery at 25 mL/hr. This nebulizer allows an auxiliary flow of gas (air, oxygen, or heliox) through the side port, which eliminates the need to recalculate the medication dose.

Photo A courtesy of Westmed, Inc. Photo B courtesy of Smiths Medical.

continuous nebulization can be provided.[36-39] Doses of albuterol between 7.5 and 15 mg/hr are effective in this case. One strategy is to use an intravenous infusion pump to deliver a premixed bronchodilator solution into a jet nebulizer. Another strategy is to use a large-volume nebulizer that delivers a consistent output of medication (Figure 14-13). The bronchodilator solution and saline are mixed in the reservoir, and the nebulizer is operated at a flow recommended by the manufacturer.

Large-volume nebulizers (Figure 14-14) are used for several applications in addition to continuous bronchodilator administration. They can be used to provide humidification of medical gases for patients with bypassed upper airways, as treatment of upper airway inflammation with cold mist for local vasoconstriction, to prevent occlusion of airway stents, and to induce sputum production for diagnostic purposes. There is little evidence to support the use of bland aerosols to hydrate airway secretions in a dehydrated patient. For delivery of humidified inspired gases, a large-volume nebulizer offers little advantage over alternative methods such as heated humidifiers.

Small-volume nebulizers used in the hospital should be cleaned and disinfected, or rinsed with sterile water and air-dried, between uses. Nebulizers for hospital use are disposable and for single patient use, and should be changed at the conclusion of the dose, every 24 hours, or when visibly soiled. Patients should be taught how to disinfect their nebulizers

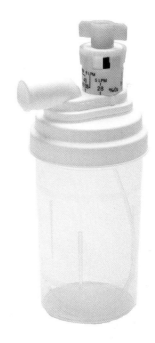

FIGURE 14-14 Large volume nebulizer for bland aerosol administration.

Courtesy of Teleflex.

used in the home. After each treatment the patient should shake the remaining solution from the nebulizer cup. The nebulizer cup should be rinsed with either sterile or distilled water and left to air dry on an absorbent towel. Once or twice a week, the nebulizer should be disassembled, washed in soapy tap water, and disinfected with either a 1.25% acetic acid mixture (1 part 5% white vinegar to 3 parts water) or a quaternary ammonium compound at a dilution of 1 ounce to 1 gallon of sterile or distilled water. The acetic acid soak should be at least 1 hour, but a quaternary ammonium compound soak needs only 10 minutes. Acetic acid should not be reused, but the quaternary ammonium solution can be reused for up to 1 week. Pneumatic nebulizers function correctly in repeated uses provided that they are cleaned after each use, rinsed, and air-dried.

Mesh Nebulizer

Mesh nebulizers are aerosol-generating devices that use a mesh or plate with multiple apertures to produce an aerosol (**Figure 14-15**).[40-44] They use a vibrating mesh (active mesh) or a vibrating horn (passive mesh) to generate an aerosol. For the vibrating mesh (e.g., Aerogen Aeroneb Go or Pari eFlow), contraction and expansion of a vibrational element produce an upward and downward movement of a domed aperture plate, which contains thousands of tapered holes. The holes have a larger cross-section on the liquid side and a smaller cross-section on the side from which the droplets emerge. The

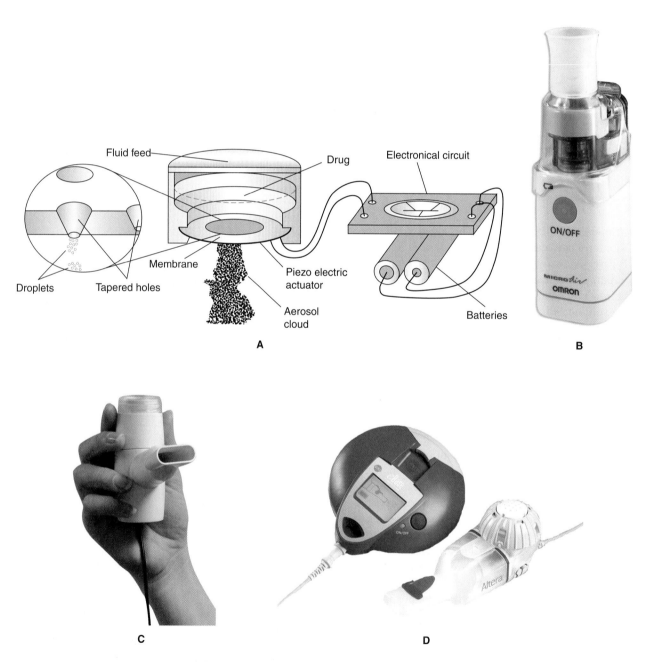

FIGURE 14-15 Mesh nebulizers. A. Principle of operation. B–D. Representative commercially available mesh nebulizers.

Art adapted from Hess DR. Aerosol delivery devices in the treatment of asthma. *Respir Care*. 2008;53:699-725. Photo B courtesy of Omron Healthcare. Photo C courtesy of Philips Healthcare, Respiratory Drug Delivery. Photo D courtesy of PARI Respiratory Equipment. "eFlow® Technology" are registered trademarks of PARI GmbH.

TABLE 14-3
Technique for Use of a Mesh Nebulizer

1. Correctly assemble the equipment.
2. Follow manufacturer's instructions to perform a functionality test prior to the first use of a new device and after each disinfection to verify proper operation.
3. Pour the solution into the medication reservoir. Do not exceed the volume recommended by the manufacturer.
4. Turn on the power.
5. Hold the nebulizer in the position recommended by the manufacturer.
6. Breathe normally with occasional deep breaths.
7. If the treatment must be interrupted, turn off the unit to avoid waste. At the completion of the treatment, disassemble and clean as recommended by the manufacturer.
8. Be careful not to touch the mesh during cleaning, because this will damage the unit.
9. Once or twice a week, disinfect the nebulizer following manufacturer's instructions.

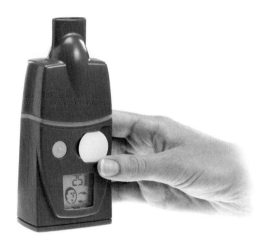

FIGURE 14-16 Adaptive aerosol delivery (AAD) system.
Courtesy of Philips Healthcare

medication is placed in a reservoir above the domed aperture plate. A pumping action extrudes solution through the holes in the plate to produce an aerosol.

In the vibrating horn system (e.g., Omron, iNeb) a piezoelectric crystal vibrates at a high frequency when electrical current is applied, and the vibration is transmitted to a transducer horn that is in contact with the solution. Vibration of the transducer horn causes upward and downward movement of the mesh plate, and the liquid passes through the apertures in the plate and forms an aerosol.

Advantages of mesh technology include a rapid rate of drug delivery, a low retained charge (dead volume), portability because a compressor is not required, and little effect of gas density (as occurs with a jet nebulizer). The mesh also results in a relatively uniform aerosol production, and the size of the holes in the mesh potentially allows manipulation of particle size and targeted drug delivery. The major disadvantage of these devices is their cost. The technique for use of a mesh nebulizer is shown in **Table 14-3**.

Mesh technology can be coupled with adaptive aerosol delivery, as in the iNeb.[45-48] The iNeb system delivers aerosol during the first half of inspiration, monitors the inspiratory time of the first three breaths, and creates

a template for nebulization during inspiration of subsequent breaths (**Figure 14-16**). This is a very efficient inhaled drug delivery system used to administer the pulmonary vasodilator iloprost.

Soft Mist Inhaler

The Respimat Soft Mist Inhaler delivers a metered dose of medication as a fine mist (**Figure 14-17**).[49-56] Medication delivered by the Respimat is stored in a collapsible bag in a sealed plastic container inside the cartridge. With each actuation, the correct dose is drawn from the inner reservoir and the flexible bag contracts accordingly. A twist of the inhaler's base compresses a spring. A tube slides into a canal in the cartridge, and the dose is drawn through the tube into a micropump. When the dose-release button is pressed, the energy released from the spring forces the solution through the uniblock and a slow-moving aerosol is released. The fine nozzle system of the uniblock is the core element of the Respimat. When the medication solution is forced through the nozzle system, two jets of liquid emerge and converge at an optimized angle, and the impact of these converging jets generates the aerosol. The aerosol produced by the Respimat moves much slower and has a more prolonged duration than an aerosol cloud from a pMDI. A dose indicator shows how many doses are left.

Ultrasonic Nebulizers

The **ultrasonic nebulizer (USN)** uses a piezoelectric crystal that vibrates at a high frequency to convert electricity to sound waves, creating standing waves in the liquid immediately above the transducer and disrupting the liquid's surface, forming a geyser of droplets (**Figure 14-18**).[15,57] A disposable medication cup is usually used, with the sound waves communicated through water acting as a couplant. Particle size is determined by frequency, and output by the amplitude of the signal. The particle size is inversely proportional to the frequency and is not user adjustable. The temperature of the solution in a USN increases by as much as 59°F (15°C) over 15 minutes.

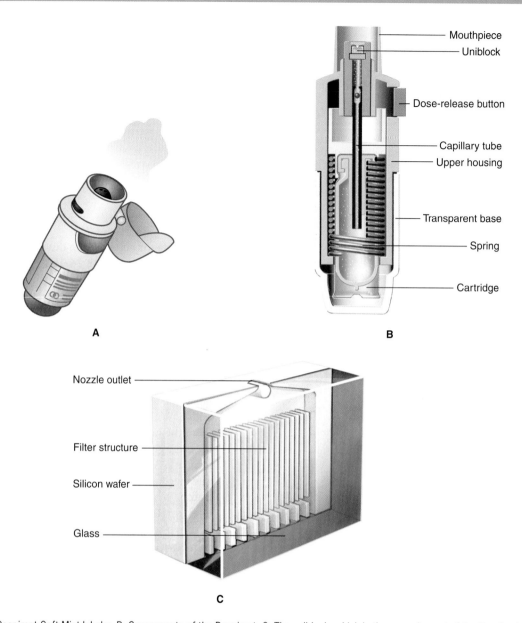

FIGURE 14-17 A. Respimat Soft Mist Inhaler. B. Components of the Respimat. C. The uniblock, which is the core element of the Respimat.
Parts B and C courtesy of Boehringer Ingelheim International GmbH, Germany.

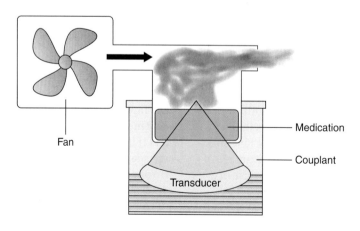

FIGURE 14-18 Schematic drawing of an ultrasonic nebulizer.
Adapted from Cohen N, Fink J. Humidity and aerosols. In: Eubanks DH, Borne RC, eds. *Principles and Applications of Cardiorespiratory Care Equipment*. Mosby; 1994.

TABLE 14-4
Technique for Use of Optineb Nebulizer

1. Correctly assemble the equipment.
2. Fill the chamber of the device with 45 mL of distilled water.
3. Insert an empty medicine cup into the chamber; make sure that the bottom tip is in the water.
4. Gently hold the medication ampule and twist off its top.
5. Squeeze the ampule's entire contents into the medicine cup.
6. Connect the device to the power source.
7. Turn on the device by pressing the ON/OFF button once. When the power is on, the display screen will show "03," and a yellow light will turn on next to the screen.
8. Hold the device so that your hands do not cover the display screen or lights and so that you can follow the visual prompts.
9. Press the START/STOP button to begin treatment.
10. The power light turns green and the device emits two short beeps.
11. While the device emits one long beep, exhale completely.
12. After the device emits a short beep, and while the inhalation indicator light is flashing green and the device emits a beep, place your lips securely around the mouthpiece and inhale deeply.
13. Repeat steps 9–12 two more times. The display screen will count down from "03" to "02" to "01".
14. Press the "ON/OFF" button to turn off the device.
15. If the treatment session requires more than one cycle of breaths (one cycle equals three breaths), press the ON/OFF button at the end of a cycle of breaths to turn the device back on and take an additional cycle of breaths.
16. Clean the accessories by hand in mild, soapy, warm water. Allow accessories to air dry. Once a week, use a clean cloth to wipe the interior of the inhalation device chamber.
17. Once a month, replace the accessories.

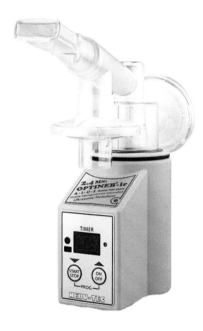

FIGURE 14-19 The Tyvaso inhalation system.
Courtesy of United Therapeutics Corporation.

Large-volume USNs, used primarily for bland aerosol therapy or sputum induction, use a blower to deliver the aerosol to the patient. Battery-powered small-volume ultrasonic nebulizers are available for aerosol drug delivery; the patient's inspiratory flow draws aerosol from the nebulizer into the lungs.

Overhydration has been associated with prolonged bland aerosol treatment by use of a USN in children and patients with renal insufficiency. The high-density aerosol from USNs may precipitate bronchospasm. An acoustic power output above 50 watts/cm^2 has been associated with disruption of the structure of some molecules.

The Optineb (**Figure 14-19**) uses an ultrasonic nebulizer to deliver treprostinil inhalation solution (Tyvaso) for the treatment of pulmonary hypertension. The device prompts the patient to use correct inhalation technique. The recommended prescribed dose is up to nine breaths per treatment session and up to four treatment sessions per day. The technique for use of the Optineb is shown in **Table 14-4**.

Drug–Nebulizer Combinations

It has been known for many years that the output of jet nebulizers can vary greatly among devices. Increasingly, the Food and Drug Administration (FDA) is approving inhaled drugs as a drug–nebulizer combination. Examples are shown in **Table 14-5**. When these drugs are prescribed, it is important the approved nebulizer is used; otherwise, appropriate dosing may not be achieved.

Pressurized Metered Dose Inhalers

A pressurized metered dose inhaler (pMDI) can be used to deliver medicated aerosol therapy. The pressurized canister of a pMDI contains a drug in the form of a

TABLE 14-5
Drug Formulations and Approved Nebulizers for That Formulation

Drug Formulation	Approved Nebulizer
Budesonide (Pulmicort Respules)	Should not be used with ultrasonic nebulizer
Tobramycin (Tobi)	Pari LC
Dornase alfa (Pulmozyme)	Hudson T Up-draft II Marquest Acorn II Pari LC Durable Sidestream, Pari Baby
Pentamadine (NebuPent)	Marquest Respirgard II
Ribavirin (Virazole)	Small particle aerosol generator
Iloprost (Ventavis)	ProDose or I-neb
Treprostinil (Tyvaso)	OptiNeb
Bronchodilator	Any nebulizer can be used

micronized powder or solution that is suspended with a mixture of propellants, surfactant, preservatives, flavoring agents, and dispersing agents (**Figure 14-20**).[6,7,58] The active drug accounts for about 1% of the contents. As much as 80% by weight of the aerosol is propellant, which in the past was a chlorofluorocarbon (CFC). Because of international agreements to ban CFCs, most pMDIs now use hydrofluoroalkenes (HFAs) such as HFA133a as a propellant.

The aerosol from a pMDI is released from the canister through a metering valve and stem that fit into an actuator boot. Because changes in the actuator design can change the characteristics and output of the aerosol, it is important to use the canister only with the boot provided. The metering valve volume varies from 30 to 100 μL and contains 20 μg to 5 mg of drug. The volume emitted by the pMDI is 15 to 20 mL after volatilization of the propellant. Lung deposition ranges from 10% to 25% of the nominal dose in adults, with intersubject variability largely due to technique.

HFA formulations are as effective as their CFC counterparts.[59,60] However, because of the redesigned

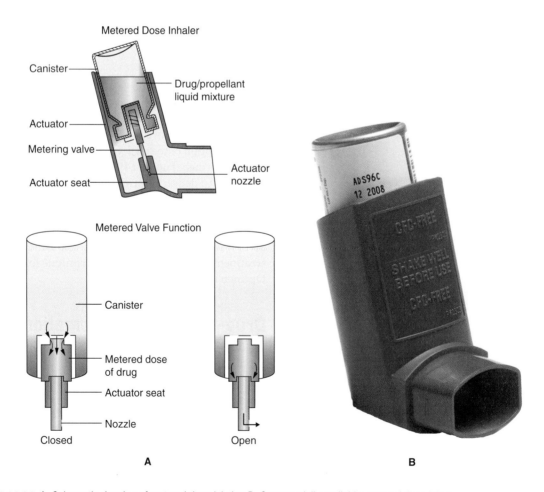

FIGURE 14-20 A. Schematic drawing of metered dose inhaler. B. Commercially available metered dose inhaler.
Art adapted from Rau JL Jr. *Respiratory Care Pharmacology*. 5th ed. Mosby; 1998. Photo © M. Dykstra/ShutterStock, Inc.

TABLE 14-6
Technique for Use of a Pressurized Metered Dose Inhaler

1. Hold the MDI in your hand to warm it.
2. Remove the mouthpiece cover.
3. Inspect the mouthpiece for foreign objects.
4. Hold the MDI in a vertical position.
5. Shake the MDI.
6. If the MDI is new or has not been used recently, prime it by shaking and pressing the canister to deliver a dose into the room. Repeat several times.
7. Breathe out normally.
8. Open your mouth and keep your tongue from obstructing the mouthpiece.
9. Hold the MDI in a vertical position, with the mouthpiece aimed at your mouth.
10. Place the mouthpiece between your lips or position it two finger widths from your mouth.
11. Breathe in slowly and press the canister down once at the beginning of inhalation.
12. Continue to inhale until your lungs are full.
13. Move the mouthpiece away from your mouth and hold your breath for 10 seconds (or as long as you comfortably can).
14. Wait at least 15 seconds between doses.
15. Repeat for the prescribed number of doses.
16. Recap the mouthpiece.
17. Rinse your mouth if using inhaled steroids.
18. Keep a diary of the number of uses so that you know when the canister is empty.
19. Clean the metered-dose inhaler once a week and as needed.

formulation, valve, and actuator, the HFA formulation has a warmer spray temperature and less impact force at the back of the throat. Moreover, storage conditions do not affect device performance. For example, Proventil HFA does not suffer a loss of dose when the inhaler is stored in an inverted position. Additionally, it is not subject to loss of dose in a cold climate, and there is less dose variability at the end of the canister's life. Because of the differences in the propellant, the HFA pMDI has a different taste. The HFA pMDI also has a different feel in the mouth because the spray emitted from the actuator has less force and a smaller plume. HFA steroid inhalers were engineered to generate aerosol particles with an average size of 1.2 μm, to more effectively reach the lower respiratory tract and have less oropharyngeal deposition, which may improve clinical outcomes. Each puff of some HFA formulations releases 4 μL of ethanol, which may be of concern for patients who abstain from alcohol. A breath alcohol level of up to 35 μg per 100 mL may be detected for up to 5 minutes after two puffs from a pMDI HFA formulation. HFA propellant may cause false positive readings in gas-monitoring systems, because the infrared spectra of HFAs overlap with common anesthetic gases. Ventolin HFA contains no excipients other than the propellant, but has a greater affinity for moisture than other HFA inhalers and is therefore packaged in a moisture-resistant protective pouch that contains a desiccant and has a limited

shelf life once it is removed from the pouch. Because clogging of HFA pMDI albuterol actuators can occur, they should be cleaned following the manufacturer's recommendations.

Effective use of the pMDI is technique dependent (**Table 14-6**). Many patients who use pMDIs, as well as health professionals who teach pMDI use, do not perform the procedure properly.[61-75] Good patient instruction can take 10 to 30 minutes and should include demonstration, practice, and confirmation of the patient's performance. Infants, young children, the elderly, and patients in acute distress may not be able to use a pMDI effectively.

The pMDI can be used as often as every 15 seconds without affecting its performance. A new pMDI or one that has not been used recently should be actuated several times before use to prime the metering chamber properly. The pMDI should always be stored with the cap on, both to prevent foreign objects from entering the boot and to reduce humidity and microbial contamination.

The pMDI should always be discarded when empty to avoid administration of propellant without medication. Although many pMDIs contain more than the labeled number of doses, drug delivery per actuation may be very inconsistent and unpredictable after the labeled number of actuations. Beyond the labeled number of actuations, propellant can release an aerosol plume that contains little or no drug, which is a phenomenon called tail-off. A practical problem for patients who use pMDIs is the difficulty of determining the number of doses remaining in the device. Floating the canister in water has been suggested as a way to determine when it is depleted, but this method is unreliable and should not be used.[76] The FDA now recommends that manufacturers integrate a dose-counting device into new pMDIs, and several pMDIs have integrated dose counters (**Figure 14-21**). Add-on devices can also be used that count the number of puffs released from a pMDI.

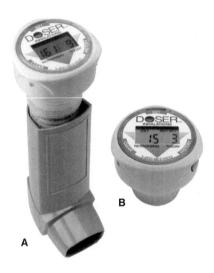

FIGURE 14-21 A. Dose counter on a hydrofluoroalkane (HFA) pressurized metered dose inhaler (Ventolin HFA). B. Doser.

Courtesy of Doser- MediTrack Products.

The Autohaler is a flow-triggered pMDI designed to reduce the need for hand–breath coordination by firing in response to the patient's inspiratory effort (**Figure 14-22**). To use the Autohaler, the patient cocks a lever on top of the unit that spring loads the canister against a vane mechanism. When the patient's inspiratory flow exceeds 30 L/min, the vane moves, allowing the canister to be pressed into the actuator, firing the pMDI. In the United States this device is available only with the β-agonist pirbuterol. The flow required to actuate the device may be too great for some small children to generate, especially during acute exacerbations of disease.

Spacers and Valved Holding Chambers

Spacers and **valved holding chambers** (**Figure 14-23**) are accessory devices that attach to the pMDI. They reduce oropharyngeal deposition of drug and, in the case of valved holding chambers (VHCs), reduce the need for hand–breath coordination.[6,7,58,77-79] These devices may reduce the pharyngeal impaction by 10-fold to 15-fold. This reduces the total body dose from swallowed medications and the risk of candidiasis with inhaled steroid administration. For the very young, very old, or others unable to use the device with a mouthpiece, a face mask can be used (**Figure 14-24**). The technique for use of a pMDI with a spacer or valved holding chamber is shown in **Table 14-7**.

A spacer is an open-ended tube or bag with sufficiently large volume to provide space for the pMDI

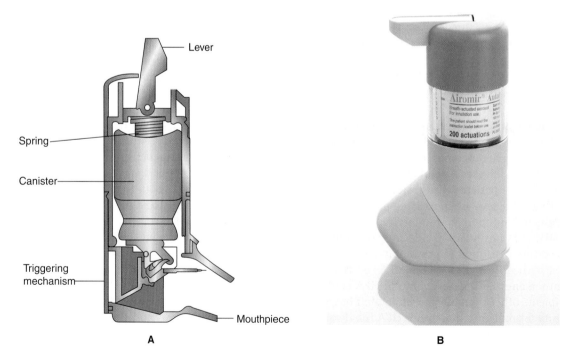

FIGURE 14-22 Breath-actuated metered dose inhaler.

Photo © Gustoimages/Science Source.

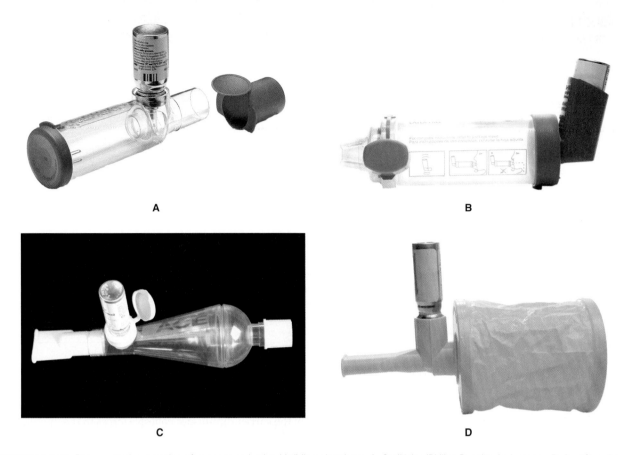

FIGURE 14-23 Representative samples of spacers and valved holding chambers. A. OptiHaler (Philips Respironics) spacer. B. AeroChamber Plus (Monaghan Medical) valved holding chamber. C. Aerosol Cloud Enhancer (ACE) (DHD Healthcare/Smiths Medical) valved holding chamber. D. InspirEase (Schering-Plough) spacer.

Photo A courtesy of Philips Healthcare. Photo B © Rob Byron/ShutterStock, Inc. Photo C courtesy of Dr. Dean Hess. Photo D © Robeo/Dreamstime.com.

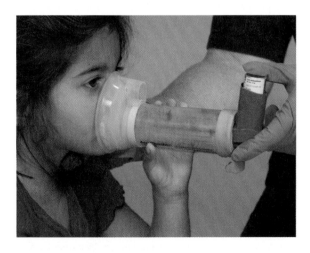

FIGURE 14-24 Valved holding chamber with face mask.

© Jones & Bartlett Learning. Courtesy of MIEMSS.

plume to expand by allowing the propellant to evaporate. A spacer should have an internal volume of more than 100 mL and provide a distance of 10 to 13 cm between the pMDI nozzle and the mouth. Spacers with internal volumes greater than 100 mL provide some

protection against early firing of the pMDI, although exhalation immediately after the actuation clears most of the aerosol from the device, wasting the dose. A valved holding chamber is usually 140 to 750 mL in volume. It allows the plume from the pMDI to expand and incorporates a one-way valve that permits the aerosol to be drawn from the chamber during inhalation only, diverting the exhaled gas to the atmosphere and not disturbing remaining aerosol suspended in the chamber.

Electrostatic charge acquired by the aerosol when generated, or present on the surface of the inhaler or add-on device, decreases aerosol delivery from VHCs.[80] A VHC made from conducting materials, such as stainless steel or aluminum, addresses this problem. Priming by firing 20 doses into a new spacer coats the inner surface with surfactant and minimizes static charge, but this is not practical, because it uses more than 10% of the doses in a new pMDI canister. Washing a nonconducting VHC with detergent is a commonly used method to reduce surface electrostatic charge, and this is now incorporated in most manufacturer instructions. Washing with detergent greatly improves drug delivery and is easy to perform. After washing, the VHC should

TABLE 14-7

Technique for Use of a Pressurized Metered Dose Inhaler with a Spacer or Valved Holding Chamber

1. Hold the MDI in your hand to warm it.
2. Assemble the apparatus and check for foreign objects.
3. Remove the mouthpiece cover.
4. Shake the MDI.
5. If the MDI is new or has not been used recently, prime the device by shaking it and pressing the canister to deliver a dose into the room.
6. Repeat several times.
7. Hold the canister in a vertical position.
8. Breathe out normally.
9. Open your mouth and keep your tongue from obstructing the mouthpiece.
10. Place the mouthpiece into your mouth (or place the mask completely over your nose and mouth).
11. Breathe in slowly through your mouth and press the MDI canister once at the beginning of inspiration.
12. If the device produces a "whistle," your inspiration is too rapid.
13. Allow 15 seconds between puffs.
14. Move the mouthpiece away from your mouth and hold your breath for 10 seconds (or as long as you comfortably can).
15. The technique is slightly different for a device with a collapsible bag:
    a. Open the bag to its full size.
    b. Remove the canister from the MDI mouthpiece and insert it into the mouthpiece attached to the collapsible bag.
    c. Press the MDI canister immediately before inhalation and inhale until the bag is completely collapsed. (If you have difficulty emptying the bag, you can breathe in and out of the bag several times to evacuate the medication.)
16. Rinse your mouth if using inhaled steroids.
17. Clean the holding chamber every 2 weeks and as needed.

not be towel-dried, which could impart electrostatic charge; instead, the device should be allowed to drip-dry in ambient air. The FDA requires manufacturers to recommend rinsing the device with clean water after washing in detergent to avoid patient contact with detergent-coated surfaces, which could result in contact dermatitis. VHCs manufactured from transparent charge-dissipative polymers have become available in recent years as an alternative to opaque conducting materials such as stainless steel or aluminum.

Accessory devices either use the manufacturer-designed boot that comes with the pMDI or incorporate a universal canister adapter to fire the pMDI canister. Different formulations of pMDI drugs operate at different pressures and have different size orifices in the boot designed by the manufacturer for use exclusively with that pMDI. Some pMDIs have a dose counter built into the boot. This type of design is incompatible with a VHC requiring the pMDI canister be removed from the boot and attached to the actuator on the VHC for use. The output characteristics of a pMDI change if an adapter with a different size orifice is used.

Particularly in young children, use of a VHC requires a face mask.[81,82] When using a face mask an adequate seal is necessary, and five to six breaths are taken through the chamber to deliver the full dose. Drug delivery is also influenced by mask dead space, VHC dead space, and the opening pressure of the inspiratory and expiratory valves.[83-86]

Dry Powder Inhalers

Dry powder inhalers (DPIs) create an aerosol by drawing air through a dose of powdered drug.[87-104] The powder contains micronized drug particles (< 5 μm

MMAD) with larger lactose or glucose particles (> 30 μm in diameter) or micronized drug particles bound into loose aggregates. Adding the larger particles of the carrier diminishes cohesive forces in the micronized drug powder so that separation into individual respirable particles (deaggregation) occurs more readily. The carrier particles thus aid delivery of the drug powder from the device. Carriers also act as fillers by adding bulk to the powder when the drug dose is very small. The drug particles usually are loosely bound to the carrier and are stripped from the carrier by the energy provided by the patient's inhalation (**Figure 14-25**). The release of respirable particles of the drug requires inspiration at relatively high flow (30 to 120 L/min). A high inspiratory flow results in pharyngeal impaction of the larger carrier particles that make up the bulk of the aerosol. The technique for use of various DPIs is shown in **Table 14-8**. Unlike the pMDI, the technique for use of a DPI is not uniform among devices.

Commercially available DPIs are either unit-dose, in which the patient loads a single-dose capsule prior to each use, or multi-dose, in which the device contains a month's prescription (**Figure 14-26**). Currently available DPIs are all passive systems, meaning that the patient must provide the energy to disperse the powder from the device. A primary advantage of DPIs is coordination of actuation with inspiration, because they are breath-actuated. A primary disadvantage of unit-dose DPIs is the time needed to load a dose for each use. Another disadvantage of DPIs is that each operates differently from the others in loading and priming.

The internal geometry of the DPI device influences the resistance offered to inspiration and the inspiratory flow required to de-aggregate the medication. Devices with higher resistance require a higher inspiratory force

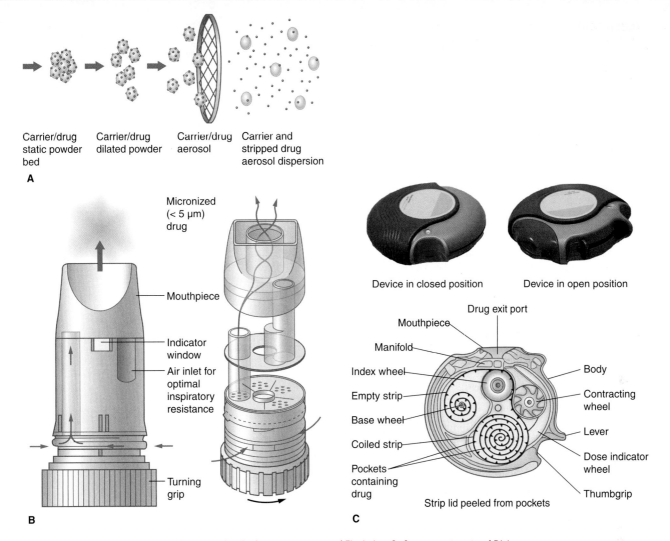

FIGURE 14-25 A. Aerosolization of dry powder. B. Component parts of Flexhaler. C. Component parts of Diskus.

Art A modified from Dhand R, Fink JB. Dry powder inhalers. *Respir Care*. 1999;44:940-951. Art B reproduced with permission from Crompton GK. Delivery systems. In: Kay AB, ed. *Allergy and Allergic Diseases*. London: Blackwell Science; 1997:1440-1450; permission conveyed through Copyright Clearance Center, Inc.

TABLE 14-8
Technique for Use of Dry Powder Inhalers

Diskus:
1. Open the device.
2. Slide the lever.
3. Breathe out normally; do not exhale into the device.
4. Place the mouthpiece into your mouth and close your lips tightly around the mouthpiece.
5. Keep device level while inhaling dose with a rapid and steady flow.
6. Remove the mouthpiece from your mouth and hold your breath for 10 seconds (or as long as you comfortably can).
7. When you exhale, be sure that you are not exhaling into the device.
8. Store the device in a cool dry place.
9. Observe the counter for the number of doses remaining, and replace when appropriate.
10. Do not clean the DPI.

Flexhaler:
1. Twist and remove cap.
2. Hold inhaler upright (mouthpiece up).
3. Turn grip right, then left, until it clicks.
4. Breathe out normally; do not exhale into the device.
5. Place the mouthpiece into your mouth and close your lips tightly around the mouthpiece.
6. Inhale dose with a rapid and steady flow; inhaler may be held upright or horizontal during inhalation.
7. Remove the mouthpiece from your mouth and hold your breath for 10 seconds (or as long as you comfortably can).

(continues)

TABLE 14-8
Technique for Use of Dry Powder Inhalers (*Continued*)

8. When you exhale, be sure that you are not exhaling into the device.
9. Replace the cover and twist to close.
10. Store the device in a cool dry place.
11. When a red mark appears at the top of the dose indicator window, there are 20 doses remaining.
12. When the red mark reaches the bottom of the window, the Flexhaler is empty and must be replaced.
13. Do not clean the DPI.

Aerolizer:
1. Remove the mouthpiece cover.
2. Hold the base of inhaler and twist the mouthpiece counterclockwise.
3. Remove capsule from foil blister immediately before use; do not store the capsule in the Aerolizer.
4. Place the capsule in the chamber in the base of the inhaler.
5. Hold the base of the inhaler and turn it clockwise to close.
6. Simultaneously press both buttons; this pierces the capsule.
7. Keep your head in an upright position.
8. Breathe out normally; do not exhale into the device.
9. Hold the device horizontal, with the buttons on the left and right.
10. Place the mouthpiece into your mouth and close your lips tightly around the mouthpiece.
11. Breathe in rapidly and as deeply as possible.
12. Remove the mouthpiece from your mouth and hold your breath for 10 seconds (or as long as you comfortably can).
13. When you exhale, be sure that you are not exhaling into the device.
14. Open the chamber and examine the capsule; if there is powder remaining, repeat the inhalation process.
15. After use, remove and discard the capsule.
16. Close the mouthpiece and replace the cover.
17. Store the device in a cool dry place.
18. Do not clean the DPI.

HandiHaler:
1. Immediately before using the HandiHaler, peel back the aluminum foil and remove a capsule; do not store capsules in the HandiHaler.
2. Open the dust cap by pulling it upward.
3. Open the mouthpiece.
4. Place the capsule in the center chamber; it does not matter which end is placed in the chamber.
5. Close the mouthpiece firmly until you hear a click; leave the dust cap open.
6. Hold the HandiHaler with the mouthpiece up.
7. Press the piercing button once and release; this makes holes in the capsule and allows the medication to be released when you breathe in.
8. Exhale normally; do not exhale into the device.
9. Place the mouthpiece into your mouth and close your lips tightly around the mouthpiece.
10. Keep your head in an upright position.
11. Breathe in slowly, at a rate sufficient to hear the capsule vibrate, until your lungs are full.
12. Remove the mouthpiece from your mouth and hold your breath for 10 seconds (or as long as you comfortably can).
13. When you exhale, be sure that you are not exhaling into the device.
14. To ensure you get the full dose, repeat the inhalation from the HandiHaler.
15. Open the mouthpiece, tip out the used capsule, and dispose of it.
16. Close the mouthpiece and dust cap for storage of the HandiHaler.
17. Do not clean the DPI.

Diskhaler:
1. Remove the mouthpiece cover.
2. Pull the tray out from the device.
3. Place the disk on the wheel (numbers up).
4. Rotate the disk by sliding the tray out and in.
5. Lift the back of the lid until fully upright so that the needle pierces both sides of the blister.
6. Breathe out normally; do not exhale into the device.
7. Place the mouthpiece into your mouth and close your lips tightly around the mouthpiece.
8. Keep the device level while inhaling the dose with a rapid and steady flow.
9. Remove the mouthpiece from your mouth and hold your breath for 10 seconds (or as long as you comfortably can).
10. When you exhale, be sure that you are not exhaling into the device.
11. Store the device in a cool dry place.
12. Replace the disk when all of the blisters have been punctured.
13. Once every week, brush off any powder remaining within the device.
14. Do not clean the DPI.

TABLE 14-8
Technique for Use of Dry Powder Inhalers (*Continued*)

Twisthaler:
1. Hold the inhaler straight up with the pink portion (the base) on the bottom.
2. Remove the cap while it is in the upright position to ensure the right dose is dispensed.
3. Hold the pink base and twist the cap in a counter-clockwise direction to remove it.
4. As the cap is lifted off, the dose counter on the base will count down by one. This action loads the dose.
5. Make sure the indented arrow located on the white portion (directly above the pink base) is pointing to the dose counter.
6. Breathe out normally; do not exhale into the device.
7. Place the mouthpiece into the mouth, with the mouthpiece facing toward you, and close your lips tightly around it.
8. Inhale the dose with a rapid and steady flow while holding the Twisthaler horizontal.
9. Remove the mouthpiece from the mouth and hold breath for 5 to 10 seconds or as long as possible.
10. Be sure not to exhale into the device.
11. Immediately replace the cap, turn in a clockwise direction, and gently press down until you hear a click.
12. Firmly close the Twisthaler to assure that the next dose is properly loaded.
13. Be sure that the arrow is in line with the dose-counter window.
14. Store the device in a cool, dry place.
15. Do not clean the DPI.

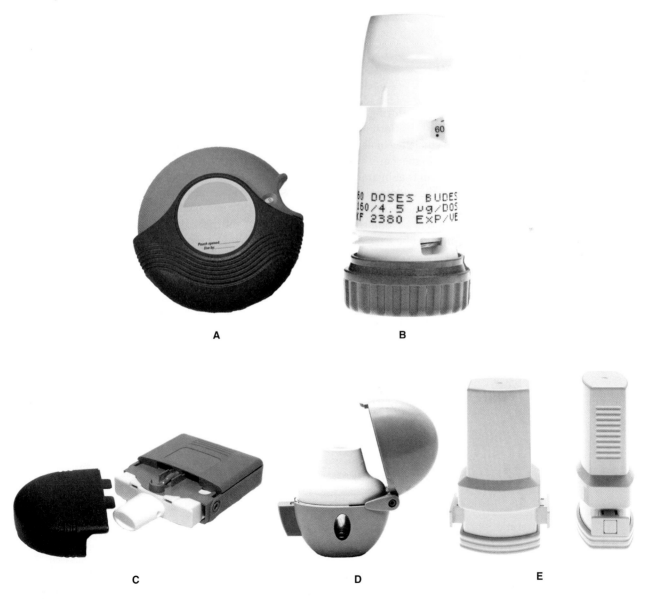

FIGURE 14-26 Multiple-dose dry powder inhalers: A. Diskus. B. Flexhaler. C. Diskhaler. Single-dose dry powder inhalers: D. Handihaler. E. Aerolizer.

to produce a dose. Inhalation through high-resistance DPIs may improve drug delivery to the lower respiratory tract compared with pMDIs, provided the patient can reliably generate the required flow rate. DPIs with several components require correct assembly of the apparatus and/or priming of the device to ensure delivery of the powder. Some DPIs require periodic brushing to remove any residual powder that has accumulated in the device.

High ambient humidity causes the dry powder to clump, creating larger particles that are not as effectively aerosolized. Air with a high moisture content is less efficient at de-aggregating particles of powder than dry air, such that high ambient humidity increases the size of drug particles in the aerosol and may reduce drug delivery to the lungs. High ambient humidity also can result from exhalation into a DPI, from bringing a DPI into a warm indoor environment from the cold outdoors causing condensation to form inside the device, or from being used in a warm, humid environment. Humidity also can accumulate if the DPI is stored with the cap off.

Aerosol Delivery During Mechanical Ventilation

A number of factors affect aerosol delivery during mechanical ventilation (**Figure 14-27**).[105-115] Until recently, the consensus was that the efficiency of aerosol delivery to the lower respiratory tract in mechanically ventilated patients was much lower than that in ambulatory patients. Aerosol impaction in the endotracheal tube can reduce the efficiency of aerosol delivery in children, but the efficiency of aerosol delivery beyond the endotracheal tube does not vary among tube sizes that

have internal diameters of 7 to 9 mm. Humidification of inhaled gas reduces aerosol deposition by approximately 40%, probably because of an increase in particle loss in the ventilator circuit. However, inhalation of dry gas can damage the airway. In addition, disconnection of the ventilator circuit, which is required to bypass the humidifier, interrupts ventilation and may increase the risk of ventilator-associated pneumonia (VAP).

Placement of the nebulizer 30 cm from the endotracheal tube is more efficient than placement between the inspiratory limb and the patient Y-piece because the inspiratory ventilator tubing acts as a spacer for the aerosol to accumulate between breaths. Addition of a spacer between the nebulizer and the endotracheal tube modestly increases aerosol delivery. Operating the nebulizer only during inspiration is more efficient for aerosol delivery than continuous aerosol generation. The technique for use of a nebulizer during mechanical ventilation is shown in **Table 14-9**.

Because the pMDI cannot be used with the actuator designed by the manufacturer, a third-party actuator is required (**Figure 14-28**). A pMDI with a spacer in the inspiratory limb of the ventilator circuit produces a fourfold to sixfold greater delivery of aerosol than pMDI actuation into a connector attached directly to the endotracheal tube or into an inline device that lacks a chamber. When an elbow adapter connected to the endotracheal tube is used, actuation of the pMDI out of synchrony with inspiratory airflow delivers very little aerosol to the lower respiratory tract. Unlike nebulizer use, dose delivery from a pMDI is relatively constant regardless of ventilator settings. The technique for use of a pMDI during mechanical ventilation is shown in **Table 14-10**.

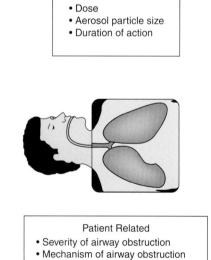

Ventilator Related
- Mode of ventilation
- Tidal volume
- Respiratory rate
- Duty cycle
- Inspiratory waveform
- Breath-triggering mechanism

Device Related—pMDI
- Type of spacer or adapter used
- Position of spacer in circuit
- Timing of pMDI actuation

Drug Related
- Dose
- Aerosol particle size
- Duration of action

Device Related—Nebulizer
- Type of nebulizer used
- Continuous/intermittent operation
- Duration of nebulization
- Position in the circuit

Circuit Related
- Endotracheal tube
- Inhaled gas humidity
- Inhaled gas density

Patient Related
- Severity of airway obstruction
- Mechanism of airway obstruction
- Presence of dynamic hyperinflation
- Patient-ventilator synchrony

FIGURE 14-27 Summary of factors affecting delivery of aerosols during mechanical ventilation.

Adapted from Dhand R, et al. Bronchodilator delivery by metered-dose inhaler in ventilator supported patients. *Eur Respir J.* 1996;9:585-595.

TABLE 14-9
Technique for Aerosol Delivery by Nebulizer During Mechanical Ventilation

1. Fill the nebulizer with the drug solution to the optimum fill volume.
2. Place the nebulizer in the inspiratory line at least 30 cm from the patient's Y-piece.
3. Ensure that the flow through the nebulizer is 6 to 8 L/min. Continuous gas flow from an external source also can be used to power the nebulizer.
4. The nebulizer may be operated continuously or only during inhalation. Some ventilators provide inspiratory gas flow to the nebulizer.
5. Adjust tidal volume as necessary.
6. Turn off the bias flow on the ventilator if possible and remove the heat and moisture exchanger.
7. Check the nebulizer for adequate aerosol generation throughout its use.
8. Disconnect the nebulizer when all the medication has been nebulized or when no more aerosol is being produced. Store the nebulizer under aseptic conditions.
9. Reconnect the ventilator circuit and reinstate the original ventilator settings.

TABLE 14-10
Technique for Use of a Pressurized Metered Dose Inhaler During Mechanical Ventilation

1. Place a spacer in the inspiratory limb of the ventilator circuit. It is preferable to use a spacer that remains in the ventilator circuit so that the circuit need not be disconnected for each bronchodilator treatment.
2. Shake the pressurized pMDI canister vigorously.
3. Actuate the pMDI to synchronize with the precise onset of inspiration by the ventilator. Actuate the pMDI only once.
4. Repeat actuations at 20- to 30-second intervals until the total dose has been delivered.

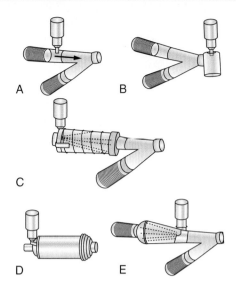

FIGURE 14-28 Devices to adapt a metered dose inhaler to a ventilator circuit. A. Inline device. B. Elbow device. C. Collapsible chamber device. D. Chamber device. E. Chamber device in which aerosol is directed retrograde into the ventilator circuit.

Modified with permission from Dhand R, et al. Bronchodilator delivery by metered-dose inhaler in ventilator supported patients. *Eur Respir J.* 1996;9:585–595.

Nebulizers placed in line in the ventilator circuit can become contaminated with bacteria, which are then carried as aerosols directly to the lower respiratory tract. The risk of VAP may be greater with a nebulizer than with a pMDI. When the collapsible chamber spacer remains in the ventilator circuit between treatments, condensate collects inside it. Care must be taken to prevent the condensate in the spacer from being washed into the patient's respiratory tract. When a noncollapsible spacer chamber is used to actuate a pMDI, it should be removed from the ventilator circuit between treatments.

With proper technique, nebulizers and pMDIs produce similar therapeutic effects in mechanically ventilated patients. The use of pMDI for routine bronchodilator therapy in ventilator-supported patients is preferred because of several problems associated with the use of nebulizers. When the gas flow driving a jet nebulizer comes from a source external to the ventilator, it produces additional airflow in the ventilator circuit. This requires adjustment of tidal volume and inspiratory flow for volume control modes. When patients are unable to trigger a breath because of the additional nebulizer gas flow, asynchrony may result in hypoventilation. Issues related to the additional gas flow from a jet nebulizer are avoided, however, with the use of a mesh nebulizer or ultrasonic nebulizer. Aerosol delivery by pMDI is easy to administer, involves less personnel time, provides a reliable dose of the drug, and is free of the risk of bacterial contamination. If a heat and moisture exchanger (HME) is in-line, either it must be removed or a specially designed HME is used that allows the HME to be bypassed during aerosol therapy (**Figure 14-29**). Aerosol therapy can be provided during noninvasive ventilation using either a nebulizer or a pMDI (**Figure 14-30**).[116]

Aerosol Delivery by Tracheostomy

Inhaled albuterol is occasionally used in nonventilated patients with a tracheostomy tube. A measurable amount of medicated aerosol can be delivered through the tracheostomy tube during spontaneous breathing, with either a nebulizer or a pMDI with spacer. Delivery of an aerosol drug into a high gas flow is inefficient for the nebulizer, and use of a T-piece for albuterol delivery is more effective than use of a tracheostomy mask. The literature shows that efficiency is greater for a pMDI with a valved holding chamber than for a nebulizer, and the pMDI is most efficient when a valved T-piece is used and the valve is placed proximal rather than distal to the spacer.[117] The proper equipment for aerosol delivery by nebulizer and pMDI for spontaneously breathing patients with a tracheostomy are shown in **Figure 14-31**.

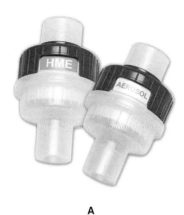
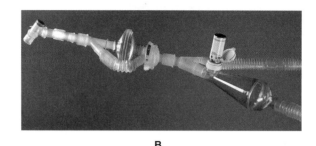

A

B

FIGURE 14-29 Devices that allow a heat and moisture exchanger to be bypassed during aerosol delivery. A. Gibeck Humid-Flo HME (Teleflex Medical). B. Portex CircuVent (Smiths Medical).

Photo A courtesy of Teleflex. Photo B courtesy of Smiths Medical.

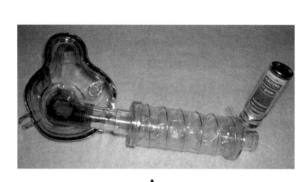
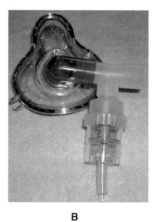

A

B

FIGURE 14-30 Insertion site for nebulizer and inhaler for use with a bilevel ventilator during NIV.

Photos courtesy of Dr. Dean Hess.

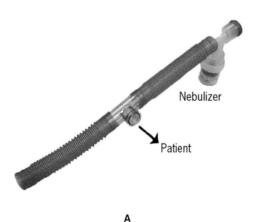
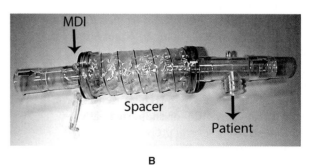

A

B

FIGURE 14-31 Equipment for aerosol delivery to tracheostomy.

Photos courtesy of Dr. Dean Hess.

Selection of an Aerosol Delivery Device

Each type of aerosol delivery device has advantages and disadvantages (Table 14-11). The choice of device often is determined by patient preference or clinician bias. In some cases the choice of device is dictated by the drug formulation. Whenever possible, patients should use only one type of aerosol delivery device. The technique for the use of each device is different, and repeated instruction is necessary to ensure that the patient uses the device appropriately. Using different devices can be confusing for patients and may reduce their compliance with therapy.

Each of the aerosol delivery devices can work equally well provided that patients can use them correctly.

Table 14-11
Advantages and Disadvantages of Various Aerosol Delivery Devices

Device	Advantages	Disadvantages
Jet nebulizer	Patient coordination is not required. Effective with tidal breathing. High doses can be given. Dose modification possible. Can be used with supplemental O_2 Can deliver combination therapies if drugs are compatible. Some are breath-actuated.	Expense. Device is not portable. Pressurized gas source required. Lengthy treatment time. Contamination is possible. Device preparation required. Not all medications are in solution form. Performance variability.
Mesh nebulizer	Patient coordination is not required. Effective with tidal breathing. High doses can be given. Dose modification possible. Some are breath-actuated. Small dead volume. Quiet. Faster delivery than jet nebulizer. Less drug lost during exhalation. Battery operated. Portable and compact. High dose reproducibility.	Expense. Contamination is possible. Device preparation required. Not all medications are in solution form.
Ultrasonic nebulizer	Patient coordination is not required. High doses possible. Small dead volume. Quiet. Faster delivery than jet nebulizer. Less drug lost during exhalation. Some are breath-actuated.	Expense. Need for electrical power. Contamination is possible. Prone to malfunction. Possible drug degradation. Does not nebulize suspensions well. Device preparation required. Potential for airway irritation.
Metered dose inhaler	Portable and compact. No drug preparation is required. Dose reproducibility is high. Device is difficult to contaminate. Treatment time is short. Some are breath-actuated. Some have a dose counter.	Patient coordination is essential. Patient actuation is required. Large pharyngeal deposition occurs. High doses are difficult to deliver. Not all medications can be used with this device. Many of these devices use CFC propellants.
Metered dose inhaler with holding chamber	Less patient coordination is required. Less pharyngeal deposition occurs.	More complex for some patients. More expensive than an MDI alone. Device is less portable than an MDI.
Dry powder inhaler	Less patient coordination is required. Propellant is not required. Breath activated. Small and portable. Short treatment time.	Requires moderate to high inspiratory flow. Some units are single dose. High pharyngeal deposition possible. Not all medications are available. High doses are difficult to deliver.

Adapted from AARC consensus statement: Aerosols and delivery devices. *Respir Care.* 2000;45:589-595; and Dolovich MB, Ahrens RC, Hess DR, et al. Device selection and outcomes of aerosol therapy: Evidence-based guidelines. *Chest.* 2005;127:335-71.

When selecting an aerosol delivery device, the following questions should be considered:[118]

1. In what devices is the desired drug available?
2. What device is the patient likely to be able to use properly, given the patient's age and the clinical setting?
3. For which device and drug combination is reimbursement available?
4. Which devices are the least costly?
5. Can all types of inhaled asthma/chronic obstructive pulmonary disease (COPD) drugs that are prescribed for the patient be delivered with the same type of device? Using the same type of device for all inhaled drugs may facilitate patient teaching and decrease the chance for confusion among devices that require different inhalation techniques.
6. Which devices are the most convenient for the patient, family (outpatient use), or medical staff (acute care setting) to use, given the time required for drug administration and device cleaning, and the portability of the device?
7. How durable is the device?
8. Does the patient or clinician have any specific device preferences?

Proper patient education is critical. Respiratory therapists, physicians, and nurses caring for patients with respiratory diseases should be familiar with issues related to performance and with the correct use of aerosol delivery devices. If the selected delivery device should fail to provide satisfactory treatment, another device should be considered.

References

1. Laube BL, Janssens HM, de Jongh FH, Devadason SG, Dhand R, Diot P, et al. What the pulmonary specialist should know about the new inhalation therapies. *Eur Respir J.* 2011;37(6):1308-1417.
2. Dolovich MB, Dhand R. Aerosol drug delivery: Developments in device design and clinical use. *Lancet.* 2011;377(9770):1032-1045.
3. Rubin BK. Air and soul: The science and application of aerosol therapy. *Respir Care.* 2010;55(7):911-921.
4. Kesser KC, Geller DE. New aerosol delivery devices for cystic fibrosis. *Respir Care.* 2009;54(6):754-767; discussion 767-768.
5. Berger W. Aerosol devices and asthma therapy. *Curr Drug Deliv.* 2009;6(1):38-49.
6. Hess DR. Aerosol delivery devices in the treatment of asthma. *Respir Care.* 2008;53(6):699-723; discussion 723-725.
7. Rau JL. Practical problems with aerosol therapy in COPD. *Respir Care.* 2006;51(2):158-172.
8. Zhou Y, Ahuja A, Irvin CM, Kracko D, McDonald JD, Cheng YS. Evaluation of nebulizer performance under various humidity conditions. *J Aerosol Med.* 2005;18(3):283-293.
9. Miller DD, Amin MM, Palmer LB, Shah AR, Smaldone GC. Aerosol delivery and modern mechanical ventilation: In vitro/in vivo evaluation. *Am J Respir Crit Care Med.* 2003;168(10):1205-1209.
10. Hess DR. Nebulizers: Principles and performance. *Respir Care.* 2000;45(6):609-622.
11. Kim IK, Saville AL, Sikes KL, Corcoran TE. Heliox-driven albuterol nebulization for asthma exacerbations: An overview. *Respir Care.* 2006;51(6):613-618.
12. Hess DR, Fink JB, Venkataraman ST, Kim IK, Myers TR, Tano BD. The history and physics of heliox. *Respir Care.* 2006;51(6):608-612.
13. Chatburn RL, McPeck M. A new system for understanding nebulizer performance. *Respir Care.* 2007;52(8):1037-1050.
14. Roth AP, Lange CF, Finlay WH. The effect of breathing pattern on nebulizer drug delivery. *J Aerosol Med.* 2003;16(3):325-339.
15. Rau JL. Design principles of liquid nebulization devices currently in use. *Respir Care.* 2002;47(11):1257-1275; discussion 1275-1278.
16. O'Riordan TG. Formulations and nebulizer performance. *Respir Care.* 2002;47(11):1305-1312; discussion 1312-1313.
17. Boe J, Dennis JH, O'Driscoll BR, Bauer TT, Carone M, Dautzenberg B, et al. European Respiratory Society guidelines on the use of nebulizers. *Eur Respir J.* 2001;18(1):228-242.
18. Bauer A, McGlynn P, Bovet LL, Mims PL, Curry LA, Hanrahan JP. Output and aerosol properties of 5 nebulizer/compressor systems with arformoterol inhalation solution. *Respir Care.* 2009;54(10):1342-1347.
19. Berg EB, Picard RJ. In vitro delivery of budesonide from 30 jet nebulizer/compressor combinations using infant and child breathing patterns. *Respir Care.* 2009;54(12):1671-1678.
20. Hess D, Fisher D, Williams P, Pooler S, Kacmarek RM. Medication nebulizer performance. Effects of diluent volume, nebulizer flow, and nebulizer brand. *Chest.* 1996;110(2):498-505.
21. Terzano C, Petroianni A, Parola D, Ricci A. Compressor/nebulizer differences in the nebulization of corticosteroids. The CODE study (Corticosteroids and Devices Efficiency). *Eur Rev Med Pharmacol Sci.* 2007;11(4):225-237.
22. Standaert TA, Bohn SE, Aitken ML, Ramsey B. The equivalence of compressor pressure-flow relationships with respect to jet nebulizer aerosolization characteristics. *J Aerosol Med.* 2001;14(1):31-42.
23. Standaert TA, Vandevanter D, Ramsey BW, Vasiljev M, Nardella P, Gmur D, et al. The choice of compressor affects the aerosol parameters and the delivery of tobramycin from a single model nebulizer. *J Aerosol Med.* 2000;13(2):147-153.
24. O'Callaghan C, White J, Jackson J, Crosby D, Dougill B, Bland H. The effects of heliox on the output and particle-size distribution of salbutamol using jet and vibrating mesh nebulizers. *J Aerosol Med.* 2007;20(4):434-444.
25. Kim IK, Phrampus E, Venkataraman S, Pitetti R, Saville A, Corcoran T, et al. Helium/oxygen-driven albuterol nebulization in the treatment of children with moderate to severe asthma exacerbations: A randomized, controlled trial. *Pediatrics.* 2005;116(5):1127-1133.
26. Hess DR, Acosta FL, Ritz RH, Kacmarek RM, Camargo CA, Jr. The effect of heliox on nebulizer function using a beta-agonist bronchodilator. *Chest.* 1999;115(1):184-189.
27. Bauer A, McGlynn P, Bovet LL, Mims PL, Curry LA, Hanrahan JP. The influence of breathing pattern during nebulization on the delivery of arformoterol using a breath simulator. *Respir Care.* 2009;54(11):1488-1492.
28. Sabato K, Ward P, Hawk W, Gildengorin V, Asselin JM. Randomized controlled trial of a breath-actuated nebulizer in pediatric asthma patients in the emergency department. *Respir Care.* 2011;56(6):761-770.
29. Harris KW, Smaldone GC. Facial and ocular deposition of nebulized budesonide: Effects of face mask design. *Chest.* 2008;133(2):482-488.

30. Smaldone GC, Berg E, Nikander K. Variation in pediatric aerosol delivery: Importance of facemask. *J Aerosol Med.* 2005;18(3): 354-363.

31. Sangwan S, Gurses BK, Smaldone GC. Facemasks and facial deposition of aerosols. *Pediatr Pulmonol.* 2004;37(5):447-452.

32. Lin HL, Restrepo RD, Gardenhire DS, Rau JL. Effect of face mask design on inhaled mass of nebulized albuterol, using a pediatric breathing model. *Respir Care.* 2007;52(8):1021-1026.

33. Rubin BK. Bye-bye, blow-by. *Respir Care.* 2007;52(8):981.

34. Ari A, Harwood R, Sheard M, Dailey P, Fink JB. In vitro comparison of heliox and oxygen in aerosol delivery using pediatric high flow nasal cannula. *Pediatr Pulmonol.* 2011;46(8):795-801.

35. Bhashyam AR, Wolf MT, Marcinkowski AL, Saville A, Thomas K, Carcillo JA, et al. Aerosol delivery through nasal cannulas: An in vitro study. *J Aerosol Med Pulm Drug Deliv.* 2008;21(2):181-188.

36. Berlinski A, Willis JR, Leisenring T. In-vitro comparison of 4 large-volume nebulizers in 8 hours of continuous nebulization. *Respir Care.* 2010;55(12):1671-1679.

37. Peters SG. Continuous bronchodilator therapy. *Chest.* 2007; 131(1):286-289.

38. Camargo CA, Jr., Spooner CH, Rowe BH. Continuous versus intermittent beta-agonists in the treatment of acute asthma. *Cochrane Database Syst Rev.* 2003(4):CD001115.

39. Rodrigo GJ, Rodrigo C. Continuous vs intermittent beta-agonists in the treatment of acute adult asthma: A systematic review with meta-analysis. *Chest.* 2002;122(1):160-165.

40. Dhand R. Nebulizers that use a vibrating mesh or plate with multiple apertures to generate aerosol. *Respir Care.* 2002;47(12):1406-1416; discussion 1416-1418.

41. Lass JS, Sant A, Knoch M. New advances in aerosolised drug delivery: Vibrating membrane nebuliser technology. *Exp Opin Drug Deliv.* 2006;3(5):693-702.

42. Waldrep JC, Dhand R. Advanced nebulizer designs employing vibrating mesh/aperture plate technologies for aerosol generation. *Curr Drug Deliv.* 2008;5(2):114-119.

43. Pitance L, Vecellio L, Leal T, Reychler G, Reychler H, Liistro G. Delivery efficacy of a vibrating mesh nebulizer and a jet nebulizer under different configurations. *J Aerosol Med Pulm Drug Deliv.* 2010;23(6):389-396.

44. Skaria S, Smaldone GC. Omron NE U22: Comparison between vibrating mesh and jet nebulizer. *J Aerosol Med Pulm Drug Deliv.* 2010;23(3):173-180.

45. Denyer J, Dyche T. The adaptive aerosol delivery (AAD) technology: Past, present, and future. *J Aerosol Med Pulm Drug Deliv.* 2010;23(Suppl 1):S1-S10.

46. Denyer J, Nikander K, Smith NJ. Adaptive aerosol delivery (AAD) technology. *Expert Opin Drug Deliv.* 2004;1(1):165-176.

47. Hardaker LE, Hatley RH. In vitro characterization of the I-neb adaptive aerosol delivery (AAD) system. *J Aerosol Med Pulm Drug Deliv.* 2010;23(Suppl 1):S11-S20.

48. Van Dyke RE, Nikander K. Delivery of iloprost inhalation solution with the HaloLite, Prodose, and I-neb adaptive aerosol delivery systems: An in vitro study. *Respir Care.* 2007;52(2):184-190.

49. Hodder R, Reese PR, Slaton T. Asthma patients prefer Respimat Soft Mist inhaler to Turbuhaler. *Int J Chron Obstruct Pulmon Dis.* 2009;4:225-232.

50. Hodder R, Price D. Patient preferences for inhaler devices in chronic obstructive pulmonary disease: Experience with Respimat Soft Mist inhaler. *Int J Chron Obstruct Pulmon Dis.* 2009;4:381-390.

51. Brand P, Hederer B, Austen G, Dewberry H, Meyer T. Higher lung deposition with Respimat Soft Mist inhaler than HFA-MDI in COPD patients with poor technique. *Int J Chron Obstruct Pulmon Dis.* 2008;3(4):763-770.

52. Anderson P. Use of Respimat Soft Mist inhaler in COPD patients. *Int J Chron Obstruct Pulmon Dis.* 2006;1(3):251-259.

53. Pitcairn G, Reader S, Pavia D, Newman S. Deposition of corticosteroid aerosol in the human lung by Respimat Soft Mist inhaler compared to deposition by metered dose inhaler or by Turbuhaler dry powder inhaler. *J Aerosol Med.* 2005;18(3):264-272.

54. Hochrainer D, Holz H, Kreher C, Scaffidi L, Spallek M, Wachtel H. Comparison of the aerosol velocity and spray duration of Respimat Soft Mist inhaler and pressurized metered dose inhalers. *J Aerosol Med.* 2005;18(3):273-282.

55. von Berg A, Jeena PM, Soemantri PA, Vertruyen A, Schmidt P, Gerken F, et al. Efficacy and safety of ipratropium bromide plus fenoterol inhaled via Respimat Soft Mist inhaler vs. a conventional metered dose inhaler plus spacer in children with asthma. *Pediatr Pulmonol.* 2004;37(3):264-272.

56. Dalby R, Spallek M, Voshaar T. A review of the development of Respimat Soft Mist inhaler. *Int J Pharm.* 2004;283(1-2):1-9.

57. Yeo LY, Friend JR, McIntosh MP, Meeusen EN, Morton DA. Ultrasonic nebulization platforms for pulmonary drug delivery. *Expert Opin Drug Deliv.* 2010;7(6):663-679.

58. Newman SP. Principles of metered-dose inhaler design. *Respir Care.* 2005;50(9):1177-1190.

59. Hendeles L, Colice GL, Meyer RJ. Withdrawal of albuterol inhalers containing chlorofluorocarbon propellants. *N Engl J Med.* 2007;356(13):1344-1351.

60. Leach CL. The CFC to HFA transition and its impact on pulmonary drug development. *Respir Care.* 2005;50(9):1201-1208.

61. Amirav I, Goren A, Pawlowski NA. What do pediatricians in training know about the correct use of inhalers and spacer devices? *J Allergy Clin Immunol.* 1994;94(4):669-675.

62. Benjaponpitak S, Kraisarin C, Direkwattanachai C, Sasisakunporn C. Incorrect use of metered dose inhaler by pediatric residents. *J Med Assoc Thai.* 1996;79(2):122-126.

63. Guidry GG, Brown WD, Stogner SW, George RB. Incorrect use of metered dose inhalers by medical personnel. *Chest.* 1992;101(1):31-33.

64. Hanania NA, Wittman R, Kesten S, Chapman KR. Medical personnel's knowledge of and ability to use inhaling devices. Metered-dose inhalers, spacing chambers, and breath-actuated dry powder inhalers. *Chest.* 1994;105(1):111-116.

65. Interiano B, Guntupalli KK. Metered-dose inhalers. Do health care providers know what to teach? *Arch Intern Med.* 1993; 153(1):81-85.

66. Jones JS, Holstege CP, Riekse R, White L, Bergquist T. Metered-dose inhalers: Do emergency health care providers know what to teach? *Ann Emerg Med.* 1995;26(3):308-311.

67. Kesten S, Zive K, Chapman KR. Pharmacist knowledge and ability to use inhaled medication delivery systems. *Chest.* 1993;104(6):1737-1742.

68. Molimard M, Raherison C, Lignot S, Depont F, Abouelfath A, Moore N. Assessment of handling of inhaler devices in real life: An observational study in 3811 patients in primary care. *J Aerosol Med.* 2003;16(3):249-254.

69. Khassawneh BY, Al-Ali MK, Alzoubi KH, Batarseh MZ, Al-Safi SA, Sharara AM, et al. Handling of inhaler devices in actual pulmonary practice: Metered-dose inhaler versus dry powder inhalers. *Respir Care.* 2008;53(3):324-328.

70. Lavorini F, Magnan A, Dubus JC, Voshaar T, Corbetta L, Broeders M, et al. Effect of incorrect use of dry powder inhalers on management of patients with asthma and COPD. *Respir Med.* 2008;102(4):593-604.

71. Melani AS. Inhalatory therapy training: A priority challenge for the physician. *Acta Biomed.* 2007;78(3):233-245.

72. O'Donnell J, Birkinshaw R, Burke V, Driscoll PA. The ability of A&E personnel to demonstrate inhaler technique. *J Accid Emerg Med.* 1997;14(3):163-164.

73. Scarpaci LT, Tsoukleris MG, McPherson ML. Assessment of hospice nurses' technique in the use of inhalers and nebulizers. *J Palliat Med.* 2007;10(3):665-676.

74. Self TH, Kelso TM, Arheart KL, Morgan JH, Umberto Meduri G. Nurses' performance of inhalation technique with metered-dose

inhaler plus spacer device. *Ann Pharmacother.* 1993;27(2): 185-187.

75. Wieshammer S, Dreyhaupt J. Dry powder inhalers: Which factors determine the frequency of handling errors? *Respiration.* 2008;75(1):18-25.

76. Rubin BK, Durotoye L. How do patients determine that their metered-dose inhaler is empty? *Chest.* 2004;126(4):1134-1137.

77. Cates CJ, Crilly JA, Rowe BH. Holding chambers (spacers) versus nebulisers for beta-agonist treatment of acute asthma. *Cochrane Database Syst Rev.* 2006(2):CD000052.

78. Cates CJ, Bestall J, Adams N. Holding chambers versus nebulisers for inhaled steroids in chronic asthma. *Cochrane Database Syst Rev.* 2006(1):CD001491.

79. Newman SP. Spacer devices for metered dose inhalers. *Clin Pharmacokinet.* 2004;43(6):349-360.

80. Mitchell JP, Coppolo DP, Nagel MW. Electrostatics and inhaled medications: Influence on delivery via pressurized metered-dose inhalers and add-on devices. *Respir Care.* 2007;52(3):283-300.

81. Rubin BK, Fink JB. The delivery of inhaled medication to the young child. *Pediatr Clin North Am.* 2003;50(3):717-731.

82. Rubin BK, Fink JB. Optimizing aerosol delivery by pressurized metered-dose inhalers. *Respir Care.* 2005;50(9):1191-1200.

83. Janssens HM, Tiddens HA. Facemasks and aerosol delivery by metered dose inhaler-valved holding chamber in young children: a tight seal makes the difference. *J Aerosol Med.* 2007;20(Suppl 1): S59-S63; discussion S63-S65.

84. Esposito-Festen J, Ates B, van Vliet F, Hop W, Tiddens H. Aerosol delivery to young children by pMDI-spacer: Is facemask design important? *Pediatr Allergy Immunol.* 2005;16(4):348-353.

85. Esposito-Festen J, Ijsselstijn H, Hop W, van Vliet F, de Jongste J, Tiddens H. Aerosol therapy by pressured metered-dose inhaler-spacer in sleeping young children: To do or not to do? *Chest.* 2006;130(2):487-492.

86. Esposito-Festen JE, Ates B, van Vliet FJ, Verbraak AF, de Jongste JC, Tiddens HA. Effect of a facemask leak on aerosol delivery from a pMDI-spacer system. *J Aerosol Med.* 2004;17(1):1-6.

87. Chrystyn H. The Diskus: A review of its position among dry powder inhaler devices. *Int J Clin Pract.* 2007;61(6):1022-1036.

88. Chougule MB, Padhi BK, Jinturkar KA, Misra A. Development of dry powder inhalers. *Recent Pat Drug Deliv Formul.* 2007; 1(1):11-21.

89. Chan HK. Dry powder aerosol delivery systems: Current and future research directions. *J Aerosol Med.* 2006;19(1):21-27.

90. Telko MJ, Hickey AJ. Dry powder inhaler formulation. *Respir Care.* 2005;50(9):1209-1227.

91. Taylor A, Gustafsson P. Do all dry powder inhalers show the same pharmaceutical performance? *Int J Clin Pract Suppl.* 2005; 149:7-12.

92. Price D. Do healthcare professionals think that dry powder inhalers can be used interchangeably? *Int J Clin Pract Suppl.* 2005;149:26-29.

93. Gustafsson P, Taylor A, Zanen P, Chrystyn H. Can patients use all dry powder inhalers equally well? *Int J Clin Pract Suppl.* 2005;149:13-18.

94. Chrystyn H. Do patients show the same level of adherence with all dry powder inhalers? *Int J Clin Pract Suppl.* 2005;149:19-25.

95. Borgstrom L, Asking L, Thorsson L. Idealhalers or realhalers? A comparison of Diskus and Turbuhaler. *Int J Clin Pract.* 2005; 59(12):1488-1495.

96. Borgstrom L, Asking L, Lipniunas P. An in vivo and in vitro comparison of two powder inhalers following storage at hot/humid conditions. *J Aerosol Med.* 2005;18(3):304-310.

97. Booker R. Do patients think that dry powder inhalers can be used interchangeably? *Int J Clin Pract Suppl* 2005;149:30-32.

98. Atkins PJ. Dry powder inhalers: An overview. *Respir Care.* 2005; 50(10):1304-1312; discussion 1312.

99. Richter K. Successful use of DPI systems in asthmatic patients—key parameters. *Respir Med.* 2004;98(Suppl B):S22-S27.

100. Newman SP. Dry powder inhalers for optimal drug delivery. *Expert Opin Biol Ther.* 2004;4(1):23-33.

101. Kamps AW, Brand PL, Roorda RJ. Variation of peak inspiratory flow through dry powder inhalers in children with stable and unstable asthma. *Pediatr Pulmonol.* 2004;37(1):65-70.

102. Bronsky EA, Grossman J, Henis MJ, Gallo PP, Yegen U, Della Cioppa G, et al. Inspiratory flow rates and volumes with the Aerolizer dry powder inhaler in asthmatic children and adults. *Curr Med Res Opin.* 2004;20(2):131-137.

103. Newman SP. Drug delivery to the lungs from dry powder inhalers. *Curr Opin Pulm Med.* 2003;9(Suppl 1):S17-S20.

104. Dhand R, Fink JB. Dry powder inhalers. *Respir Care.* 1999; 44:940-951.

105. Ari A, Atalay OT, Harwood R, Sheard MM, Aljamhan EA, Fink JB. Influence of nebulizer type, position, and bias flow on aerosol drug delivery in simulated pediatric and adult lung models during mechanical ventilation. *Respir Care.* 2010;55(7):845-851.

106. Ari A, Areabi H, Fink JB. Evaluation of aerosol generator devices at 3 locations in humidified and non-humidified circuits during adult mechanical ventilation. *Respir Care.* 2010;55(7):837-844.

107. Guerin C, Fassier T, Bayle F, Lemasson S, Richard JC. Inhaled bronchodilator administration during mechanical ventilation: How to optimize it, and for which clinical benefit? *J Aerosol Med Pulm Drug Deliv.* 2008;21(1):85-96.

108. Dhand R, Sohal H. Pulmonary drug delivery system for inhalation therapy in mechanically ventilated patients. *Expert Rev Med Device.* 2008;5(1):9-18.

109. Dhand R, Guntur VP. How best to deliver aerosol medications to mechanically ventilated patients. *Clin Chest Med.* 2008; 29(2):277-296, vi.

110. Dhand R. Aerosol delivery during mechanical ventilation: From basic techniques to new devices. *J Aerosol Med Pulm Drug Deliv.* 2008;21(1):45-60.

111. Dhand R. Inhalation therapy in invasive and noninvasive mechanical ventilation. *Curr Opin Crit Care.* 2007;13(1):27-38.

112. Dhand R. Inhalation therapy with metered-dose inhalers and dry powder inhalers in mechanically ventilated patients. *Respir Care.* 2005;50(10):1331-1334; discussion 1344-1345.

113. Dhand R. Basic techniques for aerosol delivery during mechanical ventilation. *Respir Care.* 2004;49(6):611-622.

114. Dhand R. New frontiers in aerosol delivery during mechanical ventilation. *Respir Care.* 2004;49(6):666-677.

115. Hess D. Aerosol delivery during mechanical ventilation. *Minerva Anestesiol.* 2002;68(5):321-325.

116. Hess DR. The mask for noninvasive ventilation: Principles of design and effects on aerosol delivery. *J Aerosol Med.* 2007;20(Suppl 1):S85-S98; discussion S98-99.

117. Piccuito CM, Hess DR. Albuterol delivery via tracheostomy tube. *Respir Care.* 2005;50(8):1071-1076.

118. Dolovich MB, Ahrens RC, Hess DR, Anderson P, Dhand R, Rau JL, et al. Device selection and outcomes of aerosol therapy: Evidence-based guidelines: American College of Chest Physicians/American College of Asthma, Allergy, and Immunology. *Chest.* 2005;127(1):335-371.

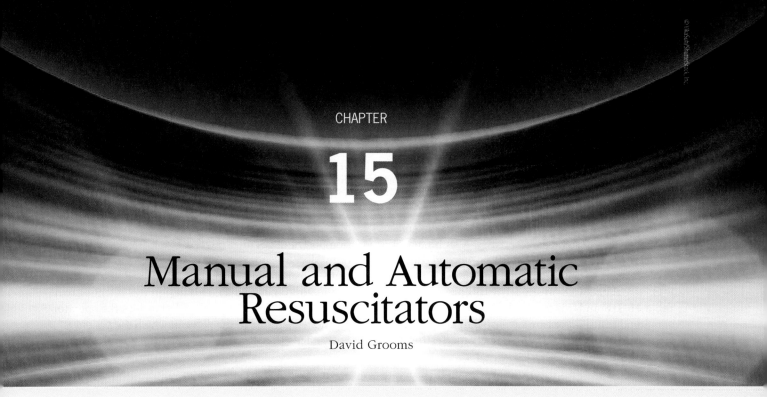

CHAPTER

15

Manual and Automatic Resuscitators

David Grooms

CHAPTER OBJECTIVES

1. Identify barriers to providing effective ventilation in association with manual resuscitator designs.
2. Describe industry standards and requirements for the development of manual resuscitators.
3. Describe the design characteristics and principles of use for flow-inflating resuscitators.
4. Describe the design characteristics and principles of use for bag-valve resuscitators.
5. Compare and contrast oxygen tube reservoirs, oxygen bag reservoirs, and oxygen supply valves for bag-valve resuscitators.
6. Describe the design characteristics and principles of use for automatic resuscitators.

KEY TERMS

Automatic resuscitator
Bag-valve resuscitators
Flow-inflating resuscitator
Gastric insufflation
Manual resuscitator

Oxygen reservoir
Pressure manometer
Pressure pop-off valve
T-piece resuscitator
Tidal volume

Introduction

Manual resuscitation is a method of providing artificial ventilation by a caregiver. This technique is often administered to patients who are unable to sustain adequate spontaneous ventilation; generally the caregiver uses a manual resuscitation device or a portable automatic resuscitator. More importantly, manual resuscitation is recognized as an essential component in providing cardiopulmonary resuscitation (CPR) following cardiac arrest. This recommendation is endorsed by the American Heart Association (AHA),

American Association for Respiratory Care (AARC), International Liaison Committee on Resuscitation (ILCOR) Advanced Life Support Task Force, and European Resuscitation Council (ERC).[1-4]

In the hospital setting, manual resuscitation is commonly provided to mechanically ventilated patients during intrahospital transport (e.g., when a transport ventilator is not available), prior to laryngoscopy performed for tracheal intubation, and for hyperinflation during tracheal suctioning. Specialized training is required for effective delivery of manual ventilation. In fact, 2010 guidelines for CPR and emergency care have de-emphasized the immediate initiation of manual ventilation in a witnessed arrest due to its procedural complexity and likelihood that the cardiac arrest is of primary cause, warranting the need for compressions. Subsequently, it is recommended for the lone rescuer, who is not a healthcare provider, to begin chest compressions and only initiate manual ventilations in two-person rescue.[1,3,4] Therefore, appropriate application of manual ventilation, coupled with consideration for hand size,[5-7] one-handed versus two-handed ventilation,[5,6,8,9] respiratory lung and chest wall mechanics,[10,11] operator fatigue,[12] **tidal volume** (V_T) and positive pressure amount,[6,8,13-16] and delivered fraction of oxygen content (F_DO_2), in association with oxygen (O_2) reservoir type,[17-20] serve as the foundation from which resuscitators have evolved to enhance resuscitation efforts.

Manual Resuscitators

Manual resuscitators have been used for over 50 years.[21] The purpose of this type of device is to provide manually applied positive pressure ventilation to a patient's airway. Although manual resuscitators are separated into three categories—flow-inflating, self-inflating, and T-piece resuscitators—the foundational concepts of breath delivery are similar. These concepts relate to the use of a mask versus a tracheal airway, the design of the manual resuscitator, the ability to minimize rebreathing of exhaled gas, and the ability to sustain a high F_DO_2. However, design principles engineered to support the foundational concepts of breath delivery often vary among these resuscitator types.

The effective use of manual resuscitators depends on the device's design characteristics. A summary of the AHA, AARC, ILCOR, and ERC proposed standards relating to the magnitude, timing, and initial F_DO_2 associated with breath delivery is presented in **Table 15-1**. Standards for the design and functionality of manual resuscitators are suggested by the AARC and are governed by the American Society for Testing and

Materials (ASTM) and the International Organization for Standardization (ISO) (**Table 15-2**).[2,22,23]

Flow-Inflating Resuscitators

Flow-inflating resuscitators, also called hyperinflation or anesthesia bags, lack a nonrebreathing valve. These devices incorporate a 15-mm inner diameter (ID) to 22-mm outer diameter (OD) patient airway or mask connector, flow control valve, **anesthesia bag**, **pressure manometer**, **pressure pop-off valve**, medication injection port, and gas inlet (**Figure 15-1**). The patient airway or mask connector is commonly designed in the form of a 90-degree angle with a 15-mm ID and 22-mm OD connector (**Figure 15-2**). This design was intended to assist in providing manual ventilation with the operator positioned parallel to the plane in which the patient is positioned. This design also allows the operator, who

TABLE 15-1
Summary of AHA, AARC, ILCOR, and ERC Suggested Breathing Patterns for Manual Resuscitation During CPR

	V_T (mL)/PIP cm H_2O	RR (bpm)	I-Time (s)	Initial Target F_DO_2
Adult	600	8–10	1.0	1.0
Pediatric	450–500	10–12	1.0	1.0
Infant/Neonate	Heart rate > 100 bpm (PIP > 20)	40–60	Variable	0.21

PIP: Positive inspiratory pressure; RR: Respiratory rate; I-time: inspiratory time; bpm: beats per minute

TABLE 15-2
ASTM/ISO/AARC Standards for Design and Functionality of Manual Resuscitators

Manual resuscitators must:

1. Have a standard 15-mm inner diameter (ID) to 22-mm outer diameter (OD) patient connector.[2,20,21]
2. Be capable of delivering F_DO_2 of 0.85–1.0 even when large volumes are delivered or when spontaneous breathing is observed.[2,20,21]
3. Operate at extreme temperatures (–292°F to 1112°F/–180°C to 600°C) and at a relative humidity of 40%–96%.[20,21]
4. Have a bag volume of approximately 1,600 mL for adults and deliver at least a V_T of 600 mL into a test lung set at a compliance of 0.02 L/cm H_2O and a resistance of 20 cm H_2O/L/sec.[2,20,21]
5. Have minimal forward and back leak and a nonrebreather valve that will function at oxygen flow rates up to 30 L/min.[2,20,21]
6. Be impossible to misassemble and easily sterilized or for single-patient use.[2]
7. Provide for measurement of exhaled tidal volume.[2]
8. Provide some indication that supplemental oxygen is being supplied (easily ascertained with bag reservoir but difficult with tube type reservoir).[2]
9. Be capable of being restored to proper function within 20 seconds after being disabled by foreign obstruction (e.g., vomitus, mucus).[2,20,21]
10. Be absent of a pressure-limiting system for adults. Pressure-release valves that limit peak inspiratory pressure to 40 ± 10 cm H_2O are required for children and suggested at 40 ± 5 H_2O for infants.[2,20,21]
11. Possess an override capability for incorporated pressure-limiting system.[20,21]
12. Be able to be restored to proper function after being dropped from a height of 1 m onto a concrete floor.[2,20,21]
13. Be designed so that pressure generated at the patient connection port is < 5 cm H_2O during exhalation at a flow of 5 L/min for patients weighing < 22 lb (< 10 kg) and 50 L/min for all others.[2]
14. Be designed so that pressure generated at the patient connection port does not exceed 5 cm H_2O during inspiration at a flow of 5 L/min for patients weighing < 22 lb (< 10 kg) and 50 L/min for all others.[2]

is most commonly positioned at the head of the patient, to rotate and position the device for assessing a proper face-mask seal and direct visualization of adequate chest rise during ventilation. The so-called "flow control valve" does not regulate the flow through the anesthesia bag. That flow is controlled by the flow of source oxygen (e.g., an oxygen flowmeter). The flow out of the bag must be equal to the source flow into the bag, or the bag would either deflate (e.g., loss of gas source) or explode (flow control valve completely closed). Instead, the flow control valve regulates the resistance of the flow out of the bag. As the valve is closed, the resistance through the valve increases; however, the flow through

the valve remains the same so that pressure drop across the valve must increase. The pressure drop is the pressure inside the bag (i.e., the continuous positive airway pressure level) minus the pressure outside the bag (atmospheric pressure). This pressure serves as the baseline pressure (above atmospheric pressure) for spontaneous breathing and also for the generation of inspiratory pressure when the bag is manually compressed so that the bag fills adequately between each breath.

Proper flow regulation is important in flow-inflating manual resuscitators to provide continuous positive airway pressure (CPAP) or positive end-expiratory pressure (PEEP) as well as ventilation.[24] The combination of the flow regulation along with the magnitude of hand squeeze delivered by the caregiver dictates the tidal volume (V_T) and associated pressure delivered during breath delivery. Flow-inflating resuscitators do not display V_T, but rather peak inspiratory pressure (PIP) with the use of a pressure manometer. This can be problematic because airway pressure has been shown to be a crude proxy for the volume of gas delivered during ventilation with a mask.[25]

Anesthesia bags are commonly attached adjacent to the flow control valve and pressure manometer. The medication injection port allows for the administration of medication directly into a tracheal airway by connection of a standard Luer lock syringe. Although the AHA suggests that if intravenous (IV) and intraosseus (IO) access cannot be established, epinephrine, vasopression, and lidocaine can be administered by the endotracheal route during CPR,[26] the ERC no longer recommends this practice.[4] Finally, the gas hose inlet is usually located between the patient connector and anesthesia bag, adjacent to the flow control valve, and allows the connection of standard clear, soft, nontoxic polyvinyl chloride (PVC) tubing to a compressed gas source.

Flow-inflating bags are also used in conjunction with anesthesia circuits and machines. This is also considered

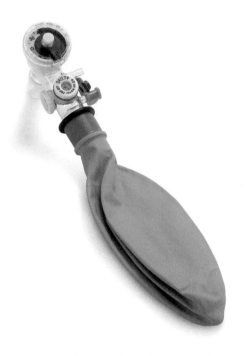

FIGURE 15-1 Flow-inflating resuscitator (Ventlab, Mocksville, NC).
Courtesy of SunMed.

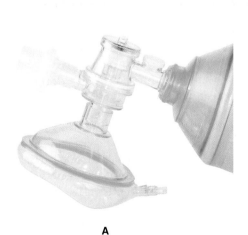

A

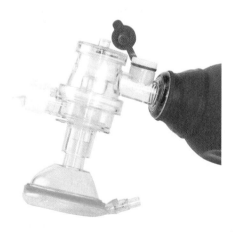

B

FIGURE 15-2 Ninety-degree angle, 15-mm inner to 22-mm outer diameter patient connector.
Photos courtesy of SunMed.

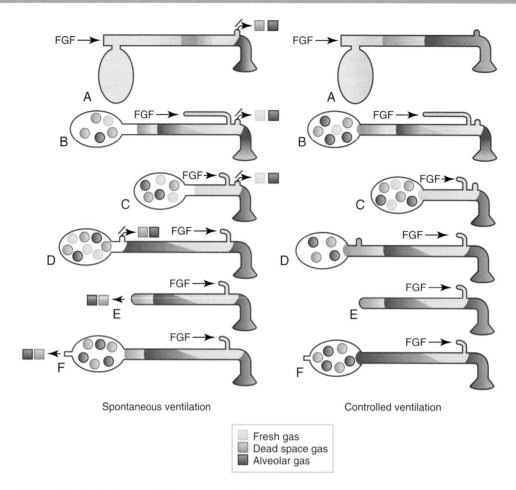

Spontaneous ventilation   Controlled ventilation

Fresh gas
Dead space gas
Alveolar gas

FIGURE 15-3 Mapleson Circuit Classification designs A through F with active and passive ventilation.

Reproduced from Bready LL, Dillman D, Noorily SH. *Decision making in anesthesiology: An algorithmic approach.* Elsevier Health Sciences; 2007, with permission from Elsevier.

a continuous-flow, semi-open breathing system, which varies in design layout based on the location of oxygen flow relative to the patient and the exhalation port. This design layout is best described by the Mapleson classification of nonrebreathing circuits,[27] which was originally designated A through E; however, it now incorporates the Jackson-Rees modification[28] of the Ayre's T-piece[29] designated as F (**Figure 15-3**). This classification is associated with the different circuit types, classified both on the basis of fresh gas flow needed to minimize rebreathing and on the capability to provide intermittent positive pressure ventilation. With respect to prevention of rebreathing, grading of the superiority/inferiority of Mapleson circuits for spontaneous ventilation is A > DFE > CB and for passive ventilation is DFE > BC > A.[30] Despite the Mapleson A system requiring a lower oxygen flow rate than the Mapleson D system to preoxygenate within 3 minutes,[31] and the Mapleson C system being more effective and subjectively easier to breathe through than a self-inflating resuscitator when used for preoxygenation,[32] the Mapleson A–C systems are not commonly used, whereas the D–F systems are still employed. However, due to the improvement in the circle system's

reliability and design, Mapleson-type breathing circuits have become less popular and are used only sporadically.

Application

Flow-inflating resuscitators are commonly used in the operating room, delivery room or neonatal intensive care unit (NICU) and for neonatal care.[33] A survey of delivery room resuscitation practices in the United States revealed that the majority of participating programs resuscitate newborns in the delivery room (83%) by providing positive pressure ventilation with flow-inflating resuscitators (51%), followed by the use of self-inflating resuscitators (40%), and thirdly T-piece resuscitators (14%).[33] In contrast, a survey sent to a neonatologist at each of 29 neonatal intensive care units in Australia and New Zealand revealed that self-inflating resuscitators were used in 22 centers (76%), flow-inflating resuscitators in 12 centers (41%), and T-piece resuscitators in 14 centers (48%).[34]

Although flow-inflating resuscitators are one of three common devices, they are not often used in adult respiratory care. Proper use of this resuscitator type requires coordination of several tasks:[35] (1) adjusting the flow of gas into the bag from the oxygen source, (2) control of outflow resistance from the anesthesia bag through the flow control valve to generate the desired CPAP level, (3) controlling the force of the manual compression of the anesthesia bag, and (4) maintaining an adequate face mask seal. Due to the complex nature of this coordination, flow-inflating resuscitators are technically more challenging in providing effective ventilation and generally require more training and practice.[36] PIP is primarily a byproduct of how hard the anesthesia bag is squeezed; however, it is also affected by the flow through the bag, the CPAP level, and the impedance of the respiratory system. Because volume is not directly measured, clinicians must rely on a manometer to monitor peak and end-expiratory pressures.

Few studies have been conducted to assess the performance of flow-inflating resuscitators in comparison to other manual resuscitators. Using an infant resuscitation mannequin, 70 participants including interns, junior and senior residents, fellows, and nurses were evaluated and demonstrated that a flow-inflating resuscitator resulted in more ventilation failures, no advantage in preventing excessive airway pressures, and less confidence among operators when compared to a self-inflating resuscitator.[37] In contrast, using a continuous pressure recording system and neonatal mannequin, 31 neonatologists, neonatal respiratory therapist, neonatal fellows, a pediatrician, pediatric residents, neonatal nurse practitioners, and neonatal nurses were evaluated to assess the ability to deliver a consistent PIP of 20 or 40 cm H_2O and a PEEP of 5 cm H_2O during a 30-second period of ventilation with the use of flow-inflating, self-inflating, and T-piece resuscitators.[38] Although the T-piece resuscitator delivered the desired pressures more accurately, the flow-inflating resuscitator delivered a lower PIP (**Figure 15-4**), higher PEEP, and quicker transition time from a PIP of 20 cm H_2O to 40 cm H_2O compared to the self-inflating resuscitator.

Anesthesia bags, used to make flow-inflating resuscitators, come in a variety of types for any clinical requirement or preference. Such examples include, but are not limited to, standard nonconductive latex, textured nonconductive latex, silicone, and most commonly, neoprene (latex protein–free) bags. These bags come in a variety of colors and range in size from 1/4-liter to 3-liter bags.

Currently Available Devices, Sizes, and Specifications

A representative list of currently available flow-inflating resuscitators is shown in **Table 15-3**.

Bag-Valve Resuscitators

The **bag-valve resuscitator**, also known as a self-inflating bag, consists of a patient connector, nonrebreathing valve, self-inflating compressible unit, oxygen entry

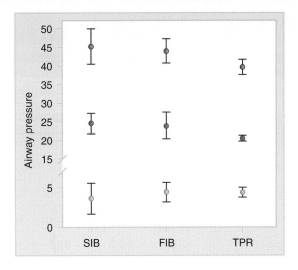

FIGURE 15-4 Comparison of pressures among three devices. The purple circle shows the average inspiratory pressure for the goal of 40 cm H_2O ± 2 standard deviations. The red circle shows the average inspiratory pressure for the goal of 20 cm H_2O ± 2 standard deviations. The blue circle shows the average PEEP ± 2 standard deviations at a goal of 5 cm H_2O. The self-inflating bag was used with the manufacturer's PEEP valve. SIB: self-inflating bag; FIB: flow-inflating bag; TPR: T-piece resuscitator.

port, and **oxygen reservoir** (**Figure 15-5**). The patient connector is similar to that of a flow-inflating resuscitator and incorporates a 90-degree-angle swivel adaptor that connects to a mask or tracheal airway. The primary function of the nonrebreathing valve is to direct flow to the patient when the compressible unit is squeezed which minimizes rebreathing of carbon dioxide (CO_2) by diverting exhaled gas to the atmosphere. A variety of valve designs are available to accomplish this, which include, but are not limited to, diaphragm/leaf valves, spring and disk valves, and duck bill valves (**Figure 15-6**). Most nonrebreathing valves are designed to control inspiratory and /or baseline pressure. Spring-loaded threshold resistors allow for the control of inspiratory and baseline pressures without the need for ancillary attachments. Other valve designs allow for the attachment of a PEEP valve to regulate baseline pressure and/or a pressure pop-off valve to limit the inspiratory pressure delivered as the bag is manually squeezed. Depending on the model, the pressure pop-off may be fixed or adjustable. This feature is more common among devices designed for infant and pediatric use. In the event that high pressures are required, there is the capability to override the pop-off valve. A port for attachment to a pressure manometer, similar to that found on the flow-inflating resuscitator, is also common.

The self-inflating compressible unit is thin walled and is about the size of a football; it often incorporates an anti-slip texture to aid the resuscitator in sustaining proper hand position and grip throughout manual

TABLE 15-3
Manufacturers, Sizes, and Specifications of Flow-Inflating Resuscitators

Manufacturer	Bag Size (L)	Elbow/Patient Connector	Mask Type	Ability to Monitor PIP
Portex	0.5–2.0	Standard/Dual swivel	Neonate; Infant	On some models
Ventlab	0.25–3.0	Standard/Dual swivel	Infant; Adult	On some models
WestMed Inc.	0.5–3.0	Standard/Dual swivel	Neonate; Infant	On some models
Teleflex Medical	0.5–1.0	Standard/Dual swivel	Neonate; Infant	On some models
Mercury Medical	0.5–1.0	Standard/Dual swivel	Neonate; Infant	On some models
Airlife	0.5–2.0	Standard/Dual swivel	Neonate; Infant	On some models
Ambu	0.5–3.0	Standard/Dual swivel	Neonate; Infant	On some models
Galemed	0.5–1.0	Standard/Dual swivel	Pediatric; Adult	On some models

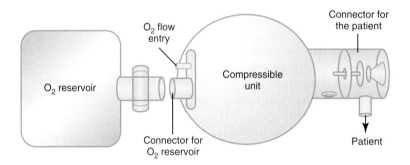

FIGURE 15-5 Schematic drawing of the basic components of a bag-valve manual resuscitator.

Reproduced with permission from Armando Carlos Franco de Godoy and Ronan José Vieira. Comparison of the F_IO_2 delivered by seven models of the self-inflating bag-mask system. *Revista Brasileira De Anestesiologia.* 2009;59(1):21-27.

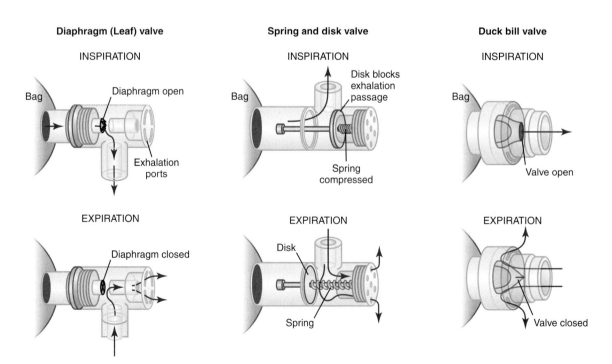

FIGURE 15-6 Nonrebreathing valves commonly used with bag-valve resuscitators.

Reproduced with permission from Branson RD, Hess DR, Chatburn RL. *Respiratory Care Equipment.* J. B. Lippincott Company;1995.

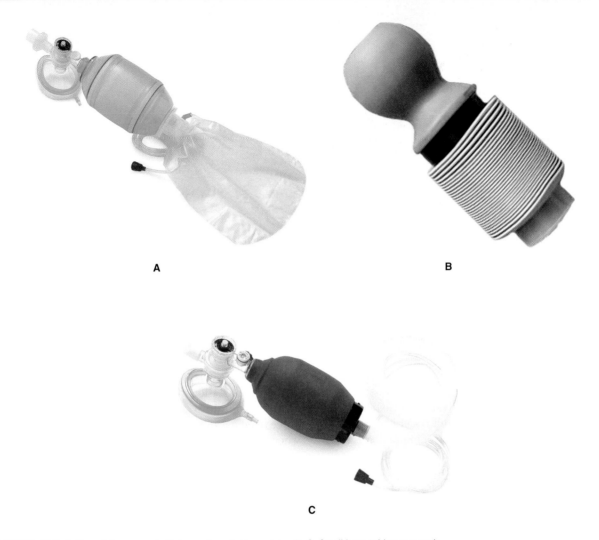

A   **B**

C

FIGURE 15-7 A. Bag style reservoir. B. Large-bore tubing reservoir. C. Small-bore tubing reservoir.
Photos courtesy of SunMed.

ventilation. The oxygen inlet is either a plastic nipple adaptor that allows standard O_2 tubing to be connected from a compressed oxygen source with the use of a medical flowmeter or incorporates a demand valve that can be manually operated or patient triggered (oxygen-powered resuscitator). Oxygen-powered resuscitators often use a high pressure hose directly connected to a 50-psi gas source, which can provide F_DO_2 of 1.0 at flows ≤ 40 L/min with inspiratory pressures limited at 60 cm H_2O. For resuscitators that incorporate an O_2 reservoir, the size and type of reservoir may vary and generally come in three different configurations: bag style, large-bore tubing, and small-bore tubing reservoirs (**Figure 15-7**). The tubing length differs among the tubing style devices. Although the reservoirs are intended to increase the F_DO_2, their configuration significantly impacts F_DO_2.[19] In a bench model evaluation of 16 adult disposable bag-mask resuscitators, bag-valve resuscitators that incorporated the bag style and large-bore reservoir provided better F_DO_2 than the small-bore design, despite one- and two-hand ventilation at rates of 12 bpm and 20 bpm (**Figure 15-8**).[19]

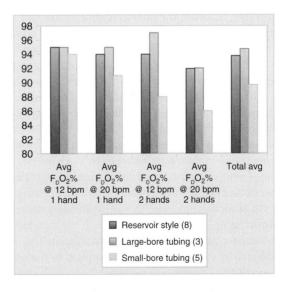

FIGURE 15-8 Average F_DO_2 delivered by bag valve resuscitators with different style reservoirs.

Data from Mazzolini DG, Marshall NA. Evaluation of 16 adult disposable manual resuscitators. *Respir Care.* 2004;49(12):1509-1514.

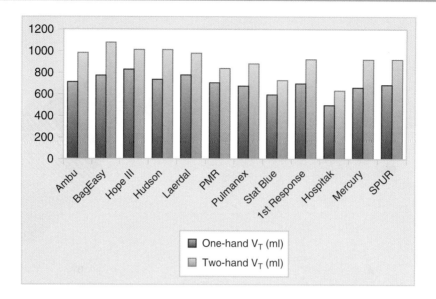

FIGURE 15-9 Variation in V_T delivery with one- and two-hand ventilation with bag valve resuscitator using a simulated lung with compliance of 0.05 L/cm H_2O and 7-mm ETT.

Data from Hess D, Spahr C. An evaluation of volumes delivered by selected adult disposable resuscitators: the effects of hand size, number of hands used, and use of disposable medical gloves. *Respir Care.* 1990;35(8):800–805.

Application

Manual resuscitation with a bag-valve resuscitator is most commonly performed in adult respiratory care. Although the AHA accepts the use of manually triggered, oxygen-powered, flow-limited resuscitators, the AARC does not recommend their use[2] due to a variety of complications and hazards associated with their use.[39-42] As a result of the increasing incidence of acute lung injury (ALI) and acute respiratory distress syndrome (ARDS),[43,44] special focus has been given to the importance of monitoring and delivery of V_T when delivering manual ventilation. Traditional standards encouraged operators to use a V_T large enough to see a chest rise; however, the increased death rates and complications associated with ALI and ARDS[45] due to biotrauma[46] and autoPEEP-associated hypotension[47] have contributed to an evolution of practices suggesting lowering V_T delivery combined with lowering respiratory rates (RR) during CPR.[48,49] Managing the correct V_T delivery is complex and is influenced by the type and design of the resuscitator as well as the technique the operator uses to compress the bag. Several studies have demonstrated inconsistent patterns in V_T delivery as a result of one- vs. two-handed ventilation (**Figure 15-9**), resuscitator type, resistance and compliance changes, and use of medical gloves,[5-9] resulting in suggestions of monitoring V_T instead of PIP. Although the standard technique for manual ventilation is to regulate the breath size by varying the pressure applied to the bag, and monitoring pressure is essential,[50] research shows that excessive V_T delivered with or without excessive PIP is injurious to preterm and term animal lungs.[51,52] This suggests that varying PIP should be performed during times when compliance changes, in particular

during resuscitation of newly born infants and after surfactant administration.[53-55] However, there is reluctance to adjust the pressure during manual ventilation when there is the propensity for lung compliance to change. This may be attributed to the inability to quantify compliance changes during manual ventilation and because pressure is a poor surrogate for gauging V_T.

Using a modified lung simulator to mimic lungs of a 3-kg neonate, 45 neonatal professionals, most of whom had participated in more than 20 resuscitations, were blinded to randomized compliance changes while using flow-inflating, self-inflating, and T-piece resuscitators. They were instructed to maintain a constant inflation volume while blinded to delivered V_T, and then subsequently with V_T displayed.[56] With only pressure displayed, subjects failed to adjust inspiratory pressure in the appropriate direction to compensate for the loss of V_T during periods of low respiratory system compliance (**Figure 15-10**). In contrast, when only V_T was displayed the subjects adjusted pressure to bring the delivered tidal volume closer to the target goal, but were only able to achieve this with a self-inflating resuscitator and only under high compliance conditions (**Figure 15-11**). The challenges in adjusting pressure to sustain a constant V_T are mirrored when trying to adjust V_T to maintain a specific pressure. One hundred and twenty medical professionals using self-inflating and T-piece resuscitators were instructed to deliver a target PIP while resultant V_T was recorded.[57] The median V_T and PIP of the self-inflating resuscitator were significantly higher compared to those for the T-piece resuscitator (**Figure 15-12**).

Resuscitation with bag-valve resuscitators may not provide an accurate V_T because of differences in the

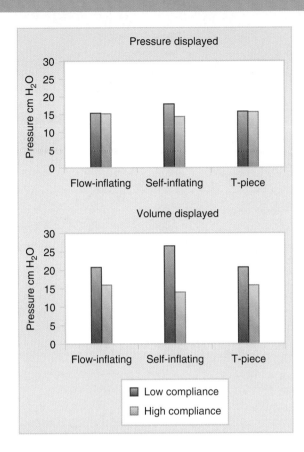

FIGURE 15-10 Mean inflation pressures (with 95% confidence limits) delivered according to subjects in response to changing compliance. Top: Pressure-only visible. Bottom: Volume-only visible.

Data from Kattwinkel J, Stewart C, Walsh B, Gurka M, Paget-Brown A. Responding to compliance changes in a lung model during manual ventilation: Perhaps volume, rather than pressure, should be displayed. *Pediatrics*. 2009;123(3):e465-e470.

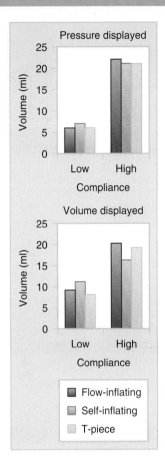

FIGURE 15-11 Mean volumes (with 95% confidence limits) delivered according to subjects in response to changing compliance. Top Pressure-only visible. Bottom Volume-only visible.

Data from Kattwinkel J, Stewart C, Walsh B, Gurka M, Paget-Brown A. Responding to compliance changes in a lung model during manual ventilation: Perhaps volume, rather than pressure, should be displayed. *Pediatrics*. 2009;123(3):735-1080.

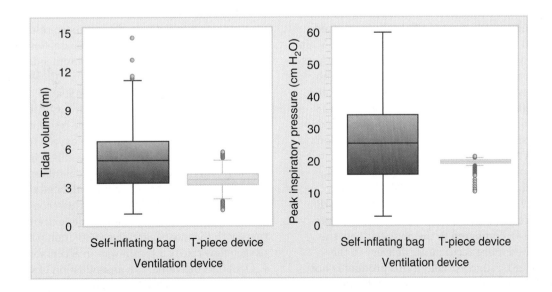

FIGURE 15-12 Comparison of applied V_T (left) and pressure (right) between both ventilation devices used.

Reproduced from Roehr CC, Kelm M, Fischer HS, et al. Manual ventilation devices in neonatal resuscitation: Tidal volume and positive pressure-provision. *Resuscitation*. 2010;81(2):202-205, with permission from Elsevier.

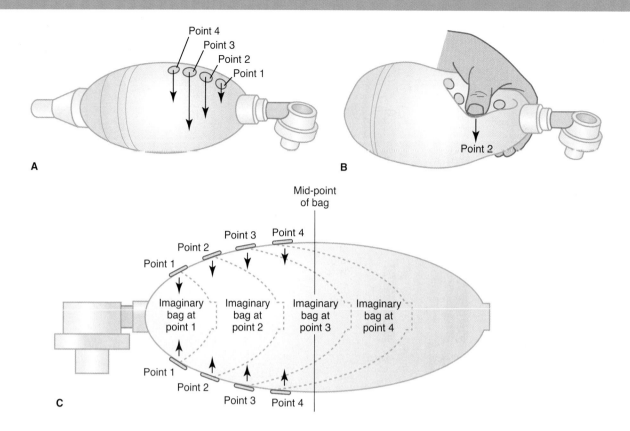

FIGURE 15-13 A. Newly designed target volume marked adult bag (TVMB). B. Compression of point 2 to deliver 200- to 300-mL target volume using the TVMB. C. Schematic representation of the TVMB (points 1–4 were marked on the surface of the adult bag and imaginary bags for each point were simulated.

Part C reproduced from Park SO, Lee KR, Baek KJ, et al. Novel target volume marked adult bag to deliver accurate tidal volume for paediatric and adolescent resuscitation. *Resuscitation*. 2011;82(6):749–754, with permission from Elsevier.

body weight or size of children.[58] Volume estimates are also difficult when visual inspection of the chest rise is obstructed (e.g., during chest compressions or specialized procedures). Therefore an emerging practice incorporating a newly created tidal volume marked bag (TVMB) has been shown to deliver accurate V_T in pediatrics and adolescent resuscitation.[59] The authors designed an adult, self-inflating, 1,600-ml bag with four compression points marked on the resuscitator bag surface (**Figure 15-13**). Fifty-three subjects (28 doctors, 17 nurses, and 8 paramedics) participated in a crossover simulation and delivered 10 ventilations using the TVMB, a standard adult bag, and a pediatric bag in each of four target V_T ranges (100–200 mL, 200–300 mL, 300–400 mL, and 400–500 mL). Compared with the standard adult bag, the TVMB showed more accurate V_T delivery for all V_T ranges (**Figure 15-14**); compared to the pediatric bag, the TVMB showed more accurate V_T delivery in the 200- to 300-mL range. Although this product is not commercially available, it provides insight into the constant consideration of manual resuscitator evolution in response to changes in clinical initiatives and patient safety.

Although minimizing delivery of excessive V_T is of utmost importance, equally important is the F_DO_2 during ventilation. This is mostly important for adults and children, because a recent meta-analysis[60] argued for a reduction in F_DO_2 used in newborn resuscitation, prompting the AHA, ERC, and Neonatal Resuscitation Program (NRP) to modify their recommendation to use room air resuscitation at birth.[1,4,61] Therefore, some resuscitators used in neonatal resuscitation do not require an oxygen reservoir for high F_DO_2. The NRP guidelines advise that with bag-valve resuscitators, a high F_DO_2 is not achieved when the oxygen reservoir is removed. Although true for some, this is in direct conflict with the design of the Laerdal infant bag-valve resuscitator (LIR). A recent study validated that this resuscitator provided high F_DO_2 at the recommended flow rates by the NRP, and only under extreme conditions with the most aggressive ventilation pattern and oxygen flow rate of 1 L/min was an acceptably low F_DO_2 of 0.53 delivered.[62] In an evaluation of seven models of adult–bag-valve resuscitators, using 15 L/min of compressed O_2, F_DO_2 was more than 0.98 with the resuscitators that did not use an attached O_2 reservoir (**Figure 15-15**).[63] Although counterintuitive, F_DO_2 does

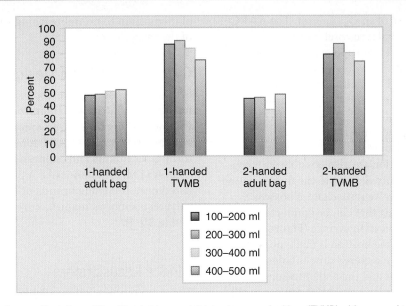

FIGURE 15-14 Percent of correctly delivered V_T with adult bag and tidal volume marked bag (TVMB) with one- and two-hand ventilation technique.

Modified from Park SO, Lee KR, Baek KJ, et al. Novel target volume marked adult bag to deliver accurate tidal volume for paediatric and adolescent resuscitation. *Resuscitation.* 2011;82(6):749–754, with permission from Elsevier.

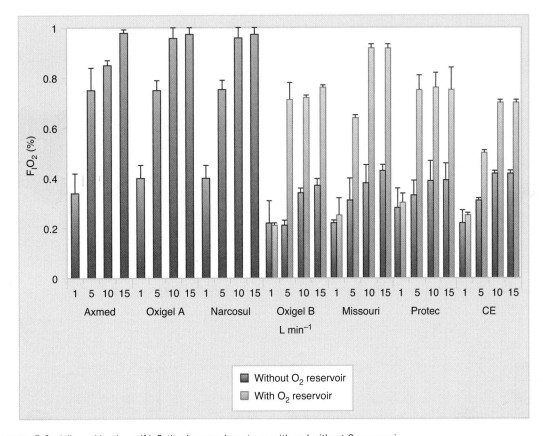

FIGURE 15-15 F_DO_2 delivered by the self-inflating bag-mask systems with and without O_2 reservoir.

Reproduced with permission from Armando Carlos Franco de Godoy and Ronan Josê Vieira. Comparison of the F_iO_2 delivered by seven models of the self-inflating bag-mask system. *Revista Brasileira De Anestesiologia.* 2009;59(1):21–27.

not solely rely on the use of an O_2 reservoir, but more importantly the flow of O_2 and the displacement of the compressible unit. Furthermore, as long as the flow rate of the gas source exceeds the delivered minute volume by the device, aspiration of room air will be minimal.

As stated previously, the design of the resuscitator coupled with reservoir type significantly affect F_DO_2. However, quantifying the appropriate F_DO_2 during manual resuscitation is impossible without the use of an oxygen analyzer. Most resuscitation processes do not incorporate the use of an O_2 analyzer. The AARC recommends that manual resuscitators be able to provide some indication that supplemental oxygen is being supplied and that it may be easier to ascertain with a bag reservoir and difficult with a tube-style reservoir.[2] Therefore, the verification for properly set oxygen flow rate is often conducted by direct visualization of the reservoir activity.

Direct medication installation and aerosolized medication administration are also possible with bag-valve resuscitator systems. Similar to the flow-inflating resuscitator, most bag-valve resuscitators possess a medication injection port that can be connected to a standard Luer lock medication syringe (**Figure 15-16**). Delivery of aerosolized medication is made possible by the incorporation of a metered dose inhaler (MDI) actuator in some models and the ability to connect a variety of handheld nebulizer and MDI devices to the 15/22-mm patient connector (**Figure 15-17**). The use of a filter can also be incorporated to minimize deposition

of medication to nonrebreathing valves and other parts of the resuscitator.

Currently Available Devices and Sizes

Self-inflating bag-valve resuscitators are manufactured for adult, pediatric, and infant/neonatal patients. The volume of these bags varies among manufacturers and ranges from 1.0 to 2.2 L for adults and from 0.2 to 1.0 L for infants and children and are required to meet ASTM/ISO standards. A 2006 global inventory listed over 100 trade brands of self-inflating bag-valve resuscitators manufactured in 10 countries (**Table 15-4**).[64]

T-Piece Resuscitators

The only commercially available **T-piece resuscitators** are the Neopuff Infant T-Piece Resuscitator (Fisher & Paykel Healthcare, East Tamaki, New Zealand;

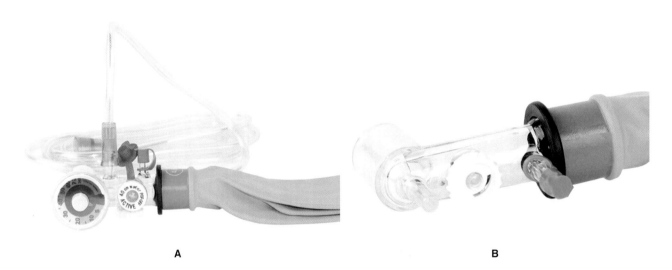

FIGURE 15-16 Medication injection port. A. Self-inflating bag (orange cap). B. Flow-inflating bag (blue cap).
Photos courtesy of SunMed.

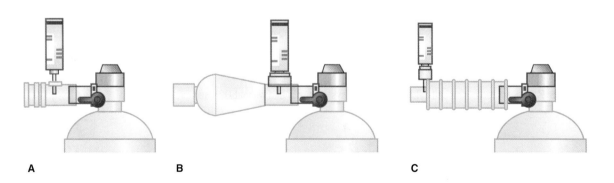

FIGURE 15-17 Metered dose inhaler devices connected to Ambu Spur II resuscitator. A. Airlife Dual Mist Spray. B. Aerosol Cloud Enhancer (ACE). C. Aerovent Collapsible Holding Chamber (CHC).

TABLE 15-4
List of Manufacturers and Self-Inflating Bag-Valve Resuscitator Systems

Country	Manufacturer	Model
Australia	L.R. Instruments	Rescu-2 Infant Set
		MR-100 Infant Set
		2297 Infant Resuscitator
Canada	O-Two Medical Technologies Inc.	Easy Grip Cold Chemical Sterilizable Resuscitator
		Easy Grip Silicone Resuscitator
		Easy Grip BVM Resuscitator
China/Taiwan	Besmed Health Business Corp.	RS-2703 Rubber Resuscitator
		BE-1303, BE-2303 Silicone Resuscitators
		BE-1703, BE-2703 PVC Resuscitators
	Enter Medical Corporation	ENT-1014 Silicone Resuscitator
		ENT-1005 PVC Resuscitator
	The Everjuan Enterprise Co., Ltd.	EM-0102-I Infant Resuscitator
		EM0101-I Infant Resuscitator
	Fortune Medical Instrument Corp.	SR-Infant #1610-0001 Silicone Resuscitator
		1690-0001 PVC Resuscitator
		1650-0001 Rubber Resuscitator
	GaleMed Corporation	Rescu-7 Silicone Resuscitator
		MR-100 Silicone Resuscitator
		MR-100 Plus Silicone Resuscitator
		Dispo-Bag Manual Resuscitator
	Headstar Medical Products	HS-9788A Silicone Resuscitator
		HR-9189A Rubber Resuscitator
		HP-9333A PVC Resuscitator
	Hsiner Co., Ltd.	HS-6311 Silicone Resuscitator
		HS-6331 Silicone Resuscitator with PEEP
		HS-6321 PVC Resuscitator
		HS-6341 PVC Resuscitator with PEEP
	Jaingxi Teli Anesthesia & Respiration Equipment Company	BE-1300 Silicone Resuscitator
		BE-1700 PVC Resuscitator
	Ningbo David Medical Device Co. Ltd.	HF-I Neonate Silicone Resuscitator

(continues)

TABLE 15-4
List of Manufacturers and Self-Inflating Bag-Valve Resuscitator Systems (*Continued*)

Country	Manufacturer	Model
China/Taiwan, cont.	Pan Taiwan Enterprise Co. Ltd.	ME6103 PVC Resuscitator
		ME6113 Silicone Resuscitator
	Shinmed (Shining World Health Care Co., Ltd.)	SW72302B Silicone Resuscitator
		SW71300C Infant Resuscitator
	Sturdy Industrial Co., Ltd.	Topster Silicone Resuscitator
		SR-013 PVC Resuscitator
		SR-023 Rubber Resuscitator
Europe	AMBU	Ambu Silicone Resuscitator
		Baby R Silicone
		SPUR II Bag and Mask Resuscitator
	Boscarol Emergency Systems	PAL30130 Newborn Non-Autoclavable Resuscitator
		PAL30240 Newborn Silicone Resuscitator
		PAL30108 Newborn Resuscitator
	Datex-Ohmeda	8570025 Silicone Resuscitator
	Dräger Medical AG & Co. KG	MR-100 Compact Silicone Resuscitator
	Farum S.A.	GO3F Silicone Resuscitator
	Laerdal Medical AS	The Bag Resuscitator
		Laerdal Silicone Resuscitator
	P.J. Dahlhausen & Co. GmbH	51.500.00.100 Silicone Resuscitator
	Spencer Italia S.r.l.	ECO B-Life Rubber Resuscitator
		B-Life Silicone Resuscitator
		Co-B Life Pediatric Manual Resuscitator
	Weinmann GmbH & Co. KG	COMBIBAG Resuscitation Bag
India	Anand Medicaids Private Limited	RG403-S2 Silicone Resuscitator
	Apothecaries Sundries Mfg. Co.	RG403-S2 Silicone Resuscitator
		RG 401 Black Rubber Resuscitator
	Atlas Surgical	AS-500 Silicone Neonate/Infant
	Bharat Enterprises	Resuscitators
	Global Products Corporation (GPC) Medical	AN 108 Silicone Resuscitator
	Hospital Equipment Manufacturing Co.	70-555-03 Silicone Resuscitator
		70-559-02 Rubber Resuscitator
	Jainsons (India) REGD.	Silicone Resuscitator for Infants

TABLE 15-4
List of Manufacturers and Self-Inflating Bag-Valve Resuscitator Systems (*Continued*)

Country	Manufacturer	Model
India, cont.	Kay & Company	Silicone Resuscitator
	Narang Medical Limited	Deluxe Quality Silicone Resuscitator
		Superior Quality Silicone Resuscitator
		Economy Quality Silicone Resuscitator
		Black Rubber Ambu-Type Bag
	Phoenix Medical Systems Pvt Ltd.	AB100 Neonatal Manual Resuscitator
	Zeal Medical	BlowSafe Mouth to Mask Resuscitator
		Silicone Infant Resuscitator
Indonesia	F2H (Frontier For Health)	Tekno Mouth-to-Mask Resuscitator
Japan	Blue Cross Emergency Co., Ltd.	IC-22, ICW-22 Silicone Resuscitators
South Africa	Adcock Ingram	Samson's Neonatal Resuscitator
United Kingdom	Albert Waeschle, Ltd.	AW Guardian Infant Resuscitator
	Intersurgical Ltd.	7150 Infant Resuscitator
	Marshall Products Ltd.	120100 Silicone Resuscitator
		150105 Infant Resuscitator
	Merlin Medical	W4456 Silicone Resuscitator
		W5556 5-Series Resuscitator
		W4446 4-Series Resuscitator
		W4477 PVC Resuscitator
	Smiths Medical	Portex 1st Response Resuscitators
	Vitalograph International	ResusBag Infant Resuscitator
United States	Allied Healthcare Products, Inc.	L554 Series
		L238 Series
		L670 Series
	Cardinal Health, Inc.	2K8010, 2K8021 Infant Resuscitators
	Engineered Medical Systems	VentiSure2 Manual Resuscitator
	Ferno-Washington, Inc.	T30511, T30511 FERNO Bag Mask Resuscitator
	Hudson RCI	Lifesaver Manual Resuscitator
	Mada Medical	4025 Infant Resuscitator
	Mercury Medical	Synthetic Rubber CPR Bag
	Nellcor	PMR 2 Resuscitation Bag
		INdGO Manual Resuscitator

(continues)

TABLE 15-4
List of Manufacturers and Self-Inflating Bag-Valve Resuscitator Systems (*Continued*)

Country	Manufacturer	Model
United States, cont.	Nellcor, cont.	Capno-Flo Resuscitation Bag
	Rescuer Products	4512 Silicone BVM Resuscitator
		Med-Rescuer BVM Resuscitator
	Rusch (Teleflex Medical Company)	Rusch Resuscitators
	Unomedical Inc.	Hospitak Mouth to Mask Resuscitator
		Pulmonary Resuscitator
	Ventlab Corporation	AirFlow Resuscitation Bags
		VN3000 Infant Resuscitators
		STAT-Check CO_2 Indicator and Resuscitation Bag
	Viasys Healthcare	Pulmanex Manual Resuscitators
	Vital Signs	Baby Blue II Infant Resuscitator
	Westmed, Inc.	BagEasy Resuscitator

Data from Coffey P, Seamans Y. *2006 global inventory of neonatal resuscitators.* Path Organization; 2006. Available at http://www.path.org/publications/files/TS_nnr_global_inventory.pdf. Accessed July 26, 2014.

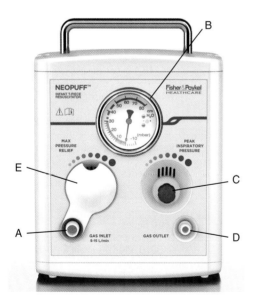

FIGURE 15-18 Fischer & Paykel Neopuff Infant T-Piece Resuscitator. A. Gas inlet. B. Pressure manometer. C. PIP control. D. Gas outlet. E. Pressure relief valve.

Courtesy of Fisher & Paykel Healthcare.

Figure 15-18) and the Neo-Tee Infant T-Piece Resuscitator (Mercury Medical, Clearwater, Florida; Figure 15-19). The Neopuff is a lightweight, standalone, manually operated, gas-powered resuscitator designed to provide ventilation at a set flow with consistent PIP

and PEEP to infants. A supply line from a compressed gas source delivering 5–15 L/min is attached to the device (Figure 15-18A). The inlet gas flows through a spring-loaded valve and allows for adjustment of inspiratory pressure (Figure 15-18C). Inspiratory pressure is displayed on the pressure manometer (Figure 15-18B). Gas exits the resuscitator through the gas outlet (Figure 15-18D). A corrugated humidified or nonhumidified circuit can be attached at this port to deliver manual ventilations with an adjustable single-use T-piece. The T-piece is constructed with three ports. One port of the T-piece is connected to the circuit, one to the patient interface (mask or endotracheal tube; **Figure 15-20**), and the last is intermittently occluded by the operator's finger to direct flow to the patient and adjust PEEP (**Figure 15-21**). There are two options for mask and endotracheal connection (15 mm female and 22 mm male). Several sizes of masks ranging from 33 mm (1.38 in) to 72 mm (2.83 in) can be attached to the circuit and can also be coupled with a single-use T-piece circuit for a complete single-use resuscitation kit.

Application

Although recent surveys demonstrate that the resuscitators of choice for neonatal resuscitation are the flow-inflating and self-inflating resuscitators,[33,34] the T-piece resuscitator is recognized as an acceptable device for neonatal resuscitation.[65] The standard method for

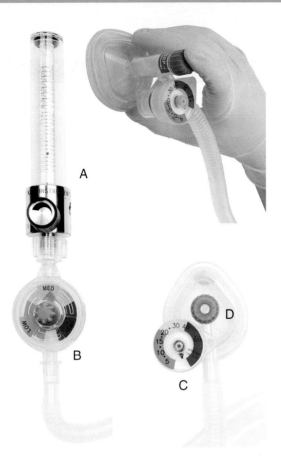

FIGURE 15-19 Neo-Tee Infant resuscitator (Mercury Medical, Clearwater Florida). A Flowmeter. B. Color-coded adjustable PIP controller with pressure relief. C. Built-in color-coded manometer. D. Variable PEEP knob with hole.

Photos courtesy of Mercury Medical.

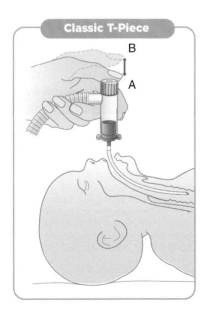

FIGURE 15-21 Breath delivery using the Neopuff T-piece resuscitator. A. Inspiration. B. Expiration.

Courtesy of Fisher & Paykel Healthcare.

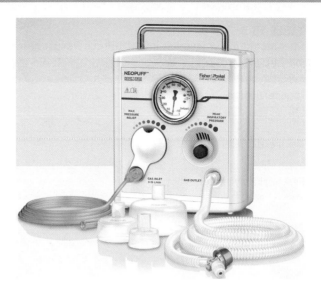

FIGURE 15-20 The Neopuff circuit, displaying the T-piece incorporated into the circuit and adjustable PEEP valve.

Courtesy of Fisher & Paykel Healthcare.

breath delivery of the Neopuff is for the operator to control inspiratory time (I-time) with the use of their finger. By simply placing a finger over the expiratory valve of the T-piece, the operator is able to divert inspiratory gas from the device down the mask or airway, facilitating ventilation. When the finger is removed from the valve, exhalation occurs with the associated PEEP set by adjustment of the valve (Figure 15-21). The recommendation for neonatal ventilation is to provide a breath rate of 40–60 bpm with initial inflation pressure of 20 cm H_2O (30–40 may be required in some term babies without spontaneous ventilation) until an improvement in heart rate occurs.[65] Although constant I-times are difficult to sustain and may be prolonged in association with lack of operator experience,[66] the major advantage of the Neopuff is its ability to deliver constant V_T and PIP, irrespective of individual, operator-dependent variables and level of experience.[57,82]

Specifications

Specifications for the Fisher & Paykel Neopuff and Neo-Tee Infant T-Piece Resuscitators are listed in **Tables 15-5** and **15-6**, respectively.

Automatic Resuscitators

Hospitals in the United States generally have sufficient numbers of ventilators, support equipment, and supplies to meet everyday demands and requirements.[67] However, they lack the ability to immediately access a sufficient number of critical care ventilators to handle mass casualty events. During such an emergency, ventilator supply within a region, including rental companies, can be rapidly depleted. In this situation, a state can request distribution of additional mechanical

TABLE 15-5
Specifications for Neopuff Infant T-Piece Resuscitator

Operating Instructions	English Language
Manometer range	–10 to 80 cm H_2O
Manometer accuracy	+/– 2.0% of full scale deflection
Max pressure relief	@ 8 L/min, 5 to 70 cm H_2O Factory set @ 40 cm H_2O
Peak inspiratory pressure (PIP)	@ 5 L/min, 2 to 70 cm H_2O @ 8 L/min, 3 to 72 cm H_2O @ 10L/min, 4 to 73 cm H_2O @ 15 L/min, 8 to 75 cm H_2O
Positive end expiratory pressure (PEEP)	@ 5 L/min, 1 to 5 cm H_2O @ 8 L/min, 1 to 9 cm H_2O @ 10 L/min, 2 to 15 cm H_2O @ 15 L/min, 4 to 25 cm H_2O
Height	250 mm (9.8 in)
Width	200 mm (7.9 in)
Depth	104 mm (4.1 in.)
Weight	1.9 kg (4.2 lb)
Delivered oxygen concentration	Up to 100% depending on gas supply
Input gas flow range	5 L/min (min) to 15 L/min (max)
Operating time (operating time calculated with the use of a 400-L cylinder)	@ 8 L/min, 50 minutes
Recommended patient body weight	Up to 10 kg (22 lb)
Storage temperature range	–10°C to 50°C (14°F to 122°F), up to 95% humidity
Operating temperature range	–18°C to 50°C (–0.4°F to 122°F), up to 95% humidity

Courtesy of Fisher & Paykel Healthcare.

TABLE 15-6
Specifications for Neo-Tee Infant Resuscitator

Delivered O_2 concentration	Up to 100%
Cycling pressure range	0 to 40 cm H_2O
Dead space	4 mL
Expiratory resistance	0.1 cm H_2O at minimum PEEP setting @ 6 L/min
Inspiratory resistance	0.2 cm H_2O at minimum PEEP setting @ 6 L/min
Input gas flow range	5–15 L/min
Operation time	Full E cylinder @ 660 L @ 5 L/min = 44 min.
Patient connection on T-piece	15 mm taper female (ISO 5356-1)
PEEP range	@ 5 L/min up to approximately 2 cm H_2O @ 8 L/min up to approximately 6 cm H_2O @ 10 L/min up to approximately 9 cm H_2O @ 15 L/min up to approximately 15 cm H_2O

Courtesy of Mercury Medical.

ventilators from the Centers for Disease Control and Prevention's (CDC's) Strategic National Stockpile (SNS).[68] The SNS maintains thousands of Puritan Bennett LP-10 and Impact Uni-vent Eagle 754 ventilators, and is considering accumulating thousands of additional ventilators. Hospitals are also developing strategies to make an increased number of ventilators available.[69,70] In the absence of the aforementioned ventilators, **automatic resuscitators** may be used to provide ventilation temporarily for some patients. As with any manual or mechanical breathing device, it is essential for the operator to maintain skill and vigilance during use.

Description

Automatic resuscitators are compact, handheld, pneumatically powered devices that deliver ventilation to a patient through a network of valves and controls that can be attached to a mask or tracheal airway. They cycle between inspiration and expiration using either pneumatic or electronic control circuits.[71] The devices vary in versatility in terms of variation of the inspiratory and expiratory patterns. Some possess the ability to use air/oxygen mixtures to conserve oxygen supplies whereas some possess demand valves to assist with patient–ventilator synchrony. These resuscitators are commonly used for mass casualty and emergency medical situations and often possess limited ability to provide the high end functionality of ventilators with which hospital clinicians may be more familiar. However, the constructs and execution of breath delivery can be accomplished with automatic resuscitators despite the absence of highly technical interfaces, breath delivery units, and graphical user interfaces. Therefore it is an option for hospitals and emergency medical services to consider developing a plan to make automatic resuscitator devices and training readily available in the event of mass casualty and unforeseeable emergencies that require immediate mechanical ventilation.

Application

The application of automatic resuscitators is different from that of manual resuscitators and transport ventilators. Manual resuscitators require the clinician to constantly engage the chosen device, and the effectiveness of the ventilation is in proportion to the direct hands-on involvement with the device. If the operator ceases to function, the device will not function. Automatic resuscitators provide the clinician with the ability to provide ventilation while not being tethered to the device. This allows the clinician to provide care to the patient outside the realm of ventilation. Due to the variation in effective ventilation provided with the use of manual resuscitators compared to that of automatic resuscitators and transport ventilators,[72,73] automatic resuscitators have become more attractive

in delivering ventilation during transport and in emergency situations. Emergency Medical Technicians-Paramedics (EMT-Ps) favor the use of automatic resuscitators because of the ease of use, time of setup, expedition of transport, and ability to accomplish more tasks, document, and provide additional patient care:[74] nurses demonstrated improved compression to ventilation ratios with the use of integrated prompts for chest compressions within an automatic resuscitator.[75] The stability of arterial blood gases of critically ill, mechanically ventilated patients has been demonstrated with the use of an automatic resuscitator during intrahospital transport.[76] Another clinical advantage of using automatic resuscitators is the ability to apply cricoid pressure with one hand and the mask with the other. Automatic resuscitators should initially be set to deliver a V_T of 6–7 mL/kg at 10 bpm.[77] In comparison to transport ventilators, automatic resuscitators lack consistency and sophistication in breath delivery (tidal volume and frequency), as well as alarm features.

Currently Available Devices

Automatic resuscitators that are currently available include the Vortran Automatic Resuscitator (VAR; Vortran Medical Technology, Sacramento, CA), CAREvent ALS, EMT, and CA (O-Two Medical Technologies, Ontario, Canada), and Pneupac VR1 resuscitator (Smiths Medical, St. Paul, MN).

Vortran Automatic Resuscitator (VAR)

The VAR, also referred to as the Sure Vent, is a disposable, single-patient-use resuscitator that is pneumatically powered by a compressed oxygen source, is pressure triggered and pressure cycled, and provides hands-free ventilator support (**Figure 15-22**). This

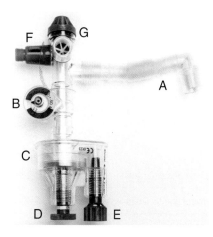

FIGURE 15-22 Vortran Automatic Resuscitator (Vortran Medical, Sacramento, CA). A. Patient connection. B. Pressure manometer. C. Control modulator. D. PIP control dial. E. Rate control. F. Gas inlet. G. Safety pop-off and entrainment.
Courtesy of VORTRAN® Medical Technology1, Inc., Sacramento, CA.

device only delivers pressure-controlled continuous spontaneous ventilation. This device is an anomaly in that the ability to manually adjust the short-term trigger rate under steady-state conditions gives the illusion that the mode is continuous mandatory ventilation (also known as Assist/Control). However, the actual trigger and cycle events are determined by the patient's respiratory system mechanics including inspiratory efforts, making the classification of all breaths spontaneous rather than mandatory. Hence, the mode is continuous spontaneous ventilation, similar to pressure support.

The flow control valve of this device opens at the trigger pressure (set by the rate control knob) and closes at the cycle pressure (set by the PIP control). The clinician connects a 50-psi compressed oxygen source either directly to the gas inlet port (F_DO_2 1.0) or to the green entrainment adaptor (F_IO_2 0.5), which will automatically deliver 40 L/min per ASTM guidelines. Oxygen can also be supplied using standard O_2 tubing from a medical gas flowmeter, which can provide 15–40 L/min.

Because the VAR is pressure triggered and cycled, if the respiratory system compliance decreases, the device markets the ability to "self-adjust" by decreasing the V_T and increasing the respiratory rate to sustain a constant minute ventilation. However, experimental data suggest that a decrease in V_T due to a decrease in respiratory system compliance would result in an overall decrease in alveolar minute ventilation, thereby potentially adversely affecting gas exchange.[78] Although an explanation was later provided by the manufacturer for these

data,[79] clinicians should be aware that changes in V_T and rate associated with changes to respiratory system mechanics are primary characteristics of all pressure-cycled devices.

Specifications
Specifications for the Vortran Automatic Resuscitator (VAR/VARi) are listed in **Table 15-7**.

CAREvent ALS, EMT, and CA

CAREvent Advanced Life Support (ALS)
The CAREvent ALS handheld resuscitator is a pneumatically powered, time-/volume-cycled resuscitator with a manually actuated automatic ventilation override button (**Figure 15-23A**). The single slider on the front of the device serves as a control for simultaneous adjustment of ventilation frequency and tidal volume, and has six preset automatic and manual override settings for patients ≥ 44 lb (≥ 20 kg) body weight. When applied during CPR, the first breath is automatically provided followed by a manually actuated breath. This stops the auto-triggered breaths for 20 seconds, allowing the rescuer to perform the recommended 30 compressions without the resuscitator attempting to provide the subsequent breath. If the manual button is not actuated, the autotriggered breath delivery will restart at the selected rate and V_T without intervention by the operator. The rescuer can remain hands free to do compressions or other related

TABLE 15-7
Specifications for the Vortran Automatic Resuscitators

	VAR-Plus	VAR
Recommended body weight	22 lb (10 kg) and above	88 lb (40 kg) and above
Ventilatory frequency	Auto-adjusting to lung capacity	Same
Adjustable PIP range	10 to 45 cm H_2O	20 to 50 cm H_2O
PEEP	One-fifth of PIP (2 to 9 cm H_2O)	One-tenth of PIP (2 to 5 cm H_2O)
Inspiratory resistance	3 ± 1 cm H_2O/L/sec	Same
Expiratory resistance	3 ± 1 cm H_2O/L/sec	Same
Dead space	4 ± 3 mL	Same
Operating environmental limits	−18 to 50°C	Same
Storage environmental limits	−40 to 60°C	Same
Patient connection	15 mm female, 22 mm male	Same
Gas inlet	DISS connection	Same
Oxygen concentration when supplied w/100% O_2	50% or 85% (Model PCM/PCE)	50% or 85% (Model RC/RCM/RCE) 85% (Model RT/RTM/RTF/RTE)

Courtesy of VORTRAN® Medical Technology1, Inc., Sacramento, CA.

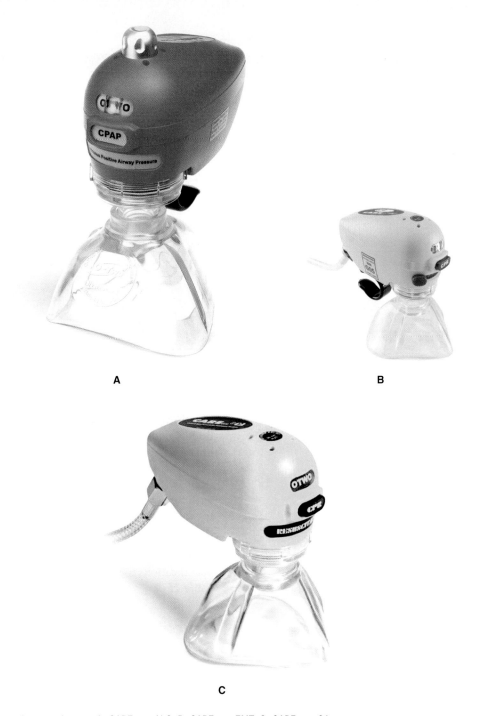

A

B

C

FIGURE 15-23 Automatic resuscitators. A. CAREvent ALS. B. CAREvent EMT. C. CAREvent CA.

Photos courtesy of O-Two Medical Technologies, Inc.

duties while ensuring adequate ventilation to the patient. The device also offers a demand feature that will allow patients to breathe spontaneously on an F_IO_2 of 1.0 at their own desired rate and V_T. The auto-trigger function will cease when spontaneous breathing is detected, and will reinitiate when spontaneous ventilation or breathing stops.

CAREvent EMT

The main differences between the CAREvent ALS and EMT are their color and the absence of a demand valve

to allow for spontaneous breathing (Figure 15-23B). All other functions mirror those of the CAREvent ALS.

CAREvent Chemical Agent (CA)

The CAREvent CA was developed to address the needs of a chemical agent release encountered within a confined industrial setting (Figure 15-23C). Whereas the CAREvent ALS and EMT lack an external control, the CAREvent CA has one external control. The rescuer simply has to turn on the oxygen/air supply, apply the mask, and secure the patient's airway. This device

TABLE 15-8
Specifications for the CAREvent ALS, EMT, and CA Automatic Resuscitators

	CAREvent ALS	CAREvent EMT	CAREvent CA
Tidal volume	150–600 mL	120–600 mL	600 mL
Frequency (6 settings) *(1 setting)	10–20 bpm	10–20 bpm	*10 bpm
Automatic flow rate range	9–18 L/min	7.2–18 L/min	18 L/min
Manual flow rate range	Per V_T setting	Per V_T setting	19 L/min
Demand breathing flow rate	0–120 L/min	NA	0–120 L/min
Demand breathing triggering pressure	–2 cm H_2O	NA	–2 cm H_2O
Storage temperature	–40°F to 140°F (–40°C to 60°C)	–40°F to 140°F (–40°C to 60°C)	–40°F to 140°F (–40°C to 60°C)
Patient dead space	8 mL	9 mL	8 mL
Weight (approx.)	16 oz	15 oz	16 oz
Dimensions (approx. in inches)	5.5 × 2.5 × 2.9	5.5 × 2.5 × 2.9	5.5 × 2.5 × 2.9
Bleed flow	NA	NA	2 L/min

Courtesy of O-Two Medical Technologies, Inc.

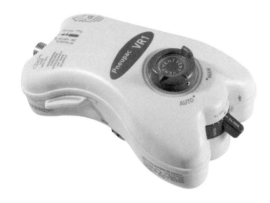

FIGURE 15-24 Pneupac VR1 automatic resuscitator.
Courtesy of Smiths Medical.

incorporates a demand valve to allow spontaneous breathing. The added feature is the 2 L/min mask purge bleed flow that purges the mask to reduce the risk of the patient drawing toxic ambient air into the mask should a leak occur.

Specifications for the CAREvent ALS, EMT, and CA automatic resuscitators are listed in **Table 15-8**.

Pnuepac VR1

The Pneupac VR1 is an oxygen-powered, handheld control unit with patient valve that includes automatic and manual modes with demand breathing (**Figure 15-24**). It incorporates a gas supply inlet and is designed as a ventilator/resuscitator that provides a single control for setting tidal volume and frequency and a demand system to support spontaneous

breathing. The patient connection is located on the underside, allowing the rescuer to hold the device upright and adjust the linked manual controls for a variety of chest compression/ventilation combinations with a single finger. It incorporates a relief valve with pneumatic alarm, is magnetic resonance imaging (MRI) compatible, and has an optional air mixture feature.

Specifications
Specifications for the Pneupac VR1 are listed in **Table 15-9**.

Indications for Ventilatory Resuscitators

Flow-inflating, self-inflating, T-piece, and automatic resuscitators all share the same indications (**Table 15-10**).[2,80-84] Choosing one over the others relies on preference for how to achieve the foundational goals of breath delivery, as highlighted previously in this chapter. Consideration should be given to the advantages and disadvantages of each resuscitator type when selecting the appropriate device for the situation in which it will be used.

Contraindications

Contraindications for ventilatory resuscitation have been outlined by the AARC and are not equipment specific (**Table 15-11**). The only absolute contraindication is documentation of a Do Not Attempt Resuscitation (DNAR) order or alternative documentation indicating

TABLE 15-9
Specifications for the Pneupac VR1 Automatic Resuscitator

Recommended body weight	22 lb (10 kg) and above
Control	Single, calibrated V_T/frequency control gives simultaneous and interdependent adjustment of the V_T and frequency.
Tidal volume and ventilatory frequency	150 mL/25 bpm 300 mL/20 bpm 450 mL/15 bpm 600 mL/12 bpm 750 mL/11 bpm 900 mL/10 bpm 1,050 mL/10 bpm
Flow range	11–32 L/min
Air mix	Optional
Pressure relief with pneumatic alarm	40 cm H_2O standard 60 cm H_2O optional
Dimensions (inches)	6.69 × 3.74 × 3.94
Weight	14.82 oz

Courtesy of Smiths Medical.

TABLE 15-10
Indications for Ventilatory Resuscitation

1. Cardiac arrest
2. Respiratory arrest
3. Presence of conditions that may lead to cardiopulmonary arrest as indicated by rapid deterioration in vital signs, level of consciousness, and blood gas values including:
   a. Airway obstruction
   b. Acute myocardial infarction with cardio-dynamic instability
   c. Life-threatening dysrhythmias
   d. Hypovolemic shock
   e. Severe infections
   f. Spinal cord or head injury
   g. Drug overdose
   h. Pulmonary edema
   i. Anaphylaxis
   j. Pulmonary embolus
   k. Smoke inhalation
   l. Defibrillation is indicated when cardiac arrest results in or is due to ventricular fibrillation
   m. Pulseless ventricular tachycardia
4. Secretion clearance
5. Improve total lung compliance
6. Assist in resolution of acute atelectasis
7. Intra-hospital and/or inter-hospital transport of patient with artificial airway

TABLE 15-11
Contraindications for Ventilatory Resuscitation

Absolute contraindication:
- Do Not Attempt Resuscitation (DNAR) order or other advanced directive indicating a person's desire to not be resuscitated in the event of cardiac arrest.[2,34]

Relative contraindication:
- Resuscitation has been determined to be futile because of the patient's underlying condition or disease.[2,34,38]
- Resuscitation efforts and defibrillation pose an immediate danger to the rescuers present.[2,86]

is the only order that allows the patient to prevent medical intervention from being provided. Allow Natural Death (AND) is becoming a preferred replacement for DNAR, and emphasizes allowing natural consequences of a disease or injury and ongoing end-of-life care.[87] A healthcare advance directive is a legally binding document in the United States that is based on the Patient Self-Determination Act of 1990.[88] This document communicates the preferences, thoughts, or wishes for healthcare decisions that might need to be made during periods of incapacity and can be verbal or written. It may be constructed based on conversations, written directives, living wills, or durable power of attorney for health care. For all these reasons, discussions regarding informed code status among physicians, patients, and family members are essential.

The only relative contraindications for manual and automatic resuscitation are the determination that resuscitation will be futile due to the patient's underlying condition or disease, and that efforts in

the patient's wish to not be resuscitated in the event of a cardiac arrest. The DNAR order was introduced nearly half a century ago, and is a medical order issued by a licensed physician or alternative authority as per local regulation, and it must be signed and dated to be valid.[85] It continues to raise questions and controversy among patients, families, and healthcare providers.[86] It

TABLE 15-12
Precautions/Hazards and/or Complications of Ventilatory Resuscitation

- Malfunctioning nonrebreathing valve
- Faulty pressure relief valves
- Inadequate oxygen delivery (F_DO_2)
- Hypoventilation and/or hyperventilation
  - *Hypoventilation:* Low V_T with inappropriately sized mask or failure to maintain adequate face/mask seal
  - *Hyperventilation:* Excessive rate and V_T delivery, especially in intubated patients
- Gastric insufflation and/or rupture
- Barotrauma
  - Excessive pressure and V_T delivery, especially in intubated patients
  - Improper setting of the pressure-relief valve
- Hypotension
  - Reduced venous return secondary to high mean intrathoracic pressure
  - Reduced venous return secondary to increased autoPEEP and hyperventilation
- Vomiting and aspiration
- Prolonged interruption of ventilation for intubation
- Loss of power

defibrillation pose an immediate danger to the rescuers present.[2,85] Healthcare providers are not obligated to provide care when scientific and social consensus agree that the treatment is ineffective. An objective criterion for medical futility was defined in 1990; it focuses on those interventions and drug therapies that provide a less than 1% chance of survival.[89] Therefore, resuscitative efforts may cease if such a criterion is identified and determined.

Precautions, Hazards and/or Complications of Manual Resuscitation

Within the complex process of ventilatory resuscitation lies the concern for potential hazards and complications that can contribute to increasing clinical deterioration (Table 15-12). The major hazards associated with the process of manual and automatic resuscitation include **gastric insufflation**, aspiration, diminished cardiac output, and inadequate ventilation due to poor technique or an improper mask fitting.[90] Coupled with this is the awareness of the most common hazards of manual resuscitators, which include a malfunctioning nonrebreathing and/or pressure-relief valve.[91]

Gastric insufflation occurs when the inflation pressure exceeds the esophageal opening pressure, allowing gas to enter the stomach. In unconscious patients it takes about 15–25 cm H_2O of pressure to open the esophagus. Unfortunately the esophageal opening pressure decreases considerably the longer the patient remains unconscious and can fall as low as 0 to 5 cm H_2O.[92] The pressure needed to produce gastric insufflations in anesthetized patients has been found to range from 10 to 35 cm H_2O with a face mask technique of ventilation, with the most frequent pressure needed for insufflation around 15 cm H_2O. Gastric insufflation can lead to gastric distention, which results in the propulsion of stomach contents to the mouth, potentially leading to aspiration. In cardiac arrest nonsurvivors, 46% were found to have full stomachs and at least 29% had evidence of pulmonary aspiration of gastric contents.[93]

Diminished cardiac output results from decreased venous return as a result of increased respiratory rate, elevated mean airway pressure, and autoPEEP. In 12 cardiac arrest victims treated in the emergency department of a United Kingdom hospital, hyperventilation was caused by excessive respiratory rate, where the respiratory rate was at least double that recommended in 9 of 12 (75%) patients while the V_T was no higher than the recommended 10 mL/kg in 9 of 12 (75%) patients.[94] In animal models, ventilator rates of 30 bpm vs. 12 bpm decreased coronary perfusion pressure and appeared to decrease survival if sustained for 4 minutes or greater.[95]

Inadequate ventilation is commonly a result of the rescuer's inability to appropriately select the correct mask type and size, while achieving an adequate face/mask seal. Using a neonatal resuscitation model, 34 participants, including neonatal consultants, fellows, residents, and nurses, were evaluated using each of four device–mask combinations using a round and anatomical mask.[25] A total of 10,780 inflations were recorded and analyzed revealing large leaks with both mask types and devices, thereby suggesting that in the hands of experienced clinicians, mask leaks are often unavoidable.

References

1. Travers AH, Rea TD, Bobrow BJ, Sayer MR, Field JM, Hazinski MF. Part 4: CPR overview: American Heart Association guidelines for cardiopulmonary resuscitation and emergency cardiovascular care. *Circulation.* 2010;122:S676-S684.
2. American Association of Respiratory Care Clinical Practice Guideline. Resuscitation and defibrillation in the healthcare setting—2004 revision and update. *Resp Care.* 2004;49(9):1085-1099.
3. Sayre MR, Koster RW, Botha M, Cave DM, Cudnik MT, Handley A, et al. Part 5: Adult basic life support: 2010 international consensus on cardiopulmonary resuscitation and emergency cardiovascular care science with treatment recommendations. *Circulation.* 2010;122(Suppl 2):S298-S324.
4. Nolan J, Soar J, Zideman D, Biarent D, Bossaert L, Deakin C, et al. European Resuscitation Council guidelines for resuscitation 2010: Section 1. Executive summary. *Resuscitation.* 2010;81:1219-1276.
5. Hess D, Goff G, Johnson D. The effect of hand size, resuscitator brand, and use of two hands on volumes delivered during adult bag-valve ventilation. *Respir Care.* 1989;34:805-810.
6. Hess D, Spahr C. An evaluation of volumes delivered by selected adult disposable resuscitators: The effects of hand size, number of hands used, and use of disposable medical gloves. *Respir Care.* 1990;35(8):800-805.
7. Hess D, Kacmarek RM. *Essentials of mechanical ventilation.* 2nd ed. St. Louis, MO: McGraw-Hill Professional; 2002.
8. Hess D, Goff G. The effects of two-hand versus one-hand ventilation on volumes delivered during bag-valve ventilation at various resistances and compliances. *Respir Care.* 1989;34:805-810.

9. McCabe SM, Smeltzer SC. Comparison of tidal volumes obtained by one-handed and two-handed ventilation techniques. *Am J Crit Care*. 1993;2(6):467-473.

10. Berney S, Denehy L. A comparison of the effects of manual and ventilator hyperinflation on static lung compliance and sputum production in intubated and ventilated intensive care patients. *Physiother Res Int*. 2002;7(2):100-108.

11. Hodgson C, Denehy L, Ntoumenopoulos G, Santamaria J, Carroll S. An investigation of the early effects of manual lung hyperinflation in critically ill patients. *Anaesth Intensive Care*. 2000;28(3):255-261.

12. Lucía A, de las Heras JF, Pérez M, et al. The importance of physical fitness in the performance of adequate cardiopulmonary resuscitation. *Chest*. 1999;115(1):158-164.

13. Lee HM, Cho KH, Choi YH, Yoon SY, Choi YH. Can you deliver accurate tidal volume by manual resuscitator? *Emerg Med J*. 2008;25(10):632-634.

14. Roehr CC, Kelm M, Proquitté H, Schmalisch G. Equipment and operator training denote manual ventilation performance in neonatal resuscitation. *Am J Perinatol*. 2010;27(9):753-758.

15. Cho YC, Cho SW, Chung SP, Yu K, Kwon OY, Kim SW. How can a single rescuer adequately deliver tidal volume with a manual resuscitator? An improved device for delivering regular tidal volume. *Emerg Med J*. 2011;28(1):40-43.

16. Lee HM, Cho KH, Choi YH, Yoon SY, Choi YH. Can you deliver accurate tidal volume by manual resuscitator? *Emerg Med J*. 2008;25(10):632-634.

17. Campbell TP, Stewart RD, Kaplan RM, DeMichiei RV, Morton R. Oxygen enrichment of bag-valve-mask units during positive-pressure ventilation: A comparison of various techniques. *Ann Emerg Med*. 1988;17(3):232-235.

18. Barnes TA, McGarry WP. Evaluation of ten disposable manual resuscitators. *Respir Care*. 1990;35(10):960-968.

19. Mazzolini DG, Marshall NA. Evaluation of 16 adult disposable manual resuscitators. *Respir Care*. 2004;49(12):1509-1514.

20. Nam SH, Kim KJ, Nam YT, Shim JK. The changes in delivered oxygen fractions using Laerdal resuscitator bag with different types of reservoir. *Yonsei Med J*. 2001;42(2):242-246.

21. Fahey DG. The self-inflating resuscitator—evolution of an idea. *Anaesth Intensive Care*. 2010;38(Suppl 1):10-15.

22. American Society for Testing and Materials. *Standard specifications for performance and safety requirements for resuscitators intended for humans*. F-920–85. Philadelphia: American Society for Testing and Materials; 1993.

23. International Organization for Standardization. *International standard ISO 8382: 1988. Resuscitators intended for use with humans*. New York: American National Standards Institute; 1988.

24. Branson RD, Hess DR, Chatburn RL. *Respiratory care equipment*. Philadelphia, PA: J. B. Lippincott; 1995.

25. O'Donnell C, Davis P, Lau R, Dargaville PA, Doyle LW, Morley CJ. Neonatal resuscitation 2: An evaluation of manual ventilation devices and face masks. *Arch Dis Child Fetal Neonatal Ed*. 2005;90(5):F392-F396.

26. Neumar RW, Otto CW, Link MS, Kronick SL, Shuster M, Callaway CW, et al. Part 8: Adult advanced cardiovascular life support: 2010 American Heart Association guidelines for cardiopulmonary resuscitation and emergency cardiovascular care. *Circulation*. 2010;122(8):S729-S767.

27. Mapleson WW. The elimination of rebreathing in various semi-closed anaesthetic systems. *Br J Anaesth*. 1954;26(5):323-332.

28. Rees GJ. Anaesthesia in the newborn. *BMJ*. 1950;2(4694):1419-1422.

29. Ayre P. Anaesthesia for hare-lip and cleft palate operations on babies. *Br J Surg*. 1937;25:131-132.

30. Bready LL, Dillman D, Noorily SH. *Decision making in anesthesiology: An algorithmic approach*. Philadelphia, PA: Elsevier Health Sciences; 2007.

31. Taha S, El-Khatib M, Siddik-Sayyid S, Dagher C, Chehade JM, Baraka A. Preoxygenation with the Mapleson D system requires higher oxygen flows than Mapleson A or circle systems. *Can J Anaesth*. 2007;54(2):141-145.

32. Stafford RA, Benger JR, Nolan J. Self-inflating bag or Mapleson C breathing system for emergency pre-oxygenation? *Emerg Med J*. 2008;25(3):153-155.

33. Leone TA, Rich W, Finer NN. A survey of delivery room resuscitation practices in the United States. *Pediatrics*. 2006;117(2):164-175.

34. O'Donnell CP, Davis PG, Morley CJ. Neonatal resuscitation: Review of ventilation equipment and survey of practice in Australia and New Zealand. *J Paediatr Child Health*. 2004; 40(4):209-212.

35. Goldsmith JP, Karotkin EH. *Assisted ventilation of the neonate*. Philadelphia, PA: Elsevier Health Sciences; 2003.

36. Kanter RK. Evaluation of mask-bag ventilation in resuscitation of infants. *Am J Dis Child*. 1987;141(7):761-763.

37. Mondolfi AA, Grenier BM, Thompson JE, Bachur RG. Comparison of self-inflating bags with anesthesia bags for bag-mask ventilation in the pediatric emergency department. *Pediatr Emerg Care*. 1997;13(5):312-316.

38. Bennett S, Finer NN, Rich W, Vaucher Y. A comparison of three neonatal resuscitation devices. *Resuscitation*. 2005;67(1):113-118.

39. Campbell TP, Stewart RD, Kaplan RM, DeMichiei RV, Morton R. Oxygen enrichment of bag-valve-mask units during positive-pressure ventilation: A comparison of various techniques. *Ann Emerg Med*. 1988;17(3):232-235.

40. Phillips GD, Skowronski GA. Manual resuscitators and portable ventilators. *Anaesth Intensive Care*. 1986;14(3):306-313.

41. Osborn HH, Kayen D, Horne H, Bray W. Excess ventilation with oxygen-powered resuscitators. *Am J Emerg Med*. 1984;2(5):408-413.

42. Paradis IL, Caldwell EJ. Traumatic pneumocephalus: A hazard of resuscitators. *J Trauma*. 1979;19(1):61-63.

43. Rubenfeld GD, Caldwell E, Peabody E, Weaver J, Martin DP, Neff M, Stern EJ, Hudson LD. Incidence and outcomes of acute lung injury. *New Engl J Med*. 2005;353(16):1685-1693.

44. Goss CH, Brower RG, Hudson LD, Rubenfeld GD. Incidence of acute lung injury in the United States. *Crit Care Med*. 2003; 31(6):1607.

45. Rubenfeld GD, Herridge MS. Epidemiology and outcomes of acute lung injury. *Chest*. 2007;131(2):554-562.

46. Dos Santos CC, Slutsky AS. The contribution of biophysical lung injury to the development of biotrauma. *Annu Rev Physiol*. 2006;68(1):585-618.

47. Franklin C, Samuel J, Hu T-C. Life-threatening hypotension associated with emergency intubation and the initiation of mechanical ventilation. *Am J Emerg Med*. 1994;12(4):425-428.

48. Doerges V, Sauer C, Ocker H, Wenzel V, Schmucker P. Smaller tidal volumes during cardiopulmonary resuscitation: Comparison of adult and paediatric self-inflatable bags with three different ventilatory devices. *Resuscitation*. 1999;43(1):31-37.

49. Handley AJ, Monsieurs KG, Bossaert LL. European Resuscitation Council guidelines 2000 for adult basic life support. *Resuscitation*. 2001;48(3):199-205.

50. Hird MF, Greenough A, Gamsu HR. Inflating pressures for effective resuscitation of preterm infants. *Early Hum Dev*. 1991;26(1):69-72.

51. Hillman NH, Moss TJM, Kallapur SG, Bachurski C, Pillow JJ, Polglase GR, et al. Brief, large tidal volume ventilation initiates lung injury and a systemic response in fetal sheep. *Am J Respir Crit Care Med*. 2007;176(6):575-581.

52. Björklund LJ, Ingimarsson J, Curstedt T, Larsson A, Robertson B, Werner O. Lung recruitment at birth does not improve lung function in immature lambs receiving surfactant. *Acta Anaesthesiol Scand*. 2001;45(8):986-993.

53. Karlberg P, Koch G. Respiratory studies in newborn infants. III: Development of mechanics of breathing during the first week of life. A longitudinal study. *Acta Paediatr*. 1962;51:121-129.

54. Davis JM, Veness-Meehan K, Notter RH, Bhutani VK, Kendig JW, Shapiro DL. Changes in pulmonary mechanics after the

administration of surfactant to infants with respiratory distress syndrome. *New Engl J Med*. 1988;319(8):476-479.

55. Kelly E, Bryan H, Possmayer F, Frndova H, Bryan C. Compliance of the respiratory system in newborn infants pre-and postsurfactant replacement therapy. *Pediatr Pulmonol*. 1993;15(4):225-230.

56. Kattwinkel J, Stewart C, Walsh B, Gurka M, Paget-Brown A. Responding to compliance changes in a lung model during manual ventilation: Perhaps volume, rather than pressure, should be displayed. *Pediatrics*. 2009;123(3):e465-470.

57. Roehr CC, Kelm M, Fischer HS, Buhrer C, Schmalisch G, Proquitté H. Manual ventilation devices in neonatal resuscitation: Tidal volume and positive pressure-provision. *Resuscitation*. 2010;81(2):202-205.

58. Berg MD, Schexnayder SM, Chameides L, Terry M, Donoghue A, Hickey RW, et al. Part 13: Pediatric basic life support: 2010 American Heart Association guidelines for cardiopulmonary resuscitation and emergency cardiovascular care. *Circulation*. 2010;122(Suppl 3):S862-S875.

59. Park SO, Lee KR, Baek KJ, Hong DY, Shim HW, Shin DH. Novel target volume marked adult bag to deliver accurate tidal volume for paediatric and adolescent resuscitation. *Resuscitation*. 2011. Available at: http://www.ncbi.nlm.nih.gov/pubmed/21397383. Accessed April 27, 2011.

60. Rabi Y, Rabi D, Yee W. Room air resuscitation of the depressed newborn: A systematic review and meta-analysis. *Resuscitation*. 2007;72(3):353-363.

61. Zaichkin J, Weiner GM. Neonatal resuscitation program (NRP) 2011: New science, new strategies. *Adv Neonatal Care*. 2011; 11(1):43-51.

62. Reise K, Monkman S, Kirpalani H. The use of the Laerdal infant resuscitator results in the delivery of high oxygen fractions in the absence of a blender. *Resuscitation*. 2009;80(1):120-125.

63. de Godoy ACF, Vieira RJ. Comparison of the FiO2 delivered by seven models of the self-inflating bag-mask system. *Revista Brasileira De Anestesiologia*.2009;59(1):21-27.

64. Coffey P, Seamans Y. *2006 global inventory of neonatal resuscitators*. Path Organization; 2006. Available at http://www.path.org/publications/files/TS_nnr_global_inventory.pdf. Accessed July 26, 2014.

65. Kattwinkel J, Perlman JM, Aziz K, Colby C, Fairchild K, Gallagher J, et al. Part 15: Neonatal resuscitation: 2010 American Heart Association guidelines for cardiopulmonary resuscitation and emergency cardiovascular care. *Circulation*. 2010;122 (18 Suppl 3):S909-S919.

66. McHale S, Thomas M, Hayden E, Bergin K, McCallion N, Molloy EJ, et al. Variation in inspiratory time and tidal volume with T-piece neonatal resuscitator: Association with operator experience and distraction. *Resuscitation*. 2008;79(2):230-233.

67. American Association for Respiratory Care. AARC guidelines for acquisition of ventilators to meet demands for pandemic flu and mass casualty incidents. Available at: http://www.aarc.org/resources/vent_guidelines_08.pdf. Accessed April 27, 2011.

68. Rubinson L, Branson RD, Pesik N, Talmor D. Positive-pressure ventilation equipment for mass casualty respiratory failure. *Biosecurity Bioterrorism: Biodefense Strat Pract Sci*. 2006;4(2):183-194.

69. Arnold JL. Disaster medicine in the 21st century: Future hazards, vulnerabilities, and risk. *Prehosp Disaster Med*. 2002;17(1):3-11.

70. Booth CM, Stewart TE. Severe acute respiratory syndrome and critical care medicine: The Toronto experience. *Crit Care Med*. 2005;33(1 Suppl):S53-S60.

71. Greaves I, Porter K, Hodgetts T, Woollard M. *Emergency care: A textbook for paramedics*. London: Elsevier Health Sciences; 2005.

72. Hurst JM, Davis K, Branson RD, Johhannigman JA. Comparison of blood gases during transport using two methods of ventilatory support. *J Trauma*. 1989;29(12):1637.

73. Auble TE, Menegazzi JJ, Nicklas KA. Comparison of automated and manual ventilation in a prehospital pediatric model. *Prehosp Emerg Care*. 1998;2(2):108-111.

74. Weiss SJ, Ernst AA, Jones R, Ong M, Filbrun T, Augustin C, et al. Automatic transport ventilator versus bag valve in the EMS setting: A prospective, randomized trial. *South Med J*. 2005;98(10):970.

75. Monsieurs KG, Regge MD, Vogels C, Calle PA. Improved basic life support performance by ward nurses using the CAREvent Public Access Resuscitator (PAR) in a simulated setting. *Resuscitation*. 2005;67(1):45-50.

76. Romano M, Raabe OG, Walby W, Albertson TE. The stability of arterial blood gases during transportation of patients using the Respii Tech PRO. *Am J Emerg Med*. 2000;18(3):273-277.

77. Deakin CD, Nolan JP, Soar J, Sunde K, Koster RW, Smith GB, Perkins GD. European Resuscitation Council guidelines for resuscitation 2010. Section 4. Adult advanced life support. *Resuscitation*. 2010;81(10):1305-1352.

78. Babic MD, Chatburn RL, Stoller JK. Laboratory evaluation of the Vortran Automatic Resuscitator Model RTM. *Respir Care*. 2007;52(12):1718-1727.

79. Piper SD. Clarification of performance characteristics of the Vortran Automatic Resuscitator. *Respir Care*. 2008;53(8):1089-1090; author reply 1090-1091.

80. Ntoumenopoulos G. Indications for manual lung hyperinflation (MHI) in the mechanically ventilated patient with chronic obstructive pulmonary disease. *Chron Respir Dis*. 2005;2(4):199-207.

81. Choi JS-P, Jones AY-M. Effects of manual hyperinflation and suctioning in respiratory mechanics in mechanically ventilated patients with ventilator-associated pneumonia. *Aust J Physiother*. 2005;51(1):25-30.

82. Branson RD. Secretion management in the mechanically ventilated patient. *Respir Care*. 2007;52(10):1328-1342; discussion 1342-1347.

83. Clarke JP, Schuitemaker MN, Sleigh JW. The effect of intraoperative ventilation strategies on perioperative atelectasis. *Anaesth Intensive Care*. 1998;26(3):262-266.

84. Dockery WK, Futterman C, Keller SR, Sheridan MJ, Akl BF. A comparison of manual and mechanical ventilation during pediatric transport. *Crit Care Med*. 1999;27(4):802-806.

85. Morrison LJ, Kierzek G, Diekema DS, Sayre MR, Silvers SM, Idris AH, et al. Part 3: Ethics: 2010 American Heart Association guidelines for cardiopulmonary resuscitation and emergency cardiovascular care. *Circulation*. 2010;122:S665-S675.

86. Loertscher L, Reed DA, Bannon MP, Mueller PS. Cardiopulmonary resuscitation and do-not-resuscitate orders: A guide for clinicians. *Am J Med*. 2010;123(1):4-9.

87. Vennemen SS, Narnor-Harris P, Perish M, Hamilton M. "Allow natural death" versus "do not resuscitate": Three words that can change a life. *J Med Ethics*. 2008;34(1):2-6.

88. Omnibus Budget Reconciliation Act of 1990, Pub. Law No. 1990;101-508.

89. Schneiderman LJ, Jecker NS, Jonsen AR. Medical futility: Its meaning and ethical implications. *Ann Intern Med*. 1990;112(12):949-954.

90. White GC. *Basic clinical lab competencies for respiratory care: An integrated approach*. Independence, KY: Cengage Learning; 2003.

91. Dorsch JA, Dorsch SE. *Understanding anesthesia equipment*. 5th ed. Philadelphia, PA: Wolters Kluwer Health/Lippincott Williams & Wilkins; 2008.

92. Margolis GS, American Academy of Orthopaedic Surgeons. *Paramedic: Airway management*. Sudbury, MA: Jones & Bartlett Learning; 2003.

93. Lawes EG, Baskett PJF. Pulmonary aspiration during unsuccessful cardiopulmonary resuscitation. *Intensive Care Med*. 1987;13(6):379-382.

94. O'Neill JF, Deakin CD. Do we hyperventilate cardiac arrest patients? *Resuscitation*. 2007;73(1):82-85.

95. Aufderheide TP, Sigurdsson G, Pirrallo RG, Yannopoulos D, McKnite S, von Briesen C, et al. Hyperventilation-induced hypotension during cardiopulmonary resuscitation. *Circulation*. 2004;109(16):1960-1965

Glossary

A

Absolute humidity The amount of water vapor contained in a given gas at a given temperature, expressed in milligrams per liter.

Accuracy The maximum difference between a measured value and the true value. Accuracy is often expressed as a percentage of the true value.

Acid A substance that produces hydrogen ions (H^+) when dissolved in water.

Acidemia Arterial pH less than reference range; indicates an increase in hydrogen ions (H^+); excess acid.

Active exhalation valve A mechanism for holding pressure in the breathing circuit by delivering the flow required to allow the patient to breathe spontaneously. This feature is especially prominent in modes like Airway Pressure Release Ventilation that are intended to allow unrestricted spontaneous breathing during a prolonged mandatory (i.e., time triggered and time cycled) pressure-controlled breath.

Active humidification The process through which devices use heat and water to add water vapor to inspired gas.

Adaptive targeting scheme A control system that allows the ventilator to automatically set some (or conceivably all) of the targets between breaths to achieve other preset targets. One common example is adaptive pressure targeting (e.g., Pressure Regulated Volume Control mode on the Maquet Servo-i ventilator) where a static inspiratory pressure is targeted within a breath (i.e., pressure-controlled inspiration), but this target is automatically adjusted by the ventilator between breaths to achieve an operator-set tidal volume target.

Aerosol therapy The application of liquid or particle suspensions to the airway in order to achieve one or more clinical objectives.

Air-entrainment mask An oxygen delivery device in which air is entrained proportional to oxygen flow. This type of mask delivers a fixed concentration of oxygen to the patient.

Airway clearance therapy Therapeutic modalities that utilize physical or mechanical means to manipulate airflow, aid in the mobilization of tracheal bronchial phlegm cephalad, and facilitate evacuation by coughing.

Airway pressure The pressure at the airway opening measured relative to atmospheric pressure during mechanical ventilation.

Airway pressure release ventilation (APRV) A form of pressure control intermittent mandatory ventilation that is designed to allow unrestricted spontaneous breathing throughout the breath cycle. APRV is applied using I:E ratios much greater than 1:1, usually relying on short expiratory times and gas trapping to maintain end expiratory lung volume rather than a preset PEEP.

Alkalemia Arterial pH greater than reference range; indicates an increase in hydroxyl ions (OH^-); excess base.

American National Standards Institute (ANSI) A private nonprofit organization that oversees the development of consensus standards for products, services, processes, systems, and personnel in the United States. These standards ensure there is consistency and standardization in the characteristics and performance of products, the terms used to define and describe products and services, and the testing of products.

American Standard Safety System (ASSS) A thread-type connection system for gas cylinders with a volume exceeding 25 cubic feet. There are only 26 connections for the 62 gases and mixtures recognized by the CGA. Although the connection type for each type of gas mixture is not unique, differences do occur in thread type and size, right- and left-handed threading, internal and external threading, and nipple-seat design.

Amperometry Measurement of current flowing through an electrochemical cell when a constant pressure is applied to the electrode.

Analyte   The compound or substance that is measured during analysis.

Angiogenesis   The formation or growth of new capillary blood vessels; an important natural process in the body used for healing and reproduction.

Anode   A positive electrode; anions (negative ions) migrate toward the anode.

Assisted breath   A breath during which all or part of inspiratory (or expiratory) flow is generated by the ventilator doing work for the patient. In simple terms, if the airway pressure rises above end expiratory pressure during inspiration, the breath is assisted.

Asynchrony   Regarding the timing of a breath, asynchrony means triggering or cycling of an assisted breath that either leads or lags the patient's inspiratory effort. Regarding the size of a breath, asynchrony means the inspiratory flow or tidal volume does not match the patient's demand. Asynchrony may lead to increased work of breathing and discomfort. Also known as dyssynchrony.

Atmosphere absolute (ATA)   A unit of barometric pressure expressed in atmospheres. One ATA is equivalent to 760 mm Hg.

Atrioventricular (AV) node   A node located in the septal wall of the right atrium that receives electrical impulses from the sinoatrial (SA) node and transmits them to the atrioventricular (AV) bundle for distribution throughout the ventricle.

Automatic resuscitator   Compact, handheld, pneumatically powered device that delivers ventilation to a patient through a network of valves and controls which can be attached to a mask or tracheal airway.

Automatic tube compensation   A feature that allows the operator to enter the size of the patient's endotracheal tube and have the ventilator calculate the tube's resistance and then generate just enough pressure (in proportion to inspiratory or expiratory flow) to compensate for the added resistive load.

autoPEEP   The positive difference between end-expiratory *alveolar* pressure (total or intrinsic PEEP) and the end-expiratory *airway* pressure (set or extrinsic).

Autotitration   A therapeutic CPAP or BiPAP device that decreases pressure when the upper airway is stable and increases pressure in response to airway events such as apnea, hypopnea, or airflow limitations.

Autotrigger   A condition in which the ventilator repeatedly initiates inspiration because the trigger sensitivity is set too sensitive (sometimes called autocycling). For pressure triggering, the ventilator may autotrigger due to a leak in the system dropping airway pressure below a pressure trigger threshold. When sensitivity is set too high, even the patient's heartbeat can cause inadvertent triggering. Autotriggering is a form of patient–ventilator asynchrony.

B

Bag-valve resuscitator   A manual resuscitator consisting of a patient connector, nonrebreathing valve, self-inflating compressible unit, oxygen entry port, and oxygen reservoir. Also known as a self-inflating bag, this type of resuscitator can be operated without a gas source.

Base   A substance that produces hydroxyl ions (OH^-) when dissolved in water.

Bilevel positive airway pressure (BiPAP)   The delivery of two levels of pressure to the airway, one during inspiration and the other a baseline or expiratory pressure. The difference in pressure, or delta P, is used to assist ventilation by augmenting tidal volume or minute ventilation.

Bio-variable targeting scheme   A control system that allows the ventilator to automatically set the inspiratory pressure or tidal volume randomly to mimic the variability observed during normal breathing. Currently this "biologically variable" targeting scheme is available in only one mode, Variable Pressure Support, on the Dräger V500 ventilator.

Blower   A machine for generating relatively large flows of gas as the direct ventilator output with a relatively moderate increase of pressure (e.g., 2 psi). Blowers are typically used on small, portable devices.

Body temperature and pressure, saturated (BTPS)   A gas volume has been expressed as if it were saturated with water vapor at body temperature (37°C) and at the ambient barometric pressure; used for measurements of lung volumes.

Bourdon gauge   A low pressure flow-metering device that utilizes a fixed-sized orifice that is always used in conjunction with a pressure-reducing valve. This type of gauge operates under variable pressures. The pressures are determined by adjusting the pressure-reducing valve.

Boyle's law   A gas law that relates a change in volume to a change in pressure at a constant temperature. This law states that if the temperature remains constant and pressure increases, volume will decrease.

Breath   A positive change in airway flow (inspiration) paired with a negative change in airway flow (expiration) associated with ventilation of the lungs. This definition excludes flow changes caused by hiccups or cardiogenic oscillations. However, it allows the superimposition of, for example, a spontaneous breath on a mandatory breath or vice versa.

Breath sequence   A particular pattern of spontaneous and/or mandatory breaths. The three possible breath sequences are: continuous mandatory ventilation,

(CMV), intermittent mandatory ventilation (IMV), and continuous spontaneous ventilation (CSV).

Breathing circuit   A system of tubing connecting the patient to the ventilator.

Bubble humidifier   A device that produces humidity by releasing the gas underwater, allowing it to bubble to the surface. Bubble humidifiers may incorporate a diffuser, which increases the surface area of contact between the water and the gas.

Buffer   A weak acid or weak base that resists changes in pH when a strong acid or strong base is added.

C

Calibration   The adjustment of an instrument's output to match a known value.

Capacity   The range or limits of measurement by an instrument.

Carbogen   A medical gas mixture of oxygen and carbon dioxide. Typically this mixture is available in 90% oxygen/10% carbon dioxide or 95% oxygen/5% carbon dioxide.

Carbon dioxide   A gas that cannot support life. It is the end product of metabolism.

Cardiac output   The volume of blood ejected from the heart's ventricles. This value is equal to the amount of blood expelled at each heartbeat multiplied by the heart rate in beats per minute.

Cathode   A negative electrode; cations (positive ions) migrate toward the cathode.

CO oximetry   Measurement of relative blood concentrations of oxyhemoglobin, carboxyhemoglobin, methemoglobin, and reduced hemoglobin through use of spectrophotometry.

Compliance   A mechanical property of a structure such as the respiratory system; a parameter of a lung model, or setting of a lung simulator; defined as the ratio of the change in volume to the associated change in the pressure difference across the system. Compliance is the reciprocal of elastance.

Compressor   A machine for moving a relatively low flow of gas to a storage container at a higher level of pressure (e.g., 20 psi). Compressors are generally found on intensive care ventilators whereas blowers are used on home care and transport ventilators. Compressors are typically larger and consume more electrical power than blowers.

Continuous mandatory ventilation (CMV)   Commonly known as Assist/Control; breath sequence for which mandatory breaths are delivered at a preset rate and spontaneous breaths are not possible between mandatory breaths.

Patient-triggered mandatory breaths may occur between machine-triggered breaths.

Continuous positive airway pressure (CPAP)   A ventilation method by which a constant distending pressure greater than atmospheric is applied to the airway throughout the respiratory cycle.

Continuous spontaneous ventilation (CSV)   A breath sequence for which all breaths are spontaneous.

Control variable   The variable (i.e., pressure or volume in the equation of motion) that the ventilator uses as a feedback signal to manipulate inspiration.

Cuff   An inflatable balloon located on the distal tip of some artificial airways (e.g., supraglottic, endotracheal, and tracheostomy tubes) that seals and protects the natural airway from aspiration and allows positive pressure to be applied to the lungs.

Cuff pressure   The pressure exerted on the airway mucosa by the artificial airway's cuff.

Cycle (cycling)   To end the inspiratory time (and begin expiratory flow).

Cycle variable   The variable (usually pressure, volume, flow, or time) that is used to end inspiration (and begin expiratory flow).

D

Dalton's law   A gas law that states the total pressure exerted by a gaseous mixture is equal to the sum of the partial pressures that comprise that mixture.

Damping   A decrease in the amplitude of an oscillation as a result of energy being drained from the system due to system impedance.

Diameter Index Safety System (DISS)   A safety system developed for low-pressure threaded connections (at 200 psi or less) between station outlets for medical gases and medical devices.

Diaphragm compressor   A portable air compressor that uses a flexible diaphragm to draw air into a chamber, compress it, and then push the air out for medical gas use. Diaphragm compressors can generate only low pressures and moderate flows and are typically used to power small volume nebulizers.

Direct-acting valve   A cylinder valve that operates by a valve stem. The valve stem itself acts directly on the valve seat to open or close it.

Driving pressure   The pressure causing delivery of the tidal volume during pressure control modes (i.e., the change in transrespiratory pressure associated with tidal volume delivery). Driving pressure may be estimated either from ventilator settings (i.e., driving pressure = inspiratory pressure above PEEP) or from the airway pressure waveform (i.e., driving pressure = end inspiratory pressure above PEEP).

Dry powder inhaler (DPI)   A device that creates aerosols by drawing a dose of dry powder medication. Most of the particles produced by this type of device are in the respirable range.

Dual targeting scheme   A control system that allows the ventilator to switch between volume control and pressure control during a single inspiration. Dual targeting is a more advanced version of set-point targeting. It gives the ventilator the decision of whether the breath will be volume or pressure controlled according to the operator-set priorities.

Durability   The ability to withstand wear, pressure, and damage.

Dynamic compliance   The slope of the pressure–volume curve drawn between two points of zero flow (e.g., at the start and end of inspiration).

Dynamic hyperinflation   The increase in lung volume that occurs whenever insufficient exhalation time prevents the respiratory system from returning to its normal resting end expiratory equilibrium volume between breath cycles. Inappropriate operator-set expiratory time may lead to dynamic hyperinflation, inability of the patient to trigger breaths, and increased work of breathing.

E

Elastance   A mechanical property of a structure such as the respiratory system; a parameter of a lung model or setting of a lung simulator; defined as the ratio of the change in the pressure difference across the system to the associated change in volume. Elastance is the reciprocal of compliance.

Elastic load   The pressure difference applied across a system (e.g., a container) that sustains the system's volume relative to some reference volume, and/or the amount of its compressible contents relative to some reference amount.

Electrocardiogram   A recording of the electrical activity of the heart.

Electrochemical cell   An anode and a cathode immersed in liquid that acts as an electrical conductor.

Electrode   Half-cell; electronic sensing device that measures pO_2, pCO_2, and/or analytes from whole blood. An electrode can also measure cardiac or skeletal muscle electrical activity.

Endotracheal tube   An artificial airway that is passed through the nose or mouth and advanced into the trachea. Endotracheal tubes protect the lower airway and may be cuffed or uncuffed depending on the size of the tube.

Endotracheal tube changer   A tube inserted into an endotracheal tube that guides the removal of the existing tube and the insertion of a new endotracheal tube.

Equation of motion for the respiratory system   A relation among pressure difference, volume, and flow (as variable functions of time) that describes the mechanics of the respiratory system.

Error   The difference between the known reference value and the measured value.

Esophageal pressure   Pressure that approximates pleural pressure. Typically this pressure is measured in the distal one third of the esophagus by a balloon catheter.

Esophageal/tracheal Combitube   A disposable double-lumen artificial airway, consisting of a cuffed, double-lumen tube that is inserted into the patient's airway to facilitate ventilation. Inflation of the cuff closes off the esophagus, minimizing the risk of pulmonary aspiration of gastric contents, and directs the flow of air during assisted ventilation into the trachea.

Exhaled nitric oxide   A marker of airway inflammation that is useful for children and adults with acute and chronic asthma.

Expiratory flow time   The period from the start of expiratory flow to the instant when expiratory flow stops.

Expiratory pause time   The period from cessation of expiratory flow to the start of inspiratory flow.

Expiratory release   A feature of home CPAP devices to enhance comfort. This feature incorporates an algorithm to reduce pressure delivered at the beginning of exhalation and return pressure to the therapeutic level just before inhalation.

Expiratory time   The period from the start of expiratory flow to the start of inspiratory flow; expiratory time equals expiratory flow time plus expiratory pause time.

F

Feedback control   Closed loop control accomplished by using the output as a signal that is fed back (compared) to the operator-set input. The difference between the two is used to drive the system toward the desired output (i.e., negative feedback control).

Fick's law of diffusion   A gas law that explains the increased oxygen diffusion to tissues when using the hyperbaric oxygen therapy occurs through increasing the partial pressure difference across tissue membranes. This law states the diffusion of a gas across a membrane is proportional to the surface area of the membrane, the concentration gradient of the gas (partial pressure difference across the membrane), and the diffusion coefficient of the gas, but is inversely related to the distance.

Flow control   Maintenance of an invariant inspiratory flow waveform despite changing respiratory system mechanics.

Flow cycling   The ending of inspiratory time due to inspiratory flow decay below a preset threshold. Also known as cycle sensitivity.

Flow restrictor   A fixed-orifice, constant-pressure, flow-metering device.

Flow target   Inspiratory flow reaches a preset value that may be maintained before inspiration cycles off.

Flow triggering   The starting of inspiratory flow due to a patient inspiratory effort that generates inspiratory flow above a preset threshold (i.e., the trigger sensitivity setting).

Flow-inflating bag   A manual resuscitator consisting of a flow control valve, bladder, pressure manometer, pressure pop-off valve, patient connection, and gas inlet. This type of device lacks a nonrebreathing valve and cannot be operated without a gas source. Also known as an anesthesia bag.

Flowmeter   A device operated by a needle valve that controls and measures gas flow according to the principles of density and viscosity.

Flush test   A procedure in which the flush valve in the infusion tubing is opened, exposing the pressure transducer to a constant high pressure from the bag, and then closed quickly, causing the pressure to drop immediately and creating a rectangular pressure waveform on the display.

Fractional distillation   The process through which oxygen and nitrogen are commercially manufactured in bulk quantities from air.

Frequency response   The relation between the input and output of a measurement system as a function of frequency.

Fusible plug   A type of pressure relief valve used for high pressure cylinders, made of a special metal alloy that will melt when the temperature of the gas reaches between 208°F and 220°F (97.8°C and 104°C). As the plug melts, all of the gas within the cylinder will escape.

G

Gastric insufflation   Air inadvertently entering the esophagus during positive pressure ventilation with a manual resuscitator or during noninvasive ventilation.

Geometric standard deviation (SD)   A measure of the magnitude of variation in particle distribution.

Gravitational sedimentation   The deposition of aerosol particles due to gravity.

H

Heat moisture exchanger (HME)   A passive humidification device that relies on the physical principles of condensation and evaporation to humidify inspired gas. HMEs may also contain a bacterial/viral filter. Also known as an artificial nose.

Heated passover humidifier   An active humidification system that relies on transfer of moisture from the surface of the liquid to the gas flowing over it.

Heliox   A gas mixture of helium and oxygen that is useful because of its low density.

Helium   An inert gas with a lower density than oxygen or air.

Henry's law   A gas law that describes the effect of pressure on the concentration of a gas in a fluid. This law states that the amount of gas dissolved in a given volume of liquid is directly proportional to the partial pressure of that gas in the gas phase.

High flow nasal cannula   A delivery device in which humidified gas is delivered to the nares at a flow of 6 L/min or greater for pediatric and adult patients and greater than 1 L/min for infants though snug-fitting nasal prongs. Depending on the delivery system, the system may also heat the humidified inspired gas to body temperature.

High flow oxygen delivery device   An oxygen delivery device capable of delivering a precise F_IO_2 at a flow rate that meets or exceeds the patient's inspiratory demand.

High frequency chest wall compression   An airway clearance technique that uses a vest or wrap to externally compress the chest wall with rapid, short expiratory flow pulses. This therapy relies on the elastic recoil of the chest wall to return the lungs to functional residual capacity.

High frequency chest wall oscillation   An airway clearance technique that uses a rigid enclosure to generate biphasic changes in transrespiratory pressure. This modality is used for airway clearance therapy and noninvasive ventilation.

Hyperbaric oxygen therapy   Treatment modality in which a patient is exposed to an oxygen-rich environment at pressures greater than that at sea level.

I

Incentive spirometer   A biofeedback device that is used to coach and/or encourage patients to take deeper breaths.

Indirect calorimetry   A technique used to determine energy requirements; it is based on measurement of oxygen consumption and carbon dioxide production.

Indirect-acting valve   A type of cylinder valve that uses a diaphragm to open and close the valve seat. Turning the valve stem causes the diaphragm to be displaced through a spring, indirectly opening the valve seat.

Inspiratory flow   The flow into the airway opening during the inspiratory time.

Inspiratory flow time　The period from the start of inspiratory flow (into the airway opening) to the cessation of inspiratory flow.

Inspiratory hold　An intentional maneuver during mechanical ventilation whereby exhalation is delayed for a preset time (inspiratory hold time) after an assisted breath. This maneuver is used to assess static respiratory system mechanics and also to increase mean airway pressure during volume control ventilation in an attempt to improve gas exchange.

Inspiratory hold (pause) time　The period from the cessation of inspiratory flow (into the airway opening) to the start of expiratory flow during mechanical ventilation.

Inspiratory pressure　General term for the pressure at the patient connection during the inspiratory phase. For pressure control modes, where the inspiratory pressure is targeted to a preset value, the term is used to designate this setting.

Inspiratory time　The period from the start of inspiratory flow to the start of expiratory flow. Inspiratory time equals inspiratory flow time plus inspiratory pause time.

Intelligent targeting scheme　A ventilator control system that uses artificial intelligence programs such as fuzzy logic, rule-based expert systems, and artificial neural networks.

Interface　The device or boundary point between the patient and a therapeutic device. Common noninvasive interfaces include nasal pillows, masks, and nasal prongs.

Intermittent mandatory ventilation (IMV)　Breath sequence for which spontaneous breaths are permitted between mandatory breaths.

Intermittent positive pressure breathing (IPPB)　The application of inspiratory positive pressure to a spontaneously breathing patient. This therapeutic modality usually is accompanied by bland or medicated aerosol therapy. Treatment times are typically 15–20 minutes in length.

Intrapulmonary percussive ventilation (IPV)　A therapeutic modality that delivers mini bursts of high flow at rates of 200 cycles per minute. Treatment times are short (15–20 minutes) and may be accompanied by the delivery of medicated aerosol therapy. This modality is used as a hyperinflation and airway clearance therapy.

J

Jet nebulizer　An aerosol device that uses a jet of compressed gas that passes through a restricted orifice, creating a low pressure area near the tip of a narrow tube to draw fluid from a reservoir, which is then sheared into droplets by the airstream.

L

Large volume jet nebulizer　An aerosol-producing device designed to humidify inspired gas and deliver that gas in quantities that sufficiently meet the patient's inspiratory demands.

Large volume nebulizer　An aerosol-producing device designed to deliver enough humidified inspired gases to provide adequate flow to meet patient inspiratory demands.

Laryngeal airway mask　A device consisting of a tube that ends in an inflatable cuff. When inflated with air the cuff seals the area around the larynx, allowing the tube to direct the airflow to the glottis.

Laryngoscope　An endoscope for examining the larynx.

Linearity　A mathematical relationship between two or more quantities in which the quantities are directly proportional to each other. A device is linear if the output versus the input can be fitted with a straight line.

Load　The pressure required to generate inspiration.

Low flow oxygen delivery device　An oxygen delivery device that is unable to meet a patient's total inspiratory demand. Therefore, during oxygen delivery air is entrained at variable proportions, depending on the patient's inspiratory flow demands. This type of device does not deliver a consistent oxygen concentration.

M

Machine cycling　Ending inspiratory time independent of signals representing the patient-determined components of the equation of motion. Examples include muscle pressure (P_{mus} [effort]), elastance, or resistance.

Machine triggering　Starting inspiratory flow based on a signal (usually time) from the machine independent of a signal indicating patient inspiratory effort. Examples include triggering based on a preset frequency (which sets the ventilatory period) or on a preset minimum minute ventilation (determined by tidal volume divided by the ventilatory period).

Mandatory breath　A breath for which the patient has lost substantial control over timing. The start and/or end of inspiration is determined by the ventilator, independent of the patient. Therefore, the machine triggers and/or cycles the breath.

Mandatory minute ventilation　A form of intermittent mandatory ventilation (IMV) in which the ventilator monitors the exhaled minute ventilation as a target variable. If the exhaled minute ventilation falls below the operator-set value, the ventilator will trigger mandatory breaths or increase the inspiratory pressure until the target is reached.

Manual resuscitator   A device that provides manually applied positive pressure ventilation to a patient's airway.

Mask interface   An interface used for noninvasive ventilation. Masks can encompass the nose only (nasal mask), the nose and mouth (oral-naso mask), or the entire face (full-face mask).

Mass median aerodynamic diameter (MMAD)   Measurement that expresses the geometric size of particles of an aerosol for medical use. Aerosol generators produce respirable particles with a MMAD of 1–5 microns.

Mechanical insufflation-exsufflation   A therapeutic modality in which positive pressure is used to inflate the lungs and negative pressure is used to generate a cough.

Mechanical ventilator   An automatic machine designed to provide all or part of the work required to generate enough breaths to satisfy the body's respiratory needs.

Methemoglobin   Abnormal hemoglobin in which the iron has been oxidized and is in the F3 or ferric state, preventing oxygen from binding to the hemoglobin.

Mode of ventilation   A predetermined pattern of interaction between a patient and a ventilator, specified as a particular combination of control variable, breath sequence, and targeting schemes for primary and secondary breaths.

Monitor   A device that displays and alerts the caregiver of an event.

Monoplace chamber   A hyperbaric chamber capable of treating a single patient.

Multiplace chamber   A hyperbaric chamber capable of treating more than one patient and that allows a healthcare professional to provide care from within the chamber.

N

Nasal cannula   A low flow, variable performance device consisting of nasal prongs. The prongs fit loosely in the nares and, when properly fit, encompass less than one-half the internal diameter of the nares.

Nasopharyngeal airway   A device to maintain or increase patency of the upper airway by creating a conduit from the tip of the nose to the hypopharynx, allowing movement of air or devices.

Nebulizer   A device that produces an aerosol, or suspension, of particles in gas.

Negative pressure ventilation   A type of assisted breathing for which transrespiratory pressure difference is generated by keeping airway pressure equal to atmospheric pressure and making body surface pressure less than atmospheric pressure.

Neonatal apnea monitor   A monitor that alerts the caregiver that an infant is not breathing. Most systems also alert caregivers of low and high heart rate occurrences.

Neurally Adjusted Ventilatory Assist (NAVA)   The name of a mode using a servo targeting scheme in which the controller sets airway pressure to be proportional to patient effort based on the voltage recorded from diaphragmatic activity from sensors embedded in an orogastric tube.

Nitric oxide   A colorless gas that plays a vital role in vascular smooth muscle relaxation, immune regulation, inhibition of platelet aggregation, and neurotransmission.

Nonrebreathing mask   An oxygen mask containing a reservoir and two or three one-way leaf valves. One or two valves are positioned over the mask ports to prevent air entrainment and one is between the mask and the reservoir bag to direct the patient's exhaled flow away from the reservoir bag and out through the ports of the mask.

O

Obstructive sleep apnea (OSA)   A sleep disorder caused by obstruction of the upper airway. It is characterized by repeated pauses in breathing during sleep (apneas) and an associated reduction in blood oxygen saturation. Obstruction is usually indicated by loud snoring and frequent, sudden, and severe snorting.

Optimum targeting scheme   A ventilator control system that automatically adjusts the targets of the ventilatory pattern to either minimize or maximize some overall performance characteristic. One example is Adaptive Support Ventilation found on the Hamilton Medical G5 ventilator.

Oropharyngeal airway   A device designed to maintain or increase patency of the upper airway by creating a conduit from the lips to the hypopharynx, allowing free movement of air or passage of devices such as a suction catheter.

Oscillatory positive expiratory pressure (OPEP)   An airway clearance device that combines positive pressure during exhalation with airway vibrations or oscillations.

Oxidation   The loss of electrons.

Oxygen   An essential gas for almost all forms of life. Oxygen gas concentration available in room air is 21%. Supplementation of oxygen gas concentrations greater than what is available in room air can be lifesaving and is considered a medical drug.

Oxygen analyzer   A device used to measure the concentration of oxygen in a gas mixture. Typically displayed as the percentage of oxygen in the gas mixture.

Oxygen blender   A device that combine the flows from air and oxygen. The ratio of the two flows is used to create the delivered F_IO_2.

Oxygen concentrator An electrically powered device capable of physically separating the oxygen in atmospheric air from nitrogen and storing high purity oxygen (approximately 95%) for delivery through low flow devices for therapeutic use.

Oxygen reservoir A bag-valve resuscitator attachment that collects oxygen from the gas source during inspiration and delivers the collected gas during inspiration to increase the F_IO_2 delivered to the patient during each manual breath.

Oxygen tent A high density aerosol device that provides oxygen in low to moderate concentrations at cool temperatures. Typically a frame and soft plastic canopy are used to enclose the patient in the device.

Oxygen-conserving device (OCD) A device that provides a flow of oxygen at the initiation of inspiration. Therefore, oxygen is only delivered when it is needed, minimizing waste during exhalation and prolonging the time oxygen is available through the portable system.

Oxyhemoglobin The chemical combination resulting from the covalent bonding of oxygen to the ferrous iron pigment in hemoglobin.

P

Partial pressure The absolute pressure exerted by one gas in a mixture of gases or in a liquid.

Partial ventilatory support The ventilator and the respiratory muscles each provide some of the work of breathing; muscle pressure adds to ventilator pressure in the equation of motion.

Passive humidification A method of humidifying inspired gases to the airway based on the physical principles of condensation and evaporation.

Patient cycling Ending inspiratory time based on signals representing the patient-determined components of the equation of motion (i.e., P_{mus} [effort], elastance, or resistance). Common examples of cycling variables are peak inspiratory pressure and percent inspiratory flow.

Patient triggering Starting inspiratory flow based on signals related to one of the patient-determined components of the equation of motion (i.e., P_{mus} [effort], elastance, or resistance). Common examples of patient trigger variables are airway pressure drop below baseline and inspiratory flow due to patient effort.

Peak airway pressure The maximum airway pressure during a mechanically assisted inspiration, measured relative to atmospheric pressure.

Peak flowmeter A monitoring device for the management of asthma that measures the patient's peak flow rate during a forceful expiratory maneuver.

Peak inspiratory pressure The inspiratory pressure that is set relative to atmospheric pressure during pressure control modes.

Pin Index Safety System (PISS) A safety system for the valve outlets of small, high pressure medical gas and gas mixture cylinders. This system uses a specific combination of two holes in the post valve just below the gas outlet for each gas or gas mixture. The regulator that connects to the gas or gas mixture will have pins that correspond to the holes to allow for proper connection.

Piston compressor A portable air compressor that uses a motor to drive a piston and compress the air for medical gas use. Piston-driven air compressors are capable of producing high pressure and flow, such as that needed for a pneumatically powered ventilator.

Pneumotachometer A transducer designed to measure the flow of respiratory gases, typically by measuring pressure differences across known resistances.

pO_2 Partial pressure of oxygen.

Polarographic oxygen analyzer A device that uses the flow of electrical current between negatively and positively charged poles to measure the oxygen concentration in a gas mixture.

Positive airway pressure (PAP) devices Devices that provide positive pressure on inspiration, expiration, or throughout the respiratory cycle of spontaneously breathing patients to provide short-term hyperinflation or airway clearance therapy.

Positive expiratory pressure (PEP) An airway clearance technique in which the patient exhales against a fixed-orifice flow resistor to aid in the movement of secretions cephalad into the larger or central airways.

Positive pressure ventilation A type of assisted breathing for which transrespiratory pressure difference is generated by raising airway pressure above body surface pressure.

Potentiometric Measurement of the voltage between a reference and measuring electrode used to measure the amount of an analyte.

Precision The degree of consistency among repeated measurements of the same quantity. Precision is commonly expressed by the standard deviation of the measurements.

Pressure control A general category of ventilator modes for which pressure delivery is predetermined by a targeting scheme such that inspiratory pressure is either proportional to patient effort or has a particular waveform regardless of respiratory system mechanics.

Pressure cycling Inspiration ends (i.e., expiratory flow starts) when airway pressure reaches a preset threshold.

Pressure manometer A device that measures pressure in a system. Typically pressure manometers are used with infant resuscitators to monitor the pressure delivered during manual ventilation.

Pressure pop-off valve A spring-loaded device that relieves pressure at a preset value. Pressure relief or pop-off valves are used with infant bag-valve resuscitators as a safety feature.

Pressure relief valve A valve designed to open at a pre-determined pressure value. Pressure relief valves are designed as safety features in cylinders and liquid and bulk gas delivery systems to prevent the pressure from exceeding the delivery system's tolerance.

Pressure support The name of a mode using a set-point targeting scheme in which all breaths are pressure or flow triggered, pressure targeted, and flow cycled.

Pressure target Inspiratory pressure reaches a preset value before inspiration cycles off.

Pressure triggering The starting of inspiratory flow due to a patient inspiratory effort that generates an airway pressure drop below end expiratory pressure larger than a preset threshold.

Pressurized metered dose inhaler (pMDI) An aerosol delivery device consisting of a pressurized canister containing a drug in the form of a micronized powder or solution that is suspended with a mixture of propellants, surfactants, preservatives, flavoring agents, and dispersal agents.

Primary breaths Mandatory breaths during CMV or IMV or spontaneous breaths during CSV.

Proportional Assist Ventilation (PAV) The name of a mode using a servo targeting scheme based on the equation of motion for the respiratory system to provide ventilatory support in which airway pressure is proportional to the patient's inspiratory effort.

Pulmonary artery catheter A catheter inserted into the vena cava and advanced through to the right side of the heart until the catheter's tip is in the pulmonary arterial tree. Typically this type of catheter is used to measure cardiac output and wedge pressure.

Pulmonary capillary wedge pressure An estimation of left atrial pressure. Normal values range from 6 to 12 mm Hg.

Pulse oximetry The process of determining the saturation of hemoglobin with oxygen using an oximeter.

Q

Quick connect adaptors An appliance that allows rapid connection and/or disconnection of a device requiring a high pressure compressed gas source from the source gas delivery system (such as a bulk gas system or high pressure cylinder).

R

Ramp A mathematical function whose value rises or falls at a constant rate. Ascending (rising) or descending (falling) functions are sometimes used for inspiratory flow in volume control modes.

Reduction The gain of electrons.

Relative humidity The relationship of the actual humidity in a gas sample and the absolute humidity that gas can hold. Relative humidity is often expressed as a percentage and calculated as (Actual humidity/Absolute humidity) × 100.

Reperfusion injury Injury to the heart, intestine, kidney, lung, and/or muscle caused by rapid flow of blood into areas previously rendered ischemic by arterial occlusion.

Reservoir cannula A type of oxygen-conserving device. One type uses a reservoir that is worn on the chest like a pendent; the other type has a reservoir that encompasses and extends beyond the nasal prongs. Reservoir cannulas enable a continuous flow of oxygen to be delivered at lower flows, conserving the amount of oxygen used with portable oxygen delivery systems, such as e-cylinders.

Resistance A mechanical property of a structure such as the respiratory system; a parameter of a lung model, or setting of a lung simulator; defined as the ratio of the change in the pressure difference across the system to the associated change in flow.

Resistive load The pressure difference applied across a system (e.g., a container) that is related to a rate of change of the system's volume and/or the flow of fluid within or through the system.

Rotary compressor A portable air compressor that uses a vane, rotating at high speeds, to entrain and compress air entering the device. This type of compressor is used by ventilator manufacturers incorporating a compressor into the ventilator design. Rotary compressors can generate pressures between 45 and 55 psi with flow rates of 60–80 L/m.

Rupture disk A type of pressure relief valve composed of a thin metal disk that will either break apart or buckle when the disk's pressure threshold is exceeded, allowing all of the gas from the high pressure cylinder to escape.

S

Secondary breaths Spontaneous breaths occurring during IMV.

Sensitivity The sensitivity setting of the ventilator is a threshold value for the trigger variable that, when met, starts inspiration.

Servo targeting A control system for which the output of the ventilator automatically follows a varying input.

Set-point targeting   A control system for which the operator sets all the parameters of the pressure waveform (pressure control modes) or volume and flow waveforms (volume control modes). Advanced volume control modes actually allow the ventilator to make small adjustments to the set inspiratory flow to compensate for such factors as patient circuit compliance.

Simple mask   A low flow, variable performance oxygen delivery device capable of delivering low to moderate oxygen concentrations.

Sinusoid   A mathematical function having a magnitude that varies as the sine of an independent variable (e.g., time). A sinusoidal function is sometimes used for inspiratory flow in volume control modes.

Spacer   A simple open-ended tube or bag that, with sufficiently large device volume, provides space for the pressurized metered dose inhaler plume to expand by allowing the propellants to evaporate.

Spirometer   A device designed to measure lung volumes and flows.

Spontaneous breath   A breath for which the patient controls the start and end of inspiration, independent of any machine settings for inspiratory time and expiratory time.

Spring-loaded device   A type of pressure relief valve used for high pressure gas cylinders. When the pressure in the cylinder exceeds the threshold, the spring will push up and unseat a valve allowing gas to escape. Once the cylinder pressure falls below the set pressure the valve is allowed to reseat, conserving the gas or gas mixture within the cylinder contents.

Suction catheter   A thin tube connected to a vacuum device used to evacuate secretions from the upper or lower airway.

Supraglottic device   An artificial airway designed to maintain airway patency and allow for administration of anesthetic gases, airway instrumentation, and the administration of manual or mechanical ventilation.

Synchronization window   A short period at the end of the expiratory time or at the end of a preset inspiratory time, during which a patient signal may be used to synchronize flow to patient effort.

Synchronized IMV (SIMV)   A form of IMV in which spontaneous breaths are permitted between or during a mandatory breath. Mandatory breath delivery is coordinated with patient effort. A synchronized breath is considered to be machine triggered.

T

T-piece resuscitator   Manually operated, gas-powered resuscitator designed to provide ventilation at a set flow with consistent positive inspiratory and expiratory pressure. Typically, this type of resuscitator is used to ventilate infants.

Tag   A mode classification. A tag can be an acronym.

Target   A predetermined goal of ventilator output. Targets can be viewed as the parameters of the targeting scheme. Within-breath targets are the parameters of the pressure, volume, or flow waveform. Between-breath targets serve to modify the within-breath targets and/or the overall ventilatory pattern.

Targeting scheme   A model of the relationship between operator inputs and ventilator outputs to achieve a specific ventilatory pattern, usually in the form of a feedback control system. The targeting scheme is a key component of a mode description.

Taxonomy   A hierarchical classification system. A taxonomy for modes of ventilation has four levels: (1) the control variable, (2) the breath sequence, (3) the targeting scheme for primary breaths, and (4) the targeting scheme for secondary breaths. These levels correspond to the levels of family, class, genus, and species of the Linnaean taxonomy used in biology.

Terminal unit   The point in a piped medical gas distribution system at which the user normally makes connections and disconnections. Also referred to as a station outlet.

Thorpe tube   A variable orifice, constant-pressure, flow-metering device consisting of a tapered transparent tube with a float. The diameter of the tube is narrower at the bottom or base. The float is suspended by flow against the force of gravity at a level determined by the rate of flow through the tube.

Tidal pressure   The change in transalveolar pressure (i.e., pressure in the alveolar region minus pressure in the pleural space, equivalent to elastance times volume in the equation of motion) associated with the inhalation or exhalation of a tidal volume.

Tidal volume   The volume of gas, either inhaled or exhaled, during a breath. The maximum value of the volume versus time waveform.

Time constant   The time necessary for inflated lungs to passively empty in response to abrupt changes in ventilatory pressure. Time constants are expressed in units of time, generally seconds, and calculated as the product of resistance and compliance.

Time control   A general category of ventilator modes for which inspiratory flow, inspiratory volume, and inspiratory pressure are all dependent on respiratory system mechanics. Because no parameters of the pressure or flow waveform are preset, the only control of the breath is the timing (i.e., inspiratory and expiratory times).

Time cycling Inspiratory time ends after a preset time interval has elapsed. The most common examples are a preset inspiratory time or a preset inspiratory pause time.

Time triggering The starting of inspiratory flow due to a preset time interval. The most common example is a preset ventilatory frequency.

Total cycle time The sum of inspiratory time and expiratory time.

Total PEEP The sum of autoPEEP and intentionally applied PEEP or CPAP. Synonymous with intrinsic PEEP.

Total ventilatory support The ventilator provides all the work of breathing; muscle pressure in the equation of motion is zero. This is normally only possible if the patient is paralyzed or heavily sedated.

Tracheostomy tube An indwelling artificial airway inserted surgically or percutaneously through an opening in the neck into the trachea. Tracheostomy tubes protect the lower airway and may be cuffed or uncuffed.

Transairway pressure Pressure at the airway opening minus pressure in the lungs (i.e., alveolar pressure).

Transalveolar pressure Pressure in the lungs minus pressure in the pleural space. Equal to transpulmonary pressure only under static conditions.

Transchestwall pressure Pressure in the pleural space minus pressure on the body surface.

Transcutaneous carbon dioxide monitor A device that measures carbon dioxide gas tensions across the skin.

Transcutaneous oxygen monitor A device that measures oxygen gas tensions across the skin.

Transpulmonary pressure Pressure at the airway opening minus pressure in the pleural space.

Transrespiratory pressure Pressure at the airway opening minus pressure on the body surface; equal to the sum of transairway pressure plus transalveolar pressure and transchestwall pressure.

Transthoracic pressure Pressure in the lungs minus pressure on the body surface; equal to the sum of transalveolar pressure and transchestwall pressure.

Transtracheal oxygen catheter A low flow oxygen device consisting of small-diameter Teflon catheter connected to a flange. Small-bore supply tubing is used to deliver oxygen directly through the catheter to the mid trachea, at the level of the second or third tracheal ring. Surgical insertion of the catheter is required; it is secured in place by a small, adjustable beaded chain.

Trigger To start inspiration.

Trigger window The period composed of the expiratory time minus a short "refractory" period required to reduce the risk of triggering a breath before exhalation is complete.

U

Ultrasonic nebulizer A device that uses the piezoelectric crystal, vibrating at a high frequency, to convert electricity to sound waves, creating standing waves in the liquid immediately above the transducer, disrupting the liquid surface, and forming a geyser of aerosolized droplets.

Undersea Medical Society (UMS) The primary scientific body governing the practice of hyperbaric medicine.

V

Valved holding chamber A device used with a pressurized metered dose inhaler that consists of a spacer with a one-way valve to prevent loss of the dose.

Ventilatory pattern A sequence of breaths (CMV, IMV, or CSV) with a designated control variable (volume or pressure) for the mandatory breaths (or the spontaneous breaths for CSV).

Ventilatory period The time from the start of inspiratory flow of one breath to the start of inspiratory flow of the next breath; inspiratory time plus expiratory time; the reciprocal of ventilatory frequency. Also called total cycle time or total breath cycle.

Vibrating mesh nebulizer An electrically powered small volume aerosol generator capable of producing particles with a mass median aerodynamic diameter of approximately 3.5 μm.

Vocalization device A device that redirects gas flow from the tracheostomy tube during exhalation through the larynx to aid in vocalization.

Volume control A general category of ventilator modes for which both inspiratory flow and tidal volume are predetermined by a targeting scheme to have particular waveforms independent of respiratory system mechanics.

Volume cycling Inspiratory time ends when inspiratory volume reaches a preset threshold (i.e., tidal volume).

Volume target A preset value for tidal volume that the ventilator is set to attain either within a breath or as an average over multiple breaths.

Volume triggering The starting of inspiratory flow due to a patient inspiratory effort that generates an inspiratory volume signal larger than a preset threshold or trigger sensitivity setting.

W

Wood's metal A fusible alloy composed of bismuth, lead, cadmium, and tin used to construct fusible plugs.

Work of breathing The general definition of work is the integral of pressure with respect to volume during an assisted inspiration.

Z

Zeroing   A calibration procedure consisting of opening a transducer to atmospheric pressure and adjusting the output reading to zero.

Zone valve   A safety valve that is placed in oxygen piping systems to enable gas flow to be shut off in the event of an emergency, such as a fire.

Index

large volume jet nebulizer, 85–88, 87*f*, 88*t*

large-volume nebulizers, 533, 533*f*

laryngeal mask airway (LMA)

    available devices, 107–109

    maximum size bronchoscope and endotracheal
        tube, 109*t*

    parts, 107, 107*f*

    sizing chart, 108*t*

    tube internal diameter and length, 108*t*

    types and manufacturers, 107

laryngeal tube suction (LTS), 102–104

laryngeal tubes, 102–104, 103*f*, 104*t*

laryngoscope, 110, 125–127

    blade styles, 122–124

    blade types, 122

    components, 120

    deconstructed, 121*f*

    Green system, 120, 121*f*

    handles types, 120

    insertion techniques, 124

    Jellicoe adapter, 120

    light source, 120

    sizes, 122, 122*t*

Laser-Flex (Covidien), 117

laser tracheal tubes, 118

leak, 454*t*, 459*t*

    compensation, 454*t*, 459*t*

    sensitivity, 459*t*

LEDs. *See* light-emitting diodes

levering tip laryngoscope blade, 124

Levey-Jennings plots, 165–166, 165*f*

Lifesaver Manual Resuscitator, 567*t*

light-emitting diodes (LEDs), 196

lighted stylet, 126, 129

linearity, 264, 265, 267

liquid oxygen systems, 3, 19–20

LIR. *See* Laerdal infant bag-valve
    resuscitator

LMA. *See* laryngeal mask airway

LMA Classic, 108

LMA Classic Excel, 108

LMA Fastrach, 109

LMA Flexible, 108

LMA, Inc., 107–109, 115

LMA North America, Inc., 126

LMA ProSeal, 108–109

LMA Supreme, 109

LMA Unique, 108

Lo-Pro/Lo-Contour, 116–117

long-term acute care (LTAC) facilities, 6

low flow oxygen delivery devices

    nasal cannula, 38–39, 39*f*

    nasal catheter, 39–40, 39*f*, 40*f*

    transtracheal catheter, 40, 40*f*

    working, 38

low-perfusion conditions, 197

low profile cuff, 116–117

lower airway devices, endotracheal tubes,
    111–120

    adjuncts, 120–129

L.R. Instruments, 565*t*

LT/LT-D, 102–104, 104*t*

LTS. *See* laryngeal tube suction

Luer lock medication syringe, 564, 564*f*

Lukens trap, 145

M

machine, 282

machine cycling, 285

machine triggering, 282

Macintosh blade, 122*t*, 123, 123*t*, 124

Mada Medical, 567*t*

Magill tip, 112, 112*f*

magnetic valve, 511

mandatory breath, 278

mandatory minute volume ventilation, Dräger Evita
    XL ventilator, 334–335

manual resuscitation, precautions, hazards and/or
    complications of, 576, 576*t*

manual resuscitators, 553–554, 554*t*

    bag-valve resuscitators, 557–564, 565*t*–568*t*

    flow-inflating resuscitators, 554–557, 558*t*

    T-piece resuscitators, 564, 568–569, 570*t*

Mapleson circuit classification, 556, 556*f*

Maquet Servo-i ventilator, 374, 374*f*

    automode, 376–378

    BiVent, 378

    features, 379–380

    manufacturer's specifications, 380, 380*t*–381*t*

    modes, 376, 377*t*

    NAVA, 378

    operator interface, 376, 376*f*

    pressure control, 378

    pressure support, 378

    SIMV, 378–379

    volume control, 379

    volume support, 379

Marshall Products Ltd., 567*t*

mask alarm, 454*t*, 460*t*

masks, 450